ADVANCED THERAPY OF INFLAMMATORY BOWEL DISEASE

THIRD EDITION

Volume II

IBD and Crohn's Disease

Advanced Therapy of Inflammatory Bowel Disease

THIRD EDITION

Volume II

IBD and Crohn's Disease

THEODORE M. BAYLESS, MD

Sherlock Hibbs Professor of Inflammatory Bowel Disease
Professor of Medicine
Director Emeritus, Meyerhoff Inflammatory Bowel Disease Center
The Johns Hopkins Hospital
Baltimore, Maryland

STEPHEN B. HANAUER, MD

Joseph B. Kirsner Professor of Medicine
Professor of Clinical Pharmacology
Chief, Section of Gastroenterology and Nutrition
University of Chicago Medical Center
Chicago, Illinois

2011
PEOPLE'S MEDICAL PUBLISHING HOUSE—USA
SHELTON, CONNECTICUT

People's Medical Publishing House-USA
2 Enterprise Drive, Suite 509
Shelton, CT 06484
Tel: 203–402–0646
Fax: 203–402–0854
E-mail: info@pmph-usa.com

PMPH-USA

11 12 13 14/PMPH/9 8 7 6 5 4 3 2 1

ISBN 13: 978–1–60795–035–6
ISBN 10: 1–60795–035–9
Printed in China by People's Medical Publishing House
Editor: Linda Mehta; Copyeditor/Typesetter: Newgen; Cover designer: Mary McKeon

Library of Congress Cataloging-in-Publication Data
Bayless, Theodore M., 1931-
  Advanced therapy of inflammatory bowel disease / Theodore M. Bayless, Stephen B. Hanauer.–3rd ed.
     p. ; cm.
  Rev. ed. of: Advanced therapy of inflammatory bowel disease / [edited by] Theodore M. Bayless, Stephen B. Hanauer. 2001.
  Includes bibliographical references and index.
  ISBN 13: 978–1–60795–035–6
  ISBN 10: 1–60795–035–9
  1. Inflammatory bowel diseases. I. Hanauer, Stephen B. II. Advanced therapy of inflammatory bowel disease. III. Title.
  [DNLM: 1. Inflammatory Bowel Diseases–therapy. WI 420]

RC862.I53A35 2011
616.3'44–dc23

2011014635

Sales and Distribution

Canada
McGraw-Hill Ryerson Education
Customer Care
300 Water St
Whitby, Ontario L1N 9B6
Canada
Tel: 1–800–565–5758
Fax: 1–800–463–5885
www.mcgrawhill.ca

Foreign Rights
John Scott & Company
International Publisher's Agency
P.O. Box 878
Kimberton, PA 19442
USA
Tel: 610–827–1640
Fax: 610–827–1671
Japan
United Publishers Services Limited
1-32-5 Higashi-Shinagawa
Shinagawa-ku, Tokyo 140–0002

Japan
Tel: 03-5479-7251
Fax: 03-5479-7307 Email: hayashi@ups.co.jp
United Kingdom, Europe, Middle East, Africa
McGraw Hill Education
Shoppenhangers Road
Maidenhead
Berkshire, SL6 2QL

England
Tel: 44–0-1628–502500
Fax: 44–0-1628–635895
www.mcgraw-hill.co.uk

Singapore, Thailand, Philippines, Indonesia, Vietnam, Pacific Rim, Korea
McGraw-Hill Education
60 Tuas Basin Link
Singapore 638775
Tel: 65-6863-1580
Fax: 65-6862-3354
www.mcgraw-hill.com.sg

Australia, New Zealand, Papua New Guinea, Fiji, Tonga, Solomon Islands, Cook Islands
Woodslane Pty Limited
Unit 7/5 Vuko Place
Warriewood NSW 2102
Australia
Tel: 61-2-9970–5111
Fax: 61-2-9970–5002
www.woodslane.com.au

Brazil
SuperPedido Tecmedd
Beatriz Alves, Foreign Trade Department
R. Sansao Alves dos Santos, 102 I
7th fl oor
Brooklin Novo
Sao Paolo 04571–090
Brazil

Tel: 55–16-3512–5539
www.superpedidotecmedd.com.br

India, Bangladesh, Pakistan, Sri Lanka, Malaysia
CBS Publishers
4819/X1 Prahlad Street 24
Ansari Road, Darya Ganj, New Delhi-110002
India
Tel: 91–11-23266861/67
Fax: 91–11-23266818
Email:cbspubs@vsnl.com

People's Republic of China
People's Medical Publishing House
International Trade Department
No. 19, Pan Jia Yuan Nan Li
Chaoyang District
Beijing 100021
P.R. China
Tel: 8610–67653342
Fax: 8610–67691034
www.pmph.com/en/

Contents

PART X: SURGERY FOR CROHN'S COLITIS

Contributors

Alessandro Armuzzi, MD, PhD [101]
Internal Medicine and Gastroenterology Unit
Complesso Integrato Columbus
Catholic University
Rome, Italy

Vivian Asamoah, MD [164]
Postdoctoral Clinical Fellow
Department of Medicine
Division of Gastroenterology
Johns Hopkins Hospital
Baltimore, Maryland

Antwan Atia [138]
Division of Gastroenterology
Feinberg School of Medicine
Northwestern University
Chicago, Illinois

Dahlia Awais, MD, MS [125]
Assistant Professor
Department of Medicine
Division of Gastroenterology
University Hospitals Case Medical Center
Cleveland, Ohio

Robert D. Baker, MD, PhD [148]
Professor of Pediatrics
Co-chief, Division of Gastroenterology
Department of Pediatrics
State University of New York
Buffalo, New York

Susan S. Baker, MD, PhD [148]
Professor
Department of Pediatrics
Digestive Diseases and Nutrition Center Women and
Children's Hospital of Buffalo
Buffalo, New York

Robert N. Baldassano, MD [113]
Professor
University of Pennsylvania, SOM
Attending Physician & Director—IBD Center
The Children's Hospital of Philadelphia
Philadelphia, Pennsylvania

Theodore M. Bayless, MD [164]
Sherlock Hibbs Professor of IBD
Professor of Medicine
Director Emeritus, Meyerhoff IBD Center
The Johns Hopkins Hospital
Baltimore, Maryland

Vishal Bhagat, MD [131]
Fellow in Gastroenterology
State University of New York
Buffalo, New York

Jason Bodzin, MD, FACS [142]
Clinical Associate Professor of Surgery
Wayne State University
Harper/University Hospital
Detroit, Michigan

Peter Bossuyt, MD [100]
Imelda GI Clinical Research Center
Imelda Hospital
Bonheiden, Belgium

Alan L. Buchman, MD, MSPH [138]
Professor
Gasroenterology and Surgery

Northwestern University Feinberg
School of Medicine
Chicago, Illinois

Robert S. Burakoff, MD, MPH [121]
Clinical Chief
Department of Gastroenterology, Hepatology, and
Endoscopy;
Director for the Center for Crohn's and Colitis
Brigham and Women's Hospital;
Associate Professor
Department of Medicine
Harvard Medical School
Boston, Massachusetts

Richard K. Burt, MD [118]
Department of Medicine
Division of Immunotherapy
Northwestern University Feinberg
School of Medicine
Chicago, Illinois

John O. Clarke, MD [117]
Division of Gastroenterology and Hepatology
Johns Hopkins Hospital
Baltimore, Maryland

Maria I. Clavell, MD [148]
Assistant Professor of Pediatrics
University of Pittsburgh School of Medicine
Pediatric Gastroenterologist
Children's Hospital of Pittsburgh
Pittsburgh, Pennsylvania

Stanley A. Cohen, MD [152]
Director, The Combined Center for IBD
Children's Center for Digestive Health Care
Emory Children's Center Adjunct
Clinical Professor of Pediatrics
Emory University School of Medicine
Atlanta, Georgia

Russell D. Cohen, MD, FACG, AGAF [111]
Associate Professor
Department of Medicine
Pritzker School of Medicine
Codirector, IBD Center
The University of Chicago Medical Center
Chicago, Illinois

Robert M. Craig, MD [118]
Professor
Department of Medicine
Division of Gastroenterology

Northwestern University Feinberg School of Medicine
Chicago, Illinois

Carmen Cuffari, MD [104]
Associate Professor
Pediatrics Gastroenterology and Nutrition
The Johns Hopkins Children's Center
Baltimore, Maryland

Sharon Dudley-Brown, PhD, FNP-BC [144]
Codirector
Gastroenterology and Hepatology Nurse Practitioner
Fellowship Program;
Assistant Professor
Schools of Medicine and Nursing
Johns Hopkins University
Baltimore, Maryland

David Edwin, PhD [153]
Associate Professor
Department of Psychiatry & Behavioral Sciences
Johns Hopkins University
Baltimore, Maryland

Paula Erwin-Toth, RN, MSN [150]
Director, Wound/Ostomy/Continence Nursing
Education
School of WOC Nursing
The Cleveland Clinic Foundation
Cleveland, Ohio

Brian G. Feagan, MD [105]
Professor of Medicine, Epidemiology and
Biostatistics
Director, London Clinical Trials Research Group
John P. Robarts Research Institute
University of Western Ontario
London, Canada

Thomas M. Fishbein, MD [139]
Professor of Surgery
Georgetown University
Director, Georgetown Transplant Institute
Georgetown University Hospital
Washington D.C.

Rosemarie L. Fisher, MD [119]
Professor of Medicine
Department of Pediatrics
Yale School of Medicine
Yale-New Haven Hospital
New Haven, Connecticut

Kimberly Frederick, MSW, LCSW [147]
VP, Patient and Professional Services

Crohn's and Colitis Foundation
New York, New York

Sobha P. Fritz, MD [152]
Assistant Professor
Department of Pediatrics
Emory University School of Medicine
Pediatric Psychologist
Children's Healthcare of Atlanta at Scottish Rite
Atlanta, Georgia

Anne M. Griffiths, MD, FRCPC [120]
Head
Division of Gastroenterology/Hepatology/Nutrition
Hospital for Sick Children;
Northridge Chair in IBD;
Associate Scientist
Program in Genetics and Genome Biology SickKids
Research Institute;
Professor
Paediatrics
University of Toronto
Toronto, ON, Canada

Juan Francisco Guerra, MD [139]
Gastroenterology Fellow
Georgetown University Hospital
Washington D.C.

Christina Ha, MD [105]
Assistant Professor
Division of Gastroenterology and Hepatology
Johns Hopkins School of Medicine
Baltimore, Maryland

Geert D'Haens, MD, PhD [100]
Imelda GI Clinical Research Center
Imelda Hospital
Bonheiden, Belgium

Smita Halder, MD, PhD [160]
Faculty of Medicine
University of Toronto
IBD Centre
Mount Sinai Hospital
Toronto, Canada

Stephen B. Hanauer, MD [107]
Professor
Department of Medicine
Chief
Clinical Pharmacology
Section of Gastroenterology,
Hepatology, and Nutrition

University of Chicago Medical Center
Chicago, Illinois

Jason W. Harper, MD [109]
Resident Physician
Department of Internal Medicine
University of Washington
Seattle, Washington

Jason Hemming, MD [119]
Gastroenterologist
Pentucket Medical Center
Haverhill, Massachusetts

Peter D.R. Higgins, MD, PhD, MSc (CRDSA) [135]
Assistant Professor
Department of Gastroenterology
Division of Gastroenterology and Hepatology;
Department of Internal Medicine
University of Michigan Medical Center
Ann Arbor, Michigan

Robert J. Hilsden, MD, PhD, FRCPC [157]
Departments of Medicine and Community
Health Sciences
University of Calgary
Calgary, AB, Canada

Daan Hommes, MD, PhD [99]
Professor of Medicine
Chief, Department of Gastroenterology and
Hepatology
Leiden University Medical Centre
Leiden, The Netherlands

Willemijntje (Sandra) Hoogerwerf, MD [155]
Department of Gastroenterology
Flagler Hospital
Saint Augustine, Florida

Sara N. Horst, MD [116]
Gastroenterology Fellow
Vanderbilt University
Nashville, Tennessee

Tracy L. Hull, MD [143]
Professor of Surgery
Department of Colon and Rectal Surgery
The Cleveland Clinic Foundation
Cleveland, Ohio

Anna Hunter, MD [113]
Fellow Pediatric GI
Hepatoloty and Nutrition

The Children's Hospital of Philadelphia
Philadelphia, Pennsylvania

Jeffrey S. Hyams, MD [114]
Head
Division of Digestive Diseases, Hepatology, and
Nutrition Connecticut Children's Medical Center
Hartford, Connecticut

Kim L. Isaacs, MD, PhD [122]
Professor
Department of Medicine
Division of Gastroenterology and Hepatology
University of North Carolina at Chapel Hill
Chapel Hill, North Carolina

Edwin R. Itenberg, DO [134]
General Surgeon
New York, New York

Howard S. Kaufman, MD, MBA [140]
Director, Colorectal Research Program
Huntington Medical Research Institutes
Pasadena, California

Judith Kelsen, MD [113]
GI, Hepatology and Nutrition Divisions
The Children's Hospital of Philadelphia
Philadelphia, Pennsylvania

Joseph B. Kirsner, MD, PhD [112]
Professor of Medicine and Clinical Pharmacology
University of Chicago
Chicago, Illinois

Jimmy Ko, MD [163]
Stanford, California

Joyce M. Koh, MD [117]
Department of Medicine
The Johns Hopkins Hospital at Bayview
Baltimore, Maryland

Burton I. Korelitz, MD [103]
Clinical Professor
Director of Research in IBD
Department of Medicine
Division of Gastroenterology
New York University School of Medicine
Lenox Hill Hospital
New York, New York

Richard A. Kozarek, MD [128]
Executive Director
Digestive Disease Institute
Virginia Mason Medical Center
Seattle, Washington

Prasanna Kumaranayake, MD [105]
Gastroenterologist
Burlington, Canada

Bret A. Lashner, MD [126]
Director, Center for IBD
Department of Gastroenterology
Cleveland Clinic
Cleveland, Ohio

Linda A. Lee, MD [165]
Assistant Professor
Department of Gastroenterology
Johns Hopkins University
Baltimore, Maryland

Scott D. Lee, MD [109]
Associate Professor
Department of Medicine;
Director, IBD Program
Division of Gastroenterology
University of Washington
Seattle, Washington

Simon Lichtiger, MD [106]
Associate Professor of Gastroenterology
Mt. Sinai Medical Center
New York, New York

Anne Lidor, MD [132]
Assistant Professor
Department of Surgery
Johns Hopkins University School of Medicine
Baltimore, Maryland

Richard P. MacDermott, MD [123]
Director, IBD Center
The Thomas Ordway Endowed Chair
Professor of Medicine
Division of Gastroenterology
The Albany Medical College
Albany, New York

Uma Mahadevan, MD [158]
Associate Professor of Medicine
Center for Colitis and CD
University of California
San Francisco, California

John K. Marshall, MD, MSc,
FRCPC, AGAF [102]
Associate Professor
Department of Medicine
Division of Gastroenterology
McMaster University
Hamilton ON, Canada

Lloyd Mayer, MD [163]
Codirector, Immunology Institute
Professor of Medicine, Clinical Immunology and
Gastroenterology
Professor, Microbiology
Mount Sinai School of Medicine
New York, New York

Genevieve B. Melton, MD [141]
Assistant Professor
Department of Surgery
University of Minnesota

Marjorie Merrick [147]
VP, Research and Scientific Programs
Crohn's and Colitis Foundation
New York, New York

Fabrizio Michelassi, MD [129]
Lewis Atterbury Stimson Professor
Department of Surgery
Weill Cornell Medical College
Surgeon in Chief
New York-Presbyterian Hospital
New York, New York

Jeffrey W. Milsom, MD [134]
Department of Surgery
Weill Cornell Medical College
New York-Presbyterian Hospital
New York, New York

Gerard E. Mullin, MD [117]
Associate Professor
Department of Medicine
Johns Hopkins School of Medicine
The Johns Hopkins Hospital
Baltimore, Maryland

Lissette Musaib-Ali, MD [127]
Internal Medicine Resident
Georgetown University Hospital
Washington Hospital Center
Washington, D.C.

Geoffrey C. Nguyen, MD, PhD, FRCP(C) [160]
Assistant Professor
Department of Medicine
University of Toronto
Toronto, ON, Canada
Adjunct Assistant Professor
Department of Medicine
Division of Gastroenterology
Johns Hopkins School of Medicine
Baltimore, Maryland

Hien T. Nguyen, MD [132]
Assistant Professor
Department of Surgery
Johns Hopkins University School of Medicine
Baltimore, Maryland

Peter Nielsen [156]
Health and Fitness Expert
Detroit, Michigan

Patrick I. Okolo III, MD, MPH [127]
Chief of Endoscopy
Johns Hopkins University School of Medicine
Baltimore, Maryland

Remo Panaccione, MD, FRCPC [108]
Director
IBD Clinic Director
Gastroenterology Research Associate
Professor
Department of Medicine
University of Calgary
Calgary, AB, Canada

Keely Parisian, MD [126]
Gastroenterology and Hepatology Fellow
Digestive Disease Institute
Cleveland Clinic
Cleveland, Ohio

P. Jay Pasricha, MC [155]
Professor of Medicine
Division of Gastroenterology and Hepatology
Stanford University School of Medicine
Stanford, California

Patrizio Petrone, MD [140]
Huntington Medical Research Institutes
Huntington Memorial Hospital
Pasadena, California

Cosimo Prantera [101]
Gastroenterology Unit
Azienda Ospedaliera S. Camillo-Forlanini
Rome, Italy

Miguel Regueiro, MD [123]
Associate Professor of Medicine
University of Pittsburgh School of Medicine
Codirector, IBD Center
Head, Clinical IBD Program
Division of Gastroenterology, Hepatology, and
Nutrition
University of Pittsburgh Medical Center
Pittsburgh, Pennsylvania

Donna K. Rode [146]
Administrative Assistant
The Johns Hopkins Hospital
Baltimore, Maryland

Peter H. Rubin, MD [124]
The Henry D. Janowitz Division of Gastroenterology
Mount Sinai Medical Center
New York, New York

Paul J. Rutgeerts, MD, PhD, FRCP [136]
Professor
Department of Medicine
University of Leuven
Leuven, Belgium

Jenny Sauk, MD [106]
Department of Gastroenterology
Mt. Sinai Medical Center
New York, New York

Lawrence R. Schiller, MD [137]
Program Director
Gastroenterology Fellowship
Baylor University Medical Center
Dallas, Texas

David A. Schwartz, MD [116]
Associate Professor of Medicine
Director, IBD Center
Division of Gastroenterology
Vanderbilt University Medical Center
Nashville, Tennessee

Marc Schwartz, MD [110]
IBD Center and Division of Gastroenterology,
Hepatology and Nutrition
University of Pittsburgh School of Medicine
Pittsburgh, Pennsylvania

Mary E. Sherlock, MB BCh BAO, FRCPC [120]
The Hospital for Sick Children
Toronto, Ontario, Canada

Cathy E. Shin, MD, FAAP, FACS [130]
Assistant Professor of Clinical Surgery
Keck School of Medicine
University of Southern California
Los Angeles, Califonia

Corey A. Siegel, MD, MS [115]
Director
IBD Center
Dartmouth-Hitchcock Medical Center
Lebanon, New Hampshire

Anne Silverman, MD [161]
Director, Gastroenterology Research
Henry Ford Hospital
Detroit, Michigan

Michael D. Sitrin, MD [131]
Professor of Medicine
State University of New York
Buffalo, New York

Sharon L. Stein, MD [129]
Assistant Professor of Surgery
Division of Colorectal Surgery
University Hospitals, Case Medical Center
Cleveland Heights, Ohio

Ryan W. Stidham, MD [135]
Department of Medicine
Division of Gastroenterology
University of Michigan School of Medicine
Ann Arbor, Michigan

Christian D. Stone, MD [98]
Associate Professor
Chief, Division of Gastroenterology
Director, IBD and Gastrointestinal Research
University of Nevada School of Medicine
Las Vegas, Nevada

Scott A. Strong, MD, FACS, FASCRS [133]
Department of Colorectal Surgery
The Cleveland Clinic Foundation
Cleveland, Ohio

Sukanya Subramanian, MD [112]
Instructor of Clinical Medicine
Columbia University
New York, New York

Glenn J. Treisman, MD, PhD [151]
Professor, Department of Psychiatry and
Behavioral Sciences
Director, AIDS Psychiatry Service
The Johns Hopkins Hospital
Baltimore, Maryland

William J. Tremaine, MD [123]
Professor
Department of Medicine
Mayo Clinic
Rochester, Minnesota

Lisa Turnbough, RN, CGRN [145]
IBD Patient Advocate
The Institute for Digestive Health and
Liver Disease

Mercy Medical Center
Baltimore, Maryland

Laura K. Turnbull, BA, MSNc   [117]
Johns Hopkins School of Nursing
Baltimore, Maryland

Anne G. Tuskey, MD   [162]
Postdoctoral Clinic Fellow
Division of Gastroenterology and Hepatology
The Johns Hopkins Hospital
Baltimore, Maryland

Eric Vasiliauskas, MD   [166]
Associate Clinical Director
IBD Center
Cedars-Sinai Medical Center
Associate Professor
Department of Medicine and Pediatrics
David Geffen School of Medicine at UCLA
Los Angeles, California

Marja J. Verhoef, PhD   [157]
Department of Community Health Sciences
University of Calgary
Calgary, AB, Canada

Georgia Vogelsang, MD   [165]
Professor
Oncology Division
Johns Hopkins University School of Medicine
Baltimore, Maryland

Akbar K. Waljee, MD, MSc   [135]
Clinical Lecturer
Department of Internal Medicine
University of Michigan Health System
Ann Arbor, Michigan

H. Richard Waranch, PhD   [154]
Assistant Professor
Medical Psychology
Johns Hopkins Medical Institutions
Private Practice in Psychology
Baltimore, Maryland

Elizabeth Wick, MD   [141]
Assistant Professor
Department of Surgery
The Johns Hopkins Hospital
Baltimore, Maryland

Douglas C. Wolf, MD   [149]
Medical Director of Research
Center for Clinical Research
Atlanta Gastroenterology Associates
Atlanta, Georgia

Mark T. Worthington, MD, AGAF   [162]
Associate Professor of Medicine
Division of Digestive Diseases
Johns Hopkins Bayview Medical Center
Baltimore, Maryland

Preface

This is the third edition of a book devoted to the details of caring for patients with Crohn's disease and ulcerative colitis.

Concern for their support and their quality of life are given equal billing with current concepts of medical and surgical care. Readers and reviewers of earlier editions appreciated the well-written "consultations" from experts who were able to clearly and concisely present their views on management on a relatively narrow and specific area while balancing risks and benefits. Evidence-based medicine is interwoven with views gained from their clinical experience. Brief editor's comments are added to some chapters to call attention to alternative views or other areas of potential interest. This format leads to a particularly useful book.

Now published in two volumes to accommodate the many advances in understanding treatment options, this set of volumes represents a ready source of information for the health care professional as well as the increasingly well-informed patient. Inflammatory bowel disease, a spectrum of diseases, is receiving increasing attention as our understanding of the genetic and luminal environmental etiologic factors increases and diagnostic tools are refined. Basic research has accelerated in this decade and is continuing to yield new, more targeted treatments than were available just a few years ago. Within the 166 chapters with authors based in 25 different countries, there is a lot of new information and approaches that should lead to ever-improving care. One envisions panels of genetic and biomarkers that will allow predictions of prognosis and selection of appropriate medications.

Volume I is on IBD and Ulcerative Colitis and Volume II is on IBD and Crohn's Disease. The first section deals with the expectations of the patient, in terms of both natural history as well as the experiences of living with these chronic and, at times, debilitating illnesses that often begin in childhood and adolescence. The average age of onset is 27 years. The section on etiology and pathogenesis includes the influence of the age of onset on the IBD phenotypes and genotypes. The 14 chapters on diagnostic and prognostic methodology highlight clinical, technical, laboratory, and imaging modalities that have sharpened our clinical acumen. There is a focus on aggravating factors in the IBD patient, including stress, infectious agents, nonsteroidal anti-inflammatory agents, and pregnancy.

The sections on therapy, first of ulcerative colitis, and in the second volume, Crohn's disease, include 55 chapters on medical therapy, including 25 chapters on immunomodulators and biologic therapies. Optimizing use of each agent and combination therapy is stressed, and mucosal healing is targeted as a goal of therapy. Maintenance therapy and prophylactic measures after Crohn's disease resection are discussed along with the risks and benefits of therapy. Subjects vary from probiotics for ulcerative colitis to stem cell transplantation for Crohn's disease.

There are 30 chapters on surgical approaches to these diseases and 20 chapters on complications including concerns about radiation exposure with some imaging modalities. The last three sections of the book include discussion of patient support services, behavioral therapy, and special situations including pregnancy and microscopic colitis.

Our goal in creating this book is to allow dissemination of the knowledge, the treatment advances and the experience at optimizing each therapy that has lessened the burden of these illnesses on the affected individuals, several million world-wide, and on society. There are good reasons to be optimistic.

T. M. Bayless, MD
S. B. Hanauer, MD

Acknowledgments

Our patients, who not only entrusted us with their care but also taught us the importance of many of the issues in this book, have provided continuous inspiration. We are grateful to the authors who generously shared their views with us and with you, the reader, and to our colleagues at the Harvey M. and Lyn P. Meyerhoff IBD Center at Johns Hopkins and at the Joseph B. Kirsner IBD Center at the University of Chicago, who have participated in the patient care and research that form many of our views of IBD management. The members, officers, and staff of the Crohn's Colitis Foundation of America and the Gastrointestinal Education and Research Foundation have helped us appreciate the multifaceted needs of patients with IBD. Our publisher, Martin Wonsiewicz of Peoples Medical Publishing House—USA (PMPH-USA), and Senior Editor, Linda Mehta, were essential to a timely and attractive publication. Kudos to Donna Rode, our administrative assistant in Baltimore who coordinated the entire effort. Our profound thanks to our wives, Jaye and Jane, and our children and grandchildren who gave up their time to permit this ambitious endeavor.

Philanthropists who "want to help people by contributing to research" (Sherlock Hibbs); who want to encourage excellence in patient care and in basic and clinical investigation (Lyn P. and Harvey M. Meyerhoff); and "venture philanthropists" (Eli and Edythe Broad) have provided pilot funds for much of our knowledge and for many of today's young IBD researchers, the leaders of tomorrow.

Dr. Bayless is grateful for the continuing support and encouragement of the Alan Guerrieri family; Alan Schecter; Atran Foundation (Leonard Atran); Barbara and David Hirshhorn; Blaine Franklin Newman IBD Nurse Advocate Fund (Zoralyn Stahl); Charles Warfield, MD; Cynthia and Peter Rosenwald; David Hutcheon, MD; David Paige, MD; Daniel Hollander, MD; Edward Wolf, MD; Francis Giardiello, MD; Frederick Krieble; Harvey and Marlene Fenster; Jane Krieger Shapiro; Joseph and Harvey Meyerhoff Family Foundation; Louise Caponegro; Marie and Ernest C. Cookerly; Marilyn Meyerhoff; Marshall Bedine, MD; Michael Weinman family; Morton and Harriett Hyatt and the Turkey Trot; Perry Hookman, MD; Philip Romano Family; Sonia Tendler; Steven Mullany; Stuart Bainum, Sr; and Stuart Bainum, Jr., Norman Blake; Ronald Hunter; and William Sikinga.

Dr. Hanauer wishes to thank his mentor, Joseph B. Kirsner, who at the age of 101 continues to inspire us all to improve the plight of our patients until we are able to unravel the etiopathogenesis and derive ultimate cures for the ulcerative colitides and Crohn's diseases; to Drs. Russell Cohen and David Rubin who direct the University of Chicago IBD Center; and, of course, to our patients who are our real heros.

Tribute

Marc Lémann, distinguished IBD specialist and a friend to so many, was born on the 27th of June 1956 in Paris and died suddenly on the 26th of August 2010 while on the beach on Reunion Island, where he spent some time during his childhood. Marc was working on a chapter for this book.

The outline of his career can be succinct. Marc gained his baccalaureate at the age of 17 in Marseille and undertook his medical studies in the Faculty of Pitié-Salpêtrière (1973–1979), before being appointed as house physician in Paris at the age of 24. He did his National Service within the Technical Assistance at Saint-Denis de La Reunion, and began his internship (1981–1985), choosing to specialize in Hepatogastroenterology. He was a registrar to Professor J.C. Chaput at the Antoine Béclère Hospital and went on to do research for 2 years (1986–1988) in the INSERM unit U290 headed by Professor J.F. Desjeux, at Saint-Lazare. After this he returned to Saint-Lazare as Assistant Head of Clinic in hepatogastroenterology and then moved to Saint-Louis (1988–1991), where he became teaching practitioner (1992–1995), hospital practitioner (1995–2000), and ultimately University Professor–Hospital Practitioner (2000–2010). When Robert Modigliani retired in 2003, Marc Lémann was appointed as his successor as the Head of Hepatogastroenterology.

This succinct outline belies the many dimensions, great breadth, and substantive achievements of his career, touched always with a personal concern for his colleagues and patients that made him unique. Marc Lémann put his medical duties before all others; he combined intuition and high-quality clinical reasoning. He treated patients as people, always sparing them time; it is no surprise that many became attached to his care. Chronic inflammatory bowel diseases (CIBD) were his main clinical specialty and his expertise was accompanied by his concern to raise the standards of care for these conditions characterized by such miserable symptoms. Marc developed clinical and translational research with his team participating in numerous trials of novel therapy. He was an instigator and novel thinker, driving many investigator-initiated trials at a time—still continuing—unlike many who pursue studies only initiated by industry. He excelled at collaboration. He was the architect of the INSERM "Avenir" team managed by

his colleague Matthieu Aliez at Saint-Louis and made digestive cancer a new interest for his team, under the management of his collaborator Jean-Marc Gornet.

Marc Lémann and Emile Sarfati, Head of General Surgery, created an exemplary and amicable medical and surgical complementarity, essential for the optimal management of CIBD and digestive cancers. In partnership with Emile Sarfati and Christophe Hennequin (radiotherapy), a committee of gastrointestinal oncology was created at Saint-Louis. Marc managed the core of the hospital, grouping together the separate but complementary specialties of endocrinology, uro-nephrology, and medical and surgical gastroenterology. This intuitive sense of how one specialty could complement—rather than compete with—another was a measure of the man. It is why his achievements are greater than the sum of the parts.

He was involved in university education, teaching at Saint-Louis and in the Faculty of Medicine at the University Paris 7–Denis Diderot. He participated in several interuniversity diplomas (CIBD, surgical coloproctology) and the EPU for gastroenterologists. His department was recognized as a training ground and center of excellence, becoming the preferred choice for DES students of hepatogastroenterology. Always prepared with care, his lectures were outstanding for their clarity and depth. He was a warm and humorous speaker, addressing the audience with a friendly tone, a smile on his face, and a twinkle in his eyes, notwithstanding a serious message. He never failed to see a paradox or recognize the irony of a situation and maintained a sense of humor that shone a searchlight on current knowledge and the ridiculous. Colleagues at all levels of expertise and seniority looked forward to his talks and were assiduous in their attendance, because there, they knew, they would find ideas and insight. Many of us practice medicine while thinking of him.

The fundamental research of Marc Lémann focused first on gastrointestinal motility and then the immunology of CIBD. Marc's work will, however, be remembered principally for his clinical research on CIBD through GETAID (group for therapeutic studies on inflammatory disorders of the digestive tract), created in 1983 by Robert Modigliani. He instigated or participated in numerous clinical trials evaluating immunosuppressant drugs and biological therapy in particular, which has revolutionized the care of patients with CIBD. He was a major player in the international trials testing new molecular targets for the treatment of CIBD. He also recognized the need to define the cumulative burden of CIBD and developed new indices, one of which has been named the Lémann Score, quantifying the extent of intestinal damage from Crohn's disease. However, his preeminent and favorite field was that of trials of therapeutic strategy: these trials, simple in concept in that they tested clinical practice, but robust in design, required a clear vision of the practical. When two-arm randomized, controlled trials were considered the state of the art, Marc designed and led therapeutic strategy trials that have become the principal drivers for changes in practice.

Marc Lémann became president of GETAID in 2002 and occupied this role in 2010. His presidency motivated an extraordinary impetus within GETAID, increasing and diversifying national and international studies, leading to high-impact publications. GETAID is now considered the prime vehicle for investigator-initiated clinical or therapeutic research on CIBD in the world. It has become a model that international colleagues want to emulate. Marc achieved this by his personality, seeking always to find the common ground for collaboration, motivating colleagues, and resolving tension to make it a force for progress. His technique was disarming, and he was often asked to explain his secret. Marc used to answer that it was the coupling between physicians and biostatisticians, internal democracy and mixing this all with friendship, without being more precise. He understood the time to be allusive and the time to be explicit. He had, as a consequence, an exceptional ability to unify and help very different people work together in a friendly atmosphere. He knew, quite simply, how to bring out the best in everyone.

Marc was a distinguished member of European and international organizations dedicated to CIBD. He contributed to the European Crohn's and Colitis Organization (ECCO) from its inception and was an elected member of the International Organization for the Study of Inflammatory Bowel Disease. Apart from being a major contributor to consensus documents on ulcerative colitis and Crohn's disease, he was the driver for a Clinical Trials Committee. Nevertheless, it was his engaging personality that resolved differences and contributed so much to the spirit of ECCO, encouraging young people and promoting collaborations. He was a leading international expert on CIBD and often invited to speak at conferences. His work resulted in 160 peer-reviewed publications, many published in major journals and others in the process of publication that will echo his memory to his many friends.

That Marc was an exceptional practitioner, a brilliant teacher and speaker, a productive researcher, and an outstanding organizer is not a matter for posthumous praise, but a faithful reflection of the man with whom we worked. We speak with loyalty of his sharp intellect, open-mindedness, powerful capacity for work, and remarkable efficiency. All who knew him spoke of his merits and engaging personality. The man was an active pessimist with a lucid irony. He cultivated and maintained friendship with the same rigorous warmth that he displayed in his work, making everyone feel like a special friend. It was his great store of medical and general knowledge that underpinned his penetrating and original thought. It is worth reading the many tributes recorded on the ECCO Web site (www.ecco.ibd.eu).

The sudden death of Marc, in the middle of his life, is a terrible bereavement for his father, his children Raphaelle and Stanislas, his brother Frederic and sisters Isabelle and Florence, and all his family. It is the loss of a very dear friend to all who worked with him. His death leaves an empty space. He is sadly missed at Saint-Louis Hospital, in the Faculty of Medicine, the world of CIBD, and in French gastroenterology. Too often we are reminded of his presence and potential, which stir sadness and regret. He was to become the next President of the French National Society of Gastroenterology.

May his children, family, friends, colleagues, and everyone know how much we loved him. He has left an indelible footprint.

Jean Frédéric Colombel, Matthieu Allez, Franck Carbonnel, Patricia Détré, Yoram Bouhnik, and the GETAID.

Editors note (TMB): We have chosen to include this tribute to a colleague in the world of IBD physician-scientists since Marc exemplifies the humanity and intelligence that we all try to bring to patient care and to asking questions. This book is meant to focus on the multiple disciplines that contribute to the well-being of the patient.

Sequential and Combination Therapy for Small Bowel Crohn's Disease

98

Christian D. Stone

A common clinical dilemma in the treatment of Crohn's disease (CD) is deciding on the initial and subsequent choice of therapies in patients with moderate to severe disease, which usually indicates that remission cannot be maintained with lower-tier medications such as antibiotics, mesalamine, and budesonide. Such patients require more aggressive therapy in the form of steroids and immunomodulators (IMM; azathioprine [AZA], 6-mercaptopurine [6-MP], or methotrexate) and/or monoclonal antibodies (biologics), such as infliximab (IFX), adalimumab, or certolizumab directed at tumor necrosis factor (TNF)-α. Despite the availability of biologics for more than a decade, in the case of IFX, and IMM for several decades, the optimal strategy for using these drugs, either as monotherapy or in combination, remains controversial. This chapter intends to provide an update on the current state of knowledge regarding these therapies for moderate to severe CD, focusing on (a) the sequential use of IMM followed by TNFα antagonists and (b) combination, or simultaneous, use of IMM and TNFα antagonists. Lastly, practical recommendations will be presented on how to use these medications in sequence or in concert.

SEQUENTIAL THERAPY IN CD

Sequential therapy refers to a traditional strategy, often depicted as "step-up" pyramid paradigm, in which the choice of medication intensifies as disease becomes more severe.[1] Patients with mild disease begin more benign therapies (budesonide, mesalamine, antibiotics) at the base of the pyramid. As disease progresses to moderate severity, the clinician can step up the pyramid by starting systemic steroids to induce short-term remission followed by other therapies such as an IMM, usually AZA or 6-MP, for long-term maintenance. If these cannot achieve a prolonged clinical remission, the next step up the pyramid is use of a TNFα antagonist. Reserving biologics until after failure of IMM represents a traditional and still popular algorithm in the treatment of CD and one that, most would

agree, follows the Federal Drug Administration's approved guidelines for use of biologics.

The bulk of the debate with traditional sequential therapy involves what to do with the IMM (which was insufficient to maintain remission) after the decision is made to begin a biologic. Generally, four possibilities exist for the fate of the IMM:

1. Discontinue the IMM before the biologic is started.
2. Continue the IMM in combination with the biologic indefinitely.
3. Continue the IMM initially, overlapping it with the biologic, then discontinue the IMM after some period of time.
4. Discontinue the biologic after induction (e.g., IFX dosed at 0, 2, and 6 weeks only), and then continue the IMM either alone or with episodic biologic dosing.

Option 4 is not a common approach inasmuch as scheduled maintenance dosing of the biologic would be considered routine with traditional sequential therapy because the IMM has already been shown to lack efficacy. However, because there are studies that employed this strategy and instances in which episodic use of the biologic may be necessary, it will be included in the following discussion.

In order to decide among the four options for IMM, the relevant studies that investigated sequential therapy and the effect of IMM must be reviewed. During the early years of the IFX experience, retrospective studies in nonfistulizing CD suggested that short-term response and duration of response were superior if patients were also taking an IMM prior to initiation of IFX.[2] This lead to the recommendation that an IMM should always be given in conjunction with IFX. Later, post-hoc analysis of the ACCENT I trial (A Crohn's Disease Clinical Trial Evaluating Infliximab in a New Long-Term Treatment Regimen) revealed that, after 54 weeks, there was a statistically significant advantage in response and remission rates to concurrent IMM with episodic IFX but no advantage if scheduled maintenance IFX was used.[3] Similarly, no differences in efficacy between patients on and off concomitant IMM were noted in the 52- and 26-week placebo-controlled trials conducted later using maintenance adalimumab[4] and certolizumab.[5]

The reason for the beneficial effect of concurrent IMM is thought to be a reduction in the immunogenicity of IFX.[6] The development of antibodies to IFX (ATI) is associated with infusion reactions that may cause intolerance leading to early discontinuation of the drug. Concomitant IMM,[3,6] as well as premedication with steroids,[7] can successfully lower the incidence of infusion reactions and increase the duration of response of IFX therapy. Development of antibodies may not be as significant a problem with the injectable TNFα antagonists, but, in general, an IMM would be expected to reduce the immunogenicity whether it was started before, or simultaneously with, a biologic. In the absence of infusion reactions, it is not clear if ATI are directly responsible for diminished efficacy or loss of response to IFX. Indeed, the presence of detectable antibodies did not correlate with lack of efficacy in the ACCENT I trial. Although there was no discernable advantage to concomitant IMM with all three biologics when given as scheduled maintenance, it should be noted that these conclusions were based on post-hoc analyses in these trials, which were not powered to examine the effect of IMM specifically.

Returning to the question at hand, what should be done with an IMM that has failed to maintain remission, leading to a decision to start a biologic with scheduled maintenance dosing? The data suggest that there should be minimal difference between options 1 and 2 in terms of response and remission rates. Option 2 would be expected to result in fewer infusion reactions with IFX up to 1 year. Beyond this, there are no studies that provide evidence of a long-term advantage to indefinite continuation of the IMM. Rather, a study from 2008 showed that any advantage to continuing the IMM does not extend beyond 6 months, which brings us to option 3—overlapping the IMM temporarily with the biologic. In the study by Van Assche et al.,[8] 80 CD subjects in remission on combination IFX + IMM for at least 6 months were randomized to either continue or discontinue IMM while maintaining IFX infusions at 5 mg/kg every 8 weeks or longer (about one-third of the subjects received "on-demand" IFX). Although specifics were not reported, most of the subjects had been taking IMM *prior to* initiating IFX. All subjects were required to have documented full clinical response to IFX. After 104 weeks, no difference between the two groups was apparent in terms of the primary end point, that is, need for rescue IFX due to disease flare or interruption of IFX because of loss of response, intolerance, or adverse event. The Crohn's Disease Activity Index scores and requirement for shortening of the IFX dosing interval also did not differ, but the group that continued IMM exhibited higher trough levels of IFX and lower serum C-reactive protein values. These results support the strategy of discontinuing the IMM 6 months after initiation of IFX in patients who had failed prior IMM monotherapy. Furthermore, they add to the growing body of evidence that IFX trough levels are a valuable indicator of long-term response to IFX.[9]

The other study of partial relevance to the current discussion is the so-called "step-up versus top-down" trial by D'Haens et al.,[10] which pitted conventional management (steroids followed by maintenance AZA, and then episodic IFX if necessary) against "combined immunosuppression" therapy (IFX induction plus maintenance AZA, and then episodic IFX if necessary) in 129 early-onset CD patients naïve to both medications. In this unblinded study, the conventional management arm approximated the traditional sequential therapy whereas the combined immunosuppressive arm represented a top-down approach using early IFX but for induction only as a bridge to AZA maintenance. After 26 weeks, 60% of the "top-down" compared to 36% of the "step-up" subjects were in steroid-free remission ($P = 0.006$). At 52 weeks, the steroid-free remission rates were 62% versus 42% ($P = 0.03$). At the end of 2 years, the difference in remission rates between the two groups was no longer statistically significant, but a greater proportion of the early combined group had complete endoscopic mucosal healing (73% vs. 30%, $P = 0.003$). The proportion of subjects who required IFX was similar in both groups. This study revealed merits to both strategies: with sequential therapy, there was increasing benefit of long-term AZA, and with "top-down" treatment several advantages of early IFX use were observed, including better mucosal healing, reduced steroid exposure, and faster remission rates. In the context of the current discussion, the "top-down" arm results are not relevant because subjects were naïve to both the AZA and IFX. The "step-up" arm, however, was representative of the fourth option for IMM listed earlier. As such, IFX induction functioned well as a bridge to maintenance AZA, though the requirement for additional episodic doses of IFX increased steadily during the trial. This result mirrors clinical experience in that patients who have previously failed IMM would not be expected to maintain long-term remission with the same IMM if they only receive induction with a biologic.

Another trial that sheds light on option 4 is the French cooperative study by Lémann et al.,[11] which examined the effect of IFX induction in 113 CD patients with steroid-dependent disease for at least 6 months, stratified into IMM-refractory and IMM-naïve groups. The subjects were randomized in double-blinded fashion to receive IFX induction (0, 2, and 6 weeks) versus placebo but no maintenance infusions. The primary end point was steroid-free remission at 24 weeks. IMM-refractory subjects (defined as those who could not maintain remission without steroids) continued either AZA or 6-MP whereas those who were IMM naïve initiated AZA or 6-MP 1 week after the first IFX infusion. Looking at all patients regardless of prior IMM use, those who received IFX had higher remission rates (57% vs. 29%, $P = 0.003$), thus IFX was effective as a bridge to continued maintenance with IMM. This observed advantage to IFX is not surprising because half of the subjects who did not receive IFX were IMM refractory and thus would not be expected to achieve a steroid-free remission at 24 weeks since they were already steroid dependent (only 26% of such patients achieved remission). Moreover, all subjects either continued low-dose or received higher-dosed steroids during the infusion phase, which may also have benefitted the response to IFX by lowering immunogenicity. In the group randomized to IFX, subjects who were IMM naïve were more likely to be in remission compared to IMM-refractory subjects (63% vs. 50%). These results confirm what is commonly appreciated in clinical practice, namely that patients who do not respond to an IMM are different from those who are IMM naïve and this must be taken into account when deciding on the next course of action. Using IFX as a bridge to maintenance with an IMM will have greater success in the IMM naïve patient. This strategy may be necessary, for instance when IFX or other TNFα antagonists cannot be obtained for maintenance or are cost prohibitive, but it is worth emphasizing that if the patient is IMM refractory (option 4), the efficacy of IMM monotherapy will certainly wane and retreatment with a biologic will be necessary in most cases.

To conclude, reviewing the four options for IMM in sequential therapy, each may be reasonable under different circumstances. Option 1 might be considered in patients who have difficulty tolerating immunosuppressives or if there is concern about the safety of double immunosuppression, to be discussed later. Option 2 allows for maximizing the efficacy of IFX long term, by lowering the incidence of infusion reactions and achieving higher trough levels. Option 3 is a middle ground approach for those who prefer the short-term gain of overlapping IMM but wish to limit possible long-term complications. Option 4 is probably not a viable long-term strategy without episodic biologic dosing, which itself is not ideal. Hence, option 4 is likely to be used more by necessity than by choice.

● COMBINED THERAPY IN CD

Study of Immunomodulator-Naïve Patients in CD Trial

This section will examine simultaneous use of an IMM and biologic, a strategy in which the debate centers mainly on CD patients who are naïve to both medications. The key question to address in such patients is "Does concomitant use of IMM and a biologic provide an advantage over a biologic alone if the patient is naïve to both and the biologic is continued as maintenance?" The recently completed Study of Immunomodulator-Naïve Patients in Crohn's Disease (SONIC) trial attempted to address this question directly. In this study, 508 subjects with moderate to severe CD and no prior exposure to either IFX or IMM were randomized in double-blind fashion to one of three arms: AZA and placebo infusions; IFX infusions plus placebo capsules; or IFX plus AZA. IFX was dosed at 5 mg/kg at 0, 2, and 6 weeks induction followed by maintenance infusions every 8 weeks. The primary end point was steroid-free remission at 26 weeks. Results from both the 26-week primary end point[12] and a 50-week extension,[13] in which 280 subjects participated, were presented in October 2008 and June 2009, respectively.

The IFX plus AZA arm was statistically superior to IFX alone at both 26 and 50 weeks. This demonstrates convincingly that a therapeutic benefit exists to concomitant AZA (and probably other IMM) plus IFX (and probably other TNFα antagonists) even when patients continue scheduled maintenance biologic dosing. Why did this occur? As stated previously, a patient who is IMM naïve differs from one who is IMM refractory. In the latter case, when a biologic is started, the concomitant use of the IMM would likely be of benefit only with regard to the reduction in immunogenicity. But if the patient is IMM naïve, he/she stands to gain from combined IMM + biologic treatment as a result of both protection from immunogenicity and improved efficacy because both drugs could provide a therapeutic effect.

Initial short-term response rates to biologics are usually in the range of 60%,[14] and by 6 to 12 months the remission rates are approximately 30% to 40% in initial responders (non–intent-to-treat analysis).[4,15] These numbers improve in patients with a shorter duration of disease prior to receiving a biologic.[16] The impressive 56% steroid-free remission rate after 26 weeks in the IFX plus AZA arm of SONIC, thus, may reflect the cumulative advantage of several factors, including a relatively early disease course (median duration of disease was about 2 years), reduction of immunogenicity with use of AZA, and a therapeutic effect of the AZA in the subset of patients who did not have a robust response to IFX.

Should the IMM and biologic both be continued indefinitely? There is little data available to guide us. The "top-down" arm of the D'Haens study,[10] which employed simultaneous IMM and IFX, unfortunately, cannot answer this question because the IFX was used episodically. The ACCENT I[15] and the van Assche[8] trials also do not apply because the majority of the subjects in these studies who received combination therapy were IMM refractory. One argument against indefinite dual therapy in CD relates to its safety. Prior *retrospective studies* suggested higher risk of opportunistic infections with combination therapy,[17] but this was not borne out in the prospective SONIC trial, where the rate of adverse events, including serious infections, was similar in all three arms. The other safety concern arises from a report of hepatosplenic T-cell lymphoma (HSTCL), which per a recent review has been diagnosed in 15 inflammatory bowel disease (IBD) patients receiving concomitant IFX (two also received adalimumab) and AZA or 6-MP.[18] Only 200 cases of this very rare and deadly lymphoma have been reported in the literature; hence, the unusually high rate observed in IBD patients, most of whom were young men, is worrisome. Whether combined immunosuppression beyond 1 year is safe in terms of lymphoma risk is not clear, but HSTCL has also been reported in 10 patients on IMM monotherapy, and, in IBD, the risk does not appear to be related to longer duration of IFX use.[18] In short, the data is insufficient at this time to make a firm recommendation regarding how long to continue dual therapy in CD if both drugs are started simultaneously.

To complete the analysis of the SONIC trial results, the final controversy to address is whether AZA/6-MP or a TNFα antagonist should be used first in moderate to severe CD. In other words, should we abandon the traditional sequential approach? In SONIC, the IFX-alone arm was superior to the AZA-alone arm with steroid-free remission rates of 30.6% versus 44.4% ($P = 0.009$) after 26 weeks. At 50 weeks, examining only the results from the 280 subjects who agreed to participate in the extension, the difference in remission rates was no longer significant (60.8% vs. 54.7%, $P = 0.32$). Despite this, both IFX arms provided consistently better results over AZA alone, including endoscopic healing rates.

However, before concluding that IFX (or another biologic) should be the first-line treatment in all patients, it is important to note several details of the SONIC trial design that may have caused the AZA-alone arm to underperform. First, the study excluded patients with less than average or intermediate activity levels of thiopurine methyltransferase (TPMT). They represent half of the patient population. They respond within

6 to 8 weeks. Such patients require dosing adjustment, but are otherwise good candidates for AZA. Second, serum levels of the therapeutic metabolite, 6-thioguanine (6-TGN), were not obtained, making it likely that some subjects did not reach a therapeutic 6-TGN range in spite of weight-based dosing at 2.5 mg/kg/day. This dose is quite reasonable at the onset of AZA therapy, but given the variability in the activity of the three enzymes (TPMT, hypoxanthine phosphoribosyltransferase, and xanthine oxidase) that metabolize AZA and compete to determine the total amount of active 6-TGN, in addition to the variability in the gut absorption of AZA, it is clear that one dose does not fit all patients. Third, some subjects in the AZA-alone arm may not have received sufficient doses of steroids to induce remission (data on steroid dosing, which was unblinded, not available at the time of this writing). SONIC investigators were allowed to dose steroids at their discretion but not more than prednisone 40 mg/day or equivalent, which could be inadequate for inducing remission in a substantial number of the subjects, whose mean weight was 70 kg. Furthermore, because two-thirds of the subjects were guaranteed to receive induction with IFX, the blinded investigators would be reluctant, understandably, to provide full induction level dosing of steroids in all subjects to cover the one-third of patients in the AZA-alone arm. Reportedly only one-third of the patients in SONIC were steroid resistant and another one-third had been offered steroids but chose the trial.

For these reasons, AZA may have underperformed and the results may not reflect the optimal use of this drug, which, given its delayed action, is to maintain remission following induction with another agent.[19,20] Other studies investigating the efficacy of AZA in CD suggest that better results could be expected. For example, the 16% mucosal healing rate at 26 weeks achieved with AZA alone in SONIC contrasts with the smaller study by D'Haens et al.,[21] in which 11 of 15 patients (73%) with ileal CD had complete or near complete healing after 24 weeks of AZA. The same investigators further demonstrated 70% healing rates with AZA in another group of ileal CD patients at 24 months.[22] A Cochrane meta-analysis of AZA calculated pooled response rates of 54% and steroid sparing in 65%.[23] Another review reported that AZA achieved remission in 71% of patients overall, though these were not necessarily steroid-free remission.[24] Thirty years ago, small controlled studies revealed steroid-sparing effects of AZA in CD in the range of 80%,[25] but no recent study has examined the efficacy of AZA using a steroid-free remission end point comparable to the one used in SONIC. Thus, it is difficult to conclude definitively that AZA would have performed better if more favorable methods had been employed. Nevertheless, statements advocating the abandonment of traditional sequential therapy in favor of IFX ± AZA as first-line therapy for all CD patients based on the SONIC data should be tempered, acknowledging that the use of AZA in the trial may have been suboptimal.

Editor's note (TMB): I share the concern that AZA use may have been suboptimal, mainly because half of the potential patients, those with less than average TPMT enzyme activity, were excluded. This group responds well (more than 70%) and quickly within 6 to 8 weeks, to modest doses of AZA (1.5 mg/kg) or of 6-MP (50 mg).

Recommendations

Universal agreement on how best to sequence or combine the use of IMM and biologics in CD is not likely. Research conducted on this issue is complex and costly, resulting in few published studies, most of which can only be accomplished by the pharmaceutical industry. Indeed, it is exceedingly difficult for independent investigators to obtain the enormous amount of funding necessary for large, long-term, randomized prospective trials using biologics. Moreover, as with all clinical trials, the studies that do exist have limitations, may not be generalizable to a broad spectrum of patients, are subject to different interpretations, and do not take into account the many social and economic factors that influence decision making between the patient and physician. In light of these realities, and considering the fact that treatment decisions are not always evidence based, the following recommendations regarding IMM and biologic use in CD can be offered.

I do not agonize, nor do I wish the patient to agonize, over whether traditional sequential steroids plus IMM or a "top-down" strategy with an early biologic should be used first in moderate to severe CD. Treatment should be individualized inasmuch as patient factors may dictate care more often than not. Moreover, inadequate response and/or adverse events with either approach should be anticipated, which will require a quick change to the alternate plan. Given this, it is critical to be familiar with—and use methods to maximize the efficacy of—all drugs in the IBD armamentarium. Most importantly, we should recognize that many of our moderate to severe CD patients deserve aggressive treatment, meaning that both IMM and biologics could stand to be started earlier and with optimal dosing.

A biologic as first-line therapy is preferred in the following cases: patients who cannot tolerate steroid induction due to significant side effects; severe perianal disease; and severe luminal disease (with or without fistulae) requiring hospitalization, where rapid onset of response is desired. In these cases, choosing a biologic as initial therapy is unlikely to generate much debate. Whether an IMM should be started simultaneously in these examples will depend on the clinical assessment of overall disease severity with severe or previously intractable disease receiving concomitant IMM for at least the first few months should be considered, bearing in mind that some patients may not tolerate combined immunosuppression.

In the ambulatory patient, without significant perianal involvement or features of aggressive disease, before deciding on traditional steroids plus IMM versus early biologic, I currently engage the patient in a discussion about the pros and cons of each approach. Any therapy is more likely to succeed and result in better adherence if the patient feels comfortable, understands the reasoning behind it, and has realistic expectations about the outcome. Encouraging dialogue also allows the patient to express any reservations that may be present about either strategy. Some patients prefer a newer, cutting-edge medication. Others are simply afraid of biologics, often borne of misconceptions about the risks of these drugs. Such fear should be discussed, allayed where appropriate, and placed in the proper context of our extensive experience with these agents and their well-recognized risks, which can be managed in experienced hands. These risks will tend to be outweighed to a greater extent by their benefits as the disease severity increases. In short, I do not advocate universally either a biologic first or an IMM first in moderate to severe CD. Rather, I make a recommendation to the patient based on the specifics of their particular disease phenotype while taking into account their individual preferences and attitude toward different treatment options.

Editor's note (TMB): I find knowing the TPMT enzyme activity helpful. If the TPMT level is less than average (13 with Mayo, 25 with Prometheus), there is a 70% likelihood of response within 6 to 8 weeks. If it is above average, only a 30% to 40% response is expected, and it might take 12 to 16 weeks (Cuffari, Bayless, Dassopoulos, et al. CHG April 2004 *Clin Gastro Hepatol.* 2004;2:410–417). If those time restraints are not acceptable, a rapid onset biologic is a better choice.

If IMM are to be used first, then I recommend aggressive use of AZA or 6-MP, ensuring that there is proper induction with weight-based steroid dosing (sometimes with antibiotics) and simultaneous initiation of full weight-based dosing of the IMM (in TPMT normal). Due to the variability in metabolism of these drugs, I strongly recommend confirmation of therapeutic levels by measuring 6-TGN levels, particularly in those who are unable to taper off of steroids. This test allows for detection of subjects who are subtherapeutic and require a dose beyond 2.5 mg/kg (for AZA) or 1.5 mg/kg (for 6-MP). In addition, checking the 6-TGN level is the only means of identifying so-called AZA/6-MP "rapid metabolizers." These patients will be unable to reach 6-TGN therapeutic levels regardless of the dose, and thus the clinician should either abandon the therapy or consider adding allopurinol.[26]

Once a therapeutic 6-TGN level has been achieved, provided sufficient time has elapsed and proper induction of remission has been achieved, if the patient still cannot maintain remission without steroids, then I consider this patient a true AZA/6-MP failure, and a biologic should then be used. In this scenario of traditional sequential therapy, if remission is achieved via the induction dosing of the biologic alone, it is reasonable to continue the IMM (at full or possibly a lower dose) for up to 6 months as noted by van Assche and others.[8,27] Whether dual therapy should continue beyond 6 months is not clear, but I contend again that this decision should be individualized with a thorough discussion of the potential risks (infection, lymphoma) and benefits (e.g., higher trough IFX levels and longer duration of therapy). The more aggressive the disease, the more likely I would advocate for dual therapy indefinitely.

Lastly, we come to the issue of combination of IMM and biologic in the patient naïve to both. Starting both agents simultaneously can result in a dilemma, for it is difficult or impossible to determine with certainty if one or both medications are contributing to the clinical response. Hence, if at a later time it becomes necessary to discontinue one of the drugs, a clinical recurrence may occur if the drug that is in fact maintaining the remission is stopped in error. There will be instances in which the biologic is not effective, therefore stopping the IMM and continuing the biologic will result in disease recurrence. Patients in this situation should be clearly distinguished from those who have already established themselves as IMM failures, in which case discontinuing the IMM after the biologic clearly induced the remission carries very little risk of disease recurrence. Again, using concurrent IMM beyond 6 to 12 months

To Optimize the Use of Either Biologics or Immunomodulators

1. Confirm active inflammatory disease (exclude large component of irritable bowel symptoms).
2. Exclude significant lumenal obstruction from fibrostenotic disease (e.g., radiographs showing prestenotic small bowel dilation). Such a finding would tend to favor surgery rather than continued medical therapy.
3. Start systemic therapies earlier and with adequate dosing to maximize their efficacy and duration of response.

To Optimize the Use of AZA/6-MP (and Methotrexate)

1. Ensure that clinical remission with steroids or another agent is induced to a sufficient degree and duration while immunomodulators (IMM) are initiated.
2. Obtain thiopurine methyltransferase (TPMT) enzyme activity or genotype and, if normal, begin full weight-based dosing. If TPMT is intermediate, begin a lower dose and monitor carefully for leukopenia.
3. Confirm therapeutic levels of azathioprine (AZA)/6-mercaptopurine (6-MP) by obtaining 6-thioguanine level, especially in patients who remain steroid dependent or have intermediate TPMT activity.
4. Allow for sufficient duration of IMM treatment at therapeutic levels (minimum of 6 weeks if the patient's symptoms allow).
5. Consider using allopurinol in conjunction with a lower dose of AZA/6-MP in "rapid metabolizers."
6. In case of intolerable idiosyncratic side effects such as nausea, rash, alopecia, or fatigue, consider change from generic to brand formulation or vice versa; likewise, consider change from AZA to 6-MP or vice versa.

To Optimize Use of Monoclonal Antibodies (Biologics)

1. In the immunomodulator (IMM)-naïve patient, start an IMM concomitantly in selected cases, whenever maximum efficacy of therapy is desired. Use combined therapy with particular caution in a younger population due to the risk of hepatosplenic T-cell lymphoma.
2. In the IMM-refractory patient, once the biologic is started, either discontinue the IMM immediately or continue for up to 6 months if there is particular desire to minimize immunogenicity with the biologic.
3. Preferentially use maintenance dosing of a biologic whenever possible.
4. Avoid disruption in dosing interval and do not lengthen the interval between dosing.
5. Elicit history of loss of response to a biologic between doses and, if found, escalate therapy early by increasing the biologic dose and/or shortening the interval.
6. Treat infusion and injection site reactions.

may not be justified when maintenance IFX or the injectable TNFα antagonists are used, though in specific patients with features of aggressive or severe disease, the benefit of reduced immunogenicity afforded by concurrent IMM use may outweigh the risk or cost. In younger patients, the risk of HSTCL must be included in the risk/benefit analysis. We have scant data with regard to IMM use with adalimumab and certolizumab, but given that their efficacy and side effect profiles have been shown to be similar to IFX, the positive and negative consequences of combining injectable biologics with IMM may likewise be similar. On the other hand, in contrast to the peak and trough pattern typical of IFX infusions, plasma levels with subcutaneous injection of TNFα antagonists have been shown to be quite stable (unpublished data from UCB, Inc.), which could lower its immunogenicity and obviate the need for concomitant IMM. If initial combination therapy is used, then I do not recommend discontinuing the biologic as a bridge to AZA/6-MP monotherapy because of the potential development of immunogenicity if the biologic is reintroduced in the future either episodically or as maintenance. Therefore, in general, whenever a decision is made to use a biologic for induction of remission, I will continue it for maintenance as long as possible.

In summary, it is critical to emphasize that clinicians should recognize when CD severity requires early IMM therapy or a biologic. Earlier, aggressive therapy regardless of the sequence of medications should increase the odds of effecting a sustained remission. There are advantages of combined therapy over monotherapy, but numerous factors, including patient preference, economic barriers, risk analysis, study limitations, the heterogeneity of the CD population, and the lack of biomarkers or pharmacogenomic profiles that can identify those who would benefit most from combined therapy or an early biologic, will continue to affect treatment decisions and challenge our ability to formulate a single therapeutic algorithm that is applicable to all patients.

Editor's note (TMB): The author has met one of the key goals of this publication: state the issues clearly, cite the evidence-based data, cite the clinical experience, and then clearly state his/her opinion. Dr. Stone, we thank you. The reader will find numerous well-founded opinions on the topic of TPMT and anti-TNFα medications. The chapters are on genomics; on IMM for UC and for CD; use of TPMT enzyme assays, symptom control, and metabolite levels in optimizing AZA/6-MP use; duration of IMM and biologic use; and risk/benefit discussions and HSTCL considerations for pediatric gastroenterologists. This is an important and timely issue and the reader will get a number of well-defined opinions. As Dr. Stone said, "There is no single therapeutic algorithm that is applicable to all patients."

References

1. Lichtenstein GR, Hanauer SB, Kane SV, Present DH. Crohn's is not a 6-week disease: lifelong management of mild to moderate Crohn's disease. *Inflamm Bowel Dis.* 2004;10(suppl 2):S2–S10.

2. Parsi MA, Achkar JP, Richardson S, et al. Predictors of response to infliximab in patients with Crohn's disease. *Gastroenterology.* 2002;123(3):707–713.

3. Hanauer SB, Wagner CL, Bala M, et al. Incidence and importance of antibody responses to infliximab after maintenance or episodic treatment in Crohn's disease. *Clin Gastroenterol Hepatol.* 2004;2(7):542–553.

4. Colombel JF, Sandborn WJ, Rutgeerts P, et al. Adalimumab for maintenance of clinical response and remission in patients with Crohn's disease: the CHARM trial. *Gastroenterology.* 2007;132(1):52–65.

5. Schreiber S, Khaliq-Kareemi M, Lawrance IC, et al.; PRECISE 2 Study Investigators. Maintenance therapy with certolizumab pegol for Crohn's disease. *N Engl J Med.* 2007;357(3):239–250.

6. Baert F, Noman M, Vermeire S, et al. Influence of immunogenicity on the long-term efficacy of infliximab in Crohn's disease. *N Engl J Med.* 2003;348(7):601–608.

7. Farrell RJ, Alsahli M, Jeen YT, Falchuk KR, Peppercorn MA, Michetti P. Intravenous hydrocortisone premedication reduces antibodies to infliximab in Crohn's disease: a randomized controlled trial. *Gastroenterology.* 2003;124(4):917–924.

8. Van Assche G, Magdelaine-Beuzelin C, D'Haens G, et al. Withdrawal of immunosuppression in Crohn's disease treated with scheduled infliximab maintenance: a randomized trial. *Gastroenterology.* 2008;134(7):1861–1868.

9. Maser EA, Villela R, Silverberg MS, Greenberg GR. Association of trough serum infliximab to clinical outcome after scheduled maintenance treatment for Crohn's disease. *Clin Gastroenterol Hepatol.* 2006;4(10):1248–1254.

10. D'Haens G, Baert F, van Assche G, et al.; Belgian Inflammatory Bowel Disease Research Group; North-Holland Gut Club. Early combined immunosuppression or conventional management in patients with newly diagnosed Crohn's disease: an open randomised trial. *Lancet.* 2008;371(9613):660–667.

11. Lémann M, Mary JY, Duclos B, et al.; Groupe d'Etude Therapeutique des Affections Inflammatoires du Tube Digestif (GETAID). Infliximab plus azathioprine for steroid-dependent Crohn's disease patients: a randomized placebo-controlled trial. *Gastroenterology.* 2006;130(4):1054–1061.

12. Sandborn W, Rutgeerts P, Reinisch W, et al. Sonic: a randomized, double-blind, controlled trial comparing infliximab and infliximab plus azathioprine to azathioprine in patients with Crohn's disease naive to immunomodulators and biologic therapy. *Am J Gastroenterol.* 2008;103:S436.

13. Sandborn WJ, Rutgeerts PJ, Reinisch W, et al. One year data from the Sonic study: a randomized, double-blind trial comparing infliximab and infliximab plus azathioprine to azathioprine in patients with Crohn's disease naive to immunomodulators and biologic therapy [abstract 751f]. *Gastroenterology.* 2009;136(5):A-116.

14. Hanauer SB, Sandborn WJ, Rutgeerts P, et al. Human anti-tumor necrosis factor monoclonal antibody (adalimumab) in Crohn's disease: the CLASSIC-I trial. *Gastroenterology.* 2006;130(2):323–333; quiz 591.

15. Hanauer SB, Feagan BG, Lichtenstein GR, et al.; ACCENT I Study Group. Maintenance infliximab for Crohn's disease: the ACCENT I randomised trial. *Lancet.* 2002;359(9317):1541–1549.

16. Sandborn WJ, Colombel JF, Panes J, Scholmerich J, McColm JA, Schreiber S. Higher remission and maintenance of response rates with subcutaneous monthly certolizumab pegol in patients with recent-onset Crohn's disease: data from PRECiSE 2 [abstract 1109]. *Am J Gastroenterol.* 2006;101:S394.

17. Toruner M, Loftus EV Jr, Harmsen WS, et al. Risk factors for opportunistic infections in patients with inflammatory bowel disease. *Gastroenterology.* 2008;134(4):929–936.

18. Mackey AC, Green L, Leptak C, Avigan M. Hepatosplenic T cell lymphoma associated with infliximab use in young patients treated for inflammatory bowel disease: update. *J Pediatr Gastroenterol Nutr.* 2009;48(3):386–388.

19. Pearson DC, May GR, Fick G, Sutherland LR. Azathioprine for maintaining remission of Crohn's disease. *Cochrane Database Syst Rev.* 2000;(2):CD000067.

20. Etchevers MJ, Aceituno M, Sans M. Are we giving azathioprine too late? The case for early immunomodulation in inflammatory bowel disease. *World J Gastroenterol.* 2008;14(36):5512–5518.

21. D'Haens G, Geboes K, Ponette E, Penninckx F, Rutgeerts P. Healing of severe recurrent ileitis with azathioprine therapy in patients with Crohn's disease. *Gastroenterology.* 1997; 112(5):1475–1481.

22. D'Haens G, Geboes K, Rutgeerts P. Endoscopic and histologic healing of Crohn's (ileo-) colitis with azathioprine. *Gastrointest Endosc.* 1999;50(5):667–671.

23. Sandborn W, Sutherland L, Pearson D, May G, Modigliani R, Prantera C. Azathioprine or 6-mercaptopurine for inducing remission of Crohn's disease. *Cochrane Database Syst Rev.* 2000; (2):CD000545.

24. Prefontaine E, Sutherland LR, MacDonald JK, Cepoiu M. Azathioprine or 6-mercaptopurine for maintenance of remission in Crohn's disease. *Cochrane Database Syst Rev.* 2009(1):CD000067.

25. Rosenberg JL, Levin B, Wall AJ, Kirsner JB. A controlled trial of azathioprine in Crohn's disease. *Am J Dig Dis.* 1975;20(8):721–726.

26. Sparrow MP, Hande SA, Friedman S, Cao D, Hanauer SB. Effect of allopurinol on clinical outcomes in inflammatory bowel disease nonresponders to azathioprine or 6-mercaptopurine. *Clin Gastroenterol Hepatol.* 2007;5(2):209–214.

27. Deshpande AR, Abreu MT. Combination therapy with infliximab and immunomodulators: is the glass half empty? *Gastroenterology.* 2008;134(7):2161–2163.

Step-Up Versus Top-Down Therapy in the Treatment of Crohn's Disease

99

Daan Hommes

INTRODUCTION

Crohn's disease (CD) is a chronic multifactorial polygenic disease, which behaves in a progressive destructive manner in most patients. Recently, it has been shown that 18.6% of CD patients experienced penetrating or stricturing complications already within 90 days after diagnosis.[1] Over the last decades, most patients ended up with developing penetrating and/or structuring complications despite therapy.[2,3] In recent years, however, the medical care for CD patients has altered significantly, aiming at avoiding these complications. The introduction of anti-TNF (antitumor necrosis factor) antibodies has impacted the outcome for patients dramatically. In addition to this antibody-based therapy, clinicians are nowadays equipped with a robust set of tools, supported by a substantial body of literature, on how to act upon diagnosing CD for the first time. There seems general consensus on the diagnostic process, using a full endoscopic work-up in combination with radiologic and histopathologic assessments. Once diagnosed, it is up to the team of inflammatory bowel disease (IBD) health professionals to fully inform and educate the patient and his/her relatives, and to install and monitor a vigorous medical regime. This chapter deals with an early intensive treatment algorithm for CD, introduced only recently.[4]

THERAPEUTIC WINDOW OF OPPORTUNITY

When a patient is diagnosed with CD, it is an important and challenging issue how to optimally treat the patient and at which point a certain therapy should be initiated. In established CD, early disease should be distinguished from late disease, since CD is characterized by progression of inflammatory disease (early disease) to a more complicated stricturing, penetrating, and fibrotic disease (late disease).[2,3] Fibrostenosis and perforations are not per se associated with early CD; usually patients with recently diagnosed CD have pure inflammatory lesions.

However, when the disease evolves, the number of complications increases and many patients will develop strictures or fistulae formation. During this stage, complications caused by tissue remodeling and fibrosis following long-standing disease are irreversible and difficult to treat with the anti-inflammatory agents. Often, surgery can not be avoided at this stage. The progression from early to late disease is accompanied by a change in mucosal cytokine profiles. Early CD is characterized by a pronounced Th1 response, whereas in late disease Th2 cytokines are predominating.[5] The concept that mucosal T-cell regulation is different in early and late disease suggests that patients with late disease respond different to therapies. The fact that disease progresses to complicated disease suggests that there is a particular time window at which therapy is most effective and favorable. This so-called "window of opportunity" is of great importance for the clinical practice since it aims to intervene with intensive therapeutic regimens in an early stage of the disease. At this point, it is most likely still possible to change the course of the disease toward a less aggressive phenotype, to control symptoms, induce mucosal healing, and to induce and maintain clinical and endoscopic remission.

THERAPEUTIC GOALS IN CD

The main treatment goals for CD patients are (1) to achieve clinical remission of steroids as quickly as possible, (2) to achieve, endoscopically assessed, mucosal healing, (3) to avoid hospitalization and surgery, and (4) to improve the quality of life. Indeed, today we are able to monitor the success of each of the treatment goals very effectively: (1) monitoring the rate of clinical remission in daily practice can be performed on a week to week basis by, for example, a specialized IBD nurse, using well defined and validated parameters of general well-being, abdominal pain, stool frequency, extraintestinal manifestations, and general symptoms like fever and weight. Next to clinical parameters, a defined set of laboratory values like CRP is recommended nowadays for monitoring. In addition, most steroid tapering schedules can be completed within 8 weeks. Intervention is required much sooner than 8 weeks should patients continue to have active disease and (2) the concepts of mucosal healing has been well accepted upon publication of a large number of studies showing the relevance of endoscopic assessments for the prediction of clinical remission.[6] Alternative biomarkers for mucosal healing are under development since endoscopy remains an invasive procedure, for instance fecal calprotectin and fecal lactoferrin.[7] It has also been shown that induction of clinical and endoscopic remission decreases the number of hospitalizations and surgeries in CD patients.[8] Similar to clinical remission, the quality of life of CD patients significantly improves upon reaching the previously discussed treatment goals.[9]

RATIONALE FOR EARLY INTENSIVE THERAPY IN CD

Historically, the step-up model of treatment for moderate-to-severe CD began with a tapered dosing schedule of steroids, lasting 8 to 12 weeks. Although early introduction of immunomodulatory therapy was also recommended in these patients, clinicians did not generally follow this practice. If patients responded to the initial course of steroid therapy, they were taken off steroids and receive no further treatment, or mesalamine or immunosuppressives were added (thiopurines or methotrexate). The anti-TNF therapy was only started if patients would fail these traditional drugs. Among the many reasons to evaluate "step-up versus top-down" were the safety concerns with the use of corticosteroids. Steroids are not very effective in the aforementioned treatment goals. In moderate to severely active CD patients, approximately 60% to 70% exhibit a symptomatic response to steroids but not for instance mucosal healing. In the long run, only a minority will achieve some benefit from steroid therapy (even with the introduction of immunomodulators) because a proportion of these patients will become resistant and others will develop steroid dependence. Furthermore, the safety profile of long-term steroid use is extremely unfavorable. Patients, particularly young adults, are at risk for Cushing's syndrome, the development of skin abnormalities, and early-onset osteoporosis. There is a large body of literature devoted to the adverse events associated with steroids, and registry data have shown increased mortality in CD patients treated with steroids alone.

The top-down approach was developed for a number of reasons. First, given the limited efficacy and safety profile of steroids, the goal of developing an algorithm that did not include them at all seemed prudent. Conversely, infliximab had maintained a relatively safe profile over the years since its introduction. So far, its use has not been associated with malignancy. Moreover, if used properly, the risk of a serious infection is minimal and clinically acceptable. It therefore seems feasible to introduce infliximab earlier in the treatment algorithm. In addition, steroids are not associated with mucosal healing, whereas recent studies of infliximab have linked it to increased mucosal healing.

Finally, and perhaps most importantly, there is the issue of IBD immunology. Considerable insight has been achieved in the immune response specific for CD. The lamina propria of patients contains T-lymphocytes that are resistant to apoptosis and thus relatively insensitive to nonspecific medications like steroids. Infliximab is capable of inducing apoptosis of this subset of T-cells, and this has been associated with clinical response as well as mucosal healing.[10] In addition, regulatory macrophages play an important role in wound healing and gut homeostasis and have anti-inflammatory properties. Induction of this cell type ($M\phi_{ind}$) by the anti-TNF antibodies infliximab and adalimumab has recently been shown in vitro.[11]

THE STEP-UP VERSUS TOP-DOWN STUDY

In a prospective, randomized controlled trial, including 130 patients with newly diagnosed CD naïve to corticosteroids, immunomodulators or anti-TNF agents, efficacy of step-up versus top-down therapy was evaluated.[4] The top-down approach involved a *treatment algorithm* starting with infliximab 5 mg/kg at weeks 0, 2, and 6 and azathioprine 2.5 mg/kg/day. Patients randomized to the step-up treatment algorithm were initially treated with corticosteroids (current standard around 1999), followed by azathioprine in case the corticosteroids were not able to control disease activity. Should this combination fail to avoid relapse, infliximab treatment was initiated. The co-primary end point in this study was clinical remission off steroids and without surgery at weeks 26 and 52. At both time points, a significant greater proportion of patients in the early combined intervention group met this end point compared to the conventional therapy group. At week 26, 39 (60.0%) of 65 patients in the top-down group were in remission without corticosteroids and without surgical resection, compared with 23 (35.9%) of 64 step-up patients, with an absolute difference of 24.1% (95% confidence interval (CI) 7.3–40.8, $P = 0.0062$). Corresponding rates at week 52 were 40/65 (61.5%) and 27/64 (42.2%) (absolute difference 19.3%, 95% CI 2.4–36.3, $P = 0.0278$). Furthermore, after 2 years, mucosal healing was observed in 73% of the patients in the early intervention group, whereas mucosal healing was seen in only 30% of the patients in the conventional treatment group. Importantly, 19% of the patients in the step-up group were still on steroids at this time point, whereas 0% of the patients in the early intervention group were receiving steroids. Also, this study showed that complete mucosal healing in patients with early-stage CD was associated with significantly higher steroid-free remission rates 4 years after therapy began.[12] Complete mucosal healing, defined as a simple endoscopic score of 0 after 2 years of therapy, was the only factor that predicted sustained, steroid-free remission 3 and 4 years after therapy was initiated; it was observed in 17 of 24 patients (70.8%) versus 6 of 22 patients with lesions detected by endoscopy (27.3%, Simple Endoscopic Score > 0) ($P = 0.036$; odds ratio (OR) = 4.352; 95% CI, 1.10–17.220). Fifteen of 17 patients with mucosal healing at year 2 maintained in remission without further infliximab infusions during years 3 and 4 ($P = 0.032$; OR = 4.883; 95% CI, 1.144–20.844). In this study, the number of side effects did not differ significantly between the two groups. Obviously, remission rates in the two groups did not differ significantly after 1 year since the two treatment algorithms were both designed to control disease and allowed intensification when disease activity persisted.

More recently, the SONIC trial evaluated the efficacy of infliximab monotherapy, azathioprine monotherapy, and the two drugs combined in 508 adults with moderate-to-severe CD who had not undergone previous immunosuppressive or biologic therapy.[13] Patients were randomly assigned to receive an intravenous infusion of 5 mg of infliximab per kilogram of body weight at weeks 0, 2, and 6 and then every 8 weeks plus daily oral placebo capsules; 2.5 mg of oral azathioprine per kilogram daily plus a placebo infusion on the standard schedule; or combination therapy with the two drugs. Of the 169 patients receiving combination therapy, 96 (56.8%) were in corticosteroid-free clinical remission at week 26 (the primary end point), as compared with 75 of 169 patients (44.4%) receiving infliximab alone ($P = 0.02$) and 51 of 170 patients (30.0%) receiving azathioprine alone ($P < 0.001$ for the comparison with combination therapy and $P = 0.006$ for the comparison with infliximab). Similar numerical trends were found at week 50. At week 26, mucosal healing had occurred in 47 of 107 patients (43.9%) receiving combination therapy, as compared with 28 of 93 patients (30.1%) receiving infliximab ($P = 0.06$) and 18 of 109 patients (16.5%) receiving azathioprine ($P < 0.001$ for the comparison with combination therapy and $P = 0.02$ for the comparison with infliximab). Thus, infliximab plus azathioprine was shown to be the superior combination for inducing remission.

● CONCLUSION

In conclusion, early intensive treatment, consisting of the combination of a thiopurine with an anti-TNF, should be considered in *all* patients who have a high risk for a complicated disease course, that is, young age at diagnosis, presentation with perianal or stricturing disease, or initial needs of steroids. If the appropriate safety measures are followed, this approach appears to be relatively safe. Treating physicians should be aware of opportunistic infections and other rare complications, and patients should be monitored carefully on a regular basis.

References

1. Thia KT, Sandborn WJ, Harmsen WS, Zinsmeister AR, Loftus EV Jr. Risk factors associated with progression to intestinal complications of Crohn's disease in a population-based cohort. *Gastroenterology.* 2010;139(4):1147–1155.

2. Louis E, Collard A, Oger AF, Degroote E, Aboul Nasr El Yafi FA, Belaiche J. Behaviour of Crohn's disease according to the Vienna classification: changing pattern over the course of the disease. *Gut.* 2001;49(6):777–782.

3. Cosnes J, Cattan S, Blain A, et al. Long-term evolution of disease behavior of Crohn's disease. *Inflamm Bowel Dis.* 2002;8(4):244–250.

4. D'Haens G, Baert F, van Assche G, et al. Early combined immunosuppression or conventional management in patients with newly diagnosed Crohn's disease: an open randomised trial. *Lancet.* 2008;371(9613):660–667.

5. Kugathasan S, Saubermann LJ, Smith L, et al. Mucosal T-cell immunoregulation varies in early and late inflammatory bowel disease. *Gut.* 2007;56(12):1696–1705.

6. Schnitzler F, Fidder H, Ferrante M, et al. Mucosal healing predicts long-term outcome of maintenance therapy with infliximab in Crohn's disease. *Inflamm Bowel Dis.* 2009;15(9):1295–1301.

7. Sipponen T, Nuutinen H, Turunen U, Färkkilä M. Endoscopic evaluation of Crohn's disease activity: comparison of the CDEIS and the SES-CD. *Inflamm Bowel Dis.* 2010;16(12):2131–2136.

8. Feagan BG, Panaccione R, Sandborn WJ, et al. Effects of adalimumab therapy on incidence of hospitalization and surgery in Crohn's disease: results from the CHARM study. *Gastroenterology.* 2008;135(5):1493–1499.

9. Schnitzler F, Fidder H, Ferrante M, et al. Long-term outcome of treatment with infliximab in 614 patients with Crohn's disease: results from a single-centre cohort. *Gut.* 2009;58(4):492–500.

10. Van den Brande JM, Koehler TC, Zelinkova Z, et al. Prediction of antitumour necrosis factor clinical efficacy by real-time visualisation of apoptosis in patients with Crohn's disease. *Gut.* 2007;56(4):509–517.

11. Vos AC, Wildenberg ME, Duijvestein M, Verhaar AP, van den Brink GR, Hommes DW. Anti-tumor necrosis factor-a antibodies induce regulatory macrophages in an Fc region-dependent manner. *Gastroenterology.* 2011;140(1):221–230.

12. Baert F, Moortgat L, Van Assche G, et al. Mucosal healing predicts sustained clinical remission in patients with early-stage Crohn's disease. *Gastroenterology.* 2010;138(2):463–8; quiz e10.

13. Colombel JF, Sandborn WJ, Reinisch W, et al. Infliximab, azathioprine, or combination therapy for Crohn's disease. *N Engl J Med.* 2010;362(15):1383–1395.

Mucosal Healing in IBD: Essential or Cosmetics?

Peter Bossuyt and Geert D'Haens

The primary goal in the management of Crohn's disease and ulcerative colitis has been to improve the symptoms of the patient. But does this end point also have an impact on the long-term outcome and disease behavior? In this review, we will focus on the importance of mucosal healing in inflammatory bowel diseases (IBDs) rather than symptomatic improvement. Which therapies can induce and maintain mucosal healing? Is mucosal healing really an important goal to achieve? What is the influence of mucosal healing on the future evolution of the disease? Is mucosal healing a relevant and reliable prognostic factor? In other words, is mucosal healing essential or just cosmetic medicine?

● CROHN'S DISEASE

Until recently, most clinical trials in the field of Crohn's disease focused on clinical outcome, using validated symptom scores such as the Crohn's disease activity index (CDAI) and the Harvey-Bradshaw index, and in pediatric populations the pediatric Crohn's disease activity index. For each of these scores, thresholds for response and remissions have been defined. Mucosal healing was rather neglected as a goal of treatment in Crohn's disease because it was considered unimportant and virtually impossible to achieve with the available treatments. An assessment of endoscopic healing in a study that was designed to validate the Crohn's disease endoscopic index of severity (CDEIS) demonstrated that high dose treatment with corticosteroids for 7 weeks led to mucosal healing in only 29% of the patients, whereas 9% clearly had deterioration of lesions.[1] It was not until it was shown that azathioprine (AZA) therapy was associated with endoscopic healing in postoperative recurrent ileitis and in primary Crohn's ileocolitis[2,3] that more attention was given to the impact of endoscopic healing. Until then, purine analogues were indeed the only drugs that had been shown to alter the course of Crohn's disease, with significant reductions in steroid need, longstanding remission, and fistula healing as a consequence.[4] The association between mucosal healing and a more favorable disease course began to be established. Currently, mucosal healing is being proposed as

an important measure of treatment efficacy and a required end point for future regulatory approval of IBD therapies, mainly due to the advent of biologic therapies. Healing has become an important parameter in the individual follow-up of patients, and has been included as a secondary or even primary end point in clinical trials with biologicals.[5]

Histologic Healing

Overall, there is a poor correlation between mucosal healing and *histologic* healing in Crohn's disease. In a somewhat older study, the improvement in Crohn's disease after drug therapy was evaluated in 38 patients with evidence of mucosal healing of the rectum. Complete histologic healing was observed in 24 patients (63%), but histologic evidence of inflammatory activity persisted in one-third of the patients despite an endoscopically normal rectum.[6]

Healing Effects of Corticosteroids in Crohn's Disease

Despite its efficacy to induce an acute clinical response, corticosteroid therapy does not appear to improve mucosal lesions or prevent postoperative endoscopic recurrence of Crohn's disease. In the studies conducted by the GETAID (Groupe d'Etudes Thérapeutiques sur les Affections Inflammatoires Digestives), oral prednisolone 1 mg/kg per day induced clinical remission in 92% of the patients within 7 weeks. Only 29% of these patients achieved endoscopic remission. A correlation between clinical severity and nature, surface, or severity of endoscopic lesions could not be established.[1,7] A small Swedish study demonstrated an excellent effect of glucocorticoids on symptoms of Crohn's disease of the small intestine but this was not accompanied by a significant reduction of endoscopically observed small intestinal lesions.[8] In a recent study in patients with steroid-dependent Crohn's ileocolitis or proximal colitis who had achieved clinical remission on conventional steroids, complete or near-complete healing was achieved in 24% of budesonide-treated (6–9 mg per day) patients after 1 year.[9] In a recent study on the impact of mucosal healing on long-term outcomes in patients receiving infliximab, a significant lower mucosal healing rate was seen in patients receiving concomitant corticosteroids.[10] The lack of healing may be the reason why steroids fail to induce long-term efficacy.

Healing Effects of Thiopurines (AZA and 6-Mercaptopurine) in Crohn's Disease

The role of AZA in mucosal healing of Crohn's disease was first demonstrated in 1997. Nineteen patients who underwent an ileocecal resection for their Crohn's disease and who subsequently developed severe recurrent ileitis were treated with AZA during at least 6 months after complete weaning of the corticosteroids. Fifteen patients were reevaluated by endoscopy or radiological examination. The immunomodulatory therapy resulted in induction and maintenance of clinical remission in all 15 patients, with complete endoscopic healing of the neoterminal ileum observed in 6 of 15 patients, near-complete healing with only superficial erosions remaining in 5 of 15 patients, partial healing in 3 of 15 patients, and unchanged inflammatory lesions in 1 patient. AZA was therefore proposed as treatment of choice in severe recurrent Crohn's ileitis.[2]

In another study by the same group, 20 patients with Crohn's colitis or ileocolitis in clinical remission, while taking AZA for at least 9 months and no corticosteroids for at least 3 months, were endoscopically evaluated. In the colon, complete to near-complete healing of the mucosa was seen in 80% of the patients; in the ileum, up to 69% of the patients had complete to near-complete healing.[3]

In a randomized, double-blind, controlled study by the GETAID, investigating the effect of AZA withdrawal on sustained remission, baseline ileocolonoscopy was performed in 54% of the patients. These patients had been in clinical remission on AZA for at least 42 months. Complete endoscopic remission defined as CDEIS = 0 was seen in 36% of the patients, although the mean CDEIS level was rather low at baseline (mean = 2.5).[11] In a Greek study looking at maintenance of mucosal healing in patients who achieved clinical remission with standard steroid treatment, AZA was also shown to achieve and maintain endoscopic remission. After one year on AZA (2–2.5 mg/kg), complete or near-complete healing was achieved in 83% of AZA-treated patients with a mean CDEIS dropping from 7 to 0.55. Multivariate logistic regression analysis identified early initiation of AZA after diagnosis (<1 year) as the only factor predicting complete endoscopic healing of Crohn's disease in this study.[9]

Healing Effects of Methotrexate in Crohn's Disease

In a pilot study on the effects of methotrexate in Crohn's colitis published in the late 1980s, 5 of 14 patients with Crohn's colitis had mucosal healing documented on colonoscopy at 12 weeks.[12] Although methotrexate proved to be an effective drug for induction and maintenance of remission,[13,14] its effect on mucosal healing was not further investigated in Crohn's disease.

Healing Effects of Anti-TNF Agents in Crohn's Disease

Several multicenter studies demonstrated the effects of the first anti-tumor necrosis factor (TNF) antibody infliximab on the mucosal lesions in Crohn's disease. "Mucosal healing," defined as disappearance of ulcers, was seen 4 weeks after a single dose of infliximab in 74% of patients, in the ileum, and in 96% of patients, in the rectum.[15] In this same study, a significant correlation between the reductions in CDAI and CDEIS was observed. A substudy of the ACCENT I project compared episodic and scheduled treatment strategies with infliximab in patients with Crohn's disease following a single induction treatment with 5 mg/kg of infliximab[16] and demonstrated that the patients randomized to "scheduled therapy" had fewer hospitalizations and surgeries and higher rates of "mucosal healing," again defined as absence of ulcers. Complete mucosal healing at week 10 was seen in 31% and 0% of the patients with scheduled and episodic treatment, respectively. At week 54, mucosal healing was seen in 50% versus in 7%. There was a direct association between the mucosal healing rates and the number of hospitalizations, with no hospitalizations needed in patients who had endoscopic remission at both week 10 and week 54. However, no consistent relationship was seen between mucosal healing and clinical remission in this study.[17] A retrospective study in 214 patients with Crohn's disease demonstrated that initiation of infliximab was associated with mucosal healing in 67.8% of responders and complete mucosal healing in 45% of all patients, with superiority of scheduled therapy versus episodic therapy. A decrease in the need for major abdominal surgery was seen, especially in patients with a scheduled treatment regimen. The concomitant use of immunomodulators except for corticosteroids had no influence on mucosal healing.[10]

In the "top-down" trial by D'Haens et al.,[18] early combined immunosuppression with three induction infusions of infliximab + AZA maintenance therapy resulted in a mucosal healing rate of 73% after 2 years, compared with 30% with conventional management. In the follow-up phase of this study, absence of mucosal lesions at year 4 was associated with higher remission rates.[19] Patients without lesions were four times as likely to be in remission without flares, without steroids and without need for infliximab at year 4.

In the recent SONIC trial, patients with active Crohn's disease who had never been exposed to biologic or immunomodulatory treatment were randomized to treatment with AZA monotherapy, infliximab monotherapy, or the combination of both. Steroids were forced to be tapered after week 14. All patients had endoscopic investigation at inclusion and at week 26, the time point of primary analysis. Mucosal healing (absence of ulcers) was observed in 44% of patients on combination treatment, 30% on infliximab monotherapy, and 16% on AZA monotherapy. The superiority of the most potent treatment was most pronounced in patients who had evidence of ulcers on the baseline endoscopy.[20]

The mucosal healing effects were also assessed for adalimumab and certolizumab pegol (CZP), two newer anti-TNF antibodies. In the EXTEND trial, 129 patients with active Crohn's disease received induction treatment with adalimumab 160 mg followed by 80 mg at week 2 and maintenance treatment with placebo or 40 mg adalimumab every 2 weeks. Endoscopies were performed at week 0, 12, and 52. At week 12, 27% of patients in the maintenance adalimumab group had complete mucosal healing, versus only 13% in the placebo maintenance group ($P = 0.056$). At week 52, 24% of patients had complete healing with adalimumab maintenance versus none with placebo maintenance ($P < 0.001$).[21] In the MUSIC study with CZP, all ($n = 89$) patients received open-label induction with 400 mg CZP every 2 weeks for three doses followed by 400 mg every 4 weeks, with endoscopies performed at week 0, 10, and 56. At week 10, a significant reduction in the CDEIS score was observed (42%, $P < 0.0001$). Four patients had complete absence of lesions at week 10, whereas 61% had a CDEIS response defined by a decrease in the score of greater than 5 points.[22]

New Ways to Investigate Mucosal Healing

Ascertainment of mucosal healing requires endoscopy, which is expensive, unpleasant for the patient, and time-consuming. New methods for the assessment of mucosal healing are emerging. Recently, a correlation was seen between the level of fecal calprotectin and fecal lactoferrin, and the endoscopic disease activity in ulcerative colitis were established.[23] It was suggested that the degree of inflammation rather than the extent of the disease determined the fecal calprotectin levels. In Crohn's ileocolitis and colitis, the Simple Endoscopic Score for Crohn's Disease (SES-CD) and histologic findings correlated significantly with fecal calprotectin and lactoferrin. A normal fecal-marker concentration was a reliable surrogate marker for endoscopically and histologically inactive Crohn's disease. This was not the fact for ileal disease.[24] The use of fecal markers in monitoring the effect of anti-TNF agents in patients with Crohn's disease was demonstrated in a recent study. Mucosal healing was associated with a significant decrease and normalization of both calprotectin and lactoferrin in an induction setting.[25]

The main problem with these biologic markers is that they are not specific for IBD. Calprotectin and lactoferrin are elevated in all situations of mucosal damage as in cases of cancer, bacterial infection, or nonsteroidal anti-inflammatory drug–induced lesions. Larger studies are needed to validate the use of fecal markers as a noninvasive surrogate of mucosal healing.

● ULCERATIVE COLITIS

Ulcerative colitis is an inflammatory condition with lesions confined to the mucosa, the most superficial layer of the colonic wall. Technically, it is easier to evaluate mucosal healing because the disease almost always involves the distal part of the colon, which is easily accessible for endoscopy. In an older trial with 5-aminosalicylic acid (5-ASA) preparations, it became clear that patients with both clinical and endoscopic remission had a higher likelihood of prolonged remission than patients with only clinical remission.[26] A study in the early 1990s demonstrated the importance of mucosal healing in the relapse rate of ulcerative colitis. The occurrence of flares within 1 year after an episode of active colitis was 4% in patients with clinical remission and mucosal healing versus 30% in patients with persistent mucosal lesions.[27] These findings were confirmed by an Italian trail, in which relapse rate at 1 year in patients achieving both clinical and endoscopic remission was 23% compared to 80% in patients with clinical remission still having endoscopic lesions.[28] In the Act 1 and 2 trials, rapid induction of mucosal healing

with infliximab was associated with a fourfold increase in clinical remission at week 30.[29] It also needs to be stated that continuously inflamed mucosa probably carries an enhanced risk of dysplasia and cancer development, because there is a highly significant correlation between the inflammation scores and the risk of colorectal neoplasia.[30]

Given its established impact on the course of the disease, endoscopic assessment has been incorporated in the evaluation of drugs for ulcerative colitis.

Healing Effects of 5-ASA in Ulcerative Colitis

Schroeder et al. assessed the effect of oral 5-ASA at a dosage of either 4.8 or 1.6 g per day versus placebo for 6 weeks in mildly to moderately active ulcerative colitis. The outcome was monitored by flexible proctosigmoidoscopy. Results showed 24% complete and 50% partial responses in those receiving 4.8 g of 5-ASA per day as compared with 5% complete and 13% partial responses in those receiving placebo.[31] Combined analysis of two recent studies with Multi Matrix system (MMX) mesalazine revealed that approximately one-third of patients treated with up to 8 weeks of MMX mesalazine had complete mucosal healing (a sigmoidoscopy score of 0) compared with 16% of those who received placebo.[32] Because 5-ASA is a topical agent, similar mucosal healing effects were seen with enemas. In a study comparing 4 g 5-ASA and 100 mg hydrocortisone enemas mucosal healing was seen in 93% versus 54%, respectively.[33]

Healing Effects of Corticosteroids in Ulcerative Colitis

The first reports of the effect of steroids on ulcerative colitis date from more than 50 years ago. In patients treated with high dose steroids (100 mg a day for 6 weeks), mucosal healing was seen in 52% of patients compared to 32% of the patients in the placebo group.[34]

Healing Effects of AZA in Ulcerative Colitis

A study comparing AZA with 5-ASA in inducing clinical and endoscopic remission demonstrated that AZA therapy was significantly more effective than 5-ASA. More than 50% of AZA-treated patients had both clinical and endoscopic remission with a therapeutic gain of approximately 35% in comparison with 5-ASA.[35] In a study with AZA in 42 patients with steroid-dependent or steroid-resistant ulcerative colitis, complete endoscopic remission was seen in 75% of patients tolerating AZA after 6 months. In the 10 patients not tolerating AZA, complete mucosal healing was established in six patients with methotrexate.[36]

Healing Effects of Anti-TNF Agents in Ulcerative Colitis

The effects of infliximab in active ulcerative colitis were extensively investigated in two large controlled trials, Act 1 and Act 2. All patients in these trials underwent endoscopic investigation at inclusion and at week 30 of the trial, which was the primary end point. Sixty to sixty-one percent of patients healed their mucosa on infliximab therapy at week 8, versus 32% on placebo ($P < 0.001$). However, it needs to be pointed out that mucosal healing in the Act trials did not mean "absence of any lesion" but rather a Mayo score of 0 or 1, allowing for milder lesions to persist. At week 30, 48% to 53% of patients had endoscopic healing on infliximab versus 27% on placebo ($P < 0.001$). Complete endoscopic healing with a Mayo score of 0 was observed in 25% at week 8 (vs. 8% on placebo) and in 28% to 31% at week 30 (vs. 9% on placebo). Moreover, patients with complete mucosal healing had a better outcome: if the mucosa was healed at week 8, the likelihood of staying in remission until week 30 was four-fold higher (43.8% vs. 9.5%). A majority of patients underwent a new endoscopic investigation at week 54 in the follow-up phase of this study, and maintenance of healing was clearly demonstrated during continued infliximab treatment.[29]

The effects of other anti-TNF agents in ulcerative colitis are currently under investigation.

Healing Effects of Antibodies to Adhesion Molecules in Ulcerative Colitis

Another biologic approach to IBDs is to inhibit the migration of leukocytes into inflamed intestinal tissue by blocking cellular adhesion molecules. Feagan and colleagues performed serial endoscopic assessments during a placebo-controlled trial of anti-$\alpha 4\beta 7$ integrin antibody (MLN-02) for active ulcerative colitis. At week 6, 28% of patients who received 0.5 mg/kg of MLN-02 were in endoscopic remission, as compared with 12% in those who received 2.0 mg per kilogram and 8% in the placebo group.[37] Further trials with this agent are ongoing.

● CONCLUSIONS

Accumulating data are supporting the importance of mucosal healing in Crohn's disease as well as in ulcerative colitis. Mucosal healing has become a reliable predictor of disease control in the era of biologic therapy, with evidence for fewer surgeries and higher remission rates in Crohn's disease. In ulcerative colitis, lower colectomy rates and longer disease control is seen after achieving mucosal healing. Newer therapies are efficacious in inducing complete and fast endoscopic remission. Whether the appearance of the mucosa should be used to guide modifications in therapeutic strategy has to be validated in further studies. Nowadays mucosal healing is no longer just cosmetics of the mucosa but an essential component of clinical practice and studies in the field of IBD.

References

1. Landi B, Anh TN, Cortot A, et al. Endoscopic monitoring of Crohn's disease treatment: a prospective, randomized clinical trial. The Groupe d'Etudes Therapeutiques des Affections Inflammatoires Digestives. *Gastroenterology.* 1992;102(5):1647–1653.

2. D'Haens G, Geboes K, Ponette E, Penninckx F, Rutgeerts P. Healing of severe recurrent ileitis with azathioprine therapy in patients with Crohn's disease. *Gastroenterology.* 1997;112(5):1475–1481.

3. D'Haens G, Geboes K, Rutgeerts P. Endoscopic and histologic healing of Crohn's (ileo-) colitis with azathioprine. *Gastrointest Endosc.* 1999;50(5):667–671.

4. Present DH. 6-Mercaptopurine and other immunosuppressive agents in the treatment of Crohn's disease and ulcerative colitis. *Gastroenterol Clin North Am.* 1989;18(1):57–71.

5. Frøslie KF, Jahnsen J, Moum BA, Vatn MH; IBSEN Group. Mucosal healing in inflammatory bowel disease: results from a Norwegian population-based cohort. *Gastroenterology.* 2007;133(2):412–422.

6. Korelitz BI, Sommers SC. Response to drug therapy in Crohn's disease: evaluation by rectal biopsy and mucosal cell counts. *J Clin Gastroenterol.* 1984;6(2):123–127.

7. Modigliani R, Mary JY, Simon JF, et al. Clinical, biological, and endoscopic picture of attacks of Crohn's disease. Evolution on prednisolone. Groupe d'Etude Thérapeutique des Affections Inflammatoires Digestives. *Gastroenterology.* 1990;98(4):811–818.

8. Olaison G, Sjödahl R, Tagesson C. Glucocorticoid treatment in ileal Crohn's disease: relief of symptoms but not of endoscopically viewed inflammation. *Gut.* 1990;31(3):325–328.

9. Mantzaris GJ, Christidou A, Sfakianakis M, et al. Azathioprine is superior to budesonide in achieving and maintaining mucosal healing and histologic remission in steroid-dependent Crohn's disease. *Inflamm Bowel Dis.* 2009;15(3):375–382.

10. Schnitzler F, Fidder H, Ferrante M, et al. Mucosal healing predicts long-term outcome of maintenance therapy with infliximab in Crohn's disease. *Inflamm Bowel Dis.* 2009;15(9):1295–1301.

11. Lémann M, Mary JY, Colombel JF, et al.; Groupe D'Etude Thérapeutique des Affections Inflammatoires du Tube Digestif. A randomized, double-blind, controlled withdrawal trial in Crohn's disease patients in long-term remission on azathioprine. *Gastroenterology.* 2005;128(7):1812–1818.

12. Kozarek RA, Patterson DJ, Gelfand MD, Botoman VA, Ball TJ, Wilske KR. Methotrexate induces clinical and histologic remission in patients with refractory inflammatory bowel disease. *Ann Intern Med.* 1989;110(5):353–356.

13. Feagan BG, Rochon J, Fedorak RN, et al. Methotrexate for the treatment of Crohn's disease. The North American Crohn's Study Group Investigators. *N Engl J Med.* 1995;332(5):292–297.

14. Feagan BG, Fedorak RN, Irvine EJ, et al. A comparison of methotrexate with placebo for the maintenance of remission in Crohn's disease. North American Crohn's Study Group Investigators. *N Engl J Med.* 2000;342(22):1627–1632.

15. D'Haens G, Van Deventer S, Van Hogezand R, et al. Endoscopic and histological healing with infliximab anti-tumor necrosis factor antibodies in Crohn's disease: A European multicenter trial. *Gastroenterology.* 1999;116(5):1029–1034.

16. Rutgeerts P, Feagan BG, Lichtenstein GR, et al. Comparison of scheduled and episodic treatment strategies of infliximab in Crohn's disease. *Gastroenterology.* 2004;126(2):402–413.

17. Rutgeerts P, Diamond RH, Bala M, et al. Scheduled maintenance treatment with infliximab is superior to episodic treatment for the healing of mucosal ulceration associated with Crohn's disease. *Gastrointest Endosc.* 2006;63(3):433–442; quiz 464.

18. D'Haens G, Baert F, van Assche G, et al.; Belgian Inflammatory Bowel Disease Research Group; North-Holland Gut Club. Early combined immunosuppression or conventional management in patients with newly diagnosed Crohn's disease: an open randomised trial. *Lancet.* 2008;371(9613):660–667.

19. Baert F, Moortgat L, Van Assche G, et al. Mucosal healing predicts sustained clinical remission in early Crohn's disease [abstract]. *Gastroenterology.* 2008;134(suppl I):A640.

20. Colombel JF, Rutgeerts P, Reinisch W, et al. Sonic: a randomized, double-blind, controlled trial comparing infliximab and

infliximab plus azathioprine to azathioprine in patients with Crohn's disease naïve to immunomodulators and biologic therapy [abstract]. *Gut.* 2008;57(suppl II):A1.

21. Rutgeerts P, D'Haens GR, Van Assche G, et al. Adalimumab induces and maintains mucosal healing in patients with moderate to severe ileocolonic Crohn's disease—first results of the extend trial [abstract]. *Gastroenterology.* 2009;136(suppl I):A116.

22. Hébuterne X, Colombel J, Bouhnik Y, et al. Endoscopic improvement in patients with active Crohn's disease treated with certolizumab pegol: first results of the MUSIC trail [abstract]. *Gut.* 2008;57(suppl II):A15.

23. Langhorst J, Elsenbruch S, Mueller T, et al. Comparison of 4 neutrophil-derived proteins in feces as indicators of disease activity in ulcerative colitis. *Inflamm Bowel Dis.* 2005;11(12):1085–1091.

24. Sipponen T, Kärkkäinen P, Savilahti E, et al. Correlation of faecal calprotectin and lactoferrin with an endoscopic score for Crohn's disease and histological findings. *Aliment Pharmacol Ther.* 2008;28(10):1221–1229.

25. Sipponen T, Savilahti E, Kärkkäinen P, et al. Fecal calprotectin, lactoferrin, and endoscopic disease activity in monitoring anti-TNF-alpha therapy for Crohn's disease. *Inflamm Bowel Dis.* 2008;14(10):1392–1398.

26. Riley SA, Mani V, Goodman MJ, Dutt S, Herd ME. Microscopic activity in ulcerative colitis: what does it mean? *Gut.* 1991;32(2):174–178.

27. Courtney MG, Nunes DP, Bergin CF, et al. Colonoscopic appearance in remission predicts relapse of ulcerative colitis. *Gastroenterology.* 1991;100:A205.

28. Meucci G, Fasoli R, Saibeni S, et al. Prognostic significance of endoscopic remission in patients with active ulcerative colitis treated with oral and topical mesalazine: preliminary results of a prospective, multicenter study. *Gastroenterology.* 2006;130:A197.

29. Rutgeerts P, Sandborn WJ, Feagan BG, et al. Infliximab for induction and maintenance therapy for ulcerative colitis. *N Engl J Med.* 2005;353(23):2462–2476.

30. Rutter M, Saunders B, Wilkinson K, et al. Severity of inflammation is a risk factor for colorectal neoplasia in ulcerative colitis. *Gastroenterology.* 2004;126(2):451–459.

31. Schroeder KW, Tremaine WJ, Ilstrup DM. Coated oral 5-aminosalicylic acid therapy for mildly to moderately active ulcerative colitis. A randomized study. *N Engl J Med.* 1987;317(26):1625–1629.

32. Sandborn WJ, Kamm MA, Lichtenstein GR, Lyne A, Butler T, Joseph RE. MMX Multi Matrix System mesalazine for the induction of remission in patients with mild-to-moderate ulcerative colitis: a combined analysis of two randomized, double-blind, placebo-controlled trials. *Aliment Pharmacol Ther.* 2007;26(2):205–215.

33. Campieri M, Lanfranchi GA, Bazzocchi G, et al. Treatment of ulcerative colitis with high-dose 5-aminosalicylic acid enemas. *Lancet.* 1981;2(8241):270–271.

34. Truelove SC, Witts LJ. Cortisone in ulcerative colitis; final report on a therapeutic trial. *Br Med J.* 1955;2(4947):1041–1048.

35. Ardizzone S, Maconi G, Russo A, et al. Randomised, controlled trial, of azathioprine and 5-aminosalicylic acid for treatment of steroid-dependent ulcerative colitis. *Gut.* 2006;55:47–53.

36. Paoluzi OA, Pica R, Marcheggiano A, et al. Azathioprine or methotrexate in the treatment of patients with steroid-dependent or steroid-resistant ulcerative colitis: results of an open-label study on efficacy and tolerability in inducing and maintaining remission. *Aliment Pharmacol Ther.* 2002;16(10):1751–1759.

37. Feagan BG, Greenberg GR, Wild G, et al. Treatment of ulcerative colitis with a humanized antibody to the alpha4beta7 integrin. *N Engl J Med.* 2005;352(24):2499–2507.

The Role of Mesalamine in Crohn's Disease

101

Cosimo Prantera and Alessandro Armuzzi

● MESALAMINE

Mesalamine (mesalazine-5-ASA) is the first-line drug for patients with ulcerative colitis (UC), whereas its use in Crohn's disease (CD) is controversial. Despite doubts on its efficacy, many gastroenterologists employ this compound in CD maintenance mainly because of its effectiveness in UC and its high safety profile.[1] However, the biological plausibility of usefulness of mesalamine in CD has to be evaluated in the light of CD pathology. CD is typified by patchy distribution and transmural inflammation, often involving all layers of the gut wall. The inflammation can extend to the extraintestinal tissues forming mesenteric abscesses. Mesalamine acts topically and cannot alleviate the inflammation of the profound tissues. This could be an epitaph for the use of mesalamine in CD, until we can find arguments to the contrary.

● 5-ASA DERIVATIVES

Sulfasalazine (SASP) was developed in the 1940s for the treatment of patients with rheumatic polyarthritis. The discovery that SASP was effective against intestinal symptoms of patients with associated UC led to its use in patients with inflammatory bowel disease (IBD). Metabolic studies in the late 1960s showed that SASP azo-bond is split by colonic bacteria releasing sulfapyridine (SP) and 5-ASA, the former functioning as a carrier molecule and the latter as the active therapeutic moiety. Subsequent 5-ASA delayed-release formulations, coated with acrylic-based resins that dissolve at specific intraluminal pH, have been developed. Asacol (Eudragit-S coated) dissolves at a pH ≥ 7 and begins to release 5-ASA in the distal ileum and right colon; Claversal, Mesasal and Salofalk (Eudragit-L coated) dissolve at a pH > 6 and begin to release 5-ASA from the mid ileum and onwards. Controlled-release formulation (Pentasa) incorporates 5-ASA into microgranules enclosed within a semipermeable membrane of ethylcellulose that dissolves when hydrated and releases 5-ASA from the duodenum to the colon in a gradual manner at all pH levels (Table 101.1).[2]

● MESALAMINE FOR INDUCING REMISSION OF CD

The National Cooperative Crohn's Disease Study (NCCDS) evaluated the efficacy of SASP, the first 5-ASA employed in CD, with the aim of inducing remission of acute flares in a double-blind,

TABLE 101.1 Properties of 5-ASA Derivatives Used in Crohn's Disease

Product	Preparation	Solubility	Site of Release
Asacol	Mesalamine coated with Eudragit S	pH ≥ 7	Distal ileum-colon
Asacol microgranular	Mesalamine encapsulated in microgranules coated with Eudragit S	pH ≥ 7	Distal ileum-right colon
Claversal, Mesasal, Salofalk	Mesalamine coated with Eudragit L	pH > 6	Jejunum-ileum-colon
Rowasa	Mesalamine coated with Eudragit L 100	pH > 6	Jejunum-ileum-colon
Pentasa	Mesalamine encapsulated in ethylcellulose microgranules	Time released	Jejunum-ileum-colon
Salazopyrin	Sulfasalazine (sulfapyridine + 5-ASA)[a]	Colonic bacteria	Colon
Dipentum	Olsalazine (5-ASA + 5-ASA)[a]	Colonic bacteria	Colon

[a]5-ASA delivery in the colon after splitting the azo-bond by colonic bacteria.

TABLE 101.2 Placebo-Controlled and Comparative Trials of 5-ASA for Active Crohn's Disease

Authors	Active Drug	Dose of 5-ASA (g/day)	Control	Period (weeks)	Sample Size (n)	Improvement or Remission (%)		P	Therapeutic Advantage of 5-ASA (%)
						5-ASA	Control		
Saverymuttu et al., 1985	Pentasa	1.5	Placebo	1.4	12	—	—	—	+50
Rasmussen et al., 1987	Pentasa	1.5	Placebo	16	67	40	30	n.s	+10
Mahida and Jewell, 1990	Pentasa	1.5	Placebo	6	40	40	35	n.s.	+5
Singleton et al., 1993	Pentasa	4	Placebo	16	310	43	18	0.01	+25
		2				24	18	n.s	+6
		1				23	18	n.s.	+5
Singleton et al., 1994	Pentasa	4	Placebo	16	232	—	—	n.s.	—[a]
		2				—	—	n.s.	—
Tremaine et al., 1994	Asacol	3.2	Placebo	16	38	60	22	0.042	+23
Wright et al., 1995	Dipentum	2	Placebo	16	91	17	49	<0.03	−32
Hanauer and Stromberg, 2004	Pentasa	4	Placebo	16	310	—	—	n.s.	—[b]
Maier et al., 1985	Salofalk	1.5	SASP	8	30	87	80	n.s.	+7
Scholmerich et al., 1990	Claversal	2	Steroid	24	62	27	66	<0.01	−39
Maier et al., 1990	Salofalk	3	Steroid + SASP	12	50	83.3	88.5	n.s.	−5.5
Martin et al., 1990	Salofalk	3		12	50	40.9	42.9	n.s.	−2
Gross et al., 1995	Salofalk	4.5	Steroid	8	34	40	56.3	n.s.	−16.3
Prantera et al., 1999	Asacol tab	4	Steroid	12	94	60	61	n.s.	−1
	Microgranular	4	Steroid			79	61	n.s.	+18
Thomsen et al., 1998	Budesonide	4	Pentasa	16	182	36	62	<0.001	−26
Colombel et al., 1999	Ciprofloxacin	4	Pentasa	6	40	55	56	n.s.	−1

[a]CDAI mean reduction of 41 ± 12 on Pentasa and of 35 ± 12 on placebo; [b]CDAI mean reduction of 72 ± 9 on Pentasa and of 64 ± 9 on placebo.

randomized, placebo-controlled trial (RCT). This landmark study showed a significant difference between SASP and placebo in patients with Crohn's colitis, whereas the difference did not reach the statistical significance when the CD was located in the small bowel.

Three grams of SASP were given to 54 patients in a successive European CD study (ECCDS). Also in this trial, SASP was more effective than placebo ($P < 0.05$), but the difference was lower than that registered in the NCCDS study. These results were confirmed by a crossover trial in which SASP was compared with Metronidazole in 78 CD patients. The better response to SASP was yet again registered in Crohn's colitis.

The efficacy shown in colitis is in line with the delivery system of SASP that splits 5-ASA from SP in the colon by bacterial action. Moreover, it is possible that SP, apart from being an inert carrier, also works in addition to the anti-inflammatory activity of 5-ASA by exerting an antimicrobial effect. A recent study has shown that the beneficial effect of SASP is in part attributable to a proapoptotic effect on lamina propria T lymphocytes with a consequent downregulation of their activation.[3]

It would seem also that higher doses of SASP are more effective: the best result being obtained in the NCCDS study that employed a mean dose of 4 g, whereas in the other two studies the dose was 3 g. High doses of SASP, however, are burdened by higher number of side effects.

Although the results of these trials were encouraging, the use of SASP in CD has been virtually abandoned. Three causes were probably the reasons of this result: the elevated number of SASP side effects, the marketing of SASP derivative mesalamine, with a consequent loss of interest of the SASP producer, and the advent of new, more potent drugs for treating IBD.

Following this, a number of mesalamines with different delivery systems were challenged against various comparators, from steroid to placebo, to test their efficacy in CD flares (Table 101.2). Seven placebo-controlled trials investigated the efficacy of mesalamine in the treatment of mildly to moderately active CD. Early trials, using low doses (1–2 g/day) of Pentasa, showed overall ineffectiveness. Subsequent studies, assessing higher doses, yielded conflicting results. Pentasa at 4 g/day was evaluated in three 16-week duration trials, involving 304 patients in the active arm and 311 in the placebo arm. A recent meta-analysis,[4] including all Pentasa trials, showed a mean Crohn's Disease Activity Index (CDAI) difference of −18 points from baseline between Pentasa and placebo ($P = 0.04$). In subgroup analysis, the difference was most evident among patients with disease duration under 7 to 8 years (−39; $P < 0.001$), duration of current disease flare under 28 days (−42; $P = 0.01$), and positive clinical benefit from prior corticosteroid use (−46; $P = 0.02$). In a placebo-controlled trial, finally, olsalazine at 2 g/day lacked therapeutic effect in the treatment of active CD; 22% of the patients withdrew from the study because of diarrhea.[5]

Mesalamine has been compared with conventional cortico-steroids in five trials. In the first study, 62 patients with mildly to moderately active CD were randomly assigned to Salofalk 2 g/day or 6-methylprednisolone for 24 weeks. The median change in CDAI was significantly higher in the corticosteroid group ($P < 0.001$). This study has been recently involved in a Cochrane review, which analyzed the efficacy of traditional corticosteroids for induction of remission in CD.[6] As far as the remission rates are concerned, other RCTs (NCCDS, ECCDS) have been included for the comparison between corticosteroid and 5-ASA deriva-tives. Other studies were excluded because they did not meet the strict Cochrane inclusion criteria. The meta-analysis reported a relative risk of 1.65 (95% confidence interval [CI] 1.33–2.03) and the AA concluded that corticosteroids are more effective than 5-ASA derivatives for inducing remission in studies with follow-up duration of over 15 weeks. The superiority of conven-tional corticosteroids in mild to moderate CD, however, has not been demonstrated in subsequent trials, in which higher doses of delayed-release mesalamine have been used. In particular, in the largest of those trials involving 94 patients with mildly to mod-erately active CD localized in the terminal ileum, patients were randomly assigned to Asacol tablets 4 g/day, Asacol microgran-ules 4 g/day or 6-methylprednisolone 40 mg for 12 weeks. Clinical remission was not significantly different among groups.

In another comparative trial, Pentasa 4 g/day was shown to be significantly less effective than budesonide 9 mg/day ($P < 0.001$) but as effective as ciprofloxacin 1 g/day in inducing clinical remission in mildly to moderately active CD.[5]

In conclusion, although mesalamine has been used as first-line treatment of mildly to moderately active CD for many years, the efficacy of this treatment has not been consistently demonstrated in comparative RCTs. Some reasons may account for the conflicting evidence: most of the studies have been performed with different designs, different patient populations, different primary endpoints, and different drug formulations. Differences in mesalamine deliv-ery systems seem to be important when the ileum and right colon are involved: pH 7-dependent could work better.

It is plausible that studies with stratification of patients into groups of adequate size, with disease affecting different anatomic regions, may identify subgroups more likely to respond.

MESALAMINE FOR MAINTAINING REMISSION OF CD

Mesalamine has been employed in maintaining remission, both when remission was drug induced and surgically induced. The two settings are different because in the latter case all the mac-roscopically diseased part of the gut has been removed, and the prevention of recurrent lesions is the main reason for using the drug. It is biologically plausible that mesalamine, which acts top-ically, could control CD inflammation starting in the mucosa.

This difference may explain why the studies on recurrence prevention after surgery worked generally better than those on relapse prevention after medically induced remission, where the lesions are usually not healed.

MESALAMINE FOR MAINTAINING MEDICALLY INDUCED REMISSION

1139 patients were enrolled in 8 RCTs that compared differ-ent mesalamine compounds against placebo (Table 101.3). The

TABLE 101.3 RCTs on Efficacy of 5-ASA for Preventing Relapse of Crohn's Disease After Medically Induced Remission

Authors	Active Drug	Dose (g/day)	Period (months)	Sample Size (n)	Relapse Rate (%) 5-ASA	Relapse Rate (%) Placebo	P	Therapeutic Advantage of 5-ASA (%)
IMSG, 1990[a,b,c]	Claversal	1.5	12	206	22.4	36.2	0.04	+13.8
Prantera et al., 1992[a,b,c]	Asacol	2.4	12	125	29.7	52.5	0.02	+22.8
Brignola et al., 1992[c]	Pentasa	2	4	44	52.4	59.1	n.s.	+6.7
Gendre et al., 1993[a,b,c]	Pentasa	2	24	161	37.5	44.4	n.s.	+6.9
Arber et al., 1995[a,b,c]	Salofalk	1	12	59	27	55	<0.05	+28
Thomson et al., 1995[a,b,c]	Claversal	3	12	207	30	30	n.s.	0
Modigliani et al., 1996[a,c]	Pentasa	4	12	129	70.8	75	n.s.	+4.2
De Franchis et al., 1997[a,c]	Claversal	3	12	117	58	52	n.s.	−6
Sutherland et al., 1997[a,b,c]	Pentasa	3	12	246	25	36	n.s.	+11
Mahmoud et al., 2001[b]	Dipentum	2	12	328	65.4	53.9	0.04	−11.5

[a]RCTs included in Ref. [7]; [b]RCTs included in Ref. [8]; [c]RCTs included in Ref. [9].

maintenance period of the studies varied from 11 to 24 months.[7] The prescribed doses went from 1 to 4 g. The 5-ASAs brand names were Pentasa in three trials, Claversal in three studies, Salofalk and Asacol in the remaining two. In the three studies with Pentasa, the differences with placebo were not statistically significant. Two out of three trials with Claversal were negative. The studies with Salofalk and Asacol showed a slightly significant difference from placebo.

A Cochrane review,[8] which analyzed the efficacy of mesalamine in maintaining medically induced remission, included seven RCTs (six of the eight described before) with a total of 1420 patients. Ten studies were excluded because they did not satisfy the strict Cochrane inclusion criteria. The meta-analysis reported an odds ratio (OR) of 1 (95% CI 0.80–1.24). The AA concluded that mesalamine formulations were not superior to placebo in maintaining medically induced remission in CD and that any further study with this regimen was not justified. A successive meta-analysis, however, suggests that the apparent lack of impact of mesalamine on the maintenance of medically induced remission in CD is open to different interpretation.[9] In fact, a modification of the criteria for including studies in the review gave a different result. The AA provided substantial motives for including some studies that were excluded from the previous meta-analysis (see Table 101.3). Nine RCTs were comprised in this systematic review involving 1305 patients. From this analysis, mesalamine worked better than placebo in maintaining medically induced remission (OR = 070 [95% CI 0.52–0.93] $P = 0.02$). But the overall therapeutic benefit of mesalamine over placebo was only 6% and the number of patients needed to treat for preventing 1 relapse (NNT) was 16. The authors of this article further examine the efficacy of different mesalamine delivery systems for the maintenance of medically induced CD remission. The delivery systems seem to make the difference. In fact, the drug which delivers mesalamine at pH 7 has the greater therapeutic efficacy than the ph 6-dependent and the controlled-release microgranules drugs. The weak point of this conclusion, however, is that only by including the study with pH 7-dependent mesalamine, showing a therapeutic benefit of 22.8% over placebo and an NNT of 5, does the meta-analysis achieve a statistically significant advantage. Although we must be wary when the outcomes depend on the results of a single trial, the result of the pH 7-dependent study could signify that diversity in delivery system has a quantifiable difference in clinical effect.

Is the above biologically plausible? Trials in relapse and recurrence prevention have reported an apparent higher success rate when CD was located in the terminal ileum. Moreover, the mucosal concentration of mesalamine in the juxta-anastomotic area is significantly lower in patients with postsurgical recurrence than in those free of recurrence. These data suggest an association between mucosal mesalamine concentrations and the clinical effectiveness of the drug. Finally, the higher success rates registered in the studies on postsurgery recurrence prevention, in comparison with the prevention of remission induced by medical therapy, could be ascribed to the differences in the pathological conditions of the two settings, the lesions not being healed in the latter situation. We must bear in mind that at the time when these studies were performed, the drugs employed for treating the flares probably did not heal the mucosa.

MESALAMINE FOR PREVENTING THE POSTSURGICAL RECURRENCE

While the benefit of mesalamine treatment for maintaining medically induced remission seems to give only a modest advantage to the treated patients, maintaining surgically induced CD remission is reasonably well established. When all the macroscopic involved bowel is removed by surgery, new lesions reappear at the anastomotic site in over 60% of patients within 1 year. In this context, mesalamine with its local action could be successfully employed.

Seven hundred and twenty-nine patients were enrolled in five RCT for prevention of clinical recurrence after surgery.[7] The doses varied from 2.4 to 4 g. A meta-analysis of these studies, only one of which reached statistical significance, has shown a 10% reduction of the risk of recurrence of symptoms. The NNT for preventing one relapse was 10.[9] Another six trials employed mesalamine in a postsurgery setting for preventing endoscopic recurrence. Also in these studies, mesalamine provided a 18% reduction of the risk of reappearance of lesions. Predictors of the better response were pH 7-dependent mesalamine, ileal location at surgery, and long disease duration.

The decision whether to treat patients with CD with mesalamine, for preventing recurrence after surgery, should be taken case by case. Mesalamine has shown a general small advantage for this purpose, and should be used in patients with ileal location and mild disease behavior. In this setting, the alternative to mesalamine is no treatment, a choice that has to be taken in agreement with the patient. However in this assessment, compliance, which is reduced in long-term treatment, must be accurately evaluated.

Editor's note (TMB): I believe postoperative recurrence studies need to be stratified by the indication for surgery. Young patients who were operated on for short duration transmurally aggressive disease have a higher recurrence rate than longer duration patients operated to reverse fixed or strictures. Sachar, et al. found no evidence of endoscopic recurrence in any of the series of patients resected for obstruction (IBD, 2009).

MISCELLANEA ON THE USE OF MESALAMINE

Enhancing 6-TGN Levels

Intriguing information comes from certain studies that have reported that mesalamine given in concomitance with azathioprine/6-mercaptopurine increases the level of 6-thioguanine nucleotide (6-TGN) which can induce leukopenia.[10] Given that azathioprine is frequently used in CD maintenance, the doctors have to be aware of this possible side effect if concomitantly mesalamine is prescribed. On the other hand, the coadministration of mesalamine and azathioprine could help patients unable to reach therapeutic level of 6-TGN because of high level of thiopurine methyltransferase.[11,12]

Chemoprevention

The hypothesis that mesalamine may be helpful in preventing colorectal cancer in colitis has been supported and refuted by several studies. Although this hypothesis is biologically plausible, a recent well conducted study in UC patients involved in a surveillance program failed to show a chemopreventive effect in rectocolonic cancer.[13] The chemopreventive value of mesalamine is currently justified in colorectal cancer high-risk groups and probably in IBD patients with incomplete mucosal healing on surveillance colonoscopy.[14] Prospective studies in high-risk populations and/or retrospective studies using large population databases may identify subgroups of patients more likely to benefit the treatment.[15]

● MESALAMINE SIDE EFFECTS

About 30% of patients using SASP experience drug-related side effects mainly related to SP. Headache, upper gastrointestinal, and allergic symptoms are the most frequently reported. Severe side effects such as toxic hepatitis, agranulocytosis, and hemolytic anemia are fortunately rare.

● CONCLUSION

Currently, the evidence is in favor of maintaining mesalamine in the CD therapeutic armamentarium, despite criticism from some authors. This conclusion is drawn by considering the following characteristics:

- Mesalamine has a very high safety profile, definitely superior to any other drug employed in IBD treatment.
- The diversity of Crohn's pathological behavior and location, together with the characteristics of the various mesalamines, could have interfered with the results of some negative studies.
- CD is usually a disease involving all the gut layers, but sometimes located only in the mucosa, especially at the beginning of its history.
- Mesalamines have different delivery systems which split the active moiety in diverse parts of the gut and, given their local action, must be employed in order to arrive at the diseased site.
- Type and location of inflammation must be defined and compared with the particular type of mesalamine to prescribe and its delivery system.
- Mesalamine can be associated with Azathioprine, increasing not only its effectiveness but also its potential side effects.
- High doses of 4.8 g or more are employed in clinical practice. It is possible that higher doses could be more effective.
- The anticarcinogenic effect of mesalamine is biologically plausible and supported by some studies.

References

1. Gearry RB, Ajlouni Y, Nandurkar S, Iser JH, Gibson PR. 5-Aminosalicylic acid (mesalazine) use in Crohn's disease: a survey of the opinions and practice of Australian gastroenterologists. *Inflamm Bowel Dis.* 2007;13(8):1009–1015.

2. Nielsen OH, Munck LK. Drug insight: aminosalicylates for the treatment of IBD. *Nat Clin Pract Gastroenterol Hepatol.* 2007;4(3):160–170.

3. Doering J, Begue B, Lentze MJ, et al. Induction of T lymphocyte apoptosis by sulphasalazine in patients with Crohn's disease. *Gut.* 2004;53(11):1632–1638.

4. Hanauer SB, Strömberg U. Oral Pentasa in the treatment of active Crohn's disease: A meta-analysis of double-blind, placebo-controlled trials. *Clin Gastroenterol Hepatol.* 2004;2(5):379–388.

5. Lim WC, Hanauer SB. Controversies with aminosalicylates in inflammatory bowel disease. *Rev Gastroenterol Disord.* 2004;4(3):104–117.

6. Benchimol EI, Seow CH, Steinhart AH, Griffiths AM. Traditional corticosteroids for induction of remission in Crohn's disease. *Cochrane Database Syst Rev.* 2008;(2):CD006792.

7. Bergman R, Parkes M. Systematic review: the use of mesalazine in inflammatory bowel disease. *Aliment Pharmacol Ther.* 2006;23(7):841–855.

8. Akobeng AK, Gardener E. Oral 5-aminosalicylic acid for maintenance of medically-induced remission in Crohn's Disease. *Cochrane Database Syst Rev.* 2005;(1):CD003715.

9. Steinhart AH, Forbes A, Mills EC, Rodgers-Gray BS, Travis SP. Systematic review: the potential influence of mesalazine formulation on maintenance of remission in Crohn's disease. *Aliment Pharmacol Ther.* 2007;25(12):1389–1399.

10. Lowry PW, Franklin CL, Weaver AL, et al. Leucopenia resulting from a drug interaction between azathioprine or 6-mercaptopurine and mesalamine, sulphasalazine, or balsalazide. *Gut.* 2001;49(5):656–664.

11. Gilissen LP, Bierau J, Derijks LJ, et al. The pharmacokinetic effect of discontinuation of mesalazine on mercaptopurine metabolite levels in inflammatory bowel disease patients. *Aliment Pharmacol Ther.* 2005;22(7):605–611.

12. Hande S, Wilson-Rich N, Bousvaros A, et al. 5-aminosalicylate therapy is associated with higher 6-thioguanine levels in adults and children with inflammatory bowel disease in remission on 6-mercaptopurine or azathioprine. *Inflamm Bowel Dis.* 2006;12(4):251–257.

13. Ullman T, Croog V, Harpaz N, et al. Progression to colorectal neoplasia in ulcerative colitis: effect of mesalamine. *Clin Gastroenterol Hepatol.* 2008;6(11):1225–30; quiz 1177.

14. Andrews JM, Travis SP, Gibson PR, Gasche C. Systematic review: does concurrent therapy with 5-ASA and immunomodulators in inflammatory bowel disease improve outcomes? *Aliment Pharmacol Ther.* 2009;29(5):459–469.

15. Rubin DT, Cruz-Correa MR, Gasche C, et al.; 5-ASA in Colorectal Cancer Prevention Meeting Group. Colorectal cancer prevention in inflammatory bowel disease and the role of 5-aminosalicylic acid: a clinical review and update. *Inflamm Bowel Dis.* 2008;14(2):265–274.

Topically Active Steroid Preparations | 102

John K. Marshall

Systemic corticosteroids are a mainstay of therapy for both ulcerative colitis and Crohn's disease. Although effective for inducing remission of moderate to severe disease, corticosteroids confer significant and cumulative adverse effects that limit their use in clinical practice. Accordingly, alternative corticosteroid formulations that reduce systemic toxicity while maintaining clinical efficacy are of considerable interest. Tixocortol pavalate, beclomethasone, and fluticasone are all such examples. However, the majority of clinical evidence and experience in managing inflammatory bowel disease has accumulated with budesonide.

Budesonide (16α,17-butylidendioxy-11β,21-hydroxy-1, 4-pregnadien-3,20-dion) is a synthetic analog of prednisolone.[1,2] Much of the efficacy of budesonide is attributed to its activation of the corticosteroid receptor. However, budesonide has also been reported to increase bile absorption and reduce bile acid synthesis in patients with collagenous colitis,[3] which may play a role in reducing secretory diarrhea.

Budesonide's 16α- and 17α-acetyl side chains help to confer an affinity for the glucocorticoid receptor that is 15 times that of prednisolone and 200 times that of hydrocortisone.[4] Although budesonide is a potent corticosteroid, its oral bioavailability is only 10% because of high first-pass hepatic metabolism.[5] Hepatic deactivation is mediated primarily by the cytochrome P450 isoenzyme CYP3A4. The major metabolites of budesonide, 6-β-hydroxybudesonide and 16-α-hydroxyprednisolone, are inactive. Of note, the administration of inhibitors of CYP3A4 such as ketoconazole and grapefruit juice in combination with budesonide should be avoided.[6]

To date, budesonide has been developed commercially as both delayed-release oral capsules and liquid suspension enemas. The most common oral formulation is a controlled ileal release preparation, wherein granules containing a matrix of budesonide and ethylcellulose are coated with Eudragit-L resin.[6] This coating dissolves above pH 5.5 to release most of the drug in the ileum and cecum. Other pH-modified release oral formulations are available, and a novel multimatrix formulation is being developed.[7]

● EFFICACY IN CROHN'S DISEASE

The primary indication for oral budesonide in the management of Crohn's disease is the treatment of mild to moderately active ileocecal disease. The efficacy of budesonide in this setting has been demonstrated in several large randomized trials. A Canadian multicentre double-blind dose-ranging trial found oral budesonide to be more effective than placebo for inducing remission of ileal, ileocolonic or proximal colonic disease over 8 weeks when administered at a dose of 15 mg or 9 mg daily but not at a dose of 3 mg daily.[8] A subsequent US multicentre trial found no difference in efficacy between budesonide given at a dose of 9 mg once daily versus 4.5 mg twice daily.[9] However, a pediatric trial found a tapering regiment beginning with budesonide 12 mg daily for 4 weeks more effective for inducing remission at 7 weeks than a regiment beginning at 9 mg daily.[2] Of note, oral budesonide 9 mg once daily was found to be superior to oral 5-aminosalicylic acid 2 g twice daily for inducing remission of active disease.[10]

Oral budesonide has been compared with conventional corticosteroids for treatment of active Crohn's disease in nine published randomized trials.[11–19] A Cochrane review of this literature concluded that conventional corticosteroids are more effective than oral budesonide, particularly among patients with more severe disease activity or more extensive colonic involvement.[20] For induction of remission, the pooled relative risk was 0.86 (95% confidence interval [CI] 0.76–0.98) in favor of conventional corticosteroids.

Just as systemic corticosteroids are not indicated for preventing relapse of inflammatory bowel disease, oral budesonide is ineffective for maintaining remission of Crohn's disease beyond 7 to 12 months. A Cochrane review[21] pooled data from eight placebo-controlled trials[22–29] to conclude that budesonide 6 mg once daily was not effective for maintaining remission over 12 months with a pooled relative risk of 1.13 (95% CI 0.94–1.35). Most of these trials evaluated patients in a medically induced remission. The only trial that evaluated budesonide for maintaining remission after surgical resection failed to demonstrate a significant benefit.[26] A single small study found budesonide 6 mg daily to be more effective than oral 5-aminosalicylic acid 3 g daily for maintaining medically-induced remission over 1 year,[30] but this observation has not been replicated.

A recent study found oral budesonide to be less effective than azathioprine for inducing mucosal healing over 1 year in patients with steroid-dependent ileocolonic Crohn's disease.[31] In this small trial, complete or near-complete healing was achieved in 83% of those on azathioprine versus only 20% of those on budesonide 6 to 9 mg daily. Not surprisingly, healing on budesonide was largely limited to the right colon.

In summary, oral budesonide should be advocated as a first-line induction therapy for patients with mild to moderate Crohn's disease limited to the terminal ileum and/or proximal colon. A standard regimen of 9 mg daily for 8 weeks is recommended, although higher doses can be considered in selected cases. There appears to be no requirement for tapering the budesonide dose after this induction regimen. There is only anecdotal evidence to support the use of budesonide enemas in rectosigmoid Crohn's disease. There is no evidence to support the use of oral or rectal budesonide to maintain clinical or endoscopic remission of Crohn's disease.

Editor's note (TMB): Despite the evidence-based conclusions cited, the average remission on 6 mg budesonide was 7 months versus 3 months on placebo. In my practice, I continue budesonide and mesalamine as maintenance in patients with moderate ileitis in clinical and laboratory remission.

● EFFICACY IN ULCERATIVE COLITIS

There is only limited anecdotal evidence to support the efficacy of oral budesonide in ulcerative colitis.[32,33] However, rectal enema formulations of budesonide have shown efficacy against placebo for the treatment of active distal disease.[34–36] A rectal foam containing budesonide was more efficacious than placebo in a single trial.[37] Budesonide enemas have also demonstrated efficacy similar to that of 5-aminosalicylic acid enemas in a multicentre single-blind trial.[38] When compared with rectal preparations of conventional corticosteroids (prednisolone or hydrocortisone), budesonide enema demonstrated similar efficacy with less suppression of endogenous cortisol production.[39–43] Given these results, rectal budesonide should be considered as an alternative to oral or rectal 5-aminosalicylic acid as a first-line therapy for mild to moderately active distal ulcerative colitis. However, there is no evidence to support the use of oral or rectal budesonide to maintain remission of ulcerative colitis.

Editor's note (TMB): I also utilize oral budesonide to lessen steroid side effects as I am tapering prednisone in patients with pancolitis.

● EFFICACY IN MICROSCOPIC COLITIS

Oral budesonide is a first-line therapy for inducing clinical and histological improvement in patients with both lymphocytic[44] and collagenous[45–47] microscopic colitis. The effect size in this population appears large, with an estimated number needed to treat to achieve clinical response of 2 for collagenous colitis and 3 for lymphocytic colitis.[48] A starting dose of 9 mg daily has

been evaluated in these trials, with total durations of therapy between 6 and 8 weeks. In contrast to its role in Crohn's disease and ulcerative colitis, budesonide also appears to be effective for maintaining remission of collagenous colitis over 6 months at a dose of 6 mg daily.[49,50] However, budesonide has not been studied specifically as a maintenance therapy in patients with lymphocytic colitis.

● SAFETY

The principal advantage of budesonide is its low systemic bioavailability. Indeed, in a systematic literature review, oral budesonide was associated with fewer corticosteroid-associated adverse effects than conventional corticosteroids in patients with Crohn's disease, with relative risk of 0.65 (95% CI 0.53– 0.80).[51] However, typical corticosteroid complications may still occur.[52]

Among the myriad adverse effect attributed to corticosteroids, particular attention has been devoted to their ability to accelerate loss of bone density in patients with inflammatory bowel disease. A small comparative study of bone markers also suggests that short-term budesonide therapy does not impair osteoblast activity.[18] However, early observational data suggested that budesonide was not associated with better bone preservation than low-dose prednisone.[53] A more recent and large randomized controlled trial found budesonide 9 mg daily to induce less loss of bone mineral density than prednisolone 40 mg daily over 2 years in corticosteroid-naive patients with Crohn's disease.[54] No such difference was seen among patients with prior corticosteroid exposure.

Editor's note (TMB): It is common practice to urge patients on maintenance budesonide to take calcium 500 mg plus vitamin D two per day and to follow bone density measurements. Also, be aware that grapefruit juice alters the metabolism of budesonide and other medication.

The low systemic bioavailability of budesonide infers a reduced capacity to suppress the hypothalamic-pituitary-adrenal axis. When compared to placebo, oral budesonide was associated with transient but measurable suppression of adrenal function in a pooled safety analysis of maintenance trials for Crohn's disease.[55] However, systematic literature reviews have demonstrated that both oral and rectal budesonide induce significantly less adrenal suppression, respectively, than conventional oral or rectal corticosteroids.[20,36] Adrenal suppression with budesonide appears to be dose related, but negligible at doses less than 9 mg daily.[8] Still, corticosteroid supplementation should be considered for patients on full-dose budesonide who require emergency surgery.

It is noteworthy that children may be more prone to adrenal suppression with budesonide than adults.[56] However, many of the key induction and maintenance trials have been conducted in pediatric populations with ostensibly good tolerability and safety.[2,15,19] These trials have used robust induction doses of 9 to 12 mg daily despite the lower average body weight of pediatric study cohorts.[2] Short-term exposure to inhaled budesonide has been associated with growth retardation,[57] but it is not clear whether oral budesonide has a similar effect. From this cumulative experience, oral budesonide does appear relatively safe for use in children as an alternative to conventional corticosteroids, but more data are needed.

The safety of medications in pregnancy and lactation is a common cause of concern among female patients of childbearing age being treated for inflammatory bowel disease. Budesonide is classified officially by the Food and Drug Administration as a Category C drug because of teratogenic and embryocidal effects seen in rats.[58] However, a published series of eight patients treated for Crohn's disease with budesonide during pregnancy did not identify any case of glucose intolerance, hypertension or fetal congenital abnormalities.[59]. Furthermore, inhaled budesonide has not been associated with an increased risk of fetal malformations in several large series of women treated with budesonide for asthma during pregnancy.[60,61] Although experience with oral budesonide during lactation is limited, fetal exposure was negligible and no adverse effect was noted among eight breastfeeding mothers on inhaled budesonide as maintenance therapy for asthma.[62] This anecdotal experience is reassuring. However, careful counseling should precede use of any medication during pregnancy or lactation.

● SUMMARY

Oral and rectal budesonide play prominent roles in the management of inflammatory bowel disease. Oral delayed-release preparations are effective for treatment of mild to moderately active ileocecal Crohn's disease, whereas rectal budesonide is effective for treating active ulcerative proctosigmoiditis. Budesonide is effective for inducing and maintaining remission of microscopic colitis. The safety profile of budesonide is good, although typical corticosteroid-associated adverse effects may arise with prolonged or high-dose therapy.

References

1. Brattsand R. Overview of newer glucocorticosteroid preparations for inflammatory bowel disease. *Can J Gastroenterol*. 1990;4:407–414.

2. Levine A, Kori M, Dinari G, et al.; Israeli Pediatric Budesonide Study Group. Comparison of two dosing methods for induction of response and remission with oral budesonide in active pediatric Crohn's disease: a randomized placebo-controlled trial. *Inflamm Bowel Dis*. 2009;15(7):1055–1061.

3. Bajor A, Kilander A, Gälman C, Rudling M, Ung KA. Budesonide treatment is associated with increased bile acid absorption in collagenous colitis. *Aliment Pharmacol Ther*. 2006;24(11–12):1643–1649.

4. Spencer CM, McTavish D. Budesonide. A review of its pharmacological properties and therapeutic efficacy in inflammatory bowel disease. *Drugs*. 1995;50(5):854–872.

5. Edsbacker S. Budesonide capsules: scientific basis. *Drugs Today*. 2000;36(Suppl.G):9–23.

6. Hofer KN. Oral budesonide in the management of Crohn's disease. *Ann Pharmacother*. 2003;37(10):1457–1464.

7. Angelucci E, Malesci A, Danese S. Budesonide: teaching an old dog new tricks for inflammatory bowel disease treatment. *Curr Med Chem*. 2008;15(24):2527–2535.

8. Greenberg GR, Feagan BG, Martin F, et al. Oral budesonide for active Crohn's disease. Canadian Inflammatory Bowel Disease Study Group. *N Engl J Med*. 1994;331(13):836–841.

9. Tremaine WJ, Hanauer SB, Katz S, et al.; Budesonide CIR United States Study Group. Budesonide CIR capsules (once or twice daily divided-dose) in active Crohn's disease: a randomized placebo-controlled study in the United States. *Am J Gastroenterol*. 2002;97(7):1748–1754.

10. Thomsen OO, Cortot A, Jewell D, et al. A comparison of budesonide and mesalamine for active Crohn's disease. International Budesonide-Mesalamine Study Group. *N Engl J Med*. 1998;339(6):370–374.

11. Rutgeerts P, Löfberg R, Malchow H, et al. A comparison of budesonide with prednisolone for active Crohn's disease. *N Engl J Med*. 1994;331(13):842–845.

12. Bar-Meir S, Chowers Y, Lavy A, et al. Budesonide versus prednisone in the treatment of active Crohn's disease. The Israeli Budesonide Study Group. *Gastroenterology*. 1998;115(4):835–840.

13. Gross V, Andus T, Caesar I, et al. Oral pH-modified release budesonide versus 6-methylprednisolone in active Crohn's disease. German/Austrian Budesonide Study Group. *Eur J Gastroenterol Hepatol*. 1996;8(9):905–909.

14. Campieri M, Ferguson A, Doe W, Persson T, Nilsson LG. Oral budesonide is as effective as oral prednisolone in active Crohn's disease. The Global Budesonide Study Group. *Gut*. 1997;41(2):209–214.

15. Escher JC; European Collaborative Research Group on Budesonide in Paediatric IBD. Budesonide versus prednisolone for the treatment of active Crohn's disease in children: a randomized, double-blind, controlled, multicentre trial. *Eur J Gastroenterol Hepatol*. 2004;16(1):47–54.

16. Van Ierssel AJ, Van der Sluys Veer A, Verspaget HW, Griffioen G, Van Hogezand RA, Lamers CB. Budesonide and prednisolone suppress peripheral blood natural killer cells in Crohn's disease. *Aliment Pharmacol Ther*. 1995;9(2):173–178.

17. Tursi A, Giorgetti GM, Brandimarte G, Elisei W, Aiello F. Beclomethasone dipropionate for the treatment of mild-to-moderate Crohn's disease: an open-label, budesonide-controlled, randomized study. *Med Sci Monit*. 2006;12(6):PI29–PI32.

18. D'Haens G, Verstraete A, Cheyns K, Aerden I, Bouillon R, Rutgeerts P. Bone turnover during short-term therapy with methylprednisolone or budesonide in Crohn's disease. *Aliment Pharmacol Ther*. 1998;12(5):419–424.

19. Levine A, Weizman Z, Broide E, et al.; Israeli Pediatric Gastroenterology Association Budesonide Study Group. A comparison of budesonide and prednisone for the treatment of active pediatric Crohn disease. *J Pediatr Gastroenterol Nutr*. 2003;36(2):248–252.

20. Seow CH, Benchimol EI, Griffiths AM, Otley AR, Steinhart AH. Budesonide for induction of remission of Crohn's disease. *Cochrane Database Syst Rev*. 2008;(3):CD000296.

21. Benchimol EI, Seow CH, Otley AR, Steinhart AH. Budesonide for maintenance of remission in Crohn's disease. *Cochrane Database Syst Rev*. 2009;(1):CD002913.

22. Greenberg GR, Feagan BG, Martin F, et al. Oral budesonide as maintenance treatment for Crohn's disease: a placebo-controlled, dose-ranging study. Canadian Inflammatory Bowel Disease Study Group. *Gastroenterology*. 1996;110(1):45–51.

23. Löfberg R, Rutgeerts P, Malchow H, et al. Budesonide prolongs time to relapse in ileal and ileocaecal Crohn's disease. A placebo controlled one year study. *Gut*. 1996;39(1):82–86.

24. Ferguson A, Campieri M, Doe W, Persson T, Nygård G. Oral budesonide as maintenance therapy in Crohn's disease—results of a 12-month study. Global Budesonide Study Group. *Aliment Pharmacol Ther*. 1998;12(2):175–183.

25. Gross V, Andus T, Ecker KW, et al. Low dose oral pH modified release budesonide for maintenance of steroid induced

remission in Crohn's disease. The Budesonide Study Group. *Gut*. 1998;42(4):493–496.

26. Ewe K, Böttger T, Buhr HJ, Ecker KW, Otto HF. Low-dose budesonide treatment for prevention of postoperative recurrence of Crohn's disease: a multicentre randomized placebo-controlled trial. German Budesonide Study Group. *Eur J Gastroenterol Hepatol*. 1999;11(3):277–282.

27. Hellers G, Cortot A, Jewell D, et al. Oral budesonide for maintenance of steroid-induced remission in Crohn's disease. *Gastroenterology*. 1999;116(2):294–300.

28. Cortot A, Colombel JF, Rutgeerts P, et al. Switch from systemic steroids to budesonide in steroid dependent patients with inactive Crohn's disease. *Gut*. 2001;48(2):186–190.

29. Hanauer S, Sandborn WJ, Persson A, Persson T. Budesonide as maintenance treatment in Crohn's disease: a placebo-controlled trial. *Aliment Pharmacol Ther*. 2005;21(4):363–371.

30. Mantzaris GJ, Petraki K, Sfakianakis M, et al. Budesonide versus mesalamine for maintaining remission in patients refusing other immunomodulators for steroid-dependent Crohn's disease. *Clin Gastroenterol Hepatol*. 2003;1(2):122–128.

31. Mantzaris GJ, Christidou A, Sfakianakis M, et al. Azathioprine is superior to budesonide in achieving and maintaining mucosal healing and histologic remission in steroid-dependent Crohn's disease. *Inflamm Bowel Dis*. 2009;15(3):375–382.

32. Löfberg R, Danielsson A, Suhr O, et al. Oral budesonide versus prednisolone in patients with active extensive and left-sided ulcerative colitis. *Gastroenterology*. 1996;110(6):1713–1718.

33. Keller R, Stoll R, Foerster EC, Gutsche N, Domschke W. Oral budesonide therapy for steroid-dependent ulcerative colitis: a pilot trial. *Aliment Pharmacol Ther*. 1997;11(6):1047–1052.

34. Danielsson A, Löfberg R, Persson T, et al. A steroid enema, budesonide, lacking systemic effects for the treatment of distal ulcerative colitis or proctitis. *Scand J Gastroenterol*. 1992;27(1):9–12.

35. Hanauer SB, Robinson M, Pruitt R, et al. Budesonide enema for the treatment of active, distal ulcerative colitis and proctitis: a dose-ranging study. U.S. Budesonide enema study group. *Gastroenterology*. 1998;115(3):525–532.

36. Marshall JK, Irvine EJ. Rectal corticosteroids versus alternative treatments in ulcerative colitis: a meta-analysis. *Gut*. 1997;40(6):775–781.

37. Bar-Meir S, Fidder HH, Faszczyk M, et al.; International Budesonide Study Group. Budesonide foam vs. hydrocortisone acetate foam in the treatment of active ulcerative proctosigmoiditis. *Dis Colon Rectum*. 2003;46(7):929–936.

38. Lémann M, Galian A, Rutgeerts P, et al. Comparison of budesonide and 5-aminosalicylic acid enemas in active distal ulcerative colitis. *Aliment Pharmacol Ther*. 1995;9(5):557–562.

39. Danielsson A, Hellers G, Lyrenäs E, et al. A controlled randomized trial of budesonide versus prednisolone retention enemas in active distal ulcerative colitis. *Scand J Gastroenterol*. 1987;22(8):987–992.

40. Danish Budesonide Study Group. Budesonide enema in distal ulcerative colitis: a randomized dose-response trial with prednisolone enema as positive control. *Scand J Gastroenterol*. 1991;26(12):1225–1230.

41. Löfberg R, Ostergaard Thomsen O, Langholz E, et al. Budesonide versus prednisolone retention enemas in active distal ulcerative colitis. *Aliment Pharmacol Ther*. 1994;8(6):623–629.

42. Tarpila S, Turunen U, Seppälä K, et al. Budesonide enema in active haemorrhagic proctitis–a controlled trial against hydrocortisone foam enema. *Aliment Pharmacol Ther*. 1994;8(6):591–595.

43. Bianchi Porro G, Prantera C, Campieri M, et al. Comparative trial of methylprednisolone and budesonide enemas in active distal ulcerative colitis. *Eur J Gastroenterol Hepatol*. 1994;6:125–130.

44. Miehlke S, Madisch A, Karimi D, et al. Budesonide is effective in treating lymphocytic colitis: a randomized double-blind placebo-controlled study. *Gastroenterology*. 2009;136(7):2092–2100.

45. Baert F, Schmit A, D'Haens G, et al.; Belgian IBD Research Group; Codali Brussels. Budesonide in collagenous colitis: a double-blind placebo-controlled trial with histologic follow-up. *Gastroenterology*. 2002;122(1):20–25.

46. Miehlke S, Heymer P, Bethke B, et al. Budesonide treatment for collagenous colitis: a randomized, double-blind, placebo-controlled, multicenter trial. *Gastroenterology*. 2002;123(4):978–984.

47. Bonderup OK, Hansen JB, Birket-Smith L, Vestergaard V, Teglbjaerg PS, Fallingborg J. Budesonide treatment of collagenous colitis: a randomised, double blind, placebo controlled trial with morphometric analysis. *Gut*. 2003;52(2):248–251.

48. Chande N, MacDonald JK, McDonald JW. Interventions for treating microscopic colitis: a Cochrane Inflammatory Bowel Disease and Functional Bowel Disorders Review Group systematic review of randomized trials. *Am J Gastroenterol*. 2009;104(1):235–41; quiz 234, 242.

49. Miehlke S, Madisch A, Bethke B, et al. Oral budesonide for maintenance treatment of collagenous colitis: a randomized, double-blind, placebo-controlled trial. *Gastroenterology*. 2008;135(5):1510–1516.

50. Bonderup OK, Hansen JB, Teglbjaerg PS, Christensen LA, Fallingborg JF. Long-term budesonide treatment of collagenous colitis: a randomised, double-blind, placebo-controlled trial. *Gut*. 2009;58(1):68–72.

51. Kane SV, Schoenfeld P, Sandborn WJ, Tremaine W, Hofer T, Feagan BG. The effectiveness of budesonide therapy for Crohn's disease. *Aliment Pharmacol Ther*. 2002;16(8):1509–1517.

52. Levine A, Watemberg N, Hager H, Bujanover Y, Ballin A, Lerman-Sagie T. Benign intracranial hypertension associated with budesonide treatment in children with Crohn's disease. *J Child Neurol*. 2001;16(6):458–461.

53. Cino M, Greenberg GR. Bone mineral density in Crohn's disease: a longitudinal study of budesonide, prednisone, and nonsteroid therapy. *Am J Gastroenterol*. 2002;97(4):915–921.

54. Schoon EJ, Bollani S, Mills PR, et al.; Matrix Study Group. Bone mineral density in relation to efficacy and side effects of budesonide and prednisolone in Crohn's disease. *Clin Gastroenterol Hepatol*. 2005;3(2):113–121.

55. Lichtenstein GR, Bengtsson B, Hapten-White L, Rutgeerts P. Oral budesonide for maintenance of remission of Crohn's disease: a pooled safety analysis. *Aliment Pharmacol Ther*. 2009;29(6):643–653.

56. Dilger K, Alberer M, Busch A, et al. Pharmacokinetics and pharmacodynamic action of budesonide in children with Crohn's disease. *Aliment Pharmacol Ther*. 2006;23(3):387–396.

57. Pedersen S, Agertoft L, Williams-Herman D, et al. Placebo-controlled study of montelukast and budesonide on short-term growth in prepubertal asthmatic children. *Pediatr Pulmonol*. 2007;42(9):838–843.

58. Kane S. Inflammatory bowel disease in pregnancy. *Gastroenterol Clin North Am*. 2003;32(1):323–340.

59. Beaulieu DB, Ananthakrishnan AN, Issa M, et al. Budesonide induction and maintenance therapy for Crohn's disease during pregnancy. *Inflamm Bowel Dis*. 2009;15(1):25–28.

60. Norjavaara E, de Verdier MG. Normal pregnancy outcomes in a population-based study including 2,968 pregnant women exposed to budesonide. *J Allergy Clin Immunol.* 2003;111(4):736–742.

61. Gluck PA, Gluck JC. A review of pregnancy outcomes after exposure to orally inhaled or intranasal budesonide. *Curr Med Res Opin.* 2005;21(7):1075–1084.

62. Fält A, Bengtsson T, Kennedy BM, et al. Exposure of infants to budesonide through breast milk of asthmatic mothers. *J Allergy Clin Immunol.* 2007;120(4):798–802.

6-Mercaptopurine and Azathioprine for Treatment of Crohn's Disease

103

Burton I. Korelitz

From a historical point of view, it is now exactly 40 years since the launch of the double blind controlled trial of 6-mercaptopurine (6-MP) for the treatment of moderate to severe Crohn's disease and 30 years since the publication of its favorable results.[1] In the past, there had been a long hiatus in the search for new drugs since adrenocorticotropic hormone and the corticosteroids had led to such dramatic responses and remissions, nurturing an attitude of complacency in research; until the realization that these drugs had no maintenance value. Recognition of the efficacy of immunosuppressives was then further delayed because physicians and patients feared that this new category of therapeutic weapons might compromise the body's immune defense mechanism as was the intention in their use in treating human kidney transplants and childhood leukemias.

The efficacy of 6-MP and azathioprine (AZA) has been demonstrated by controlled trials,[1,2] meta-analysis,[3] and long-term experiences for both Crohn's disease[4] and ulcerative colitis.[5,6] For patients with Crohn's disease, sufficient indication for starting 6-MP has been the severity of manifestations according to the location of the disease. This is summarized in Table 103.1, which also includes failures of other drugs to affect remission and prevention of postoperative recurrence. This conforms in principle to the "top-down versus bottom-up" approach championed by Hommes et al.,[7] but recognizes that clinical judgment for management of each Crohn's disease patient must supercede any list of rules.

The decision whether or not to start immunosuppressives for the original manifestations (or to prevent postoperative recurrence) should be guided by the previous untreated severity of disease and the failure of previous drug therapy. If treatment with sulfasalazine or one of the aminosalicylic acid (5-ASA) products has already been started and the patient has responded, perhaps 6-MP need not yet be introduced. If the patient has been treated with corticosteroids and has a dramatic response, then starting a 5-ASA drug might be sufficient. In less sever cases, this is likely to be uncomplicated by fistulization, abscess formation, or obstruction. To start 6-MP under these favorable circumstances, it must be remembered that it still requires commitment to long-term therapy, alteration of lifestyle by necessity of getting blood counts (frequently at the outset), risk of the early complications of an allergic reaction, and the frustration of early failure. It often takes 3 weeks to 6 months for success to be achieved. On the other hand, to procrastinate and delay because of the potentially long "incubation period" is an error, since brief introduction or reintroduction of steroids might be sufficient until the goal of immunosuppression is accomplished. The commitment to starting the treatment with biologicals is easier because of the likelihood of rapid response, even in the ailing patients.[8] Here too, the commitment is a long one but at least is supported by early satisfaction.

For Crohn's disease in children and adolescents where the prognosis for irreversible damage from complications is still greater than for adults, pediatric gastroenterologists often recommend 6-MP as the first-line drug without waiting for exacerbation or the risk of irreversible complications due to the disease or treatment with prolonged steroid therapy.[9]

6-MP: HOW TO BEGIN?

Patient education regarding medication safety, side effects, risks, and benefits is essential. The literature and the discussion must emphasize the need, the clinical relevance, and the frequency of blood drawings. A monitor sheet should ideally be used by the clinician on which the results of the white blood cell (WBC), hemoglobin, hematocrit, and platelets are written along with the directions the patient should follow with regard to their 6-MP dose and when the next complete blood count (CBC) should be done. We allow time for the patient and the family to read the literature we have prepared and provide ample opportunity to ask any questions.

Checking a CBC and liver function tests before and soon after starting therapy is beneficial. This allows the clinician to

TABLE 103.1 Considerations for Starting Treatment with 6-MP/AZA in Crohn's Disease

Location of Crohn's disease	Most severe manifestations	Least severe manifestations
Ileitis	Small bowel obstruction, abdominal, mass, symptomatic fistulization	Incidental finding
Ileocolitis	Diarrhea, dehydration, fever, weight loss, perirectal disease, same as for ileitis	Mild diarrhea, and/or mild abdominal pain
Colitis	Diarrhea, blood loss, fistulization, perirectal disease, same as for ileocolitis	Mild diarrhea and/or mild abdominal pain
Anorectal	Abscesses, fistula, stricture	Present but not incapacitating
Upper GI tract	Pain, obstruction, vomiting	Biopsy only or found by imaging
Failure of other drug therapies	No response to 5-ASA drugs, failure of steroids, failure of biologicals given without 6-MP or AZA	Asymptomatic with or without drug therapy
Prevention of postop recurrence (ileocolic anastomosis)	Severity of disease preoperatively	

GI, gastrointestinal; 5-ASA, 5-aminosalicylic acid; 6-MP/AZA, 6-mercaptopurine or azathioprine.

follow the WBC count trend throughout the therapy as well as to evaluate any development of liver abnormalities that may coincide with the therapy.

The starting dose of 6-MP is usually 50 mg orally, once a day, and is not dependent on the patient's weight.

PATIENT INSTRUCTIONS TO ENSURE COMPLIANCE WITH 6-MP

Close follow-up with the patient on 6-MP is essential to treatment success and serves to minimize the risks of adverse events with therapy. Over the first 3 weeks, CBC evaluations should occur weekly. Dose adjustments should occur if there is evidence of leukopenia (WBCs <3500), thrombocytopenia, or new onset anemia. Concurrent treatment with intravenous or oral steroids will elevate the total WBC count, coincidentally providing added safety. After 2 or 3 weeks of stable WBC values, the duration between blood drawings for the CBC can be extended to 2-week intervals and shortly thereafter monthly and then longer. These guidelines assume that the patient is tolerating the starting dose.

If within this early period the patient is not improving or relapses and steroids have to be reintroduced, the dose of 6-MP should be raised at the same time. The steroids, if used at all, should be considered a rescue therapy. When practical, they should be administered intravenously and should be terminated after clinical relief has been secured. This serves to reduce the risk of steroid dependence. With any increase in dose of 6-MP the CBCs should again be performed weekly for 3 weeks.

THE ROLE OF LEUKOPENIA IN ACCELERATING RESPONSE TO 6-MP THERAPY

Patients developing leucopenia (<5000) coincident with 6-MP treatment are able to achieve remission of inflammatory bowel disease (IBD) and significant improvement faster than patients who were nonleukopenic.[10] The mean time to achieve remission is much shorter for leukopenic (<5000) than for nonleukopenic patients. There is also a lower rate of recurrence and a longer remission than in those who do not develop leukopenia. Candy et al.[2] reported similar findings. This does not mean that the dose of 6-MP should be increased purposefully to achieve leukopenia, but if a moderate leukopenia occurs and is not progressive there are therapeutic advantages in maintaining it even if CBCs have to be done more often. This clinical observation contrasts with the experience where introduction of 6-MP was followed by a severe and sustained leukopenia.[11] These patients suffered consequences of 6-MP toxicity with fever, usually high, and moderate to severe bone marrow suppression. All however, recovered and had a prolonged remission. Perhaps these are the patients with low or absent blood cell levels of the enzyme thiopurine methyltransferase. In all five patients, the course described occurred prior to the availability of serological tests for enzymes and 6-MP metabolites.[12,13]

ALLERGIC REACTIONS TO IMMUNOSUPPRESSIVES

Early adverse reactions to 6-MP are due to myelosuppression, susceptibility to infections, nausea and vomiting, and malaise.[14] These are almost always reversible. Less common are the hypersensitivity reactions like fever, skin rash, arthralgias, myalgias, and pancreatitis, which occur during the first month of treatment or might be delayed in those on steroid therapy and occur when the steroids are reduced or stopped. Desensitization has been successful in many cases by reintroduction of the 6-MP in tiny doses and gradually increasing it, or by switching to AZA with and without starting it at tiny doses.[15] This has been overlooked as a therapeutic procedure. Many of these patients then enjoy prolonged remissions. Unfortunately, desensitization when the allergic reaction is pancreatitis, has been infrequently successful.

MALIGNANCIES IN PATIENTS TREATED WITH 6-MP

There is a continued exploration of a potential association between neoplasms and immunosuppressive drugs. The increased risk of colon cancer remains attributable to the chronic inflammation of Crohn's colitis as it is in ulcerative colitis, and indeed 6-MP therapy might, according to a recent French study, be responsible for a reduction in risk of colon cancer. This, however, is not the case for lymphomas where a small but significant increase in risk has been demonstrated.[16]

Editor's note (TMB): The risk-benefit discussions in a subsequent chapter list 2 per 10,000 patient years for Crohn's disease and 4 per 10,000 patient years for Crohn's disease patients on AZA or 6-MP. A 2009 French study published in *Lancet* suggested an increased risk in Crohn's disease death on AZA.

Perhaps a more substantial cause and effect relationship exists in the development of basal cell and squamous cell carcinomas of the skin in patients with prolonged immunosuppressive therapy. There is also evidence to support the increased risk of lymphomas and other hematological malignancies in patients who have a sustained leukopenia after treatment with 6-MP.[17]

REASONS FOR TEMPORARY CESSATION OF 6-MP/AZA

It is advisable to stop 6-MP temporarily if a patient develops marked leukopenia (WBC <3500) or thrombocytopenia. Blood tests should be followed weekly or sooner to monitor for normalization. Rarely is treatment with a granulocyte stimulating factor necessary. When restarting 6-MP in this setting, the dose should be decreased by at least 50%. Later, the patient might adapt and tolerate a better dose.

If a patient experiences an allergic reaction including pancreatitis, 6-MP should be discontinued. The patient can later be rechallanged with the medication at significantly lower doses. This can sometimes be accomplished by switching to AZA. If desensitization is attempted for pancreatitis, the serum amylase should still be followed even if clinical symptoms do not recur.

Less often than leukopenia, the patient on 6-MP or AZA may develop thrombocytopenia. If the fall is progressive, the drug might have to be stopped, but often the platelet count stabilizes at a safe level.

Rarely does an anemia due to 6-MP or AZA occur and when it does, it is accompanied by leukopenia and thrombocytopenia. Pancytopenia due to an immunosuppressive drug is an indication for stopping that drug.

HOW LONG TO CONTINUE THERAPY AFTER SUCCESS WITH 6-MP/AZA?

Historically, many patients who have responded to drug therapy and are symptom-free on maintenance 6-MP or AZA want to stop the drug out of lingering fear of later toxicity. Bouhnik et al.[18] initially concluded thatin relation to Crohn's disease, after 4 years of maintenance treatment, the prognosis is no different whether the drug is continued or stopped. This finding was contrary to our findings at Lenox Hill Hospital where rarely did an exacerbation of Crohn's disease occur early after stopping 6-MP and in most cases,

recurrence was later.[19] For those who stopped the drug, they experienced gradual return of disease symptoms and then a full-blown exacerbation as compared to the patients who continued the use. Very recently, the same French group[18] has agreed and confirmed that the results favor statistically on continuing AZA for Crohn's disease rather than stopping it.[20] It is therefore our recommendation that the drug should be continued indefinitely in patients with IBD once there is an indication to start it in the first place. In some cases it would be appropriate to reduce the dose.

Editor's note (TMB): There is a separate chapter on duration of immunomodulator (IMM) and anti-tumor necrosis factor therapy confirming a high relapse rate. However, the chapter on mucosal healing suggests that prolonged remissions, often trials with complete mucosal healing, such as in Crohn's colitis, might allow a clearance in IMM therapy.

PREGNANCY AND 6-MP/AZA

The issue of 6-MP/AZA before and during pregnancy prevails, since the most common years of onset of Crohn's disease and ulcerative colitis are during the ages of greatest fertility and Crohn's disease occurs more often in females than in males. Furthermore, consideration of continuing immunosuppressives during pregnancy is markedly diluted as an issue since pregnancy usually takes emotional priority over treatment of the disease in female IBD patients who want to stop all medications and often the obstetrician is encouraging them to do so.

The evidence favoring continuing 6-MP/AZA during pregnancy is based on the following:

1. The largest reported study on pregnancy and adverse outcomes possibly attributed to 6-MP from Mount Sinai has concluded that these drugs are safe.[21]
2. Most adverse reactions to 6-MP/AZA occur early, soon after the drug is started. Therefore the coincidence of any other toxicity to 6-MP in pregnancy most likely must be attributed to active disease.[22]
3. If the most virulent factor with toxic complications during pregnancy is active Crohn's disease and if the patient is in a remission just achieved by the drug, it should not be stopped. On the other hand, in a study from Lenox Hill Hospital there was a 23% incidence of spontaneous abortions (vs. 13% in IBD controls), a 3% incidence of ectopic pregnancies (compared with none in IBD controls), and finally an abnormal amniocentesis in two patients (and none in the IBD controls).[23]

Editor's note (TMB): There are three other chapters on pregnancy and IBD with information on use of IMMs.

4. The controversy about the outcome of pregnancy when the father has taken 6-MP for IBD at or before the time of conception is also attributable to a Lenox Hill study. It revealed an incidence of 3/50 spontaneous abortions and congenital anomalies in 2/50, but 4/5 complications occurred when the father had taken the 6-MP during the 3 months before impregnation.[24] Comparing these results to the subset of male patients in the Mount Sinai study,[21] where 10/81 of the wives had spontaneous abortions (still higher) and 4/81 had "major congenital abnormalities" (also higher) with 2/4 aborted.

Statistically speaking, no one is yet certain of the risk or the safety of immunosuppressives taken before or during pregnancy and therefore no conclusion should yet be drawn. Logically there must be a compromise solution:

1. Given that the most important issue is active Crohn's disease at conception, if the patient has already been started on the immunosuppressive drug it should be continued and the dose even increased if the clinical severity of the disease warrants it.
2. If the IBD is in remission and it has been for months or for years, the author finds no contraindication to stopping the drug at or before the diagnosis of pregnancy since our experience has shown that any exacerbation is not likely to occur immediately or for that matter even for months, by which time the pregnancy may be ended or at least the fetus is protected through the first trimester when theoretically it would be most susceptible to any danger. Should an exacerbation occur earlier in the pregnancy, the choice may be made to reintroduce the drug.
3. The risk of toxicity to the pregnancy when the father is the one who has the IBD and is taking 6-MP/AZA raises a special consideration. If the male has been in remission, it might be prudent to stop the drug for 1 to 3 months before conception. Since the timing of the pregnancy is so infrequently controlled, this opportunity does not occur often.

Editor's note (TMB): In the chapter on conception by Mahadevan, it is suggested that AZA/6-MP be considered as an issue if infertility seems to be due to sperm adequacy and activity.

4. Decisions whether to continue 6-MP/AZA in pregnant women and their husbands who are taking the drug for IBD require rigorous clinical judgment. For example, if the woman has been in remission for a long time, it seems reasonable to stop the drug until delivery since recurrence is very unlikely. If recurrence does develop, then the drug can be restarted at that time. If either the pregnant female patient or the husband with IBD have active Crohn's disease or have been in remission only briefly following a severe attack, the author recommends continuing the drug. This is an area where rules should not be rigid.

MANAGING 6-MP/AZA IN RELATION TO INFLIXIMAB AND OTHER BIOLOGICALS

Although not related to the primary focus of this chapter, some of the most challenging therapeutic decisions have been raised since the publication of articles suggesting that once a patient with Crohn's disease is in clinical remission while being treated with both infliximab and 6-MP/AZA, there is no advantage to continuing the immunosuppressive drug.[25,26] These studies do not adequately allow for the duration of treatment with the 6-MP, when it was started in reference to infliximab, or the duration and dose of infliximab required to bring the patient into remission. Furthermore, it does not allow for the conclusions of the Study of Immunomodulator Naïve Patients in Crohn's Disease (SONIC), which demonstrated that the therapeutic efficacy of the combination of infliximab and 6-MP/AZA is greater than either drug alone.[27]

The following are the author's suggested options for changing therapy for Crohn's disease in regard to either 6-MP or AZA alone, infliximab or other biological, and 6-MP/AZA and a biological together.

THERAPEUTIC OPTIONS

No Response or Beginning Failure with 6-MP/AZA Alone

1. Increase the dose if WBC or platelets permit.
2. Add a biological.
3. Add a 5-ASA product (this is a particularly good opportunity to add a once daily dose product for compliance reasons).
4. Surgery, usually the last resort, but influenced by location and specific complications of Crohn's disease.

Editor's note (TMB): The following chapter has information on using allopurinol and lowering the AZA/6-MP dose to ¼ when the 6-thioguanine nucleotide level is well below therapeutic and the 6-methylmercaptopurine level is near or over 5000.

THERAPEUTIC OPTIONS

No Response or Failure with a Biological

1. Increase the dose.
2. Decrease the interval between infusions or injections.
3. Add 6-MP or AZA.
4. Add a 5-ASA product.
5. Change the biological.
6. Rescue therapy with intravenous corticosteroids.
7. Surgery, usually the last resort, but influenced too by location and specific complications of Crohn's disease.

THERAPEUTIC OPTIONS

Failure with Combined Therapy of Immunosuppressives and Biological

1. Increase the dose of the immunosuppressive if WBC or platelet counts permit.
2. Decrease the interval between infusions or injections.
3. Add a 5-ASA product.
4. Rescue therapy with intravenous corticosteroids.
5. Stop biological if degree of immunogenicity is high and accompanied by allergic symptoms such as joint pains.
6. Stop 6-MP or AZA if complications suspected of being attributed to these drugs are evident, such as nausea, malaise, fever, worsening liver, or pancreatic function tests.
7. Surgery.

THERAPEUTIC OPTIONS

Eliminating 6-MP/AZA after Remission with Combined Therapy of Immunosuppressives and Biologicals

1. Complications of drug or disease.
2. Reduce the dose—especially for persistent leukopenia.
3. Patients' fear of late complications.

4. In some cases of pregnancy or anticipated pregnancy.
5. Continuation influenced by earlier severity of the disease.

● THERAPEUTIC OPTIONS

Eliminating Biologicals (when used alone) after Remission

1. Fear of complications.
2. Lack of compliance.
3. Now substitute 6-MP/AZA.
4. First extend interval for infusion or injection.
5. First reduce the dose.
6. Add a 5-ASA product if not already done.

● THERAPUETIC OPTIONS

Eliminating the Biological or Immunosuppressive after Remission with Both

1. To be considered preferably only after 1 full year of maintenance therapy and full dose of both after remission achieved.
2. First reduce dose of the biological and extend the interval.
3. Eventually eliminate the 6-MP/AZA if the clinician is more impressed with current literature recommending this versus stopping the biological.
4. The author's preference is to eliminate the biological and continue the 6-MP/AZA.
5. Reduce the dose of 6-MP/AZA and subsequently reduce the dose of the biological as well.

Editor's note (TMB): Several chapters discuss these controversial issues. Patients who demonstrate incomplete response to AZA/6-MP before the institution of the biologic or cyclosporine may experience different issues than the patient in which MM was stated de novo with the biologic, as in the SONIC and the Top-Down studies.

References

1. Present DH, Korelitz BI, Wisch N, Glass JL, Sachar DB, Pasternack BS. Treatment of Crohn's disease with 6-mercaptopurine. A long-term, randomized, double-blind study. *N Engl J Med.* 1980;302(18):981–987.

2. Candy S, Wright J, Gerber M, Adams G, Gerig M, Goodman R. A controlled double blind study of azathioprine in the management of Crohn's disease. *Gut.* 1995;37(5):674–678.

3. Pearson DC, May GR, Fick GH, Sutherland LR. Azathioprine and 6-mercaptopurine in Crohn disease. A meta-analysis. *Ann Intern Med.* 1995;123(2):132–142.

4. Korelitz BI, Adler DJ, Mendelsohn RA, Sacknoff AL. Long-term experience with 6-mercaptopurine in the treatment of Crohn's disease. *Am J Gastroenterol.* 1993;88(8):1198–1205.

5. Adler DJ, Korelitz BI. The therapeutic efficacy of 6-mercaptopurine in refractory ulcerative colitis. *Am J Gastroenterol.* 1990;85(6):717–722.

6. George J, Present DH, Pou R, Bodian C, Rubin PH. The long-term outcome of ulcerative colitis treated with 6-mercaptopurine. *Am J Gastroenterol.* 1996;91(9):1711–1714.

7. Hommes D, Baert F, Van Assche G. The ideal management of Crohn's disease: Top-Down versus step up strategies, a randomized controlled trial. *Gastroenterology.* 2006;130:A108.

8. Bhatia JK, Korelitz BI, Panagopoulos G, et al. A prospective open-label trial of Remicade in patients with severe exacerbation of Crohn's disease requiring hospitalization: a comparison with outcomes previously observed in patients receiving intravenous hydrocortisone. *J Clin Gastroenterol.* 2007;41(7):677–681.

9. Markowitz J, Grancher K, Kohn N, Lesser M, Daum F. A multicenter trial of 6-mercaptopurine and prednisone in children with newly diagnosed Crohn's disease. *Gastroenterology.* 2000;119(4):895–902.

10. Colonna T, Korelitz BI. The role of leukopenia in the 6-mercaptopurine-induced remission of refractory Crohn's disease. *Am J Gastroenterol.* 1994;89(3):362–366.

11. Lobel EZ, Korelitz BI, Vakher K, Panagopoulos G. Prolonged remission of severe Crohn's disease after fever and leukopenia caused by 6-mercaptopurine. *Dig Dis Sci.* 2004;49(2):336–338.

12. Cuffari C, Théorêt Y, Latour S, Seidman G. 6-Mercaptopurine metabolism in Crohn's disease: correlation with efficacy and toxicity. *Gut.* 1996;39(3):401–406.

13. Dubinsky MC, Lamothe S, Yang HY, et al. Pharmacogenomics and metabolite measurement for 6-mercaptopurine therapy in inflammatory bowel disease. *Gastroenterology.* 2000;118(4):705–713.

14. Warman JI, Korelitz BI, Fleisher MR, Janardhanam R. Cumulative experience with short- and long-term toxicity to 6-mercaptopurine in the treatment of Crohn's disease and ulcerative colitis. *J Clin Gastroenterol.* 2003;37(3):220–225.

15. Korelitz BI, Zlatanic J, Goel F, Fuller S. Allergic reactions to 6-mercaptopurine during treatment of inflammatory bowel disease. *J Clin Gastroenterol.* 1999;28(4):341–344.

16. Kandiel A, Fraser AG, Korelitz BI, Brensinger C, Lewis JD. Increased risk of lymphoma among inflammatory bowel disease patients treated with azathioprine and 6-mercaptopurine. *Gut.* 2005;54(8):1121–1125.

17. Disanti W, Rajapakse RO, Korelitz BI, Panagopoulos G, Bratcher J. Incidence of neoplasms in patients who develop sustained leukopenia during or after treatment with 6-mercaptopurine for inflammatory bowel disease. *Clin Gastroenterol Hepatol.* 2006;4(8):1025–1029.

18. Bouhnik Y, Scemama G, Lemann R, et al. Effect of immunosuppressive therapy withdrawal on the course of Crohn's disease in patients successfully maintained in prolonged remission using Azathioprine or 6-mercaptopurine. *Lancet.* 1996; 347:215–219.

19. Kim PS, Zlatanic J, Korelitz BI, Gleim GW. Optimum duration of treatment with 6-mercaptopurine for Crohn's disease. *Am J Gastroenterol.* 1999;94(11):3254–3257.

20. Treton X, Bouhnik Y, Mary JY, et al.; Groupe D'Etude Thérapeutique Des Affections Inflammatoires Du Tube Digestif (GETAID). Azathioprine withdrawal in patients with Crohn's disease maintained on prolonged remission: a high risk of relapse. *Clin Gastroenterol Hepatol.* 2009;7(1):80–85.

21. Francella A, Dyan A, Bodian C, Rubin P, Chapman M, Present DH. The safety of 6-mercaptopurine for childbearing patients with inflammatory bowel disease: a retrospective cohort study. *Gastroenterology.* 2003;124(1):9–17.

22. Baiocco PJ, Korelitz BI. The influence of inflammatory bowel disease and its treatment on pregnancy and fetal outcome. *J Clin Gastroenterol.* 1984;6(3):211–216.

23. Zlatanic J, Korelitz BI, Rajapakse R, et al. Complications of pregnancy and child development after cessation of treatment with 6-mercaptopurine for inflammatory bowel disease. *J Clin Gastroenterol.* 2003;36(4):303–309.

24. Rajapakse RO, Korelitz BI, Zlatanic J, Baiocco PJ, Gleim GW. Outcome of pregnancies when fathers are treated with

6-mercaptopurine for inflammatory bowel disease. *Am J Gastroenterol.* 2000;95(3):684–688.

25. Van Assche G, Magdelaine-Beuzelin C, D'Haens G, et al. Withdrawal of immunosuppression in Crohn's disease treated with scheduled infliximab maintenance: a randomized trial. *Gastroenterology.* 2008;134(7):1861–1868.

26. Lichtenstein GR, Diamond RH, Wagner CL, et al. Clinical trial: benefits and risks of immunomodulators and maintenance infliximab for IBD-subgroup analyses across four randomized trials. *Aliment Pharmacol Ther.* 2009;30(3):210–226.

27. SandbornW, Rutgeerts P, Reinisch W, et al. SONIC: A randomized, double-blind, controlled trial comparing infliximab and infliximab plus Azathioprine to Azathioprine in patients with Crohn's disease naive to immunomodulators and biologic therapy. Presentation to the American College of Gastroenterology, Orlando, Florida, October 6, 2008.

Optimizing Azathioprine Therapy in IBD Patients

104

Carmen Cuffari

Critical-dose drugs are therapeutic agents that demonstrate a wide interpatient variability in drug metabolism. These inherent differences in pharmacokinetics are perceived to influence patient responsiveness to therapy and patient susceptibility to drug-induced cytotoxicity. 6-Mercaptopurine (6-MP) and its prodrug, azathioprine (AZA), are two examples of critical-dose drugs that are well known for their immunosuppressive and lymphocytotoxic properties in the management of patients with inflammatory bowel disease (IBD). These antimetabolite drugs have been shown to suppress disease activity in 40% to 70% of patients with Crohn's disease.[1] Although the overall risk of 6-MP-induced toxicity is low, not all patients achieve disease remission despite presumed therapeutic drug dosing, thereby suggesting that inherent differences in either drug metabolism or immune modulation may influence clinical responsiveness to therapy. Herein, we will review the use of AZA and 6-MP in the management of patients with IBD. Furthermore, the application of pharmacogenetic and 6-MP metabolite testing will also be discussed based on an analysis of the literature. Several recommendations will be provided on applying this technology in clinical practice.

Editor's note (TMB): Optimizing AZA 6-MP use is discussed in other chapters as well as the arguments on combination of new therapy with biologics.

PHARMACOGENETICS OF 6-MERCAPTOPURINE

Pharmacogenomics deals with influence of genetic variation on drug response by correlating gene expression with a drug's efficacy or toxicity. Although the terms "pharmacogenomics" and "pharmacogenetics" tend to be used interchangeably, "pharmacogenetics" is generally regarded as the study or clinical testing of genetic variation that gives rise to differing response to drugs, as it applies to either a single or at most a few gene polymorphisms.

Over the past 20 years, much has been learned about the pharmacogenetics of AZA and 6-MP metabolism in the clinical management of patients with leukemia and in IBD. Although most of our understanding has to do with the polymorphisms of thiopurine methyl tranferase (TPMT) enzyme activity,[2,3] studies have now also introduced potential polymorphisms in intracellular

antimetabolite transport that influence clinical response despite presumed therapeutic drug dosing and metabolite levels.[4]

Once absorbed into the plasma, AZA is rapidly converted to 6-MP by a nonenzymatic reaction. 6-MP is then taken up by a variety of actively replicating cells and tissues, including erythrocytes, T- and B-cell lymphocytes, as well as the bone marrow. The uptake of 6-MP is believed to be a rapid process. Once inside the cell, the metabolism of 6-MP occurs intracellularly along the competing routes catalyzed by hypoxanthine phosphoribosyl transferase and thiopurine S-methyltransferase (TPMT), giving rise to 6-thioguanine nucleotides (6-TGn) and 6-methyl-mercaptopurine (6-MMP), respectively (Fig. 104.1). 6-TGn is the active ribonucleotide of 6-MP that functions as a purine antagonist inducing lymphocytotoxicity and immunosuppression.[5]

An apparent genetic polymorphism has been observed in TPMT activity in both the Caucasian and African American population. Negligible activity was noted in 0.3% and low levels (<5 U/mL of blood) in 11% of individuals. TPMT enzyme deficiency is inherited as an autosomal recessive trait, and to date, 10 mutant alleles and several silent and intronic mutations have been described. In patients with the heterozygous TPMT

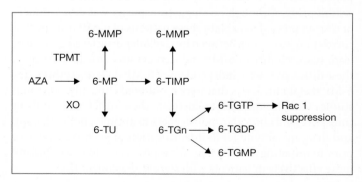

FIGURE 104.1 • Cellular metabolism of 6-MP. AZA, azathioprine; 6-MP, 6-mercaptopurine; 6-TIMP, 6-thioinosine mono-phosphate; 6-MMP, 6-methyl mercaptopurine; 6-TU, 6-thiouric acid; 6-TGn, 6-thioguanine nucleotide; 6-TGM (D), (T)P, 6-thioguanine mono, (di), (tri) phosphate; TPMT, thiopurine methyl transferase; XO, xantine oxidase.

genotype, 6-MP metabolism is shunted preferentially into the production of 6-TG nucleotides.[6] Although 6-TG nucleotides are thought to be lymphocytotoxic, and beneficial in the treatment of patients with leukemia and lymphoma, patients with low (<5) TPMT activity are at risk for bone marrow suppression by achieving potentially toxic erythrocyte 6-TGn levels on standard doses of 6-MP.[7] Despite low TPMT enzyme activity levels, therapeutic erythrocyte 6-TGn metabolite levels can still be achieved without untoward cytotoxicity by lowering the dose of 6-MP 10- to 15-fold.[8] 6TGn are active ribonucleotides that collectively function, as purine antagonists, incorporating into DNA, thereby interfering with in ribonucleotide replication.[9,10]

One of these 6TGn ribonucleotides, 6-TGTP, induces the apoptosis of both peripheral blood and intestinal lamina propria T-cell lymphocytes through the inhibition of Rac-1, a GTPase that inhibits apoptosis. The specific blockade of CD-28 dependent Rac 1 activation by 6-TGTP is the proposed molecular target of 6-MP and its prodrug AZA (Fig. 104.1). The intracellular build-up of this specific 6-TGn metabolite may also show specific inherent polymorphisms in its enzymatic production that may explain refractoriness to AZA therapy despite presumed therapeutic 6-TGn metabolite levels.[11]

Recent studies have also proposed that there may also exist pharmacogenetic differences in the intracellular transport of 6-MP in peripheral blood lymphocytes that could potentially affect responsiveness to antimetabolite therapy in patients with IBD. There was an inherent variability in transport of 6-MP in imortalized lymphocytes derived from patients with IBD. In these studies, 7 inward and 8 outward transporters were tested. One patient demonstrated the least amount of intracellular transport of 6-MP that correlated with the lowest susceptibility to 6-MP cytotoxicity. In this particular patient, multiple inward transporters, including CNT-1, CNT-3, ENT-3, and ENT-4, were notably low in expression. Interestingly, this patient was refractory to 6-MP therapy despite presumed therapeutic drug dosing and erythrocyte 6-TG metabolite levels. In comparison, a second patient exhibited robust 6-MP transport and an increased susceptibility to 6-MP cytotoxcity, and a decreased expression of CNT-1 and ENT-3, but an increased level of expression of another inward transporter, such as ENT-4. This patient maintained a steroid-free disease remission on conventional doses of azathioprine. Although no single transporter was either under- or over-expressed to explain these patterns of 6-MP transport, a correlation was shown between intracellular drug levels and the in vitro susceptibility to 6-MP-induced cytotoxicity. Interestingly, these differences were independent of 6-MP dose or erythrocytes 6-MP metabolite levels that were monitored clinically.[4] Ongoing studies will also attempt to correlate these differences in drug transport with clinical responsiveness to antimetabolite therapy and drug metabolite levels. Identification of such transporters prior to initiating therapy may allow physicians to tailor therapy more effectively in patients with steroid-dependent IBD.

CLINICAL APPLICATION OF METABOLITE TESTING

In patients with IBD, the aim is to optimize antimetabolite therapy to improve overall clinical response, including response time while minimizing the risk of untoward side effects. Ulcerative colitis and Crohn's disease are also regarded as critical disease states that are often difficult to manage clinically. Although 6-MP and AZA have proven clinical efficacy in the induction and maintenance of remission in patients with steroid-dependent disease, therapeutic responsiveness to therapy ranges from 40% to 70% and independent of drug dose. Indeed, the wide therapeutic dosing range used in clinical practice today, as well as the variation in clinical response time, would suggest that pharmacokinetic differences in drug metabolism may also influence clinical responsiveness to therapy.[1,12–16] A true separation between immunosuppression and cytotoxicity has yet to be defined since the dosing of 6-MP and AZA has been based largely on clinical outcome. Indeed, the wide range in AZA dose used in clinical practice would suggest that a safe and established therapeutic dose has yet to be determined. As a consequence, the clinician must always remain aware of potential adverse effects, including allergic reactions, hepatitis, pancreatitis, bone marrow suppression, and lymphoma, while attempting to achieve an optimal therapeutic response.[17]

The measurement of erythrocyte 6-TG and 6-MMP metabolite levels by means of high-pressure liquid chromatography has now become a useful clinical tool for documenting patients' compliance to therapy. Erythrocyte 6-TG metabolite levels showed a strong inverse correlation between with disease activity in adolescent patients with Crohn's disease. Although a wide range of erythrocyte 6-TG levels was associated with clinical responsiveness to therapy, patients with 6-TG levels > 250 pmol/8×10^8 RBCs were uniformly asymptomatic. Moreover, the lack of clinical response was clearly associated with low erythrocyte 6-TG metabolite levels. In one patient, noncompliance was easily suspected in view of very low erythrocyte 6-TG levels and was subsequently confirmed by the patient.[18] To date, a number of studies in both the pediatric and adult literature have supported the notion of a therapeutic drug monitoring in patients with IBD (Table 104.1). However, a uniform consensus has not yet been reached on account of the absence of well-controlled clinical trial (Table 104.1). Nevertheless, a meta-analysis

TABLE 104.1 Clinical Responsiveness to 6-MP and AZA Therapy Based on Threshold (235–250*) Erythrocyte 6-TGn Metabolite Levels

Study	Patients (Response)	6-TGn Response Threshold		Odds Ratio
		Above	Below	
Dubinsky[19]	92 (30)	0.78	0.40	5.0
Gupta[20]	101 (47)	0.56	0.43	1.7
Belaiche[21]	28 (19)	0.75	0.65	1.6
Cuffari[22]	82 (47)	0.86	0.35	11.6
Achar[23]	60 (24)	0.51	0.22	3.8
Lowry[24]	170 (114)	0.64	0.68	0.9
Goldenberg[25]	74 (14)	0.24	0.18	1.5

*pmoles/8×10^8 RBCs.

has shown that higher metabolite levels correlated with a more favorable clinical response, despite no clearly defined therapeutic window of efficacy and toxicity based on 6-MP metabolite levels. The lone prospective clinical trial that was heralded to finally provide consensus on the value of metabolite testing was closed due to limited patient recruitment.

TPMT TESTING

Low and Intermediate (<5 U/mL Blood) TPMT

Eleven percent of the population are considered heterozygous carriers of the TPMT-deficient allele and potentially at risk for drug-induced leukopenia. In the patient who is homozygous recessive with absent TPMT enzyme activity, there is the added risk of severe, irreversible bone marrow suppression. There have been a number of similar cases of irreversible bone marrow suppression both in patients with IBD on maintenance AZA therapy and in patients with leukemia on standard doses of 6-MP.

A number of secondary malignancies, including acute myelogenous leukemia and brain tumors, have been insinuated to be related to the use of maintenance 6-MP therapy in patients with leukemia and the heterozygous TPMT genotype. Although 6-TG and 6-MMP metabolites were not measured in these patients, it may be assumed that these patients were potentially exposed to high-maintenance 6-TG metabolite levels despite presumed therapeutic 6-MP dosing and were thus overly immunosuppressed.

In IBD, patients with Crohn's disease and a "mutant" TPMT allele incurred significant drug-induced leukopenia on standard doses of AZA therapy and were compelled to discontinue treatment. In contrast, patients with the wild-type allele achieved a good clinical response while on AZA therapy without untoward cytotoxicity. Unfortunately, this would suggest that all patients with the heterozygote allele are at an increased risk for drug toxicity and should not be prescribed AZA or 6-MP therapy. However, this would exclude 11% of the population who could potentially benefit from 6-MP therapy. It has been shown in prospective open-labeled clinical trials that by identifying these patients prior to initiating AZA therapy and adopting a moderate dosing (1 mg/kg/day) most patients can achieve a favorable clinical response while avoiding potential bone marrow suppression. These patients must be monitored carefully with serial complete blood counts (CBCs).[3]

High (>16 U/mL Blood) TPMT

The genetic polymorphism in TPMT activity observed in the general population may also have far-reaching implications regarding patient responsiveness to therapy and clinical response time. Fifty per cent of the population are considered to be "normal" (>13) metabolizers of 6-MP and AZA and in theory would require standard (2.5 mg/kg of AZA) large doses of drug in order to achieve any therapeutic drug benefit. In these patients, 6-MP metabolism is shunted away from 6-TG production and into the formation of 6-MMP[26] (Fig. 104.1). In patients with leukemia, high TPMT activity is associated with an increased risk for disease recurrence. The same was also shown in a pediatric study of children with IBD. In that study, the patients either remained refractory to therapy or corticosteroid dependent despite a presumed therapeutic drug dosing regimen.

In a prospective open-labeled study in adults, just 20% of patients with erythrocyte TPMT levels >16 U/mL of blood responded to AZA therapy despite therapeutic presumed drug dosing (2 mg/Kg/day). In comparison, 30% of patients with TPMT levels between 12- and 16-U/mL blood responded to therapy. These were also more likely to require higher dosages (2 mg/kg/day) of AZA from the outset in order to optimize their erythrocyte 6-TGn metabolite levels.

In comparison, patients with TPMT activity levels <12 U/mL blood achieved high (>250) mean erythrocyte 6-TG levels after 16 weeks of induction AZA. This occurred even though both groups received a similar dosage of AZA. In this patient population, 69% patients achieved a favorable clinical response with therapeutic erythrocyte 6-TGn metabolite levels after 4 months of continuous AZA therapy.[3]

High hepatic TPMT activity may draw most of the 6-MP from the plasma, thereby limiting the amount of substrate available for the bone marrow and peripheral leukocytes. This concept of rapid AZA metabolism interfering with therapeutic response could explain the low response rate in a published controlled trial in Crohn's disease that compared high dose oral (2 mg/Kg/day) AZA therapy with and without initiating a short course of high-dose intravenous (40 mg/Kg) AZA therapy. That study was confined to individuals with above 13 enzyme to TPMT levels, that is, "normal levels of TPMT enzyme activity" so that the intravenous AZA treatment group could be studied safely. Even at 2 mg/kg/day of oral AZA therapy, only 20% of these rapid metabolizers in both groups achieved clinical remission, a clinical response that is lower than that reported in most consecutive patient publications.[27]

Furthermore, "normal" (>13) erythrocyte TPMT levels may also explain the rather low clinical response noted in the AZA treatment arm of the SONIC trials. In this study, despite presumably optimized induction dosages (2.5 mg/kg/day) of AZA, just 30% of patients responded to therapy, lower than what has been generally concluded from the Cochran meta-analyses of AZA therapy in treating patients with IBD.[28]

CLINICAL APPLICATION OF TPMT TESTING

Leukopenia and hepatoxicity can occur soon after commencing antimetabolite therapy. Most physicians will monitor CBC and serum aminotransferases weekly or biweekly and then monthly during the first 3 months of initiating therapy. Although TPMT measurement has been shown to predict leukopenia in up to 20% of patients, TPMT monitoring may be used clinically to increase the level of physician comfort in prescribing antimetabolite therapy in titrations of potential toxicity as well clinical response time.

Knowing the TPMT status in a patient can aid in utilizing a variable AZA dosing strategy.[3] Furthermore, in the event TMPT is not present, then those patients should not receive AZA therapy. Those with very low (<5) TPMT activity can be effectively treated with 1 mg/kg/day while, as in all groups, monitoring CBC and liver function tests. Patients with TPMT activity between 5 and 12 U/mL blood have an increased likelihood of responding to a

TABLE 104.2 Clinical response to metabolite profiles. 6-MMp, 6-methyl mercaptopurine; 6-TGn, 6-thioguanine nucleotide

	Metabolite Profiles	Clinical Impression	Therapeutic Decision
Group A	Absent/very low (<50)	Nonadherence	Patient education
	6-TGn absent 6-MMP		
Group B	Low (<250) 6-TGn	Subtherapeutic dose	Dose titration
	Low (<2500) 6-MMP		
Group C	Low (<250) 6-TGn	Rapid-metabolizer	Switch therapy vs. allopurinol
	High (>5700) 6-MMP		
Group D	High (>400) 6-TGn	Thiopurine resistant	Switch therapy
	High (>5700) 6-MMP		Methotrexate or biologic

more moderate dosing strategy, such as 1.5 mg/kg/day. In patients with above-average (>12) TPMT activity, AZA therapy should be started at 2.0 mg/Kg/day in order to achieve a favorable clinical response. However, higher dosages, such as 2.5 mg/kg/day may be needed for those with very high (>16) TPMT enzyme activity.

● METABOLITE TESTING

Although TPMT testing may guide the physician's initial dosing practices, metabolite testing may help explain patient refractoriness to therapy despite presumed therapeutic dosing (Table 104.2). Patients who are clearly noncompliant (group A) with low metabolite (6TGn, 6-MMP) levels should receive education and have the need for improved adherence to therapy reinforced. Patients who are nonresponding and clearly subtherapeutic (group B) should have their dose of AZA titrated to improve overall clinical response. Following a CBC and comprehensive metabolic panel every 2 weeks for 8 weeks can be reassuring. This approach can be highly effective in improving overall clinical response while avoiding unnecessary toxicity. In a study of 25 adult patients refractory to AZA and low (<250) erythrocyte 6-TGn metabolite levels, 18 were pushed into clinical remission by having their dose of AZA increased by 25 mg/day.[22] Among patients who are deemed rapid metabolizer (group C) the possibility of changing the pharmacokinetic through the addition of allopurinol (100 mg) and increasing the AZA dose by three fourths may be considered.[29] However, the physician will need to be aware of the potential risk of toxicity. CBC and LFT should be measured every 2 weeks and metabolite panel at 8 weeks.

Lastly, those patients clearly refractory to AZA despite therapeutic drug dosing should be considered for alternative therapies (Group D).

Editor's note (TMB): If the WBC is more than 7000 in a refractory patient, I feel comfortable increasing the AZA dose by 25 mg and checking CBC and LFT every 2 weeks for the next 8 weeks. When the WBC is 6000 or less, I depend on 6-TGN levels.[23]

● COMBINATION THERAPY

It has been the practice in many institutions, including our own, to initiate maintenance anti-TNFα therapy in patients who have shown clear refractoriness to either long-term 6-MP or AZA therapy. All of the studies, including ACCENT, CHARM, and PRECISE, have not shown any potential role of combining anti-TNFα with antimetabolite therapy. Moreover, the increasing concern of hepatic T-cell lymphoma has led many physicians to consider discontinuing either 6-MP or AZA with the introduction of biologicals. Although all anti-TNFα have antigenic properties, thereby rendering patients susceptible to HACA formation, those patients on infliximab therapy are most vulnerable. The concurrent use of immunosuppressive therapy permits a favorable clinical response to maintenance infliximab therapy, presumably due to the prevention of HACA antibody formation. In one study, 75% (12 of 16) of patients on concurrent 6-MP maintained a favorable clinical response, compared to 50% (9/18) of those on nonconcurrent immunosuppressive therapy. In the ACCENT 1 study, only 18% of the patients on neither concurrent prednisone nor immunosuppressive drug therapy developed HACA, compared to just 10% of patients on concurrent AZA or methotrexate therapy.

In our experience at The Johns Hopkins Hospital with adult patients with IBD on combination therapy, high 6-TGn levels associated with an improved clinical responsiveness to maintenance anti-TNF therapy. Patients in remission had higher (>300) median erythrocyte 6-TGn metabolite levels compared to patients (<100) with either a partial clinical response or ongoing corticosteroid dependency. Interestingly, patients with anti-TNF-associated side effects (SE) also had low (<100) median 6-TGn levels. Although the concurrent use of either AZA or 6-MP may allow for a more protracted clinical response, the precise mechanism of action is unclear. Whether this purported benefit would justify the increased risk of hepatic T-cell lymphoma is debatable, especially because adalimumab and certolizumab have proven efficacy of salvaging patients refractory to infliximab. More important, TPMT and 6-MP metabolite levels have shown no correlation with the 12 reported cases of hepatic T-cell lymphoma.

● CONCLUSIONS

6-MP and AZA have proven efficacy in the maintenance of disease remission in patients with IBD. The application of pharmacogenetic and metabolite testing in clinical practice may improve the overall clinical response to antimetabolite therapy reduce the risk of antimetabolite-induced side effects. The careful monitoring of complete blood counts, and when refractory, erythrocyte 6-TG metabolite levels are indicated in patients with either low (<5) or above-average (>16) TPMT levels.

Editor's note (TMB): The issues of duration of immunomodulator therapy is covered in another chapter, including the arguments on combination immunomodulator therapy, as well as "top-down" therapy. References to additional recent articles are included in other chapters.

References

1. Pearson DC, May GR, Fick GH, Sutherland LR. Azathioprine and 6-mercaptopurine in Crohn disease. A meta-analysis. *Ann Intern Med.* 1995;123(2):132–142.

2. Lennard L. The clinical pharmacology of 6-mercaptopurine. *Eur J Clin Pharmacol.* 1992;43(4):329–339.

3. Cuffari C, Dassopoulos T, Turnbough L, Thompson RE, Bayless TM. Thiopurine methyltransferase activity influences clinical response to azathioprine in inflammatory bowel disease. *Clin Gastroenterol Hepatol.* 2004;2(5):410–417.

4. Cuffari C, Conklin L, Li X. 6-MP transport in human lymphocytes: Correlation with drug induced apoptosis in patients with IBD. *Journal of Crohn's and Colitis.* 2010;4:32.

5. Alves S, Prata MJ, Ferreira F, Amorim A. Screening of thiopurine S-methyltransferase mutations by horizontal conformation-sensitive gel electrophoresis. *Hum Mutat.* 2000;15(3):246–253.

6. Weinshilboum RM, Sladek SL. Mercaptopurine pharmacogenetics: monogenic inheritance of erythrocyte thiopurine methyltransferase activity. *Am J Hum Genet.* 1980;32(5):651–662.

7. Evans WE, Horner M, Chu YQ, Kalwinsky D, Roberts WM. Altered mercaptopurine metabolism, toxic effects, and dosage requirement in a thiopurine methyltransferase-deficient child with acute lymphocytic leukemia. *J Pediatr.* 1991;119(6):985–989.

8. Bostrom B, Erdmann G. Cellular pharmacology of 6-mercaptopurine in acute lymphoblastic leukemia. *Am J Pediatr Hematol Oncol.* 1993;15(1):80–86.

9. Christie NT, Drake S, Meyn RE, Nelson JA. 6-Thioguanine-induced DNA damage as a determinant of cytotoxicity in cultured Chinese hamster ovary cells. *Cancer Res.* 1984;44(9):3665–3671.

10. Fairchild CR, Maybaum J, Kennedy KA. Concurrent unilateral chromatid damage and DNA strand breakage in response to 6-thioguanine treatment. *Biochem Pharmacol.* 1986;35(20):3533–3541.

11. Tiede I, Fritz G, Strand S, et al. CD28-dependent RAC1 activation is the molecular target of azathioprine in primary human CD4+ T lymphocytes. *J Clin Invest.* 2003;111:1133–1145.

12. Kornbluth A, Sachar DB, Salomon P. Crohn's disease. In Sleisenger MH, Fordtran JS, eds. *Gastrointestinal Diseases.* Philadelphia, PA: W.B. Saunders; 1998:1708–1734.

13. Ewe K, Press AG, Singe CC, et al. Azathioprine combined with prednisolone or monotherapy with prednisolone in active Crohn's disease. *Gastroenterology.* 1993;105(2):367–372.

14. Korelitz BI, Adler DJ, Mendelsohn RA, Sacknoff AL. Long-term experience with 6-mercaptopurine in the treatment of Crohn's disease. *Am J Gastroenterol.* 1993;88(8):1198–1205.

15. Present DH, Korelitz BI, Wisch N, Glass JL, Sachar DB, Pasternack BS. Treatment of Crohn's disease with 6-mercaptopurine. A long-term, randomized, double-blind study. *N Engl J Med.* 1980;302(18):981–987.

16. O'Brien JJ, Bayless TM, Bayless JA. Use of azathioprine or 6-mercaptopurine in the treatment of Crohn's disease. *Gastroenterology.* 1991;101(1):39–46.

17. Present DH, Meltzer SJ, Krumholz MP, Wolke A, Korelitz BI. 6-Mercaptopurine in the management of inflammatory bowel disease: short- and long-term toxicity. *Ann Intern Med.* 1989;111(8):641–649.

18. Cuffari C, Théorêt Y, Latour S, Seidman G. 6-Mercaptopurine metabolism in Crohn's disease: correlation with efficacy and toxicity. *Gut.* 1996;39(3):401–406.

19. Dubinsky MC, Lamothe S, Yang HY, et al. Pharmacogenomics and metabolite measurement for 6-mercaptopurine therapy in inflammatory bowel disease. *Gastroenterology.* 2000;118(4):705–713.

20. Gupta P, Gokhale R, Kirschner BS. 6-mercaptopurine metabolite levels in children with inflammatory bowel disease. *J Pediatr Gastroenterol Nutr.* 2001;33(4):450–454.

21. Belaiche J, Desager JP, Horsmans Y, Louis E. Therapeutic drug monitoring of azathioprine and 6-mercaptopurine metabolites in Crohn disease. *Scand J Gastroenterol.* 2001;36(1):71–76.

22. Cuffari C, Hunt S, Bayless T. Utilisation of erythrocyte 6-thioguanine metabolite levels to optimise azathioprine therapy in patients with inflammatory bowel disease. *Gut.* 2001;48(5):642–646.

23. Achar JP, Stevens T, Brzezinski A, Seidner D, Lashner B. 6-Thioguanine levels versus white blood cell counts in guiding 6-mercaptopurine and azathioprine therapy. *Am J Gastroenterol.* 2000;95:A272.

24. Lowry PW, Franklin CL, Weaver AL, et al. Leucopenia resulting from a drug interaction between azathioprine or 6-mercaptopurine and mesalamine, sulphasalazine, or balsalazide. *Gut.* 2001;49(5):656–664.

25. Goldenber BA, Rawsthorne p, Berstein CN. The utility of 6-thioguanine metabolite levels in managing patients with inflammatory bowel disease. *Am J Gastroenterol.* 2004;99:1744–1748.

26. Dubinsky MC, Yang H, Hassard PV, et al. 6-MP metabolite profiles provide a biochemical explanation for 6-MP resistance in patients with inflammatory bowel disease. *Gastroenterology.* 2002;122(4):904–915.

27. Sandborn WJ, Wolf DC, Targan SR, et al. Lack of effect of intravenous administration on time to respond to azathioprine for steroid-treated Crohn's disease. North American Azathioprine Study Group. *Gastroenterology.* 1999;117:527–535.

28. Colombel JF, Sandborn WJ, Reinisch W, et al. Infliximab, azathioprine, or combination therapy for Crohn's disease. *N Eng J Med.* 2010;362:1383–1395.

29. Sparrow MP, Hande SA, Friedman S, et al. Effect of allopurinol on clinical outcomes in inflammatory bowel disease non-responders to azathioprine or 6-mercaptopurine. *Clin Gastroenterol Hepatol.* 2007;5:209–214.

Methotrexate in Crohn's disease | 105

Christina Ha, Prasanna Kumaranayake, and
Brian G. Feagan

Glucocorticoids may be effective for the induction of remission in inflammatory Crohn's disease (CD); however, they have no role as a maintenance strategy. Their adverse effect profile is substantial particularly with prolonged and repeated steroid courses. Therefore, identifying treatment alternatives for patients dependent or refractory to steroid therapy is necessary early in the course of disease management. Recent therapeutic advances in the medical management of CD, particularly with the introduction of biologic agents, have provided additional steroid sparing options for patients with moderate to severe disease activity. The thiopurines, azathioprine (AZA) and 6-mercaptopurine (6-MP), are often used as first-line steroid-sparing agents for maintenance of steroid-induced remission in CD. Although the efficacy of these immunomodulators for maintaining remission in pediatric and adult CD is well established based on results from randomized clinical trial data, many patients will exhibit either nontolerance or nonresponse to these agents prompting the need for a different treatment option.[1-3]

Methotrexate (MTX), originally developed as a treatment for leukemia, is a competitive antagonist of folic acid. It inhibits dihydrofolate reductase with resultant interference of DNA synthesis leading to apoptosis. During an initial experience with MTX in oncology, it was serendipitously recognized that some leukemic children who had concomitant psoriasis and rheumatoid arthritis (RA) had improvement in their conditions. Subsequent controlled trials using MTX in RA and other chronic inflammatory diseases have demonstrated efficacy as a steroid-sparing agent.[4-6] There has been growing literature about the emerging role of MTX as an effective treatment for CD based on randomized clinical trial data combined with multiple observations from cohort studies over the past decade.

PHARMACOLOGY

The mechanism of the anti-inflammatory properties of MTX is not clearly defined; however, inhibition of dihydrofolate reductase is not presumed to be the primary mediator as supplementation with folic acid does not reduce clinical efficacy.[7] In vitro, a number of immunosuppressive properties have been demonstrated including suppression of proinflammatory molecules, decreased cytotoxic T-cell function, and reductions in neutrophil activity.[8]

MTX can be administered by the oral, subcutaneous, intramuscular, or intravenous routes.[9] Although the drug is highly bioavailable at doses of 15 mg or less, absorption may be erratic with higher oral doses.[10] Among patients with stable CD, the bioavailability of MTX, dosed between 15 and 25 mg by mouth weekly, was 73% lower than patients given similar subcutaneous doses of MTX.[11] Following absorption, MTX is concentrated in the liver, kidneys, and synovium with a steady-state volume of distribution of approximately 1 L/kg. The parent molecule is transported into cells by an energy-dependent process. In the liver, the hepatic aldehyde converts MTX to the major metabolite, 7-hydroxy-MTX. The drug is excreted through the kidneys by glomerular filtration with both tubular secretion and reabsorption. As a result, other organic acids such as aminosalicylic and nonsteroidal anti-inflammatory drugs may interfere with renal tubular secretion and increase serum MTX levels. Therefore, MTX should be used with caution among patients with chronic renal failure as they may be at an increased risk of drug toxicity. However, therapeutic drug monitoring of MTX has no demonstrated utility in RA patients.[12]

ADVERSE EVENT PROFILE

The most common adverse events associated with MTX therapy include nausea and vomiting, bone marrow suppression with leukopenia, hypersensitivity pneumonitis, fatigue, headache, and hepatotoxicity with potential hepatic fibrosis.[13]

Editor's note (TMB): If clinical adverse events are an issue, administering methotrexate as a split-dose regimen may be helpful. If fatigue is a prominent complaint, consider nighttime dosing or weekend dosing.

Although low-dose MTX was first established as an effective treatment for severe psoriasis in the early 1960s, an unacceptably high incidence of hepatic toxicity was noted. Among 104 patients with psoriasis treated daily with MTX for cumulative doses of 20 to 25 mg weekly over an average duration of 3.4 years, 23% of patients showed significant pathologic changes of cirrhosis or active hepatitis on liver biopsy.[14] Subsequent pharmacokinetic investigations found daily drug administration results in high hepatic polyglutamic folic acid and MTX concentrations.[15] Because MTX is a folate analogue, the drug accumulates in the liver and causes toxicity. However, MTX dose not accumulate if sufficient time is allowed for renal excretion between dosing.[16] As a result, weekly MTX dosing schedules were adopted leading to significant reductions in the incidence of drug-related hepatotoxicity. Among patients with inflammatory bowel disease (IBD), there is little evidence of significant hepatotoxicity with MTX. Transient elevations of liver enzymes are commonly seen among IBD patients treated with MTX; however, they frequently normalize while on therapy and rarely necessitate drug discontinuation.[17,18]

The American Rheumatology Association recommends liver biopsy if liver enzymes are consistent elevated or decreasing serum albumin over the course of 1 year[19]; however, the role of routine liver biopsy among IBD patients remains to be determined. Among 20 CD patients treated with cumulative doses of MTX greater than 1500 mg who received liver biopsies, 19 of the 20 patients had only mild histologic abnormalities. Although elevated liver enzymes were present in 30% of the study patients, they were not predictive of chronic hepatic fibrosis.[20] Another study compared MTX-naïve and -exposed CD patients with cumulative doses of greater than 1500 mg using noninvasive transient elastograph scanning to assess liver fibrosis and found similar values for liver fibrosis. Overall, significant liver fibrosis was rare in the MTX-exposed CD patients. There were also no correlations between elevated liver enzymes and hepatic fibrosis.[21] MTX should be used with caution, however, among patients with additional risk factors for hepatotoxicity including alcohol use, abnormal baseline liver enzymes, concomitant diabetes mellitus, and obesity.[22]

Because of potential bone marrow suppression, routine monitoring of complete blood counts is necessary while on MTX in addition to serial liver enzyme measurements. Folic acid supplementation is routinely given to patients while on MTX due to reduced hepatic folate stores. MTX does not impact female fertility, but can cause sterility in men.[23,24] MTX is also a teratogen, Food and Drug Administration pregnancy category X, and should not be given to women of childbearing potential[25] or during breastfeeding due to potential effects of immunosuppression, growth abnormalities, and carcinogenesis among babies.[26]

● INDUCTION OF REMISSION IN CD

There have been five randomized controlled trials of MTX in chronic, active steroid-dependent CD. However, the variability in MTX administration and dosing among these studies as well as the varying end points defining clinical remission makes the determination of true therapeutic efficacy challenging. In the North American Crohn's Study Group (NACSG) study, 141 patients with chronically active steroid-dependent disease received 25 mg of intramuscular MTX weekly or placebo. Following 16 weeks of treatment, 39% of MTX-treated patients were in steroid-free remission, defined as a Crohn's Disease Activity Index (CDAI) score of less than 150, compared to only 19% of the placebo group ($P = 0.025$) with associated improvements in quality of life and cumulative steroid exposure.[27]

Another randomized placebo-controlled Israeli multicenter trial of steroid-dependent CD patients with moderately active disease, defined as a Harvey-Bradshaw Index score of more than 7, comparing oral MTX (12.5 mg/week) and 6-MP (50 mg/day) to placebo found similar proportions of patients entering remission and experiencing relapse among treatment groups. However, more MTX-treated patients had significant improvements in abdominal pain and general well-being with reductions in steroid dosing.[28] In another study, fewer patients treated with oral MTX (15–22.5 mg weekly) experienced disease exacerbations compared to placebo (46% vs. 80%), although these differences were not statistically significant at 1 year.[29]

Two other trials comparing therapeutic efficacy of MTX versus thiopurines found similar rates of steroid-free remission, defined as complete steroid withdrawal and CDAI less than 150. Maté-Jiménez et al. randomized three groups of steroid-dependent IBD patients to receive 6-MP (1.5 mg/kg/day), oral MTX (15 mg/week), or 5-aminosalicylates (3 g/day). The remission rates among 6-MP (94%) and MTX (80%) treated patients were similar as were the adverse event rates requiring study withdrawal (MTX 13.3% vs. 6-MP 6.7%).[30] Ardizzone et al. compared a combination of intravenous followed by oral MTX (25 mg weekly) to AZA 2 mg/kg/day for steroid-dependent CD. At 3 and 6 months, steroid-free remission rates were similar between the MTX and AZA cohorts, although there were more adverse events among the MTX-treated patients (44%) compared to the AZA group (7%). However, most of these drug-related adverse events were minor and there were no differences in drug-related study withdrawals between treatment groups.[31] Based on the clinical trial data, MTX appears to have demonstrable efficacy as an induction agent when used at doses of 25 mg intramuscularly weekly, but the efficacy of lower doses or oral administration may be less robust.[32]

Editor's note (TMB): These trials follow the groundbreaking open-label trial by Kozarek et al. using weekly subcutaneous injections methotrexate 25 mg demonstrating not only clinical response to methotrexate but also potential for mucosal healing, which set the stage for the NACSG study.[33]

Although clinical trial data support the utilization of MTX as a steroid-sparing agent for moderately severe CD, it is often used as a second-line agent for patients who are either nonresponders or intolerant to thiopurines. Prospective clinical trials investigating the role of MTX for thiopurine failures are not widely available, but data from retrospective studies suggest therapeutic efficacy with remission rates of 77% to 79% after 12 to 16 weeks of MTX 25 mg weekly. There were high numbers of adverse events reported (39–79%), most commonly liver enzyme abnormalities, nausea, and vomiting with 10% to 33% of treated patients requiring medication discontinuation due to sustained drug-related symptoms.[17,34]

● MAINTENANCE OF REMISSION IN CD

A placebo-controlled maintenance study of 76 patients demonstrated that low-dose intramuscular MTX (15 mg weekly) is an effective maintenance strategy for patients achieving remission after 16 to 24 weeks of treatment with MTX 25 mg weekly. At the end of the 40-week study of initial MTX responders, more MTX-treated patients (65%) were maintained in remission compared with 39% of placebo patients ($P = 0.015$). MTX-treated patients were less likely to require prednisone (28% vs. 58%) and had lower disease activity. Over half of the patients who relapsed were able to be reinduced into remission with higher dosing of MTX (25 mg/week) and maintained in steroid-free remission by week 40. Adverse events were common, including nausea and vomiting (40%), cold-like symptoms (25%), abdominal pain (18%), headache (18%), joint pain (12%), and fatigue (12%). However, only one patient had to discontinue therapy due to adverse events during the study.[35]

In another randomized controlled trial, CD patients in steroid-free remission after 30 weeks of oral induction MTX therapy (15 mg weekly) were enrolled into a maintenance study using oral MTX dosed at 10 mg weekly. By week 76, the majority (67%) of patients continuing MTX maintained steroid-free remission.[30] Oren et al. compared remission rates using a lower dose of oral MTX (12.5 mg weekly) versus 6-MP 50 mg daily and placebo. Although the number of MTX-treated patients entering remission was lower compared to other published studies (38%), 90% of these patients maintained remission on the same low-dose MTX regimen at 9 months.[28]

There are currently no published prospective studies of the long-term efficacy of MTX; however, as with other medications used to treat CD, the durability of response appears to wane over time. A retrospective study of CD patients in complete remission on MTX had relapse rates of 29%, 41%, and 48% by years 1, 2, and 3, respectively.[36] A meta-analysis of published retrospective studies of MTX maintenance therapies also revealed a gradual loss of remission over time with maintenance of remission rates of 53% and 43% by 24 and 36 months.[34]

COMBINATION THERAPY WITH BIOLOGIC AGENTS

In a 50-week double-blind, multicenter randomized controlled trial, biologic-naïve steroid-dependent CD patients were randomized to receive conventional induction and maintenance therapy with infliximab (IFX) with placebo injections weekly or MTX 25 mg weekly. The primary outcomes were failure to achieve steroid-free clinical remission (CDAI<150) at week 14 and maintain remission at week 50. At week 14, clinical remission rates were similar between the placebo + IFX-treated (77%) and MTX + IFX-treated patients (76%). By week 50, maintenance of remission rates were also similar between the two treatment arms (placebo + IFX, 57% vs. MTX + IFX, 56%). There were also no differences in the infectious adverse events (59% MTX, 62% placebo).[37] However, MTX-treated patients were less likely to develop antibodies to IFX compared to patients receiving IFX monotherapy (4% vs. 20%, $P = 0.01$).[38] Although combination therapy with MTX may not have had superior remission rates for luminal CD, combination therapy may have a role in perianal CD. A prospective French multicenter study of patients with severe perianal fistulizing CD receiving combination therapy with surgery, IFX, and MTX

25 mg weekly showed complete fistula closure rates of 74% by week 14 with 50% of patients maintaining complete response at 1 year.[39]

Editor's note (TMB): In the COMMIT trial, patients with longer disease duration (more than 12 years) had a less robust response to infliximab, fitting with the concept of early aggressive combination therapy for moderate to severe disease.

EFFICACY IN PEDIATRIC CD

Therapeutic efficacy of MTX in pediatric CD is largely based on observational and retrospective studies of children classified as immunomodulator intolerant or failures. A multicenter retrospective cohort study of 60 children treated with MTX (53% thiopurine failures, 47% thiopurine intolerant) described steroid-free clinical remission rates of 42% at both 6 and 12 months. Additional outcome measurements demonstrated increases in height velocities at 1 year following MTX introduction.[40] A similar retrospective study of 61 pediatric CD patients in France, all prior thiopurine nonresponders or intolerant, yielded similar results with complete remission rates of 49% and 45% at 6 and 12 months, respectively.[41] Adverse events were common in both studies with 24% to 50% of children experiencing at least one adverse event, most commonly nausea and elevated liver enzymes; however, only 10% to 13% of patients had to discontinue therapy.[40, 41] Although there are no prospective randomized controlled trials using MTX as a first- or second-line therapy in pediatric CD, the available published data suggests reasonable efficacy as an alternative treatment strategy for patients who cannot take thiopurines.

Editor's note (TMB): The reader is referenced to the chapter on a pediatric gastroenterologist's view of the risk of hepatosplenic T-cell lymphoma, particularly among younger males on combination therapy with anti-tumor necrosis factor agents.

CONCLUSION

MTX is a relatively effective therapy for chronically active CD, and is a reasonable therapeutic alternative among patients who are unable to tolerant thiopurine therapy prior to initiation of biologic therapy. The role of MTX as a combination treatment for CD remains to be determined. Although therapeutic efficacy was no different between patients receiving IFX monotherapy and combination therapy, MTX-treated patients had lower levels of antibodies to IFX, which may impact durability of remission.

The data presently available directly comparing thiopurines and MTX largely support therapeutic equivalence for induction and maintenance of remission. However, the varied dosing schedules and routes of administration for MTX impact the generalizability of these trial and observational data. Although the majority of available studies support the relative safety of MTX for CD particularly with respect to hepatotoxicity and liver fibrosis, in clinical practice MTX tends to be only second-line therapy after thiopurines and/or biologics. Additional controlled trials, both in the pediatric and adult setting, are needed to determine the role of MTX, particularly in the biologic era in the management of CD.

References

1. Present DH, Korelitz BI, Wisch N, Glass JL, Sachar DB, Pasternack BS. Treatment of Crohn's disease with 6-mercaptopurine. A long-term, randomized, double-blind study. *N Engl J Med.* 1980;302(18):981–987.

2. Prefontaine E, Sutherland LR, Macdonald JK, Cepoiu M. Azathioprine or 6-mercaptopurine for maintenance of remission in Crohn's disease. *Cochrane Database Syst Rev.* 2009;(1): CD000067.

3. Markowitz J, Grancher K, Kohn N, Lesser M, Daum F. A multicenter trial of 6-mercaptopurine and prednisone in children with newly diagnosed Crohn's disease. *Gastroenterology.* 2000;119(4):895–902.

4. Klippel JH, Decker JL. Methotrexate in rheumatoid arthritis. *N Engl J Med.* 1985;312(13):853–854.

5. Black RL, O'Brien WM, Vanscott EJ, Auerbach R, Eisen AZ, Bunim JJ. Methotrexate therapy in psoriatic arthritis; double-blind study on 21 patients. *JAMA.* 1964;189:743–747.

6. Weinblatt ME, Coblyn JS, Fox DA, et al. Efficacy of low-dose methotrexate in rheumatoid arthritis. *N Engl J Med.* 1985;312(13):818–822.

7. Morgan SL, Baggott JE, Vaughn WH, et al. Supplementation with folic acid during methotrexate therapy for rheumatoid arthritis. A double-blind, placebo-controlled trial. *Ann Intern Med.* 1994;121(11):833–841.

8. Cronstein BN, Naime D, Ostad E. The antiinflammatory mechanism of methotrexate. Increased adenosine release at inflamed sites diminishes leukocyte accumulation in an *in vivo* model of inflammation. *J Clin Invest.* 1993;92(6):2675–2682.

9. Jundt JW, Browne BA, Fiocco GP, Steele AD, Mock D. A comparison of low dose methotrexate bioavailability: oral solution, oral tablet, subcutaneous and intramuscular dosing. *J Rheumatol.* 1993;20(11):1845–1849.

10. Hillson JL, Furst DE. Pharmacology and pharmacokinetics of methotrexate in rheumatic disease. Practical issues in treatment and design. *Rheum Dis Clin North Am.* 1997;23(4):757–778.

11. Kurnik D, Loebstein R, Fishbein E, et al. Bioavailability of oral vs. subcutaneous low-dose methotrexate in patients with Crohn's disease. *Aliment Pharmacol Ther.* 2003;18(1):57–63.

12. Bannwarth B, Péhourcq F, Schaeverbeke T, Dehais J. Clinical pharmacokinetics of low-dose pulse methotrexate in rheumatoid arthritis. *Clin Pharmacokinet.* 1996;30(3):194–210.

13. Lichtenstein GR, Abreu MT, Cohen R, Tremaine W; American Gastroenterological Association. American Gastroenterological Association Institute technical review on corticosteroids, immunomodulators, and infliximab in inflammatory bowel disease. *Gastroenterology.* 2006;130(3):940–987.

14. Malatjalian DA, Ross JB, Williams CN, Colwell SJ, Eastwood BJ. Methotrexate hepatotoxicity in psoriatics: report of 104 patients from Nova Scotia, with analysis of risks from obesity, diabetes and alcohol consumption during long term follow-up. *Can J Gastroenterol.* 1996;10(6):369–375.

15. Hall PD, Jenner MA, Ahern MJ. Hepatotoxicity in a rat model caused by orally administered methotrexate. *Hepatology.* 1991;14(5):906–910.

16. Lewis JH, Schiff E. Methotrexate-induced chronic liver injury: guidelines for detection and prevention. The ACG Committee on FDA-related matters. American College of Gastroenterology. *Am J Gastroenterol.* 1988;83(12):1337–1345.

17. Domènech E, Mañosa M, Navarro M, et al. Long-term methotrexate for Crohn's disease: safety and efficacy in clinical practice. *J Clin Gastroenterol.* 2008;42(4):395–399.

18. Fournier MR, Klein J, Minuk GY, Bernstein CN. Changes in liver biochemistry during methotrexate use for inflammatory bowel disease. *Am J Gastroenterol.* 2010;105(7):1620–1626.

19. Kremer JM, Alarcón GS, Lightfoot RW Jr, et al. Methotrexate for rheumatoid arthritis. Suggested guidelines for monitoring liver toxicity. American College of Rheumatology. *Arthritis Rheum.* 1994;37(3):316–328.

20. Te HS, Schiano TD, Kuan SF, Hanauer SB, Conjeevaram HS, Baker AL. Hepatic effects of long-term methotrexate use in the treatment of inflammatory bowel disease. *Am J Gastroenterol.* 2000;95(11):3150–3156.

21. Laharie D, Zerbib F, Adhoute X, et al. Diagnosis of liver fibrosis by transient elastography (FibroScan) and non-invasive methods in Crohn's disease patients treated with methotrexate. *Aliment Pharmacol Ther.* 2006;23(11):1621–1628.

22. Sandborn WJ. A review of immune modifier therapy for inflammatory bowel disease: azathioprine, 6-mercaptopurine, cyclosporine, and methotrexate. *Am J Gastroenterol.* 1996; 91(3):423–433.

23. Schilsky RL, Lewis BJ, Sherins RJ, Young RC. Gonadal dysfunction in patients receiving chemotherapy for cancer. *Ann Intern Med.* 1980;93(1):109–114.

24. Sussman A, Leonard JM. Psoriasis, methotrexate, and oligospermia. *Arch Dermatol.* 1980;116(2):215–217.

25. Kozlowski RD, Steinbrunner JV, MacKenzie AH, Clough JD, Wilke WS, Segal AM. Outcome of first-trimester exposure to low-dose methotrexate in eight patients with rheumatic disease. *Am J Med.* 1990;88(6):589–592.

26. American Academy of Pediatrics Committee on Drugs. The transfer of drugs and other chemicals into human milk. *Pediatrics.* 1994;93:137–150.

27. Feagan BG, Rochon J, Fedorak RN, et al. Methotrexate for the treatment of Crohn's disease. The North American Crohn's Study Group Investigators. *N Engl J Med.* 1995;332(5):292–297.

28. Oren R, Moshkowitz M, Odes S, et al. Methotrexate in chronic active Crohn's disease: a double-blind, randomized, Israeli multicenter trial. *Am J Gastroenterol.* 1997;92(12):2203–2209.

29. Arora S, Katkov W, Cooley J, et al. Methotrexate in Crohn's disease: results of a randomized, double-blind, placebo-controlled trial. *Hepatogastroenterology.* 1999;46(27):1724–1729.

30. Maté-Jiménez J, Hermida C, Cantero-Perona J, Moreno-Otero R. 6-mercaptopurine or methotrexate added to prednisone induces and maintains remission in steroid-dependent inflammatory bowel disease. *Eur J Gastroenterol Hepatol.* 2000;12(11):1227–1233.

31. Ardizzone S, Bollani S, Manzionna G, Imbesi V, Colombo E, Bianchi Porro G. Comparison between methotrexate and azathioprine in the treatment of chronic active Crohn's disease: a randomised, investigator-blind study. *Dig Liver Dis.* 2003;35(9):619–627.

32. Alfadhli AA, McDonald JW, Feagan BG. Methotrexate for the induction of remission in refractory Crohn's disease. *Cochrane Database Syst Rev.* 2004;(4):CD003459.

33. Kozarek RA, Patterson DJ, Gelfand MD, Botoman VA, Ball TJ, Wilske KR. Methotrexate induces clinical and histologic remission in patients with refractory inflammatory bowel disease. *Ann Intern Med.* 1989;110(5):353–356.

34. Hausmann J, Zabel K, Herrmann E, Schröder O. Methotrexate for maintenance of remission in chronic active Crohn's disease:

long-term single-center experience and meta-analysis of observational studies. *Inflamm Bowel Dis.* 2010;16(7):1195–1202.

35. Feagan BG, Fedorak RN, Irvine EJ, et al. A comparison of methotrexate with placebo for the maintenance of remission in Crohn's disease. North American Crohn's Study Group Investigators. *N Engl J Med.* 2000;342(22):1627–1632.

36. Lémann M, Zenjari T, Bouhnik Y, et al. Methotrexate in Crohn's disease: long-term efficacy and toxicity. *Am J Gastroenterol.* 2000; 95(7):1730–1734.

37. Feagan BG, McDonald JW, Panaccione R, et al. A randomized trial of methotrexate in combination with infliximab for the treatment of Crohn's disease. *Gastroenterology.* 2008; 135(1):294–295.

38. Feagan BG, McDonald JW, Panaccione R, et al. Methotrexate for the prevention of antibiodies to infliximab in patients with Crohn's disease. *Gastroenerology.* 2010;138:S167–S168.

39. Roumeguère P, Bouchard D, Pigot F, et al. Combined approach with infliximab, surgery, and methotrexate in severe fistulizing anoperineal Crohn's disease: results from a prospective study. *Inflamm Bowel Dis.* 2011;17(1):69–76.

40. Turner D, Grossman AB, Rosh J, et al. Methotrexate following unsuccessful thiopurine therapy in pediatric Crohn's disease. *Am J Gastroenterol.* 2007;102(12):2804–2812; quiz 2803, 2813.

41. Uhlen S, Belbouab R, Narebski K, et al. Efficacy of methotrexate in pediatric Crohn's disease: a French multicenter study. *Inflamm Bowel Dis.* 2006;12(11):1053–1057.

Cyclosporine and Tacrolimus in the Treatment of Crohn's Disease

106

Jenny Sauk and Simon Lichtiger

In the mid-1980s, the chronic use of corticosteroids in the treatment of Crohn's disease was found to be ineffective and littered with potential adverse effects. Immunomodulators were incorporated as maintenance agents. However, their slow onset of action precluded their use as induction agents. Armed with the success of cyclosporine in patients with ulcerative colitis, several trials examined cyclosporine's effect in patients with Crohn's disease.

CYCLOSPORINE—MECHANISM OF ACTION

Cyclosporine (CSA), a lipophilic polypeptide used as a potent immunosuppressant in organ transplantation, inhibits both humoral and cellular responses. Not only does it block Interleukin-2 production by T-helper lymphocytes but also inhibits T-cell activation by binding to cyclophilin, a cyclosporine-binding protein, forming a cyclosporine-cyclophilin complex.[1] This complex binds to and inhibits calcineurin, a cytoplasmic phosphatase involved in T-cell activation. Cyclosporine also indirectly affects B-cell function by blocking the T-helper cells' production of interferon gamma and B-cell-activating factors.

CYCLOSPORINE FORMULATION AND DOSING

There are two oral formulations of cyclosporine, sandimmune and cyclosporine microemulsions (Neoral and Gengraf). Bioavailability of the oral liquid preparation and gelatin capsules range from 15% to 35%. Limitations to the absorption of oral cyclosporine include Crohn's disease as well as short-bowel syndrome and decreased contact with the small-bowel mucosa or rapid transit times.[2] Bile is also required for cyclosporine absorption; therefore, biliary diversion can lead to malabsorption of the drug.

The microemulsion preparations (Neoral and Gengraf) were designed to improve bioavailability and to remove the necessity of bile for absorption of cyclosporine. They contain polyethylene glycol, medium chain triglycerides, castor oil, and low-molecular-weight glycols. Compared to standard oral cyclosporine, the microemulsions have 150% more bioavailability. No studies have looked at microemulsion preparations for Crohn's disease, but in ulcerative colitis several suggest that Neoral may have a better sustained response rate than cyclosporine.

When analyzing the clinical trials for cyclosporine, it is important to assess the results in light of the dosages used. Oral cyclosporine can be divided into high dose (and greater than 5 mg/kg/day) or low dose (less than 5 mg/kg/day). This categorization was based on studies suggesting decreased biopsy-proven nephropathy at doses equal or lower than 5 mg/kg/day. Four controlled trials have demonstrated intravenous cyclosporine's effectiveness in treating severely ill patients with ulcerative colitis at 2 to 4 mg/kg/day. The controlled trials in Crohn's disease used lower doses of cyclosporine than in the ulcerative colitis trials, and only oral, formulations of cyclosporine.

TACROLIMUS—MECHANISM OF ACTION

Tacrolimus is a compound isolated from *Streptomyces tsukubaensis*, which binds to an intracellular protein called the FK binding protein. This complex inhibits the binding of calcineurin with its cytoplasmic receptors, inhibiting the transcription of the *IL-2* gene, which is required for T-cell activation.[3] In addition, there is suppression of inflammatory mediators, including IL-2, IL-3, IL-4, and TNF. As opposed to CSA, tacrolimus is well absorbed by the gastrointestinal tract; therefore, it can be utilized in patients with small-bowel Crohn's. Although tacrolimus has been used to prevent rejection in liver transplant in patients with primary sclerosing cholangitis, which is associated with ulcerative colitis, it was also noted that the primary IBD improved. Tacrolimus has a rapid onset of action resulting in clinical improvement within 5 days of administration. In addition, several case reports as well as small controlled trials have used tacrolimus topically in perianal Crohn's disease. Although the results of these studies were equivocal, low blood levels were obtained with the preparation. Initial systemic dosing is 0.1 to 0.2 mg/kg/day, adjusting the dosage in order to achieve blood levels of 5 to 10 ng/mL.

● UNCONTROLLED TRIALS—CYCLOSPORINE

There have been numerous uncontrolled trials using both intravenous and oral cyclosporine in both enteric and fistulizing Crohn's disease. Egan et al.[4] reported on the treatment of refractory Crohn's disease with parenteral CSA, and a Cochrane review[5] summarized the beneficial effect of cyclosporine in patients with steroid refractory disease. We reported[6] the beneficial effects of parenteral CSA on perianal disease. Loftus et al.[7] pooled the data from the trials with a total of 227 patients and found a mean response rate of 64%. The mean initial oral cyclosporine dose was 10 mg/kg/day. In patients who achieve a clinical response, the effect of cyclosporine was rapid. However, long-term remission was only achieved in 29% of patients. In many of the studies, azathioprine, 6-MP, or methotrexate were not used in maintaining remission. While no controlled trials have examined the effect of CSA on fistulizing Crohn's disease, 12 uncontrolled trials revealed that high-dose cyclosporine could beneficially impact the course of disease. The overall short-term fistula closure rate was 77%. However, long-term closure after discontinuation of cyclosporine was only 40%. This reinforces the fact that cyclosporine is an induction agent. Interpretation is limited, as studies have not been homogeneous in terms of patient selection, dose of CSA, length of treatment, and therapeutic end points.

● TACROLIMUS—UNCONTROLLED TRIALS

Similar to treatment with CSA, uncontrolled trials of tacrolimus have dominated the literature. Though these trials have confirmed the utility of tacrolimus in steroid-refractory disease, conclusions are clouded by the use of different doses, different end points, and treatment goals. However, in more than 100 patients treated with tacrolimus, it appeared to be associated with both short- and long-term benefit. In the largest study,[8] a mix of patients with steroid, immunomodulator, or biologic refractory disease were treated with either oral or parenteral tacrolimus. Authors aimed for a trough level of 10 to 15 ng/mL. After attaining clinical remission, maintenance therapy was administered in order to maintain trough levels of 5 to 10 ng/ mL. Though all initially improved, only 63% were in remission at 4 months, and 37% of these required further treatment with either steroids or infliximab. In another long-term retrospective study,[9] aiming for trough levels of 4 to 8 ng/ mL, therapeutic end point was defined by a modified subjective clinical activity index. In this trial, 90% of patients responded within thirty days; however, inclusion medications as well as a subjective improvement scale dilute interpretation of this trial. There have also been patients with fistulizing disease who have responded to tacrolimus. In several of these trials, there was a subgroup of patients with either perianal or enterocutaneous disease who responded to tacrolimus. Several small trials have reported on the beneficial effect of topical tacrolimus on perianal disease as well as its effect on pyoderma gangrenosum associated with Crohn's disease. Its topical or local effect was independent of a therapeutic serum concentration.

● CONTROLLED CLINICAL TRIALS OF CSA IN CROHN'S DISEASE

Controlled trials have shown that low-dose oral CSA (less than 5 mg/kg/day) is ineffective either for inducing or maintaining remission in Crohn's disease. The cyclosporine study group of Great Britain[10] and Ireland studied 146 patients with active ileitis, ileocolitis, or colitis, all resistant to standard therapy. Patients were randomized to either placebo or 5 mg/kg/day of oral cyclosporine. Treatment success was defined as "freedom from symptoms or clinically significant improvement plus successful withdrawal or reduction of prednisolone to the original or lower dose." Treatment failure was defined as death due to Crohn's disease, surgery for complications, the development of a new fistula or abscess, continued disease activity, or obvious deterioration necessitating other treatment or discontinuation of treatment due to side effects. At 3 months there was no significant difference between active agent and placebo.

Three hundred and five patients in the Canadian Crohn's Relapse Prevention Trial[11] with either active Crohn's disease or Crohn's disease in remission were randomized to oral cyclosporine with a mean dose of 4.8 mg/kg/day versus placebo. Patients were stratified according to disease activity, with active disease defined as a CDAI of greater than 150. The primary outcome was worsening Crohn's disease defined by a 100-point increase in the CDAI from baseline. After 18 months of treatment, there was no significant difference in the number of patients who achieved or maintained remission in the cyclosporine group (40% vs. 48%, P = NS). The European trial of cyclosporine in Crohn's disease[12] randomized 182 patients with active Crohn's disease who had been treated with greater than 20 mg of steroids for at least 2 months prior to entry. Patients were stratified by CDAI and were randomized to receive either oral CSA (5 mg/kg/day) or placebo. Treatment success was defined as CDAI of less than 150. After 4 months, there was no difference in remission rates between the treatment and placebo group (35% vs. 27%), and at 12 months, only 20% of patients in both groups maintained clinical remission. Only one controlled trial[13] used a higher dose of oral cyclosporine (7.6 mg/kg/day) for patients with active Crohn's disease. Seventy one patients were randomized to oral cyclosporine versus placebo. At 3 months there was a statistically significant difference in the number of patients who achieved clinical remission in the treatment group versus the placebo group (59% vs. 32%, P = 0.03). Although these findings were significant, the modified clinical grading scale utilized in the study was not validated. Using this modified CDAI after 12 weeks, cyclosporine was no more effective than placebo for the maintenance of remission in Crohn's disease. Furthermore, patients who achieved remission did so within 2 weeks, but only 11% of patients maintained remission after CSA was discontinued. Based on these four trials, a Cochrane review analyzing cyclosporine use for the induction and maintenance remission in Crohn's disease concluded that it was ineffective.

CONTROLLED TRIALS—TACROLIMUS

The largest controlled trials of tacrolimus in Crohn's disease are in patients with fistulizing disease. Sandborne et al.[14] in a prospective trial examined tacrolimus' effect in 48 patients with either perianal or enterocutaneous Crohn's disease. Patients were randomized to either placebo or 0.2 mg/kg/day of tacrolimus. Primary end point was defined as fistula improvement, with the secondary end point reflecting complete closure of the fistula. Although the secondary end point was not met, oral TCA was effective in the improvement of perianal disease as defined as 50% decline in fistula drainage. A large controlled trial[15] examined the effect of topical tacrolimus applied to active perianal fistula. Nineteen patients were randomized to either 1 g of tacrolimus (1 mg/g in Orabase ointment (0.1%)) twice daily or to a placebo ointment. Ointment was applied to the external opening of fistula as well as the neighboring indurated skin. Compliance was assessed by weighing the balance of the tube at each visit. In this trial the primary end point was partial closure, with the secondary end point being complete closure for a period of 2 months. There was little that delineated fistulas from ulcerating disease, and patients were not randomized with consideration of concomitant steroids, agents that are thought to be contraindicated in the treatment of active fistulous disease. Although each subgroup was small, topical tacrolimus was minimally more effective than placebo. Tacrolimus blood levels were undetectable in the vast majority of patients, whether they improved or not. Both the topical and enteral trials were approximately 3 months in duration. Earlier trials of systemic tacrolimus in Crohn's disease as well as the topical effect on psoriasis and pyoderma gangrenosum may have shown long-term benefits, as patients followed for 6 to 24 months had prolonged periods of remission.

SAFETY OF CYCLOSPORINE IN INFLAMMATORY BOWEL DISEASE

In the Cochrane review of cyclosporine in Crohn's disease,[5] cyclosporine is associated with significantly higher rates of adverse effects when compared to placebo. However, given the dose of cyclosporine in these studies, the adverse effects were not severe and included paresthesias, hypertrichosis, hypertension, diarrhea, tremor, and increased creatinine level. The concern of cyclosporine use is nephrotoxicity from vasoconstriction of the afferent arterioles, which usually reverses within 2 weeks of cyclosporine cessation.

Sternthal et al.[16] studied adverse effects in 111 IBD patients of whom 40% had Crohn's disease. In this series patients were initially treated with intravenous cyclosporine at 4 mg/kg/day for 10 days and then transitioned to oral cyclosporine at 8 mg/kg/day for an average of 9 months. Major adverse effects included nephrotoxicity unresponsive to dose adjustment in 5.4% of patients, serious infections in 6.3%, seizures in 3.6%, and death in 1.8% of patients. This review reported higher adverse events than in other studies. However, mean blood level and duration of therapy were much longer than in other IBD trials.

Nephrotoxicity

In another study of 192 patients with autoimmune disease, renal biopsies were obtained in the majority of patients; 21% had histologic evidence of cyclosporine-induced nephrotoxicity. However, the mean CSA dose in these patients was 9.3 mg/kg/day, which is much higher a dose than was used in patients with IBD. Careful monitoring of the serum creatinine is recommended with dose reduction for serum creatinine values greater than 30% above the patient's baseline. Although patients are treated with intravenous cyclosporine, serum creatinine should be checked at least every other day.

Seizures

Risk factors for seizures include low cholesterol level and hypomagnesemia. With a cholesterol level at less than 120 mg/dL and serum magnesium at less than 1.5 mg/dL, the risks for seizure increase. Each can be repleted prior to initiation of treatment and can be checked while patients receive cyclosporine on an every-other-day basis.

Although serious infectious complications have not been reported for low-dose oral cyclosporine, high-dose or intravenous cyclosporine has been associated with infectious complications in IBD patients. In particular, opportunistic infections have been reported in patients remaining on 6-MP while receiving simultaneous corticosteroids. While patients are on 6-MP with cyclosporine and corticosteroids, prophylaxis with Septra for Pneumocystis carinii should be given.

SAFETY OF TACROLIMUS

Similar to CSA, tacrolimus produces nephrotoxicity by producing arteriole constriction that is reversible in the vast majority of patients. Again, close monitoring of blood pressure as well as BUN and creatinine as well as potassium is required. In most series, the incidence of renal disease is less than that of CSA. However, both require careful monitoring of the aforementioned. Antibiotic prophylaxis may be necessary, as most patients are on concomitant immunomodulators or steroids. Unlike CSA, there have been several reports of non-Hodgkin's lymphoma in patients treated with tacrolimus, with most of these thought to be EBV associated lymphomas. Therefore, initiation of tacrolimus in the setting of an acute EBV illness should be postponed until an adequate antibody response is attained. Even in those patients who develop a lymphoma, once the tacrolimus was stopped, 90% of the lymphomas regressed spontaneously, without any therapy.

CONCLUSION

The use of cyclosporine or tacrolimus in the treatment of Crohn's disease is not as effective as its use in the treatment of ulcerative colitis. Both can be adopted as bridge therapy to immunomodulators in patients resistant to either steroids or biologic therapy. Whether this can be explained by the primary role of TNF-in the pathogenesis of Crohn's disease, as opposed to the role of interleukins in the pathogenesis of ulcerative colitis, is not known. Trials illustrated in this chapter showed equivocal benefit of both drugs; though there may be a role for calcineurin inhibitors in the induction of remission in Crohn's disease, its use as maintenance agents has not been proven. Adverse effects may be minimized by careful monitoring, and most adverse effects are reversible with a decrease in dosage. In the "era of biologics," the use of these agents in Crohn's disease may eventually become a historical footnote.

References

1. Hess AD, Tutschka PJ, Santos GW. Effect of cyclosporin A on human lymphocyte responses in vitro. *J Immunol*. 1982;128(1):355–359.

2. Brynskov J, Freund L, Campanini MC, Kampmann JP. Cyclosporin pharmacokinetics after intravenous and oral administration in patients with Crohn's disease. *Scand J Gastroenterol*. 1992;27(11):961–967.

3. Liu J, Farmer JD Jr, Lane WS, Friedman J, Weissman I, Schreiber SL. Calcineurin is a common target of cyclophilin-cyclosporin A and FKBP-FK506 complexes. *Cell*. 1991;66(4):807–815.

4. Egan LJ, Sandborn WJ, Tremaine WJ. Clinical outcome following treatment of refractory inflammatory and fistulizing Crohn's disease with intravenous cyclosporine. *Am J Gastroenterol*. 1998;93(3):442–448.

5. Cyclosporine for induction of remission in Crohn's disease. Cochrane database of systematic review 2005, issue 2. #CD000297.

6. Present DH, Lichtiger S. Efficacy of cyclosporine in treatment of fistula of Crohn's disease. *Dig Dis Sci*. 1994;39(2):374–380.

7. Loftus CG, Egan LJ, Sandborn WJ. Cyclosporine, tacrolimus, and mycophenolate mofetil in the treatment of inflammatory bowel disease. *Gastroenterol Clin North Am*. 2004;33(2):141–69, vii.

8. Ierardi E, Principi M, Francavilla R, et al. Oral tacrolimus long-term therapy in patients with Crohn's disease and steroid resistance. *Aliment Pharmacol Ther*. 2001;15(3):371–377.

9. Baumgart DC, Pintoffl JP, Sturm A, Wiedenmann B, Dignass AU. Tacrolimus is safe and effective in patients with severe steroid-refractory or steroid-dependent inflammatory bowel disease–a long-term follow-up. *Am J Gastroenterol*. 2006;101(5):1048–1056.

10. Jewell DP, Lennard-Jones JE. Oral cyclosporine for chronic active Crohn's disease: a multicenter controlled trial. *Eur J Gastroenterol Hepatol*. 1994;6:499–505.

11. Feagan BG, McDonald JW, Rochon J, et al. Low-dose cyclosporine for the treatment of Crohn's disease. The Canadian Crohn's Relapse Prevention Trial Investigators. *N Engl J Med*. 1994;330(26):1846–1851.

12. Stange EF, Modigliani R, Peña AS, Wood AJ, Feutren G, Smith PR. European trial of cyclosporine in chronic active Crohn's disease: a 12-month study. The European Study Group. *Gastroenterology*. 1995;109(3):774–782.

13. Brynskov J, Freund L, Rasmussen SN, et al. A placebo controlled double blind, randomized, trial of cyclosporine therapy in active Crohn's disease. *N Engl J Med*. 1989;321:845–850.

14. Sandborn WJ, Present DH, Isaacs KL, et al. Tacrolimus for the treatment of fistula in patients with Crohn's disease: a randomized placebo control trial. *Gastroenterology*. 2003;125:380–388.

15. Hart AL, Plamondon S, Kamm M. Topical tacrolimus in the treatment of perianal Crohn's disease, exploratory randomized control trials. *Inflammatory Bowel Disease*. 2007;13:245–253.

16. Sternthal MB, Murphy SJ, George J, Kornbluth A, Lichtiger S, Present DH. Adverse events associated with the use of cyclosporine in patients with inflammatory bowel disease. *Am J Gastroenterol*. 2008;103(4):937–943.

De Novo Anti-TNF Therapy in Crohn's Disease: Evidence-Based Results and Clinical Experience

107

Stephen B. Hanauer

Infliximab was the first biologic therapy approved by the Food and Drug Administration for the treatment of Crohn's disease in 1998. Subsequently, in the United States, adalimumab, certolizumab pegol, and natalizumab have also been approved for the treatment of Crohn's disease. When considering who to select for biologic therapy, it is important to consider the clinical trial evidence for each agent, the importance of class effects for biologics, and the individual patient's clinical situation including their disease phenotype, disease activity, disease duration, and response or refractoriness to prior therapies.[1–3] In addition, it is essential to "prepare" candidates for biological therapy by considering the potential risks associated with mono- or combination immunosuppressive therapy.[4]

INFLIXIMAB

Infliximab was initially evaluated for patients with lumenal Crohn's disease with moderate to severe clinical activity according to the Crohn's Disease Activity Index (CDAI) despite ongoing therapy with aminosalicylates, corticosteroids, and/or immunosuppressives. Both the trials for induction of response/remission[5] and maintenance therapy[6] demonstrated that infliximab was superior to placebo for the reduction in signs and symptoms and induction of clinical remission (CDAI < 150). Subsequent trials with infliximab for the treatment of draining fistula in Crohn's disease also demonstrated reductions in the number of draining fistula or complete cessation of drainage from all fistula[7] and maintenance of response to fistula,[8] independent of whether patients were receiving concomitant aminosalicylates, antibiotics, corticosteroids, or immunosuppressives.

ADALIMUMAB AND CERTOLIZUMAB

Subsequently, induction and maintenance trials with adalimumab[9,10] and certolizumab pegol[11–13] demonstrated efficacy in patients with lumenal Crohn's disease, and post-hoc analyses of the maintenance trials also suggested benefits for adalimumab[14] and certolizumab pegol at maintaining fistula closure; although the data are not as strong.[15]

DISEASE DURATION AFFECTS RESPONSE RATE

Several consistent, secondary outcomes from the clinical trials with infliximab, adalimumab, and certolizumab pegol were observed in secondary analyses. When assessed, patients with shorter disease duration had better absolute benefits than patients with longer disease duration although relative advantages versus placebo were maintained. In other words, patients with shorter disease duration had improved, overall, outcomes. These findings were also confirmed in the REACH study with infliximab in children.[16] Corticosteroid tapering was not "enforced" over the duration of the trials and so, despite the reduced steroid requirements, the proportion of patients in steroid-free remission was very modest, approximately 20%. Finally, results were based, primarily, on clinical outcomes assessed by the CDAI, which is more of a subjective assessment of "well-being" than a measure of inflammatory disease burden.

IMMUNOGENICITY

Another important outcome that is discussed in the chapter on maintenance therapy is that the immunogenicity of these agents became apparent at an early phase of clinical trials; probably, because infliximab, the first anti-tumor necrosis factor (TNF) to be evaluated in Crohn's disease, is a chimeric antibody with the greatest risk of immunogenicity.[1] Low-induction doses and episodic therapy leads to the development of antibodies to all of the individual anti-TNF antibodies. The immunogenicity appears to be less with adalimumab and certolizumab, partially because experience with infliximab led to avoidance of episodic treatment arms with the latter agents. With all anti-TNF antibodies, high-dose induction therapy followed by regularly scheduled maintenance therapy has reduced the development of antibodies that are associated with acute and delayed infusion reactions with infliximab, and loss of response to all agents. In addition, combination therapy with immunosuppressives also reduces immunogenicity associated with all of the anti-TNF monoclonal antibodies. In contrast, however, in the long-term clinical trials with infliximab (ACCENT I, ACCENT II), adalimumab (CLASSIC II and CHARM), and certolizumab (PRECiSE), there were no differences in outcome for patients receiving combination therapy compared to those receiving monotherapy with the biologic agent, alone.[17] These observations, along with the findings of increased infectious complications associated with multiple immunosuppressive agents[18] and the risk of lymphomas, in particular hepatosplenic T-cell lymphomas in young males, led to a several-year span where clinicians were avoiding combination therapy.[19]

As additional trials and clinical experience have evolved, the issue of combination therapy was obfuscated by failure to randomize immunosuppressive-naïve versus immunosuppressive-refractory patients at entry.

● COMBINATION THERAPY TRIALS

To prospectively assess the advantage of combination therapy with infliximab and an immunosuppressive, two recent trials with different methodologies were performed. In the COMMIT trial (Combination of Maintenance Methotrexate-Infliximab Trial), patients receiving induction steroid therapy were randomized to receive combination infliximab and methotrexate, or monotherapy with infliximab. There were no differences in the proportion of patients in remission who were off steroids at 14 or 52 weeks.[20]

SONIC

In contrast, the SONIC (Study of Biologic and Immunomodulator Naïve Patients in Crohn's Disease) trial randomized a group of immunosuppressive-naïve patients to receive either azathioprine monotherapy, infliximab with azathioprine, or infliximab monotherapy. Importantly, the average duration of disease was 2 years. Thirty-one percent of patients receiving azathioprine monotherapy achieved the primary study outcome of corticosteroid-free clinical remission at 26 weeks compared with 57% of patients receiving the combination ($P = 0.001$) and 44% of patients receiving infliximab monotherapy ($P = 0.009$). In addition, 44% of patients on the combination ($P = 0.001$) and 30% on infliximab monotherapy ($P = 0.022$) demonstrated mucosal healing compared with 17% of patients receiving azathioprine alone.[21] The reconciliation of these two trials appears to be the

differences in induction regimens and suggests that aggressive therapy with two agents, infliximab with steroids or infliximab with immunosuppressives, is superior to treatment with monotherapy.

Editor's note (TMB): The chapters on azathioprine discuss the 30%-remission rate in SONIC compared to 50% to 70% response rate with azathioprine or 6-*mercaptopurine* in other trials. All of the patients in SONIC had thiopurine methyltransferase levels above average (13 Mayo units), and remission rates of 25% to 40% have been found in that population of rapid metabolizers (Sandborn WJ, et al. *Gastroenterology.* 1999;117:527–535; Cuffari C, et al. *Clin Gastro Hepatol.* 2004;2:410–417).

Thus, the largest evidence base for biologic therapy in Crohn's disease is for treatment of clinically active Crohn's disease (with or without perianal fistulae) with anti-TNF agents in adult patients who have been refractory to "conventional" (nonbiological) therapies. Smaller studies also demonstrated a similar efficacy and safety profile for infliximab in children with chronic, active Crohn's disease despite ongoing therapies with nonbiological agents.[16] However, once the registration trials were completed and the anti-TNF biologics were marketed for moderate to severe refractory disease, additional goals of earlier interventions and the potential for disease modification (prevention of transmural progression of Crohn's disease to strictures and fistula) began to evolve.[22]

Editor's note (TMB): There is very little evidence that immunomodulators or anti-TNF agents will prevent the development of fixed stenosis and obstruction.[32] The chapter on stenosing Crohn's disease reviews this topic.

The initial clinical trials for anti-TNF biologic agents enrolled patients with chronic, active Crohn's disease refractory to conventional agents. The average duration of Crohn's disease in all of these trials was greater than 7 years. Nevertheless, infliximab, adalimumab, and certolizumab pegol demonstrated clinical improvement compared to placebo in subgroup analyses including disease duration. However, despite the advantage over placebo, absolute response rates with active treatment (and placebo) declined with increasing disease duration.[15,23,24] Additional analyses of these trials also demonstrated, overall, reductions in 1-year rates of surgery and hospitalization with infliximab and adalimumab although the results for these outcomes were not analyzed according to duration of disease.[25]

More recent trials have begun to explore the utility of anti-TNF strategies in Crohn's disease for patients with earlier onset disease based on cohorts of patients who had either never received corticosteroids or immunosuppressives.[21,26] However, the primary outcomes were assessed according to either early intervention with infliximab compared to corticosteroids[26] or the comparison of infliximab alone compared to combination therapy with azathioprine in immunosuppressive-naïve patients.[21] Additional trials have evaluated the role of anti-TNF agents in pediatric Crohn's disease[27] where results appeared superior to those in adult studies.

● EARLY INTERVENTION

In contrast to rheumatoid arthritis, clinical trials have yet to evaluate the specific benefits of biologic therapy in early onset Crohn's disease. Nevertheless, there has been a great deal of speculation regarding early intervention and the potential benefits of initiating patients with a poor prognosis at diagnosis on early aggressive therapy with immunomodulation or biologic therapies.[22,28–30] In particular, because the toxicities associated with Crohn's disease therapy have been, primarily, associated with either corticosteroids[31] or multiple immunosuppressives,[18] the avoidance of corticosteroids with earlier intervention with biologic agents has received more speculation than controlled trial assessment.

"Top-Down Therapy"

The concept of "top-down" therapy with anti-TNF biologic therapies has derived from similar clinical data and experience in rheumatoid arthritis where early intervention (in appropriate candidates with risk factors for a progressive course) prevents the development or progression of structural damage (joint erosions and joint space narrowing). Until recently, it was not possible to prospectively identify patients who will experience a "severe" or "progressive" clinical course, and in whom the potential benefits of a top-down approach might justify the increased risk and expense Table 107.1. However, there is increasing evidence that certain patient factors are predictive of a more complicated disease course, including (a) disease presentation at a young age, (b) fistulizing or obstructing presentations early in the course of active disease, (c) deep ulcerations, (d) the need for corticosteroids, and (e) high titers of serologic markers such as antineutrophilic cytoplasmic antibody and anti-*Saccharomyces cerevisiae* antibody (see chapter on disease course). It remains to be determined whether these factors will be predictive of a response (or not) to anti-TNF therapies. Nevertheless, the observations that patients with earlier disease have better outcomes and that anti-TNF therapies have not benefited patients with preexistent strictures[32] and that maintenance treatment reduces hospitalizations and surgeries[10,33] have encouraged the concept or potential for disease modification.

Currently, the only anti-TNF biologic that has been tested earlier in the course of Crohn's disease has been infliximab. In two comparative effectiveness trials in adult patients with Crohn's disease, infliximab induction followed by azathioprine maintenance therapy was superior to conventional "step-up" therapy with corticosteroids, initially, followed by azathioprine at inducing steroid-free remissions for steroid-naïve patients[26] and, in the "SONIC" trial, the combination of infliximab with azathioprine was more effective than infliximab or azathioprine monotherapies at inducing and maintaining steroid-free

TABLE 107.1 Patients Who Might Be Considered for Top-Down Therapy
a. Disease presentation at a young age
b. Fistulizing or obstructed presentations early in disease course
c. Deep ulcerations
d. Need for corticosteroids
e. High titers of serologic markers, e.g., ASCA, etc.

ASCA, anti-*Saccharomyces cerevisiae* antibody.

remissions and at inducing "mucosal healing" for immunosuppressive-naïve patients.[21] The latter trial demonstrated that the benefits of biologic therapy were more pronounced in patients with symptoms combined with evidence of inflammatory disease activity such as an elevated C-reactive protein (CRP) or demonstrable ileocolonic ulcerations. In contrast, patients with no mucosal lesions or normal CRP when initiating anti-TNF therapy fared no better than patients treated with placebo. Of note, in the SONIC trial with "early" intervention in immunosuppressive-naïve patients, the risks of infection were actually lower in the group of patients receiving combination therapy suggesting that effective treatment of Crohn's disease and minimization of steroids actually reduce infectious risks.

● COMPARISON OF ANTI-TNF AGENTS

Despite the strong evidence of benefit for the three, marketed, anti-TNF biological agents, there are no head-head trials between these agents to compare and contrast efficacy (speed of onset, maintenance of response, loss of response), safety, convenience, or compliance. The earliest assessments of therapy have been at 2 weeks but end points for induction studies have been at 4 to 6 weeks with individual agents. All of the agents have been effective at the earliest time frames that were assessed. The induction dosing for each agent has also been selected to minimize immunogenicity and provides serum levels that are higher than maintenance levels. It has been challenging to identify a "target" blood level to achieve or maintain effectiveness for any of the agents as TNF production may change through the course of disease, and it is possible that higher concentrations are necessary in induction versus maintenance of remission. Nevertheless, we have been impressed by the correlation of serum concentrations (or lack thereof) with clinical responses, particularly during maintenance therapy.[34,35] At present, there is only one commercial assay in the United States for determination of infliximab levels (and antibodies to infliximab) although proprietary assays have demonstrated similar correlations between blood concentrations of adalimumab and certolizumab pegol.[36,37]

● LOSS OF RESPONSE

We use concentrations of infliximab and antibodies to infliximab, primarily, when assessing loss of response to maintenance therapy. It is important to understand the concepts of antibody/antigen excess in determining the timing of assays. Immediately after infusions or injections there will be antigen excess, and no antibodies to the biologics are likely to be identified so it is best to wait approximately 4 weeks after infliximab to measure infliximab or antibodies to infliximab levels. Similar to Afif,[35] we have found that, at approximately 4 weeks after an infusion if a patient has lost response and there are antibodies to infliximab present, these patients should be switched to an alternative anti-TNF agent. Clinical studies with both adalimumab and certolizumab pegol have enrolled patients who have failed infliximab with reasonable recovery of response. In contrast, patients without antibodies to infliximab and low infliximab levels respond to higher doses or shortened intervals of infusions. The unfortunate patients who have lost response to infliximab despite "therapeutic" infliximab levels are unlikely to respond to an alternative anti-TNF.

Editor's note (TMB): There is a separate chapter on switching anti-TNF agents and another on duration of therapy with immunomodulators and with anti-TNF agents.

● MODES OF ADMINISTRATION

The different modes of administration and dosing for infliximab (infusions) versus adalimumab and certolizumab pegol (injections) make it difficult to compare cost, convenience, or compliance between agents. Despite "similar" efficacies and side effects, there is no "one size fits all" for anti-TNF therapy, and some patients prefer intravenous infusions every 8 weeks whereas others prefer to self-medicate on a biweekly or monthly schedule. We do emphasize that each of these agents requires individualized dose modifications. We assess responses to treatment according to clinical and laboratory (CRP) on a short-term basis (usually after 4–8 weeks of treatment) and long-term basis using endoscopy in attempt (not always successful) to achieve mucosal healing.

Response Loss

It is most important, on a long-term basis, to appreciate that *maintenance* therapies *prevent* signs and symptoms. Hence, patients who become symptomatic between doses require dose adjustments. Approximately 50% of our patients need either increased doses or shorter intervals between administrations, independent of the choice of anti-TNF therapy. Patients who do not respond or have short-term (less than a few weeks) response to dosing should be assessed for antibodies to the agent. At present, this is only possible with commercial assays for infliximab (Prometheus Labs, San Diego, California), but one can gain a clinical sense base on the nature or response. Patients with infusion/injection site reactions who lose response most often have antibodies against the monoclonal and can be switched to an alternative anti-TNF. Patients who lose response at the end of a cycle should receive intensified doses or shorter intervals between infusions/injections. Patient who have lost response and do not respond, at all, to a subsequent dose most often have lost response to the anti-TNF mechanism and are likely to require therapy with an alternative mechanism of action.

Editor's note (TMB): It is not known whether measuring trough levels of infliximab will help decide when it might be reasonable to lower the dosage from 10 mg/kg back to 5 mg/kg in the patient who is doing well for a prolonged period. This issue of decreasing the dosage of infliximab is discussed in the chapter on "Optimizing Anti-TNF Therapy in IBD." As discussed in the chapter on arthritis in inflammatory bowel disease (IBD) patients, measuring antibodies to infliximab may be useful in the patient whose symptoms are worse after an infusion or, as stated in this chapter, a patient who is losing effectiveness of infliximab.

● WHO SHOULD RECEIVE COMBINATION THERAPY?

The issues of who should receive combination therapy with an immunosuppressive and how long to maintain combination treatment have not been adequately addressed in clinical trials. Because patients who have already failed therapy with an immunosuppressive have not benefited, long term, from maintenance of combination therapy and are at risk for increased infections, we often terminate the immunosuppressive after 6 to 12 months, particularly in young men (susceptible to hepatosplenic T-cell lymphomas). The approximate 10% to 15% benefit of combination therapy for steroid- and immunosuppressive-naïve patients leads us to advocate this approach for most immunosuppressive-naïve patients initiating anti-TNF therapy. In the short term, that is, less than 6 months, the infectious complications are less with the more effective therapy for Crohn's disease. Again, in young men, we discontinue thiopurines after 6 to 12 months, after which immunogenicity is less of an issue. The majority of patients, however, are committed to long-term combination therapy. Although small clinical trials have demonstrated the potential to stop either the biologic[38] or immunosuppressive[39] agent in patients who were responding to combination therapy, withdrawal of the biologic agent led to substantial failure of treatment over 1 year whereas withdrawal of the immunosuppressive led to a decline in concentrations of infliximab and increases in CRP levels suggesting impending loss of clinical response.

● SUMMARY

The results of these trials and extensive experience emphasize that, when considering initiating biologic therapy, it is critical to confirm the presence of active inflammation (e.g., elevated CRP or evidence of ulcerations at endoscopy or alternative imaging). The *indications* for biologic therapy include objective evidence for active disease that is steroid refractory, steroid dependent, or steroid intolerant; as an alternative to steroids for patients with objective evidence of active disease who have previously been steroid refractory, steroid dependent, or steroid intolerant; or as "top-down" therapy as an alternative to corticosteroids for patients presenting with features predictive of a bad prognosis (early onset, extensive disease, perianal or fistulizing disease, cigarette smokers, or individuals with an early need for steroids).[2]

When considering the introduction of biological therapies for IBD, it is essential to consider, comprehend, and convey[40] the safety issues with mono- or combination therapy with steroids and conventional immunosuppressives (thiopurines or methotrexate). The most common risks associated with corticosteroids, conventional immunosuppressives, and biologic agents are infections. Hence, biological therapy should not be initiated in patients with evidence of active infection or abscess. Further, due to the risk of common and opportunistic infections and the impact of immunosuppression on responses to vaccines, it is important to make certain that patients receive appropriate vaccinations, in particular, avoiding any live vaccines, *before* initiating immunosuppressive therapies.[3,4] In addition, because TNF is critical for defense against intracellular pathogens, skin testing with purified protein derivative (PPD) or quantification of interferon-γ released from sensitized lymphocytes in whole blood incubated overnight with PPD from *M. tuberculosis* and control antigens (e.g., QuantiFERON), and a chest radiograph, should be performed before initiating biological therapy.

Therapeutic monitoring for infectious complications is important throughout the course of biologic therapy, and treatment should be held in the presence of active infections. The most serious safety concern to date with anti-TNF use is the rare development of lymphomas[41] and, in particular, hepatosplenic T-cell lymphoma in young patients treated with concomitant immunomodulator therapy.[42] Autoimmune phenomena (e.g., development of anti-dsDNA antibodies) occur in less than 10% of patients treated with anti-TNF agents but antibody concentrations are usually low and transient, with only rare reports of drug-induced lupus-like syndromes. The incidence of anti-antinuclear antigen/dsDNA antibodies with certolizumab appear to be lower than with infliximab and adalimumab, potentially due to differences in lymphocyte/macrophage apoptosis induced by the monoclonal antibodies versus pegylated antibody fragments.[43] Patients who have developed lupus-like syndromes with infliximab have tolerated either a "drug holiday" (during which anti-DNA titers decline) or a switch to certolizumab.

Anti-TNF antibodies may exacerbate heart failure and should not be administered to patients with advanced heart failure. Neurologic events, such as demyelinization of peripheral nerve bundles and optic neuritis, have been observed with anti-TNF treatments and the presence of demyelinating disorders is another contraindication to anti-TNF therapy.

Women anticipating pregnancy during anti-TNF therapy can safely continue treatment although infliximab and adalimumab are recognized to cross the placenta most efficiently during the third trimester. These agents are discontinued at 20 weeks, as discussed in the chapters on therapy during pregnancy in the Special Situation Section of this volume. Certolizumab is less likely to cross the placenta. Although no adverse effects of anti-TNF therapy on the fetus have been confirmed, infants exposed to anti-TNF antibodies will have delayed clearance of the antibody and may not respond as well to vaccinations. Live vaccines are contraindicated to infants exposed to anti-TNF antibodies in utero for 3 to 6 months.[44]

Editor's note added in proof (TMB): Ustekinemab: In a May 2011 DDW abstract (#592, A145) W.J. Sandborn et al. described a Phase IIB study of ustekinemab, a mAb to IL12/23 p40 in patients with CD who had failed one to three anti-TNF agents; one-third were primary anti-TNF failures. The response rate to the highest dose, 6 mg/kg IV, was 39.7% versus 23.5% in the placebo at 8 weeks. At 22 weeks, 69.4% of the responders at 8 weeks were still responding versus 42.5% of placebo. This suggests the possibility of a new therapeutic pathway for patients unresponsive to anti-TNF therapies.

References

1. Clark M, Colombel JF, Feagan BC, et al. American gastroenterological association consensus development conference on the use of biologics in the treatment of inflammatory bowel disease, June 21–23, 2006. *Gastroenterology.* 2007;133(1):312–339.

2. Dignass A, Van Assche G, Lindsay JO, et al.; European Crohn's and Colitis Organisation (ECCO). The second European evidence-based Consensus on the diagnosis and management of Crohn's disease: Current management. *J Crohns Colitis.* 2010;4(1):28–62.

3. D'Haens GR, Panaccione R, Higgins PD, et al. The London Position Statement of the World Congress of Gastroenterology on Biological Therapy for IBD with the European Crohn's and Colitis Organization: when to start, when to stop, which drug to choose, and how to predict response? *Am J Gastroenterol.* 2011;106(2):199–212; quiz 213.

4. Kane S. Preparing the patient for immunosuppressive therapy. *Curr Gastroenterol Rep.* 2010;12(6):502–506.

5. Targan SR, Hanauer SB, van Deventer SJ, et al. A short-term study of chimeric monoclonal antibody cA2 to tumor necrosis factor alpha for Crohn's disease. Crohn's Disease cA2 Study Group. *N Engl J Med.* 1997;337(15):1029–1035.

6. Hanauer SB, Feagan BG, Lichtenstein GR, et al.; ACCENT I Study Group. Maintenance infliximab for Crohn's disease: the ACCENT I randomised trial. *Lancet.* 2002;359(9317):1541–1549.

7. Present DH, Rutgeerts P, Targan S, et al. Infliximab for the treatment of fistulas in patients with Crohn's disease. *N Engl J Med.* 1999;340(18):1398–1405.

8. Sands BE, Anderson FH, Bernstein CN, et al. Infliximab maintenance therapy for fistulizing Crohn's disease. *N Engl J Med.* 2004;350(9):876–885.

9. Hanauer SB, Sandborn WJ, Rutgeerts P, et al. Human anti-tumor necrosis factor monoclonal antibody (adalimumab) in Crohn's disease: the CLASSIC-I trial. *Gastroenterology.* 2006;130(2):323–33; quiz 591.

10. Colombel JF, Sandborn WJ, Rutgeerts P, et al. Adalimumab for maintenance of clinical response and remission in patients with Crohn's disease: the CHARM trial. *Gastroenterology.* 2007;132(1):52–65.

11. Sandborn WJ, Feagan BG, Stoinov S, et al.; PRECISE 1 Study Investigators. Certolizumab pegol for the treatment of Crohn's disease. *N Engl J Med.* 2007;357(3):228–238.

12. Schreiber S, Khaliq-Kareemi M, Lawrance IC, et al.; PRECISE 2 Study Investigators. Maintenance therapy with certolizumab pegol for Crohn's disease. *N Engl J Med.* 2007;357(3):239–250.

13. Schreiber S, Rutgeerts P, Fedorak RN, et al.; CDP870 Crohn's Disease Study Group. A randomized, placebo-controlled trial of certolizumab pegol (CDP870) for treatment of Crohn's disease. *Gastroenterology.* 2005;129(3):807–818.

14. Colombel JF, Schwartz DA, Sandborn WJ, et al. Adalimumab for the treatment of fistulas in patients with Crohn's disease. *Gut.* 2009;58(7):940–948.

15. Peyrin-Biroulet L, Deltenre P, de Suray N, Branche J, Sandborn WJ, Colombel JF. Efficacy and safety of tumor necrosis factor antagonists in Crohn's disease: meta-analysis of placebo-controlled trials. *Clin Gastroenterol Hepatol.* 2008;6(6):644–653.

16. Hyams J, Crandall W, Kugathasan S, et al.; REACH Study Group. Induction and maintenance infliximab therapy for the treatment of moderate-to-severe Crohn's disease in children. *Gastroenterology.* 2007;132(3):863–73; quiz 1165.

17. Kozuch PL, Hanauer SB. General principles and pharmacology of biologics in inflammatory bowel disease. *Gastroenterol Clin North Am.* 2006;35(4):757–773.

18. Toruner M, Loftus EV Jr, Harmsen WS, et al. Risk factors for opportunistic infections in patients with inflammatory bowel disease. *Gastroenterology.* 2008;134(4):929–936.

19. Hanauer SB. Risks and benefits of combining immunosuppressives and biological agents in inflammatory bowel disease: is the synergy worth the risk? *Gut.* 2007;56(9):1181–1183.

20. Feagan BG, Panaccione R, Sandborn WJ, et al. Effects of adalimumab therapy on incidence of hospitalization and surgery in Crohn's disease: results from the CHARM study. *Gastroenterology.* 2008;135(5):1493–1499.

21. Colombel JF, Sandborn WJ, Reinisch W, et al.; SONIC Study Group. Infliximab, azathioprine, or combination therapy for Crohn's disease. *N Engl J Med.* 2010;362(15):1383–1395.

22. Peyrin-Biroulet L, Loftus EV Jr, Colombel JF, Sandborn WJ. The natural history of adult Crohn's disease in population-based cohorts. *Am J Gastroenterol.* 2010;105(2):289–297.

23. Schreiber S, Colombel J-F, Bloomfield R, et al. Increased response and remission rates in short-duration Crohn's disease with subcutaneous certolizumab pegol: an analysis of PRECiSE 2 Randomized Maintenance Trial Data. *Am J Gastroenterol.* 2010;105:1574–1582.

24. Etchevers MJ, Ordás I, Ricart E. Optimizing the use of tumour necrosis factor inhibitors in Crohn's disease: a practical approach. *Drugs.* 2010;70(2):109–120.

25. Assasi N, Blackhouse G, Xie F, et al. Patient outcomes after anti TNF-alpha drugs for Crohn's disease. *Expert Rev Pharmacoecon Outcomes Res.* 2010;10(2):163–175.

26. D'Haens G, Baert F, van Assche G, et al.; Belgian Inflammatory Bowel Disease Research Group; North-Holland Gut Club. Early combined immunosuppression or conventional management in patients with newly diagnosed Crohn's disease: an open randomised trial. *Lancet.* 2008;371(9613):660–667.

27. Rosh JR. Use of biologic agents in pediatric inflammatory bowel disease. *Curr Opin Pediatr.* 2009;21(5):646–650.

28. Rutgeerts P, Vermeire S, Van Assche G. Biological therapies for inflammatory bowel diseases. *Gastroenterology.* 2009;136(4):1182–1197.

29. Peyrin-Biroulet L, Loftus EV Jr, Colombel JF, Sandborn WJ. Early Crohn disease: a proposed definition for use in disease-modification trials. *Gut.* 2010;59(2):141–147.

30. Vermeire S, van Assche G, Rutgeerts P. Review article: altering the natural history of Crohn's disease—evidence for and against current therapies. *Alimentary Pharmacology & Therapeutics.* 2007;25(1):3–12.

31. Lichtenstein GR, Feagan BG, Cohen RD, et al. Serious infections and mortality in association with therapies for Crohn's disease: TREAT registry. *Clin Gastroenterol Hepatol.* 2006;4(5):621–630.

32. Lichtenstein GR, Olson A, Travers S, et al. Factors associated with the development of intestinal strictures or obstructions in patients with Crohn's disease. *Am J Gastroenterol.* 2006;101(5):1030–1038.

33. Lichtenstein GR, Yan S, Bala M, Blank M, Sands BE. Infliximab maintenance treatment reduces hospitalizations, surgeries, and procedures in fistulizing Crohn's disease. *Gastroenterology.* 2005;128(4):862–869.

34. Steenholdt C, Bendtzen K, Brynskov J, Thomsen OØ, Ainsworth MA. Cut-off levels and diagnostic accuracy of infliximab trough levels and anti-infliximab antibodies in Crohn's disease. *Scand J Gastroenterol.* 2011;46(3):310–318.

35. Afif W, Loftus EV Jr, Faubion WA, et al. Clinical utility of measuring infliximab and human anti-chimeric antibody concentrations in patients with inflammatory bowel disease. *Am J Gastroenterol.* 2010;105(5):1133–1139.

36. Lichtenstein GR, Thomsen OØ, Schreiber S, et al.; Precise 3 Study Investigators. Continuous therapy with certolizumab pegol maintains remission of patients with Crohn's disease for up to 18 months. *Clin Gastroenterol Hepatol.* 2010;8(7):600–609.

37. Karmiris K, Paintaud G, Noman M, et al. Influence of trough serum levels and immunogenicity on long-term outcome of adalimumab therapy in Crohn's disease. *Gastroenterology.* 2009;137(5):1628–1640.

38. Treton X, Bouhnik Y, Mary JY, et al.; Groupe D'Etude Thérapeutique Des Affections Inflammatoires Du Tube Digestif (GETAID). Azathioprine withdrawal in patients with Crohn's disease maintained on prolonged remission: a high risk of relapse. *Clin Gastroenterol Hepatol.* 2009;7(1):80–85.

39. Van Assche G, Magdelaine-Beuzelin C, D'Haens G, et al. Withdrawal of immunosuppression in Crohn's disease treated with scheduled infliximab maintenance: a randomized trial. *Gastroenterology.* 2008;134(7):1861–1868.

40. Siegel CA. Review article: explaining risks of inflammatory bowel disease therapy to patients. *Aliment Pharmacol Ther.* 2011;33(1):23–32.

41. Siegel CA, Marden SM, Persing SM, Larson RJ, Sands BE. Risk of lymphoma associated with combination anti-tumor necrosis factor and immunomodulator therapy for the treatment of Crohn's disease: a meta-analysis. *Clin Gastroenterol Hepatol.* 2009;7(8):874–881.

42. Kotlyar DS, Osterman MT, Diamond RH, et al. A systematic review of factors that contribute to hepatosplenic T-cell lymphoma in patients with inflammatory bowel disease. *Clin Gastroenterol Hepatol.* 2011;9(1):36–41.e1.

43. Wong M, Ziring D, Korin Y, et al. TNFalpha blockade in human diseases: mechanisms and future directions. *Clin Immunol.* 2008;126(2):121–136.

44. Mahadevan U, Cucchiara S, Hyams JS, et al. The London Position Statement of the World Congress of Gastroenterology on Biological Therapy for IBD with the European Crohn's and Colitis Organisation: pregnancy and pediatrics. *Am J Gastroenterol.* 2011;106(2):214–223; quiz 224.

Switching Anti-TNF Agents: Evidence-Based Results and Clinical Experience

108

Remo Panaccione

Inflammatory bowel disease (IBD) is a chronic inflammatory condition of the intestinal tract for which there is no medical cure. Thus, the current aim of treatment is focused on inducing and maintaining remission while keeping up the highest achievable quality of life. The introduction of biologic agents, in the form of anti-tumor necrosis factor (TNF)-α therapy, has significantly advanced IBD therapy and greatly expanded the range of options to patients and physicians. Infliximab, a chimeric monoclonal antibody directed against TNFα, was first approved by the US Food and Drug Administration (FDA) in 1998 for the treatment of adult patients with Crohn's disease (CD). This was followed shortly thereafter by European approval in 1999. Since its initial approval, infliximab has subsequently been approved for maintenance of moderate to severe CD, induction and maintenance of fistulizing CD, pediatric CD, as well as induction and maintenance of moderate to severe ulcerative colitis (UC). A decade's worth of experience as well as the approval of other anti-TNFα drugs for CD, such as the fully human monoclonal antibody adalimumab and the pegylated Fab fragment certolizumab pegol, has firmly established this class of agents as an invaluable part of the present therapeutic armamentarium. In the United States, natalizumab, an anti-adhesion molecule, is also approved for the treatment of moderate to severe CD in patients who have failed or are intolerant to conventional therapy and at least one anti-TNFα agent. The data supporting the use of all these agents can be found in other chapters.

This chapter will review specific issues regarding the switching of patients from one anti-TNFα agent to another, the reasons this may occur, and a general approach to the "switch" patient with a focus on avoiding the "premature" switch.

● CLINICAL SCENARIOS TO SWITCH OR NOT TO SWITCH

There are several clinical scenarios where the practicing physician may be faced with a decision to switch anti-TNF agents.

These include patient and physician preference, a primary non-response to an initial anti-TNF, secondary loss of response, intolerance to one agent, or dose interruption. In most cases, it is preferable to optimize and preserve the initial anti-TNF rather than switch. Once a decision is made to switch from one anti-TNF to another anti-TNF, there is no need for a washout period and patients should be treated with a full induction dosing regimen of the new agent.

Patient and Physician Preference

With the approval of the subcutaneously administered anti-TNF agents, adalimumab and certolizumab pegol, an increasingly popular question from both patients and physicians is whether there is role for empiric switching from infliximab to one of the subcutaneous preparations in patients who have responded to infliximab and are doing well clinically. The reason that is often cited is convenience for the patient. There are no controlled data on empiric switching within the anti-TNF class, and although this practice would seem logical and harmless at first glance *it is ill advised*. It is well known that all of these agents are associated with immunogenicity and one of the key factors in sensitizing an individual is the episodic use of an anti-TNF agent. In essence, empiric switching because of patient or physician preference sets up a scenario whereby a patient loses response to the alternate agent after the switch—the environment being set for sensitization to the original agent—thereby burning two bridges. Given the fact that most patients are treated with anti-TNF therapy because they have failed traditional nonbiologic therapy, the risk is too great to advocate empiric switching. Empiric switching from the subcutaneous preparations to the intravenous preparation is less common but is equally ill advised for similar reasons.

Primary Nonresponse to a First Anti-TNF

Despite the shift in treatment paradigms ushered in by the arrival of infliximab as a treatment option for CD and the recent approvals of adalimumab and cetolizumab pegol, it is important to remember that one-third of patients will not respond to anti-TNF therapy.[1–3] Patients exposed to anti-TNF therapy who have failed to respond are referred to as primary nonresponders. In clinical trials, this is defined as failure to achieve a 70- or 100-point drop in Crohn's Disease Activity Index score; in clinical practice, this may be established by the physician's global assessment. It is important to have an approach to these patients.

There are several points to make about primary nonresponse. First, it is important to exclude alternative causes of symptoms, including strictures, fistulas, abscesses, bile salt diarrhea, steatorrhea, small bowel bacterial overgrowth, irritable bowel syndrome, and concomitant infection with *Clostridium difficile* or cytomegalovirus. Second, it is important to insure that the patient has had the appropriate induction dosing and has had an adequate length of time to respond to drug. In regard to this, initial dosing of anti-TNF agents, the author would give full induction dosing with infliximab 5 mg/kg at weeks 0, 2, and 6 before determining whether the patient has responded. Some have advocated increasing the dose to 10 mg/kg for the week 6 dose before deeming a patient a primary nonresponder. In the case of adalimumab, beginning with 160 mg at week 0 and then 80 mg at week 2 gives the most robust initial response and is the FDA-approved induction dosing. The European Medicines Agency–approved labeling is for 80 mg followed by 40 mg, but this may not be adequate for a proportion of patients. Although these two regimes represent "induction" dosing, further data suggests that patients will continue to respond out to week 12 and therefore it is suggested to wait at least 12 weeks before deeming that a patient is a nonresponder to adalimumab.[4] In the case of certolizumab pegol, 400 mg given at week 0 and week 2 as induction followed by 400 mg every 4 weeks over 12 weeks are the timelines suggested for certolizumab pegol before patients are considered to be primary nonresponders.

If true primary nonresponse is documented, the decision is whether there is a role to switch to an alternate anti-TNF. It is generally accepted that primary nonresponse could result from a different underlying pathobiology in which TNF is not a dominant component of the inflammatory cascade. If this indeed is true then these patients should be best treated with switching to a biologic with an alternate mechanism of action such as natalizumab. Natalizumab is effective for induction and maintenance of remission in moderate to severe CD and has demonstrated efficacy in anti-TNF primary nonresponders.[5] Unfortunately, natalizumab has been associated with an increased risk of progressive multifocal leukoencephalopathy (PML).[6] For this reason, its use is restricted to patients who have failed anti-TNF biologics, and it must be administered as monotherapy. Despite the rationale for switching out of the anti-TNF class in primary nonresponders, many gastroenterologists attempt therapy with a second or even a third anti-TNF agent primarily because of physicians' and patients' concerns regarding the risk of PML with natalizumab. The data supporting this practice are very limited.[7,8] However, this strategy is used often with surprising results.

This may underscore our incomplete understanding of exactly how each of these agents actually works.

Secondary Nonresponse to Anti-TNF

Among patients who do respond initially to anti-TNF therapy, 40% to 50% will lose response over the subsequent 12 months.[9–11] After 12 months it is estimated that 10% to 15% of patients will experience secondary loss of response on a yearly basis. Treatment options in this patient population include escalating the dose (increasing dose or shortening interval), switching within the anti-TNF class, and switching out of class.

As with primary nonresponders, patients with secondary loss of response should be evaluated for alternative causes of symptoms. In addition, drug-related factors can occur, including the formation of neutralizing antidrug antibodies and/or altered clearance of the drug (leading to decreased or absent serum concentrations of the drug).[12] Furthermore, some patients will have therapeutic concentrations of the drug and loose response, which suggest biologic escape mechanisms. A logical approach to these patients is critical.

In patients who are secondary nonresponders, it is important to assess for antidrug antibodies and drug concentrations when available. At this time the only commercially available assays for antibodies and drug concentrations are with infliximab. It is hoped that commercially available assays for the other two agents will become available in order to facilitate decision making. The availability of drug concentrations and antibodies gives an initial insight into whether drug-related factors are at work. It is also important to reevaluate these patients to insure that there is objective evidence of inflammation that is causing the recurrent symptoms. This means ruling out infection with stool studies and looking for biochemical markers or stool markers of inflammation such as an elevated C-reactive protein, elevated erythrocyte sedimentation rate, increased platelet count, or abnormal fecal calprotectin. In addition, a structural reassessment of the disease state with ileocolonoscopy, wireless capsule endoscopy, or cross-sectional imaging (computed tomography enterography or magnetic resonance enterography) should be undertaken. In a recent study from the Mayo Clinic, approximately 50% of patients with absent antibodies and detectable infliximab levels had no evidence of active inflammation demonstrating that symptoms were arising from other etiologies.[13]

Patients who have previously responded to an anti-TNF agent and then lost response can be treated with dose escalation or switching within the anti-TNF class. For infliximab, where commercial assays for measuring both serum concentration and antibodies to infliximab (ATIs) are available, dose escalation from 5 mg/kg to 10 mg/kg or shortening of the dosing interval from every 8 weeks to every 4 to 6 weeks may be preferred for patients who are negative for ATIs and who have low or undetectable infliximab serum concentrations. The decision on which strategy to use largely depends on the clinical scenario. Patients who have recurrent symptoms shortly after an infusion benefit most from dose escalation whereas patients who are well controlled for the majority of the dosing cycle and then have increased symptoms prior to the next infusion benefit most from shortening the interval. A small proportion of infliximab patients will benefit from a combination of both strategies. Dose escalation with infliximab has been shown to be of benefit in up to 80% of patients who lose response to this agent.[14] For adalimumab, dose escalation from 40 mg every other week to 40 mg weekly has been shown to be of benefit in up to 50% of patients who lose response.[15] For certolizumab pegol, patients who lose response can be treated with a single extra 400 mg dose of certolizumab pegol at 2 weeks, changing the dosing regimen from 400 mg every 4 weeks to 200 mg every 2 weeks, or escalating the certolizumab pegol dose from 400 mg every 4 weeks to 400 mg every 2 weeks.[16] The latter treatment strategy is more widely employed. Overall, it is important to individualize the strategy based on the patient symptoms.

Patients who are positive for ATIs should be switched within the anti-TNF class to another agent.[17,18] The literature supporting this strategy is switching from infliximab to either adalimumab or certolizumab pegol. Only one controlled trial, Guaging Adalimumab Efficacy in Infliximab Nonresponders (GAIN), has been performed in patients with secondary loss of response.[17] The GAIN trial demonstrated that adalimumab was more effective than placebo in patients who initially responded to infliximab and then lost response or became intolerant to the drug. More recently, the results of a similar open-label trial with certolizumab pegol, WELCOME, demonstrated similar results in patients losing response or intolerant to infliximab.[18] Although the available data is with switching from infliximab to adalimumab or certolizumab, it is likely that similar results would be obtained with switching from adalimumab or certolizumab pegol to another one of the drugs within the class.

Intolerance to Anti-TNF

The development of intolerance to an anti-TNF is another reason why a decision may need to be made to switch to another anti-TNF. It is important to assess the degree and severity of the intolerance before switching. It may be better to employ strategies to overcome or limit the adverse event rather than switch too early. In many instances, infusion or injection reactions may be mild or transient. In a study by Cheifetz et al.,[19] approximately 50% of infusion reactions were characterized as mild and were transient. Minor infusion reactions (transient rash, flushing, minor chest pain, or dyspnea) may be abrogated with slowing down the infusion or premedication with corticosteroids, antihistamine, or acetaminophen. It is important once again to determine if the patient has developed antibodies associated with the reaction as antibody-associated reactions tend to worsen over time and lead to loss of response. More severe reactions such as alteration in vital signs, severe chest pain, dyspnea, or anaphylactoid reactions are all valid reasons to abandon therapy and switch within class. Therefore, patients who have previously responded to an anti-TNF agent and then develop intolerance (treatment-limiting acute or delayed infusion reactions or injection site reactions) should switch within the anti-TNF class to another agent.[17,18]

Skin Reactions

Over a decade of anti-TNF use has demonstrated that many patients will develop anti-TNF–associated skin disease. This may range from folliculitis, psoriaform lesions (pseudopsoriasis),

palmar-plantar pustulosis, or new onset psoriasis. These eruptions have been described with all anti-TNF agents. The use of topical agents and the aid of a dermatology opinion is very valuable and often patients will not need to switch to another anti-TNF.[20]

Rheumatological Complications

Rheumatological complaints on anti-TNF therapy are not uncommon. They range from nonspecific arthralgias, arthritis, psoriatic arthritis, lupus-like syndrome, and documented drug-induced lupus and have been described with all three drugs within the class. Many patients on anti-TNF, particularly infliximab and adalimumab, will develop antinuclear antibodies and anti—double stranded DNA antibodies (anti-dsDNA).[21] In itself, this is not a reason to switch anti-TNF agents as the clinical relevance of these antibodies remains unknown. It is imperative to get the opinion of a rheumatologist. In seronegative arthralgias and arthritis, symptomatic treatment should be tried before a switch is made. In cases where drug-induced lupus has been made, the original anti-TNF should be discontinued and a switch made. Given the fact that certolizumab pegol is not associated with apoptosis and this may be one of the mechanisms by which patients develop drug-induced lupus a switch to certolizumab is the most logical choice, but successful switches to adalimumab have been described. The return of drug-induced lupus with a second agent should lead to discontinuation of the class.

Postoperative Switching

With over a decade of use of anti-TNF in CD, many patients will be exposed to anti-TNF and still require surgery. Many times this will lead to dose interruption of variable lengths of time ranging from weeks to years. There are several clinical considerations that need to be taken into account. Important questions to ask before deciding to go to an alternate anti-TNF include when the anti-TNF was originally introduced (i.e., was it introduced when the patient already had a stricture that led to surgery), whether the patient had an initial response and then lost response, whether the patient developed a complication that led to surgery, and when the last dose of the last anti-TNF was taken. Any dose interruption may be associated with the development of antibodies. If the clinical scenario suggests that the patient was responding to the original anti-TNF and went to surgery for a CD-related complication, the preference would be to go back to the original agent. The measurement of drug antibodies once again may be useful. If it appears that the patient lost response requiring surgery or antibodies can be documented then switching is preferred.

UC and Switching Anti-TNF

Presently, the only anti-TNF agent approved for the treatment of moderate to severe UC is infliximab. A small experience in switching from infliximab to adalimumab in patients with UC has been described with results similar to the CD experience.[22] Most of what was discussed here for CD will likely apply to UC.

Editor's note (TMB): We await data on whether higher doses will be needed in some UC patients.

● CONCLUSIONS

Despite the impact that anti-TNF therapy has had on the management of IBD, physicians are faced with decisions regarding the optimal introduction and use of this class of medication. Optimization of anti-TNF includes recognizing the clinical scenarios where switching is appropriate versus dose adjustment. Central to this is the proper evaluation and reevaluation of patients on anti-TNF therapy to rule out alternative causes of symptoms and to insure symptoms are arising from inflammation. Premature switching does not benefit the physician or the patient.

Editor's note added in proof (TMB): Ustekinemab: In a May 2011 DDW abstract (#592, A145) W.J. Sandborn et al. described a Phase IIB study of ustekinemab, a mAb to IL12/23 p40 in patients with CD who had failed one to three anti-TNF agents; one-third were primary anti-TNF failures. The response rate to the highest dose, 6 mg/kg IV, was 39.7% versus 23.5% in the placebo at 8 weeks. At 22 weeks, 69.4% of the responders at 8 weeks were still responding versus 42.5% of placebo. This suggests the possibility of a new therapeutic pathway for patients unresponsive to anti-TNF therapies.

References

1. Targan SR, Hanauer SB, van Deventer SJ, et al. A short-term study of chimeric monoclonal antibody cA2 to tumor necrosis factor alpha for Crohn's disease. Crohn's Disease cA2 Study Group. *N Engl J Med.* 1997;337(15):1029–1035.

2. Hanauer SB, Sandborn WJ, Rutgeerts P, et al. Human anti-tumor necrosis factor monoclonal antibody (adalimumab) in Crohn's disease: the CLASSIC-I trial. *Gastroenterology.* 2006;130(2):323–33; quiz 591.

3. Schreiber S, Khaliq-Kareemi M, Lawrance IC, et al.; PRECISE 2 Study Investigators. Maintenance therapy with certolizumab pegol for Crohn's disease. *N Engl J Med.* 2007;357(3):239–250.

4. Panaccione R, Sandborn WJ, Colombel J-F, et al. Response with continued adalimumab therapy for up to 12 weeks in patients with Crohn's disease who were non-responders at week 4. *Can J Gastroenterol.* 2009;23(suppl SA).

5. Targan SR, Feagan BG, Fedorak RN, et al.; International Efficacy of Natalizumab in Crohn's Disease Response and Remission (ENCORE) Trial Group. Natalizumab for the treatment of active Crohn's disease: results of the ENCORE Trial. *Gastroenterology.* 2007;132(5):1672–1683.

6. Van Assche G, Van Ranst M, Sciot R, et al. Progressive multifocal leukoencephalopathy after natalizumab therapy for Crohn's disease. *N Engl J Med.* 2005;353(4):362–368.

7. Lofberg R, Louis E, Reinisch W, et al. Adalimumab effectiveness in TNF-antagonists-naive patients and in infliximab nonresponders with Crohn's disease: results from the care study [abstract 1069]. *Am J Gastroenterol.* 2008;103(S1):S418.

8. Allez M, Vermeire S, Mozziconacci N, et al. The efficacy and safety of a third anti-TNF monoclonal antibody in Crohn's disease after failure of two other anti-TNF antibodies. *Aliment Pharmacol Ther.* 2010;31(1):92–101.

9. Hanauer SB, Feagan BG, Lichtenstein GR, et al.; ACCENT I Study Group. Maintenance infliximab for Crohn's disease: the ACCENT I randomised trial. *Lancet.* 2002;359(9317):1541–1549.

10. Colombel JF, Sandborn WJ, Rutgeerts P, et al. Adalimumab for maintenance of clinical response and remission in patients with Crohn's disease: the CHARM trial. *Gastroenterology.* 2007;132(1):52–65.

11. Sandborn WJ, Feagan BG, Stoinov S, et al.; PRECISE 1 Study Investigators. Certolizumab pegol for the treatment of Crohn's disease. *N Engl J Med.* 2007;357(3):228–238.

12. Hanauer SB, Wagner CL, Bala M, et al. Incidence and importance of antibody responses to infliximab after maintenance or episodic treatment in Crohn's disease. *Clin Gastroenterol Hepatol.* 2004;2(7):542–553.

13. Afif W, Loftus EV Jr, Faubion WA, et al. Clinical utility of measuring infliximab and human anti-chimeric antibody concentrations in patients with inflammatory bowel disease. *Am J Gastroenterol.* 2010;105(5):1133–1139.

14. Rutgeerts P, Feagan BG, Lichtenstein GR, et al. Comparison of scheduled and episodic treatment strategies of infliximab in Crohn's disease. *Gastroenterology.* 2004;126(2):402–413.

15. Sandborn WJ, Colombel JF, Rutgeerts P, et al. Benefits of dosage adjustment with adalimumab in Crohn's disease: an analysis of the CHARM trial. *Gastroenterology.* 2008;134:A-347.

16. Lichtenstein GR, Mitchev K, D'Haens G. Re-induction with certolizumab pegol following disease exacerbation during maintenance therapy is effective to regain response and remission. *Gastroenterology.* 2008;133:A-488.

17. Sandborn WJ, Rutgeerts P, Enns R, et al. Adalimumab induction therapy for Crohn disease previously treated with infliximab: a randomized trial. *Ann Intern Med.* 2007;146(12):829–838.

18. Vermeire S, Abreu MT, D'Haens G, et al. Efficacy and safety of certolizumab pegol in patients with active Crohn's disease who previously lost response or were intolerant to infliximab: Open-label induction preliminary results of the WELCOME study. *Gastroenterology.* 2008;134:A-67.

19. Cheifetz A, Smedley M, Martin S, et al. The incidence and management of infusion reactions to infliximab: a large center experience. *Am J Gastroenterol.* 2003;98(6):1315–1324.

20. Kerbleski JF, Gottlieb AB. Dermatological complications and safety of anti-TNF treatments. *Gut.* 2009;58(8):1033–1039.

21. Vermeire S, Noman M, Van Assche G, et al. Autoimmunity associated with anti-tumor necrosis factor alpha treatment in Crohn's disease: a prospective cohort study. *Gastroenterology.* 2003;125(1):32–39.

22. Afif W, Leighton JA, Hanauer SB, et al. Open-label study of adalimumab in patients with ulcerative colitis including those with prior loss of response or intolerance to infliximab. *Inflamm Bowel Dis.* 2009;15(9):1302–1307.

Optimizing Anti-TNF Therapy | 109

Jason W. Harper and Scott D. Lee

Since the introduction of the antitumor necrosis factor (anti-TNF) monoclonal antibody, infliximab, for clinical use in moderate-to-severe Crohn's disease (CD) in 1998, the management of CD and ulcerative colitis (UC) has undergone dramatic changes. The clinical use of anticytokine antibodies (included under the more general heading of biologic agents) has rapidly expanded. Currently there are four biologic agents for the treatment of inflammatory bowel disease (IBD). This includes three anti-TNF agents: infliximab, adalimumab, and certolizumab. Natalizumab is the other available biologic agent, and unlike the anti-TNF molecules, natalizumab's molecular target is the alpha-4 integrin (involved in inflammatory cell-to-cell adhesion), and its use is not the subject of this chapter. Other chapters have addressed the issue of the appropriate use of biologics and their safety. We will specifically address the issue of optimizing the response rates and long-term maintenance of response with anti-TNF therapy in IBD patients. This includes identifying optimal patients in whom to initiate biologics, adjusting the dose for patients who appear to be losing response, and minimizing antibody formation.

INDUCTION THERAPY

Choice of Agent

Of the three available anti-TNF monoclonal antibodies—infliximab, adalimumab, and certolizumab—the choice of initial agent will vary depending on a number of parameters. With regard to differences in clinical efficacy in inducing remission in patients, there is no evidence to suggest that any of the anti-TNF agents are superior to the others. To date, there has been no trial comparing head-to-head response rates in treatment-naïve patients between the three agents, but data from clinical trials involving each agent versus placebo have indicated similar rates of response. Therefore, the choice of agent is guided more by dosing convenience, cost to the patient, and individual clinical experience.

Patient Selection

There are no specific demographics that have been identified to predict response to anti-TNF therapy. In general, age, sex,

duration of disease, severity of disease, surgical history, location of disease, family history, serological markers, and smoking history have not predicted response rates for anti-TNF therapy. In addition, previous use of biologic therapy and concomitant medications do not have an effect on the likelihood of response for induction therapy.

Currently, as we do not have predictors of response to anti-TNF therapy in IBD or any parameters that we can modify to increase response rates, it is prudent to ensure that patients do not have a complication, such as a fibrostenotic stricture or an abscess, which will not respond to any currently available medical therapy prior to the initiation of anti-TNF therapy.

MAINTENANCE THERAPY

Current evidence suggests that anti-TNF therapy is the most efficacious maintenance therapy available. At its inception, anti-TNF therapy was used on an as-needed basis to treat the symptoms of refractory CD; however, when used episodically, symptoms would recur quickly. With all of the available anti-TNF therapies, the pivotal maintenance trials[1–3] have shown unequivocal superiority of scheduled maintenance therapy versus episodic therapy with regard to long-term outcomes. These outcomes have included maintenance of response, remission, discontinuation of steroids, decreased hospitalization, and need for surgical intervention. Unfortunately, even with scheduled maintenance, a significant number of patients who initially respond to anti-TNF therapy will lose response or become intolerant to that therapy. Unlike induction therapy, there are several characteristics associated with loss of response. Given the need for long-term maintenance of response, it is important to understand how to best optimize long-term response rates.

Choice of Agent

As with induction therapy, there are no head-to-head trials between any of the available anti-TNF agents comparing maintenance of response and remission rates; however, there is no evidence to date that shows any of the available agents to be superior to the others at maintaining response or remission in patients who have initially responded to induction therapy. In addition, the route of administration (subcutaneous vs. intravenous) does not appear to affect the likelihood of maintenance of response. As with induction therapy, the choice of agent should be guided more by dosing convenience, cost to the patient, and individual clinical experience.

Patient Selection

Most patient demographics, including age, sex, severity of disease, location of disease, and serological markers, do not predict long-term response. However, there are several patient characteristics that correlate with long-term response including: duration of disease, previous anti-TNF exposure, antibody formation, episodic therapy, and concomitant medications.

Duration of Disease

Several studies have shown that patients with a shorter duration of disease will have a higher likelihood of maintaining response. It is theorized that treating patients early on in their disease course prevents the development of irreversible damage, such as strictures and abscesses, which then allows longer maintenance of response. Alternatively, those patients with longer duration of disease may already have bowel damage that may not be amenable to medical therapy and that, over time, will inevitably continue to cause recurrent symptoms and complications. In general, it appears that patients diagnosed 2 or fewer years prior to treatment have the highest likelihood of maintaining remission.

Previous Anti-TNF Exposure

In both pivotal studies evaluating adalimumab and certolizumab for the treatment of CD[1,3] a portion of the patients enrolled had previously lost response or become intolerant to infliximab. Although there was no difference in initial response, this group that had previously experienced anti-TNF therapy also had a significantly lower likelihood of maintaining response than biologic-naïve patients. The cause of this lesser response is not understood; however, it does not appear to be dependent on the patient's antibody status to the previous anti-TNF agents. Unfortunately, within this group of biologic experienced patients, there are no clinical predictors for loss of response that clinicians can utilize to identify the group of patients who will have an optimal response to the second anti-TNF agent. Therefore, though this group as a whole is less likely to maintain response, we do not hesitate to give a second anti-TNF agent as a therapeutic trial, as this is the only strategy currently available to determine whether the patient will respond to the second anti-TNF therapy.

Antibody Formation

In clinical trials, up to 40% to 50% of patients eventually become refractory to the biologic agents. Formation of antibodies to the specific anti-TNF therapy are thought to play a pivotal role in this loss of response.[4,5]

All of the anti-TNF therapies have been associated with formation of antibodies regardless of the route of delivery or degree of humanization. In addition, the rate of antibody formation

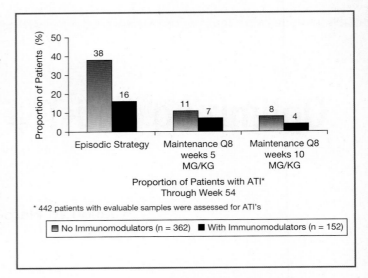

FIGURE 109.1 • Results from ACCENT 1: Effect of infliximab dose and concomitant use of immunomodulators on ATI formation. From Hanauer et al.[2,5]

is similar among all of the agents. Interestingly, there are several factors that appear to affect the rate of antibody formation (Fig. 109.1), and further discussion on minimizing the risk of antibody development is outlined as follows.

Only serum tests to assess antibodies to infliximab (ATI) and serum infliximab levels are available commercially. Unfortunately, there are no available serum tests to evaluate antibodies or serum levels to adalimumab or certolizumab. When a patient is having an increase in symptoms while being treated with infliximab, if the patient's insurance carrier will pay for the testing, we will often check for ATIs and infliximab levels. If a patient has ATIs and low serum levels, we will often consider changing to another anti-TNF agent. If the patient is ATI negative and has low serum levels, we will alter his or her maintenance dose (see dose modification section). If patients are ATI negative and have therapeutic infliximab levels, we will consider switching the class of medications rather than starting another anti-TNF agent.

Episodic Therapy

Interruption of scheduled maintenance anti-TNF therapy or episodic therapy has consistently been associated with higher rates of antibody formation. The rates have been noted to be as high as 60% when patients are treated with episodic therapy.[4] This is much higher compared to consistently lower rates, in the range of 8% to 12%, observed in patients treated with scheduled maintenance therapy.[2,3] The formation of these antibodies is associated with loss of response and adverse reactions to anti-TNF therapy. Prior to starting a patient on anti-TNF therapy we typically discuss the importance of maintenance therapy with the patient. If a patient plans not to use a biologic on a consistent maintenance basis, we often will consider other therapy or consider using another immunosuppressant along with the anti-TNF agent (see concomitant medication considerations), in order to give the patient the highest likelihood of continued response. In general, we recommend avoiding episodic therapy.

Concomitant Medication Considerations

Although the pivotal maintenance trials have demonstrated no clinical benefit from concomitant administration of immunosuppressants such as azathioprine and methotrexate, they have established a consistent reduction in antibody formation rate.[2,3] In addition, the combination of anti-TNF therapy and azathioprine has been associated with higher serum concentrations of anti-TNF therapy when compared to patients not on combination therapy.[6] In studies of rheumatoid arthritis, the concomitant use of oral methotrexate at doses as low as 7.5 mg per week with biologic therapy was found to be beneficial in overall patient response and lowering the risk of antibody formation. In addition, this dual-treatment regimen has not been associated with a significant increase in infections or tumors.

Although it has been shown that oral methotrexate can increase a patient's response and decrease the likelihood of antibody formation, the combination of infliximab and methotrexate at 25 mg subcutaneously per week has not similarly been shown to increase the maintenance of remission over a 1-year period compared to infliximab monotherapy.[7] Although there was no benefit observed with the addition of subcutaneous methotrexate in the COMMIT study, there was importantly no significant increase in infections or malignancy.

Finally, the SONIC trial[8] demonstrated that combination therapy (with an anti-TNF and azathioprine) in a group of patients who were azathioprine and anti-TNF naïve was superior to either therapy alone at maintaining remission for up to 1 year (Fig. 109.2).

From a safety standpoint, concomitant immunosuppression does not appear to significantly increase the risk of adverse events in IBD patients.[8,9] Although the results of the SONIC trial are in contrast to previous evidence that combination therapy offered no therapeutic benefit, one has to keep in mind that this is the only trial to date that specifically looked at an adult group of patients who were all naïve to azathioprine and anti-TNF therapy. There has been another trial known as the REACH study, which examined infliximab in pediatric CD patients who received at least 8 weeks of immunomodulator therapy before receiving infliximab. In this study, 80% of patients achieved response; however, SONIC remains the only trial that specifically enrolled adult CD patients who were naïve to both azathioprine and anti-TNF treatment.

The majority of patients in previous pivotal trials had been tried on azathioprine and had failed to achieve remission. Our clinical assessment regarding the use of combination therapy incorporates whether the patient has previously been on azathioprine. If the patient is naïve to azathioprine we usually recommend combination therapy on the basis of evidence that this group has a significantly higher likelihood of achieving remission without any increase in risk.

Given these facts, we typically will consider concomitant immunosuppression in patients who we feel are at high risk for complications from their IBD or at high risk for loss of response to anti-TNF therapy. This group includes patients with

1. perianal disease
2. a history of multiple surgeries
3. previous biologic loss of response or intolerance
4. a history of noncompliance and hence at risk for episodic therapy
5. incomplete response to anti-TNF therapy as evidenced by ongoing disease on endoscopy, laboratory testing (elevated C-reactive protein, persistent anemia, hypoalbuminemia, or ongoing thrombocytosis), or radiographic evidence of active disease.

Within this group of patients, certain other considerations factor into our decision of using concomitant immunosuppression. This includes avoiding methotrexate in women who are of child-bearing potential, given that methotrexate is a category X (contraindicated and clearly causative of poor fetal outcomes) medication with regard to pregnancy. In addition, if possible we avoid combination therapy with azathioprine in young men (age less than 30) because of the occurrence of hepatospleno T-cell lymphomas in association with this combination in young male IBD patients.[10]

For the majority of patients who we have started on combination therapy, we continually assess the need for concomitant immunosuppression. If there are any infectious adverse events that we feel are related to this combination we usually choose to discontinue the immunosuppressant agent rather than the biologic. The discontinuation of the biologic can, as noted previously, result in higher rates of antibody formation. Conversely, there is little risk in discontinuing the immunosuppressant.

If patients are in complete remission after 12 months on dual therapy, we will consider discontinuing the concomitant immunosuppressant but will carefully monitor for any signs of subclinical (laboratory abnormalities without symptoms) or clinical evidence of recurrence of disease activity. For those patients who have few remaining medical therapeutic maintenance options should they lose response to the current anti-TNF therapy (they have lost response or become intolerant to other available medications), we will usually continue concomitant

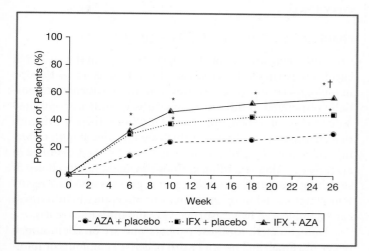

FIGURE 109.2 • Results from SONIC: Biologic therapy with dual immunosuppression is superior at maintaining corticosteroid-free remission up to 26 weeks. From Colombel et al.[8]

immunosuppression indefinitely unless the patient has an adverse event related to this therapy.

There has been recent interest in discontinuing the anti-TNF therapy in those patients who have achieved remission with combination therapy. Although the use of concomitant immunosuppression lowers the risk of antibody formation, we typically do not advocate this approach, as currently there is no substantial evidence with regards to the outcomes of such a strategy. In addition, though concomitant immunosuppression lowers the risk of antibody formation, there still is risk associated with intermittently using biologics in this group of patients. A previous chapter discusses sequential and combination therapy in Crohn's disease as well as the appropriate prophylactic therapy for PCP if patients are on triple immunosuppression with corticosteroids.

Dose Modification

As noted previously, a significant number of patients will have loss of response to anti-TNF therapy over time despite maintenance dosing. If disease complications (stenoses, perforating disease, and malignancy) and development of infection have been eliminated as the cause of loss of response, the most common practice to recapture response is modification of the maintenance dose. This can be achieved with dose escalation (increase of the dose at the same dosing interval) of the anti-TNF agent or by shortening the interval (giving the patient a standard maintenance dose earlier than the standard interval). The majority of patients with either strategy will have recapture of response.[1,2]

With patients losing response to infliximab we typically increase their maintenance dose from 5 mg/kg to 10 mg/kg rather than shortening their dosing interval.[2] We opt for dose escalation with infliximab because dose escalation does not require the patient to come in more frequently for therapy. This strategy is, therefore, potentially less inconvenient (fewer infusions and trips to the infusion suite or hospital) and potentially lower cost, as some of the cost with infliximab is due to the actual infusion cost. Although there are no formal studies addressing how to manage these patients if they respond to dose modification, after a 6- to 12-month interval we attempt to reduce the dose back to the 5-mg/kg maintenance dose. If the patient loses response again, we will reinstitute the 10-mg/kg dose and maintain this indefinitely until loss of response or the patient has adverse reaction that requires cessation of the medication. Other physicians will shorten the interval for those patients who have lost response. Our experience with interval shortening suggests that this strategy works, but for the reasons previously mentioned, we prefer dose escalation for those patients who have lost response.

For patients losing response to adalimumab, we will change the maintenance dose from 40 mg every 2 weeks to 40 mg every week.[1] As with infliximab, after 6 months we will try to change the dose back to 40 mg every other week. If patients have a recurrence of symptoms, we will continue 40 mg every week as a maintenance dose indefinitely. We have had anecdotal success with increasing the dose beyond 40 mg every week; however, cost considerations often require that we switch agents. Another strategy for managing adalimumab loss of response is to change

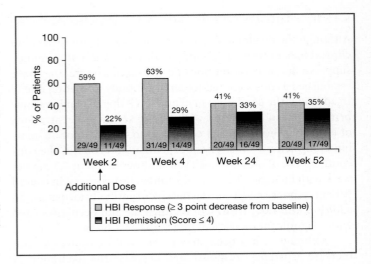

FIGURE 109.3 • Results from PRECiSE: Additional dosing with certolizumab pegol is effective at recapturing and maintaining response. From Sandborn et al.[11]

the dose to 80 mg every other week. This is also a reasonable strategy, but the majority of published safety and efficacy analyses are with the aforementioned 40-mg-every-week approach.

For those patients losing response to certolizumab, we will give an extra dose of 400 mg 2 weeks after their last dose (Fig. 109.3).[11]

If patients regain response, we will continue on the standard maintenance dose of 400 mg every 4 weeks. If the patient continues to experience shortened duration of response, despite the additional dose, we will change his or her dose from 400 mg every 4 weeks to 200 mg every 2 weeks. Although the total net dose is equivalent in both strategies, splitting the dose to 200 mg every 2 weeks appears to increase the trough levels of certolizumab, and, anecdotally, we have had success with splitting the dose in this manner. If the patient fails these modifications, we will give the patient 400 mg every 2 weeks. As with the other biologics if the patient has improved, after 6 to 12 months we will try to return to the standard maintenance dose of 400 mg every 4 weeks.

Switching Anti-TNF Therapy

Currently there are no data to suggest that any of the anti-TNF agents are particularly better than the others as initial therapy in biologic-naïve patients. However, in those patients who initially responded to infliximab and subsequently discontinued it due to loss of response or adverse reactions, there is evidence that adalimumab and certolizumab are effective at both inducing and maintaining remission (Fig. 109.4).[12,13] As mentioned in an earlier section regarding antibody formation, our choice of switching to another anti-TNF agent in patients who have recurrent symptoms while on infliximab or intolerance to infliximab can be influenced by measuring ATIs and infliximab levels.

Unfortunately, for those patients who are on adalimumab or certolizumab and have a return of active symptoms or intolerance to either medication, we currently have to empirically make choices regarding using another anti-TNF agent. For most patients losing response or developing intolerable side effects to

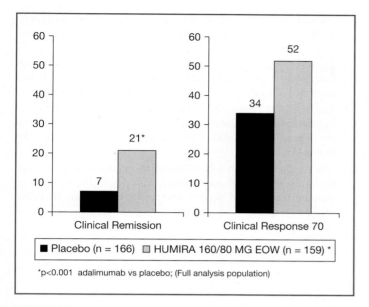

FIGURE 109.4 • Results from GAIN: Adalimumab is effective at inducing and maintaining response in an infliximab-refractory patient population. From Sandborn et al.[12]

adalimumab or certolizumab, we most often will try another anti-TNF agent, and anecdotally we have been successful when using another anti-TNF agent with this group.

For those patients who develop adverse events such as neurologic symptoms, a lupus-like syndrome, or psoriasiform rash while on anti-TNF therapy, we will often consult the appropriate subspecialist to have the patient evaluated regarding the presence of another autoimmune condition (multiple sclerosis, lupus, or psoriasis). If it is felt that the condition is a result of the anti-TNF agent, we will usually discontinue the current therapy, and if the symptom resolves, very cautiously consider another anti-TNF therapy with careful monitoring. In the situation that the adverse event recurs, we advocate switching the class of medications to treat the patient's IBD, though we have had some clinical success when switching within the anti-TNF class for some of these adverse events.

In general, we discourage switching between other anti-TNF therapies for convenience reasons. This practice has not been extensively evaluated, and it is known that a significant number of patients who respond to one anti-TNF therapy will not respond to another anti-TNF agent. A recent study, not yet published, revealed that more than 50% of patients doing well on infliximab, but switched to adalimumab later, had a flare of disease.[14] For this reason and because episodic dosing is associated with antibody formation, we prefer not to discontinue an anti-TNF agent if the patient has a good response and no adverse events.

When we do switch a patient from one anti-TNF agent for loss of response, in general we do not have a long washout period if the patient has active disease. Our rationale is that most of these patients likely have low levels of the previous anti-TNF agent, or if the agent is present and the patient has symptoms, the patient's immune system no longer is affected by the presence or absence of TNF.

Future Approaches to Optimizing Anti-TNF Therapy

Future studies will hopefully help clarify unanswered questions regarding how physicians should use anti-TNF therapy. Hopefully we will be able to define or develop patient characteristics that will predict which patients will be most likely to respond to induction therapy. In addition, the optimal dosing strategy regarding those patients who have a flare of symptoms while on standard maintenance therapies is still unknown. Finally, though we have definitive evidence that early intervention with anti-TNF therapies is the most efficacious medical strategy to keep patients in long-term remission, we need further studies to show that this strategy clearly changes the natural history of the disease. This will include decreasing hospitalizations, the use of prednisone, and surgery, while not resulting in a significant increase in number of infections or tumors.

Recommendations

Once the decision to use an anti-TNF therapy has been made in the biologic naïve patient, the initial choice of medication is based on patient and physician discussion regarding out-of-pocket cost and the route of delivery. We usually counsel our patients that we advocate long-term maintenance therapy if there is an initial response. For those patients with more severe disease, or those we feel are at risk for antibody development, we will often start azathioprine or methotrexate along with the anti-TNF agent chosen. For patients who are losing response or develop adverse reactions to an anti-TNF agent, we will often switch to another agent and use the standard induction regimen. For adverse events that are thought to be due to the type of therapy (class effect), rather than the specific therapy, we will consider switching class of medication or very cautiously try another anti-TNF agent. Lastly, when a patient on combination therapy does not initially respond completely, we find it often useful to optimize the immunomodulator, azathioprine, or methotrexate, before escalating the anti-TNF dosage.

References

1. Colombel JF, Sandborn WJ, Rutgeerts P, et al. Adalimumab for maintenance of clinical response and remission in patients with Crohn's disease: the CHARM trial. *Gastroenterology.* 2007;132(1):52–65.

2. Hanauer SB, Feagan BG, Lichtenstein GR, et al. Maintenance infliximab for Crohn's disease: the ACCENT I randomised trial. *Lancet.* 2002;359(9317):1541–1549.

3. Schreiber S, Khaliq-Kareemi M, Lawrance IC, et al. Maintenance therapy with certolizumab pegol for Crohn's disease. *N Engl J Med.* 2007;357(3):239–250.

4. Baert F, Noman M, Vermeire S, et al. Influence of immunogenicity on the long-term efficacy of infliximab in Crohn's disease. *N Engl J Med.* 2003;348(7):601–608.

5. Hanauer SB, Wagner CL, Bala M, et al. Incidence and importance of antibody responses to infliximab after maintenance or episodic treatment in Crohn's disease. *Clin Gastroenterol Hepatol.* 2004;2(7):542–553.

6. Lémann M, Mary JY, Duclos B, et al. Infliximab plus azathioprine for steroid-dependent Crohn's disease patients: a randomized placebo-controlled trial. *Gastroenterology.* 2006;130(4):1054–1061.

7. Feagan B, McDonald J, Ponich T, et al. A randomized trial of methotrexate (MTX) in combination with infliximab (IFX) for the treatment of Crohn's disease (CD). *Gastroenterology.* 2008;134:682C.

8. Colombel JF, Sandborn WJ, Reinisch W, et al.; SONIC Study Group. Infliximab, azathioprine, or combination therapy for Crohn's disease. *N Engl J Med.* 2010;362(15):1383–1395.

9. Tourner M, Loftus EV Jr, Harmsen WS, et al. Risk factors for opportunistic infections in patients with inflammatory bowel disease. *Gastroenterology.* 2008;134:929–936.

10. Clark M, Colombel JF, Feagan BC, et al. American gastroenterological association consensus development conference on the use of biologics in the treatment of inflammatory bowel disease, June 21–23, 2006. *Gastroenterology.* 2007;133(1):312–339.

11. Sandborn WJ, Schreiber S, Hanauer SB, Colombel JF, Bloomfield R, Lichtenstein GR; PRECiSE 4 Study Investigators. Reinduction with certolizumab pegol in patients with relapsed Crohn's disease: results from the PRECiSE 4 Study. *Clin Gastroenterol Hepatol.* 2010;8(8):696–702.e1.

12. Sandborn WJ, Rutgeerts P, Enns R, et al. Adalimumab induction therapy for Crohn disease previously treated with infliximab: a randomized trial. *Ann Intern Med.* 2007;146(12):829–838.

13. Sandborn WJ, Abreu MT, D'Haens G, et al. Certolizumab pegol in patients with moderate to severe Crohn's disease and secondary failure to infliximab. *Clin Gastroenterol Hepatol.* 2010;8(8):688–695.e2.

14. Van Assche GA. Switch to adalimumab in patients with Crohn's disease controlled by maintenance infliximab: the Prospective Randomized Switch Study. Abstract Presentation, Digestive Disease Week, New Orleans, May 2010.

Experience with Long-Term Anti-TNF Therapy

110

Marc Schwartz and Miguel Regueiro

Treatment of Crohn's disease (CD) and ulcerative colitis (UC) has evolved over the past decade. The anti-tumor necrosis factor alpha (anti-TNFα) agents have significantly impacted the management of patients with inflammatory bowel disease (IBD) and may impact the natural course of disease. Currently, the three anti-TNF medications used for the treatment of IBD are infliximab, adalimumab, and certolizumab. All three of these medications effectively induce and maintain remission of CD and infliximab of UC. Although the evidence-based data rely on results of randomized trials of 1 year or less, many physicians opt to continue anti-TNF treatment beyond 1 year. There are a paucity of long-term prospective data evaluating the efficacy of anti-TNF therapy for IBD. As such, the experience with anti-TNF agents beyond 1 year is largely anecdotal or based on clinical experience. This chapter will review the experience of anti-TNF therapy at 1 year and beyond, and will focus on several aspects of long-term treatment; (a) 1-year maintenance data from pivotal trials, (b) maintenance (and loss of response) beyond 1 year, (c) dose intensification, and (d) postoperative maintenance of remission. Evidence-based data will be provided where possible, but this review will include open label experience and expert opinion to supplement areas lacking clinical trial experience.

● ONE-YEAR EXPERIENCE

For purposes of this review, long-term experience with anti-TNF therapy will be defined as treatment for at least 1 year. There are several large randomized controlled trials (RCTs) with 1-year efficacy and maintenance endpoints. All three anti-TNF agents have been approved by the Food and Drug Administration for reducing the signs and symptoms of active CD through induction and maintenance regimens. Infliximab was the first anti-TNF agent to show induction and maintenance benefit in active CD. In the infliximab maintenance trial, patients who responded to a single infusion of infliximab 5 mg/kg were then randomized to receive placebo, infliximab 5 mg/kg, or infliximab 10 mg/kg for

1 year.[1] There was a statistically higher clinical remission (defined by a Crohn's Disease Activity Index (CDAI) < 150) rate at 54 weeks in those patients maintained on 5 mg/kg (28%) or 10 mg/kg (38%) of infliximab compared with placebo (15%; $P = 0.021$ and 0.01, respectively). In addition, the median time to loss of response was significantly greater in infliximab treated patients compared with placebo; 38 weeks in patients maintained on infliximab 5 mg/kg and more than 54 weeks in those receiving infliximab 10 mg/kg compared to 19 weeks in placebo ($P = 0.002$ and $P = 0.0002$, respectively). A similar 1-year CD maintenance trial was conducted with adalimumab.[2] Patients who responded to open-label induction with adalimumab 80 mg (week 0) and 40 mg (week 2) were randomized to placebo, adalimumab 40 mg every other week (eow) or 40 mg weekly. The 56-week clinical remission rate was significantly higher in the adalimumab eow and adalimumab weekly group compared with placebo (36%, 41%, and 12%, respectively; $P < 0.001$). Finally, certolizumab has been shown to be effective in the induction and maintenance of clinical response to 26 weeks, but there are no published data on 1-year maintenance of remission.[3]

One-year maintenance of fistula closure has also been assessed. Only infliximab has been evaluated in a prospective clinical trial with fistula closure as a primary endpoint.[4] CD patients with perianal or enterocutaneous fistula who responded to three dose infliximab 5 mg/kg induction were randomized to infliximab 5 mg/kg every 8 weeks or placebo for 1 year. At 54 weeks, there were significantly more patients with complete closure of fistula in the infliximab treated group compared with placebo (38% vs. 22%, $P = 0.02$). As part of the previously referenced adalimumab maintenance trial, fistula closure was identified as a secondary endpoint.[2] In this study, CD patients who had enterocutaneous or perianal fistula were evaluated for fistula closure at 56 weeks. The adalimumab (40 mg eow and weekly combined) maintained patients had a significantly higher rate of continued fistula closure at 56 weeks compared to placebo (30% vs. 13%; $P = 0.043$). Similarly, certolizumab was superior to placebo in closing fistula in CD patients, but this was assessed as a secondary endpoint at 26 weeks only.

Infliximab is the only biologic agent assessed in RCTs for the treatment of UC and pediatric CD. In the UC trials, patients were randomized to a three dose induction of placebo, infliximab 5 mg/kg or infliximab 10 mg/kg followed by every 8-week maintenance for 1 year.[5] At 54 weeks, the rates of remission, defined as a Mayo score ≤2, were significantly higher in the 5 mg/kg and 10 mg/kg infliximab groups compared to placebo (46%, 44%, 20%, respectively; $P < 0.001$ for both infliximab groups vs. placebo). Infliximab has also been assessed for the treatment of pediatric CD. The primary endpoint of the study was 10-week clinical response after a three dose induction of infliximab with secondary endpoints being 1-year clinical response and remission. Responders to three dose induction with infliximab 5 mg/kg were randomized to every 8-week or every 12-week 5 mg/kg infliximab for 1 year (no placebo arm). At 54 weeks, 56% of the patients receiving every 8-week infliximab were in remission, defined as pediatric CDAI ≤ 10, compared with 24% of every 12-week infliximab ($P < 0.01$).[6] In an open label trial of adalimumab in pediatric CD, the results were similar with 65% of patients in remission at 48 weeks.[7]

The maintenance data from the 1-year anti-TNF agents in CD and UC have paralleled the authors' experience. In our practice, we have found that one-third to one-half of our IBD patients are in complete clinical remission and have no signs or symptoms of active CD or UC after 1 year of anti-TNF treatment. Approximately two-thirds to three-quarters of our patients have significant improvement with tolerable IBD-related symptoms on anti-TNF treatment at 1 year. It has also been our experience that the earlier in the course of IBD the anti-TNF agent is administered, the better the 1-year outcome, similar to the pediatric CD trial results. It has been our practice to continue anti-TNF therapy long-term for those patients who have had clinical improvement at 1 year.

● LONG-TERM EXPERIENCE: BEYOND 1 YEAR

Since there are no RCTs of the anti-TNF therapies in IBD with duration longer than 1 year, we must rely on several observational studies from single centers and regional registries for information on the durability of response. As the first anti-TNF therapy with efficacy in IBD to become available, infliximab is the subject of most of the long-term data.

In ACCENT I, CD response was measured 2 weeks (by CDAI) after a single dose of infliximab.[1] Responders were randomized to placebo or infliximab maintenance. Of the responders at 2 weeks, 46% had "lost response" by 6 months and 57% by 1 year. At 6 weeks and—even more so—at 12 weeks, stable responders have usually become apparent. The use of 2-week response as inclusion criteria for a course of maintenance therapy probably led many transient, weak, or placebo responders to be included, whereas some slow, durable responders were excluded. This categorization of response resulted in a significant overestimate of early loss of response. The ACT I study of infliximab for UC with a similar protocol produced similar results with a 51% response rate at 6 months, which only fell to 45% at 12 months.[5] This monumental loss of response during the first 6 months of the study is not consistent with the authors' experience and most other studies. Instead, it is, most likely, a result of unusual methodology.

In a community GI practice, 198 patients received infliximab for CD with an initial clinical response rate of 88%. Of those 174 initial responders, the long-term response rate was 78% at 3 years. While the durability of the response was severely reduced in smokers, the use of concomitant immunomodulator therapy did not prolong the response.[8]

At Boston's Beth Israel Hospital, 100 CD patients on infliximab had 2-year follow-up and 36 patients had 5-year follow-up with clinical remission rates of 65% and 58%, respectively. Concomitant immunomodulator therapy resulted in statistically fewer surgeries and numerically greater clinical remission at 5 years.[9]

By far, the largest cohort with long-term follow-up comes from Belgium where 614 CD patients treated with infliximab were followed, beginning in 1994, for a median of 55 months.[10] The initial response rate was 89%. Of the 547 initial responders (defined by symptom improvement), three similarly sized treatment cohorts arose. One-third were treated with episodic infliximab dosing for the duration of follow-up, which was common during the early use of infliximab, another third received scheduled dosing for the duration of follow-up, and the final third started on episodic dosing, but eventually switched to scheduled dosing. Three hundred and forty seven patients (63%) continued to have clinical benefit at the end of follow-up, whereas 200 patients (37%) discontinued infliximab because of loss of response (22%) or side effects (13%). Long-term outcomes were much better in patients who had an initial response to IFX. Only 42% of the initial responders required hospitalization compared to 67% of primary nonresponders. While 60% of the patients on episodic IFX dosing maintained a clinical benefit for a median of 79 months, 75% of subjects receiving scheduled infusions were still on medication at the end of follow-up. The rate of loss of response was similar between the episodic and scheduled treatment groups, but the rate of side effects, most notably hypersensitivity reactions, leading to discontinuation was dramatically higher in the episodic treatment (17% vs. 6%, $P = 0.0001$). Rates of hospitalization (26% vs. 47%, $P < 0.001$) and major abdominal surgery (20% vs. 30%, $P = 0.02$, at 72 weeks) were significantly lower in patients who were treated with scheduled dosing, either from initiation of therapy or after previous episodic therapy. Major abdominal surgery was frequent in both infliximab primary nonresponders (18%) and patients with loss of response (16%). In contrast, only 3% of patients with sustained clinical benefit required surgery.

One hundred and seventeen patients with perianal fistulae were among the 854 subjects in the CHARM study of maintenance adalimumab. Thirty-eight (32%) patients without fistula drainage after 12 months of randomization received open-label adalimumab for an additional year. Maintenance of fistula healing was at least 74%, because 7 of the 10 patients who dropped out of the study, did so for reasons other than loss of response.[11]

In a single center experience of 99 infliximab treated patients with perianal CD, the complete response rate was significantly higher at the end of follow-up than after three induction doses of 5 mg/kg infliximab.[12] Healing of ulceration improved from 42% to 72% ($n = 94$), anal stricture healing jumped from 18% to 55% ($n = 22$), and fistula resolution went from 32% to 55% ($n = 31$) at a median follow-up of 175 weeks. This study highlights the fact that the response of perianal and fistulizing disease to anti-TNF therapy can be slower than luminal disease due to the presence of scar tissue formation, infection, and destruction of normal anatomy. In studies of anti-TNF therapy for luminal CD, response peaks at 3 to 6 months before beginning a slow decline, but response of perianal and fistulizing disease may continue to increase for several months. In the CHARM study, response in perianal CD was 30% at 6 months and 33% at 12 months, in contrast to a drop from 44% to 38% in luminal disease over the same time period.

The only long-term experience with anti-TNF therapy in pediatrics was assembled by the Pediatric IBD Collaborative Research Group Registry with 87 CD patients on infliximab with at least two years of follow-up.[13] After 2 years, 72/87 (83%) patients were still on infliximab and 63/72 (88%) had a clinical response (21% mild disease/67% inactive disease). Beyond 2 years, 65 of 72 (90%) patients continued on treatment until the end of follow-up. Overall, of the 121 patients with a follow-up time of 1 to 3 years, only 21 discontinued therapy.

A review of 16 studies, including several discussed separately in this chapter, found that loss of response occurred at a rate of 10% to 15% per year in patients treated with maintenance infliximab.[14] A majority of the patients who lost response re-entered remission after infliximab dose intensification. Rates of response loss for adalimumab and certolizumab have not been assessed in CD, but in the authors' experience, are similar to the rate for infliximab.

Most of the patients who respond to induction anti-TNF therapy do so in the first 6 months of therapy. For those who do respond to induction therapy, durability of response and side effect profile are a primary concern. Although the use of episodic dosing of infliximab, extrapolated to adalimumab and certolizumab, can maintain remission, there is a higher rate of discontinuation as a result of side effects and loss of response.

In the authors' experience, the frequency of response loss and hypersensitivity reactions with episodic anti-TNF therapy is prohibitive, even on concomitant immunomodulators, so this approach is not recommended. If anti-TNF therapy remains effective, we continue treatment for a long term, as we have found that disease recurrence is likely if therapy is discontinued.

There is significant variation in practice when it comes to the use of a concomitant immunomodulator with anti-TNF therapy. Although there is conflict in the evidence, there is a scientific basis for improved induction of response and prolonged duration of effectiveness when immunomodulator therapy is added to an anti-TNF. Concern about adverse effects is what prevents many from pursuing this route. These include both the side effects from long-term use of methotrexate (pulmonary fibrosis, hepatitis, thyroid disease) and azathioprine (leucopenia, hepatitis, and cancer), as well as the rare, but fatal cases of hepatosplenic T-cell lymphoma.

There are several approaches to this dilemma, which span the spectrum from single agent anti-TNF therapy to full-dose two-agent therapy. In the patient who is already on, but failing an immunomodulator, we favor initiating anti-TNF therapy while the immunomodulator remains at full dose. If remission is induced, then we taper the azathioprine down to approximately 1 mg/kg and continue at that dose as long as remission is maintained. For methotrexate, we will often switch to 10 mg of weekly oral therapy instead of continuing weekly 25 mg injections. It is crucial to assess disease activity using clinical, radiographic, and endoscopic means in order to assure that the patient's regimen has resolved any inflammation.

If a patient is not on an immunomodulator when the decision is made to start anti-TNF therapy, we prefer to start the two drugs together, and as described above, taper the immunomodulator to a low dose if remission is achieved. Many patients have had prior intolerance or side effects from immunomodulator therapy. In these patients, we initiate and maintain scheduled anti-TNF monotherapy.

● DOSE INTENSIFICATION FOR LOSS OF RESPONSE

The anti-TNF medications are parenterally administered antibodies. Consequently, they induce the formation of neutralizing antibodies, which increases the likelihood of hypersensitivity reactions and loss of response. Loss of response, also referred to as secondary nonresponse, is a failure in maintaining a previously attained induction endpoint, as opposed to primary nonresponse, in which the medication is ineffective from the start and fails to reach induction endpoints.

Dose intensification is the first intervention for patients who experience a loss of response to anti-TNF therapy. This can be implemented by an increase in dose, a decrease in dosing interval, or both. Regueiro et al.[15] followed 108 CD patients who had received at least 1 year of infliximab therapy. After 2.5 years of treatment, 54% of the patients required dose intensification, 76% were able to remain on infliximab until the end of follow-up. Out of 108 patients, only 13 discontinued therapy over the course of 30 months. Although the study was not powered to measure risk factors for dose intensification, age less than 25 had a protective effect against dose intensification (43% reduction, P value = 0.05)

A similar cohort from Milwaukee included 153 patients with infliximab exposure for at least 1 year.[16] After 4 years, ~22% of the patients had discontinued the therapy. The 50% to 60% rate of dose intensification was similar in patients whether they eventually continued or discontinued therapy. Neither of the studies measured antibodies to infliximab (ATI) nor found that active tobacco use or concomitant immunomodulator use affected the need for dose intensification, although they conflicted as to whether there was a detrimental effect of previous episodic infliximab exposure on durability of response.

The adalimumab maintenance trial CLASSIC II included an open-label arm with 204 patients who failed to enter clinical remission after two 40 mg doses of medication or placebo.[17] At 1-year follow-up or at the time of the last visit, 44% of the study subjects required dose intensification by decreasing the dosing interval from eow to every week. Three-quarters of the patients who received dose intensification reestablished a clinical response and 42% entered clinical remission. The rates of response and remission were similar between the patients who remained on standard dosing and those who required dose intensification. Long-term follow-up from the Belgian cohort, described previously, found that only 22% of initial responders to infliximab stopped therapy at 55 months, even though more than half required dose intensification.[10]

These studies highlight the fact that although loss of response to anti-TNF therapy occurs in 10% to 15% of patients annually, as suggested in a recent review article, approximately two-thirds of those with a loss of response will regain a durable response after dose intensification.

The authors will switch to another anti-TNF agent when a patient fully loses response despite dose intensification. Our strategy for dose intensification of anti-TNF therapy is as follows. For infliximab, we usually increase the dose from 5 to 10 mg/kg first, followed, if necessary by a decrease in the dosing interval. Although a dose increase is no more effective than an interval decrease when a patient loses response, it is more convenient for the patient. Ultimately, if a patient is on 10 mg/kg of infliximab every 6 weeks with continued symptoms, we recommend switching to adalimumab or certolizumab. Typically, we do not measure ATI in the setting of loss of response but rely on clinical signs and symptoms of CD recurrence.

Our strategy for adalimumab dose intensification is to switch from 40 mg eow to once weekly dosing. Although rare, we do have patients who we have escalated to 80 mg weekly adalimumab. In the case of certolizumab, if loss of response occurs with maintenance on every 4-week certolizumab then we decrease the interval to every 2 weeks.

● POSTOPERATIVE CD

A majority of patients with moderate or severe CD will undergo abdominal surgery at some point. Ileocolonic resection is the most common bowel resection in CD. Postoperative recurrence is at least 80% within 2 years without medical therapy. Antibiotics, 5-aminosalicylates, and immunomodulators have been studied in just a few RCTs. There is mixed evidence for the use of mesalamine and antibiotics. A meta-analysis of three RCTs found that azathioprine, despite subtherapeutic dosing, is more effective than placebo, yet, after 1 year of treatment severe endoscopic recurrence was 20% to 30%.[18]

The ability of anti-TNF therapy to induce mucosal healing in IBD has led to optimism that it may be capable of blocking the recurrence of inflammation after resection of CD. Sorrentino et al.[19] first illustrated the potential benefit of infliximab in the postoperative setting with an open-label study of 23 patients. Three-quarters of the patients in each group underwent ileal or ileocolonic resection and three-quarters of each group were nonsmokers. Seven patients received infliximab (5 mg/kg) and low-dose oral methotrexate (10 mg/week) beginning 2 weeks after surgery. Sixteen patients received 2.4 g of mesalamine per day. Two years after surgery, the mesalamine group had a 75% endoscopic recurrence rate, whereas none of the infliximab/methotrexate treated patients had recurrence.

Recently, the first RCT of anti-TNF therapy for postoperative prophylaxis was published.[20] Within 4 weeks of ileocolonic resection, patients were randomized to infliximab (5 mg/kg) or placebo. Patients were permitted to continue immunomodulators and 5-aminosalicylates, but steroids and antibiotics were discontinued. Approximately 35% of the patients in each group had previously received infliximab. The treatment group contained more smokers and fewer patients on immunomodulators. One year after surgery, 10/11 (91%) infliximab treated patients were free of endoscopic recurrence compared to only 2/13 (15%) receiving placebo. ($P = 0.0006$)

After 1 year of randomized treatment, open-label infliximab was offered to all patients.[21] Three of the treatment patients who were in remission 1 year after surgery opted to discontinue infliximab. All three of these patients had significant endoscopic recurrence 1 year after discontinuing infliximab, which was 2 years after surgery. Seven of the patients who had an endoscopic recurrence on placebo 1 year after surgery opted for open-label infliximab. All of them had endoscopic improvement of CD with five (71%) having an endoscopic remission 1 year after starting infliximab, which was 2 years after surgery. During the 48 annual endoscopies that were performed during the RCT and open-label follow-up, 88% of the patients on anti-TNF therapy were in endoscopic remission compared to only 22% of patients not on an anti-TNF. A multicenter RCT is being planned to confirm the efficacy of infliximab in the postoperative setting.

The authors approach for the management of postoperative CD is to use 6-mercaptopurine or azathioprine for those patient with a moderate risk for recurrence, that is, >10 cm inflammatory stricture but no fistula, and reserve infliximab (or anti-TNF therapy) for the high-risk patient, that is, penetrating disease and multiple prior surgeries. Regardless of the initial postoperative treatment, the authors perform ileocolonoscopy 6 to 12 months after surgery to assess for endoscopic recurrence. Continuing advances in noninvasive biomarkers and imaging may soon make invasive testing unnecessary to measure CD recurrence. If a patient is maintained in remission on postoperative anti-TNF therapy after 1 year we recommend continuing therapy, if there is disease recurrence then dose intensification or switching to another anti-TNF is an option.

● CONCLUSION

Infliximab and adalimumab have proven efficacy for the maintenance of IBD beyond 1 year. Although there are less data on the long-term use with certolizumab, the maintenance benefit will likely be similar to the other two anti-TNFs. While there is no regimen which prevents loss of response and hypersensitivity reactions to anti-TNF therapy, scheduled dosing and, probably, concomitant immunomodulator therapy minimizes these events. Despite dose intensification, a small percentage of patients each year lose response or discontinue therapy due to side effects. Infliximab appears effective in maintaining surgical remission in the postoperative setting. Although the optimal duration of anti-TNF usage is currently not known, the authors recommend continuing treatment beyond 1 year for those patients who have maintained remission.

References

1. Hanauer SB, Feagan BG, Lichtenstein GR, et al.; ACCENT I Study Group. Maintenance infliximab for Crohn's disease: the ACCENT I randomised trial. *Lancet.* 2002;359(9317):1541–1549.

2. Colombel JF, Sandborn WJ, Rutgeerts P, et al. Adalimumab for maintenance of clinical response and remission in patients with Crohn's disease: the CHARM trial. *Gastroenterology.* 2007;132(1):52–65.

3. Schreiber S, Khaliq-Kareemi M, Lawrance IC, et al.; PRECISE 2 Study Investigators. Maintenance therapy with certolizumab pegol for Crohn's disease. *N Engl J Med.* 2007;357(3):239–250.

4. Sands BE, Anderson FH, Bernstein CN, et al. Infliximab maintenance therapy for fistulizing Crohn's disease. *N Engl J Med.* 2004;350(9):876–885.

5. Rutgeerts P, Sandborn WJ, Feagan BG, et al. Infliximab for induction and maintenance therapy for ulcerative colitis. *N Engl J Med.* 2005;353(23):2462–2476.

6. Hyams J, Crandall W, Kugathasan S, et al.; REACH Study Group. Induction and maintenance infliximab therapy for the treatment of moderate-to-severe Crohn's disease in children. *Gastroenterology.* 2007;132(3):863–73; quiz 1165.

7. Viola F, Civitelli F, Di Nardo G, et al. Efficacy of adalimumab in moderate-to-severe pediatric Crohn's disease. *Am J Gastroenterol.* 2009;104(10):2566–2571.

8. Rudolph SJ, Weinberg DI, McCabe RP. Long-term durability of Crohn's disease treatment with infliximab. *Dig Dis Sci.* 2008;53(4):1033–1041.

9. Moss AC, Kim KJ, Fernandez-Becker N, Cury D, Cheifetz AS. Impact of concomitant immunomodulator use on long-term outcomes in patients receiving scheduled maintenance infliximab. *Dig Dis Sci.* 2010;55(5):1413–1420.

10. Schnitzler F, Fidder H, Ferrante M, et al. Long-term outcome of treatment with infliximab in 614 patients with Crohn's disease: results from a single-centre cohort. *Gut.* 2009;58(4):492–500.

11. Colombel JF, Schwartz DA, Sandborn WJ, et al. Adalimumab for the treatment of fistulas in patients with Crohn's disease. *Gut.* 2009;58(7):940–948.

12. Bouguen G, Trouilloud I, Siproudhis L, et al. Long-term outcome of non-fistulizing (ulcers, stricture) perianal Crohn's disease in patients treated with infliximab. *Aliment Pharmacol Ther.* 2009;30(7):749–756.

13. Hyams JS, Lerer T, Griffiths A, et al.; Pediatric Inflammatory Bowel Disease Collaborative Research Group. Long-term outcome of maintenance infliximab therapy in children with Crohn's disease. *Inflamm Bowel Dis.* 2009;15(6):816–822.

14. Gisbert JP, Panés J. Loss of response and requirement of infliximab dose intensification in Crohn's disease: a review. *Am J Gastroenterol.* 2009;104(3):760–767.

15. Regueiro M, Siemanowski B, Kip KE, Plevy S. Infliximab dose intensification in Crohn's disease. *Inflamm Bowel Dis.* 2007;13(9):1093–1099.

16. Gonzaga JE, Ananthakrishnan AN, Issa M, et al. Durability of infliximab in Crohn's disease: A single-center experience. *Inflamm Bowel Dis.* 2009;15(12):1837–1843.

17. Sandborn WJ, Hanauer SB, Rutgeerts P, et al. Adalimumab for maintenance treatment of Crohn's disease: results of the CLASSIC II trial. *Gut.* 2007;56(9):1232–1239.

18. Peyrin-Biroulet L, Deltenre P, Ardizzone S, et al. Azathioprine and 6-mercaptopurine for the prevention of postoperative recurrence in Crohn's disease: a meta-analysis. *Am J Gastroenterol.* 2009;104(8):2089–2096.

19. Sorrentino D, Terrosu G, Avellini C, Maiero S. Infliximab with low-dose methotrexate for prevention of postsurgical recurrence of ileocolonic Crohn disease. *Arch Intern Med.* 2007;167(16):1804–1807.

20. Regueiro M, Schraut W, Baidoo L, et al. Infliximab prevents Crohn's disease recurrence after ileal resection. *Gastroenterology.* 2009;136(2):441–50.e1; quiz 716.

21. Regueiro M, Kip K, Schraut W, et al. Long-term follow-up of patients enrolled in the randomized controlled trial (RCT) of infliximab (INF) for prevention of postoperative Crohn's disease (CD) [abstract 1232]. Presented at the 74th American College of Gastroenterology Annual Scientific Meeting; October 2009; San Diego, CA.

Duration of Therapy of Immunomodulators and Biologics in Crohn's Disease

111

Russell D. Cohen

Crohn's disease is a chronic relapsing condition that is thought to develop from an inappropriate immune response from a dysregulated immune system in a genetically susceptible host. Therapeutic interventions to date have centered mainly upon agents shown to mechanistically impact various pathways of the human inflammatory response with the exception of agent trials targeting elimination or control of various microorganisms (i.e., bacteria, viruses, fungi, atypical organisms) suspected to be either the etiology or the driving force behind the disease. The inability to clearly identify an infectious causative agent and the failure of the anti-infective agents to convincingly "cure" the disease in controlled clinical trials have refocused attention on agents that attenuate the defective immune response.

Foremost among the immune-regulating therapies are the agents commonly referred to as "immunomodulators" (i.e., 6-mercaptopurine, azathioprine, methotrexate, cyclosporine, tacrolimus) as well as the "biological therapies" (infliximab, adalimumab, certolizumab, and natalizumab). The efficacy of these agents is covered elsewhere in this textbook; large controlled trials validate the use of biologics, whereas the immunomodulators were either studied in small trials or supported by expert experience and opinion. These agents have been adopted for use in patients with Crohn's disease worldwide.

One of the main controversies in this debate concerns the duration of therapy that is required once committing to these drug therapies. The question, simply stated is, "Are these lifelong therapies?" Unlike the relatively innocuous mesalamine products, there is an undercurrent of concern over the safety of long-term use of immune-modulating drugs, particularly regarding the risk of developing neoplasms. The early age of onset of Crohn's disease raises the specter of decades upon decades of exposure to these agents—much longer than any clinical trials evaluate. The absence of long-term data leaves both the patient and the physician in unchartered territory, and is clearly a topic area where guidance is needed.

This chapter explores the use of continuing long-term therapy with the immunomodulators and biologics in patients with Crohn's disease, review the existing data supporting or refuting continuous use, and provide further insight and guidance for patient care today.

IMMUNOMODULATORS

The Purine Analogues

The purine analogues, azathioprine and 6-mercaptopurine, are the most common immunomodulators used in Crohn's disease. Thioguanine's use is controversial and will not be covered in this section. Azathioprine is converted to 6-mercaptopurine in the liver and henceforth they share the same subsequent metabolism. While intolerances may vary between the two agents, for the purposes of therapeutic efficacy, the two are referred to interchangeably, as adequate studies comparing the two drugs have not been widely publicized.

The purine analogues are believed to be effective in both the induction and remission of Crohn's disease, in both adults and children, although induction studies have typically included a coinduction corticosteroid that is gradually tapered off over the ensuing weeks to months. Multiple studies looking at the long-term remission in Crohn's disease with the purine analogues have been published, as well as Cochrane Database Systematic Reviews. In all of these instances, patients who have responded to these agents experience high rates of relapse upon discontinuation of therapy. (Fig. 111.1).

One of the earliest, if not the first, azathioprine withdrawal trial was a British double-blinded placebo-controlled study in which 51 Crohn's patients in "good health" on 2 mg/kg/day of azathioprine were randomized to continue therapy, or were provided a placebo. Relapse rates at 6 and 12 months were 0% and 5% for patients on therapy, vs. 25% and 41% on placebo, respectively. Safety evaluation revealed one death in a patient on azathioprine after nearly 11 years of therapy.[1]

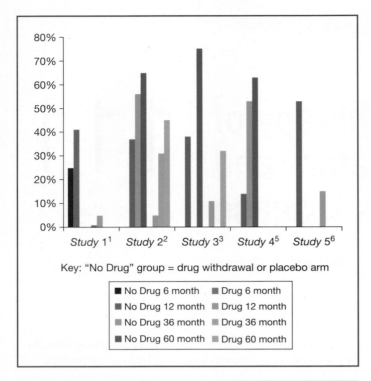

FIGURE 111.1 • Failure to maintain clinical response once purine analogues are discontinued. Relapse rates over time in Crohn's disease patients who initially responded to and were continued on azathioprine or 6-mercaptopurine ("Drug") compared with those who stopped therapy or were randomized to the placebo arm in withdrawal studies ("No Drug").

The Oxford group subsequently presented retrospective data from a 30-year period (1968–1999) comparing maintenance of remission in a mixed group of 662 Crohn's and ulcerative colitis patients treated with azathioprine.[2] The proportion of patients remaining in remission after 1, 3, and 5 years of therapy were 95%, 69%, and 55% whereas the rates at the same time points in those who had stopped therapy were 63%, 44%, and 35%, respectively. Safety evaluations revealed leukopenia in 4.6% of patients; only two patients had significant pancytopenia. Nine patients developed sepsis that was likely related to therapy; one patient had cytomegalovirus hepatitis, one with herpes zoster, and two with "generalized warts."

The French group at Hôpital Saint-Lazare evaluated 199 Crohn's patients treated with either azathioprine or 6-mercaptopurine for more than 6 months, who had all achieved at least 6 months of remission without corticosteroids, and compared time to relapse between those who were maintained on therapy versus those who stopped drug for reasons other than relapse.[3] The cumulative probability of relapse at 1 and 5 years was 11% and 32% for those who stayed on therapy, versus 38% and 75% for those who stopped. Predictors for relapse among those who stayed on therapy were female gender, younger age, and longer time to achieve remission (>6 months). For those who stopped therapy, relapse was predicted by male gender, younger age, and duration of remission of <4 years. The investigators reported that after 4 years, the risk of relapse remained similar. Safety evaluation revealed 18 events of leukopenia (only three required cessation of therapy), hepatic nodular regenerative hyperplasia

in one patient, and the diagnosis of the following tumors, each in one patient: malignant melanoma, cutaneous basal cell carcinoma, renal carcinoma, and a brain lymphoma.

The French consortium GETAID, which included some of the same investigators, conducted a randomized double-blind controlled withdrawal study in Crohn's disease patients who were in clinical remission for at least 42 months on azathioprine.[4] At 18 months, only 3 of the 40 patients maintained on azathioprine relapsed, compared to 9 of the 43 patients in the placebo group, with Kaplan–Meier estimates of relapse of 8% vs. 21%, respectively. Predictors of relapse include elevated C-reactive protein (CRP) (>20 mg/L), less time free of corticosteroids (<50 months), and hemoglobin levels below 12 g/dL. The recommendations were that azathioprine therapy should be continued beyond three and one-half years.

The GETAID group subsequently published a long-term follow-up evaluation in 66 Crohn's disease patients in remission for a mean of 64 months after a mean 68 months of azathioprine, who subsequently stopped therapy.[5] After a median follow-up of 55 months, nearly one-half (32 of 66) patients had relapsed, with cumulative probabilities of relapse at 1, 3, and 5 years of 14%, 53%, and 63%, respectively. Predictors of relapse were elevated CRP (≥20 mg/L), hemoglobin level <12 g/dL, and neutrophil count ≥4 × 10⁹/L. The conclusions of the GETAID investigators is that azathioprine should not be interrupted if it is well tolerated.

A smaller Danish study randomized 29 Crohn's patients with inactive Crohn's disease after a median of 37 months of azathioprine to continue or withdraw from therapy.[6] After 12 months, the relapse rates were 15% in patients continuing therapy vs. 53% in those who stopped therapy. These differences were more pronounced in patients who had received at least 1.60 mg/kg/day of therapy, with relapse rates of 11% for those on drug vs. 67% in those who discontinued azathioprine.

The Cochrane Database of Systematic Reviews had released an initial evaluation of azathioprine's use in maintenance of Crohn's disease in 2000,[7] which was subsequently updated in 2009 for azathioprine and 6-mercaptopurine.[8] In the original work, data was abstracted from five randomized double-blinded placebo-controlled trials. The Peto odds ratio (OR) for maintaining remission was 2.16 (95% confidence interval: 1.35–3.47), with a number needed to treat (NNT) of 7. The odds for withdrawal due to adverse events was 4.36 (1.63–11.67), with a number needed to harm (NNH) of 19. The 2009 update included seven studies on azathioprine and one on low-dose 6-mercaptopurine. The Peto OR for remission maintenance with azathioprine was 2.32 (1.55–3.49) with a NNT of only 6; for 6-mercaptopurine the OR was 3.32 (1.40–7.87) with a NNT of 4. The odds of withdrawal due to azathioprine were 3.74 (1.48–9.45), with a NNH of 20. Both analyses concluded that azathioprine was effective in maintenance of remission, and is corticosteroid sparing.

Purine Analogs Plus Biologic Therapy

Withdrawal of the purine analogues in Crohn's disease patients who have subsequently been started on a biological therapy has received much attention lately, in part due to the recent reports of rare hepatosplenic T-cell lymphomas[9,10] and the hypothesized increase in risk of progressive multifocal leukoencephalopathy[11,12] in patients on dual immunosuppression. The Belgian group randomized 80 patients with controlled Crohn's disease after at least 6 months of combination therapy of infliximab plus either azathioprine, 6-mercaptopurine, or methotrexate to either continue or stop the immunomodulator, while staying on infliximab therapy.[13] This 2-year open-label trial did not reveal any differences in the need to change infliximab dosing schedule or to stop therapy. The Crohn's Disease Activity Index, Inflammatory Bowel Disease Questionnairescores, and endoscopic outcomes were similar between the two groups. However, CRP levels were higher in the patients who discontinued the immunomodulator, whereas serum trough infliximab levels were lower raising the possibility of a decrease in efficacy over time in the patients on monotherapy with infliximab. Important safety signals included a renal cell cancer in a patient on dual immunosuppression, and a sudden cardiac death on a patient on monotherapy.

Adverse Events

Major adverse events from the previously cited trials were rare, and discussed above. Additional studies have looked at long-term safety of the purine analogues in Crohn's disease patients. The New York group reported on 396 patients (276 with Crohn's disease) who were treated with 6-mercaptopurine for a mean of 34 months (38 months for Crohn's; range 1–130 months).[14] Follow-up was recorded in 90% of patients at a mean of 60 months. Pancreatitis occurred in 3.3% of patients; whereas bone marrow depression was reported in "many" requiring temporary cessation or dose lowering, the authors found that only eight patients (2.2 %) had bone marrow suppression requiring hospitalization, all but one case in Crohn's disease. Infectious complications were seen in 7.4%; most common were hepatitis (but only two had confirmed infectious hepatitis), herpes zoster, and pneumonia. Neoplasms were found in 3.1%, one was a histiocytic lymphoma (fatal; patient had 9 months of 6-mercaptopurine prior to diagnosis), one a melanoma, two basal cell carcinomas, and the others were solid tumors occurring in one patient each.

Methotrexate

Methotrexate is widely used in rheumatoid arthritis, psoriasis, and other inflammatory conditions. Its use in Crohn's disease has traditionally been limited to patients who are allergic or intolerant to the purine analogues. There is far less published on the long-term use of methotrexate in Crohn's disease, and formal withdrawal trials have yet to be performed or widely published.

The largest published placebo-controlled withdrawal trial to date was the North American Crohn's Study Group trial, whereby 76 Crohn's patients who had entered remission with weekly methotrexate 25 mg delivered intramuscularly were randomized in a double-blind fashion to either continue methotrexate 15 mg intramuscularly weekly or receive placebo injections.[15] The study was limited to 40 weeks, and revealed relapse rates of 35% in the drug group vs. 61% in those who received placebo. There were no serious safety issues that arose during this short trial.

● BIOLOGICAL THERAPIES

Anti-TNF Therapies

Large-scale formal withdrawal trials have not been conducted for the anti-tumor necrosis factor (TNF) agents to date. Some information on relapse rates after short-term (i.e., induction) therapy can be gleaned from the large clinical trials, all of which have shown a rapid, dramatic drop off in patient response and remission once the biological agent is replaced by placebo (Fig. 111.2).

Infliximab

One of the earliest Crohn's trials, commonly referred to as the "Rutgeerts trial,"[16] randomized responders to an initial blinded dose of infliximab (at 5 mg, 10 mg, or 20 mg/kg) or placebo from the initial "Targan trial"[17] to receive four additional doses of either infliximab (at 10 mg/kg) or placebo every 8 weeks, with final results measured 8 weeks after the last dose (at week 44). The proportion of patients receiving infliximab who were in clinical remission increased from the time of the first infusion (37.8%) to 52.9% by week 44, whereas those who received placebo showed a decrease from 44.4% to 20% at the same time period. In the safety analysis, there was one B-cell duodenal lymphoma in a patient who was receiving placebo-retreatment after a single infliximab infusion 9½ months earlier.

The ACCENT-I trial was a 573 patient luminal Crohn's disease trial whereby responders to an initial 5 mg/kg dose of infliximab were randomly assigned to receive additional blinded infusions of drug (at 5 or 10 mg/kg) or placebo at weeks 2 and 6, and then every 8 weeks thereafter until week 46.[18] Remission rates at week 30 were higher in the patients who received 5 mg/kg (39%) or 10 mg/kg (45%) than those receiving placebo (21%). By week 54, the rates were 28%, 38%, and 14%, respectively. Safety signals included six tumors; two were in patients who had received placebo maintenance (one epithelial-cell skin cancer; one natural killer cell lymphoma) and four were in patients who had received infliximab maintenance (one basal cell skin; one hypernephroma; one breast cancer, and one bladder cancer). There were two patients with sepsis (one died), one myocardial infarction, and one case of tuberculosis; all were patients who were in infliximab-treatment arms.

The ACCENT-II trial of perianal and perineal fistulas differed from the previous trials in that the induction regimen was the standard three dose load (infliximab 5 mg/kg at week 0, 2, and 6) after which the responders (defined as at least a 50% decrease in the number of draining fistulas) were randomized to receive five additional doses of drug at 5 mg/kg or placebo every 8 weeks.[19] A response was maintained at week 54 in 46% of those who continued to receive infliximab, versus 23% who were withdrawn from therapy and received placebo. Complete response (an absence of draining fistulas) was maintained in 36% vs. 19%, respectively. Safety events of note were one case of cutaneous nocardiosis and one cytomegalovirus infection, both during induction. During the maintenance phase, new fistula-related abscesses were seen in 12% of patients receiving infliximab and 17% of those receiving placebo.

Editor's note (TMB): This led many physicians to have setons placed through the fistula prior to biologic induction. The setons were withdrawn at 4 to 6 weeks in responders. In the chapter on perianal fistulas, use of cutting setons for superficial fistulas is discussed.

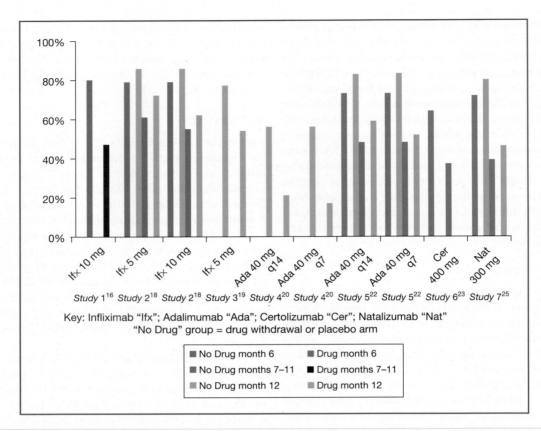

FIGURE 111.2 • Failure to maintain clinical response once biological therapies are discontinued. Relapse rates over time in Crohn's disease patients who initially responded to and were continued on a biological therapy ("Drug") vs. those who stopped therapy or were randomized to the placebo arm in withdrawal studies ("No Drug").

Adalimumab

Similar to the scenario with infliximab, virtually all of the information that we have regarding adalimumab "withdrawal" is based upon the patients who received induction doses of adalimumab, followed by randomization to the placebo arm in the maintenance study. There have been no formal withdrawal studies or large-center experiences published to date.

In the CLASSIC-II trial,[20] 55 patients who attained remission after two open-label doses of adalimumab 40 mg at weeks 0 and 2 (after an initial two doses in the placebo-controlled dose-ranging CLASSIC-I trial)[21] were randomized to receive either drug or placebo ($n = 18$) out to 56 weeks. Remission rates had fallen off by week 56 in the placebo-treated group (44%) as compared to the patients who received 40 mg of active drug dosed weekly (83%) or every other week (79%).

In the CHARM trial,[22] 499 patients who had responded to an initial open-label induction of adalimumab (80 mg at week 0, 40 mg at week 2) were randomized to receive either drug or placebo ($n = 170$) out to 56 weeks. The response rates (measured by CR-100) fell off dramatically within the first 6 months in the patients receiving placebo (only 27% responding) as compared to 52% of patients receiving weekly or twice-monthly 40 doses of adalimumab. By 56 weeks, the placebo rate fell to only 17%, as compared to 41% to 48% for the active drug patients.

The safety data from the patients who received active drug in these 1-year studies did not reveal any alarming events during the maintenance period. In the CLASSIC-II trial, there were six

abdominal abscesses, one patient who developed pneumonia and sepsis, another patient had parvovirus and nocardiosis, whereas a different patient had viral meningitis. In the CHARM study, there were eight abscesses (although five placebo patients also had abscesses), one case of pneumonia, and no cancers or other concerning serious events. During the postrandomization open-label trial that followed, there were two cases of tuberculosis, both in patients who had normal tuberculosis skin test and chest x-rays at baseline.

Certolizumab Pegol

Certolizumab's data is strikingly similar to the other two anti-TNF agents; a rapid fall off in patient response and remission rates once the open-label drug is switched over to placebo, at rates far faster than that seen with active drug maintenance.

In the PRECISE-2 trial,[23] 428 patients who had responded to an initial open-label induction of certolizumab pegol (400 mg at weeks 0, 2, and 4) were randomized to receive either drug or placebo ($n = 212$) out to 26 weeks. The response rates (measured by CR-100) declined to only 36% the patients receiving placebo versus 63% in those who were receiving monthly injections of active drug. Among the patients who received active drug during the maintenance phase, there was one case of tuberculosis (negative tuberculosis skin test at screening), one pneumonia, one pyelonephritis, and one perianal abscess; there were no cancers or other concerning safety events.

The PRECISE-1 trial[24] did not have an initial open-label induction, so "relapse rates" with placebo are not comparable.

However, the safety data from this 6-month 662 patient study is helpful in accessing risk associated with therapy. There were two cancers: one was a metastatic lung cancer in a patient who also had hypertension and died from an acute myocardial infarction. The other was a rectal cancer that was diagnosed just 20 days after study initiation. Of note, the placebo group also had two cancers (cervical and Hodgkin's). Notable infectious events included abscesses in six patients (four were perianal); there were three abscesses in the placebo group.

Natalizumab

Natalizumab is the first biological agent approved for Crohn's disease that does not work primarily through inhibition of TNF. The clinical trial data shows a similar pattern to the other biologics; once patients were switched from an open-label induction to the placebo, they experienced rapid disease recurrence.

In the ENACT trials,[25] 905 patients randomly received either natalizumab 300 mg or placebo infusions at weeks 0, 4, and 8 (ENACT-1). The responders at week 10 were then randomized to either 300 mg of natalizumab or placebo every 4 weeks through week 56 (ENACT-2). The patients receiving placebo experienced a rapid drop off in sustained response rates at week 36 (28% vs. 61% natalizumab) which continued to plummet by week 60 (20% vs. 54% natalizumab). The safety analysis with the drug over this course of time revealed no tumors, no hematological malignancies, no atypical infections, and two perianal abscesses (two also seen in the placebo group). One patient who dropped out of the study enrolled in the open-label extension study and subsequently died from progressive multifocal leukoencephalopathy associated with the JC virus.[11]

Editor's note (TMB): The risk of PML with natalizumab is detailed in Volume One chapter on viral infections complicating IBD.

● CONCLUSIONS

The urge to stop effective medications in patients with chronic relapsing inflammatory diseases must be balanced against the drug's safety, likelihood of relapse if therapy is terminated, and projected success in reattaining a durable response or remission with reintroduction of the pharmacological agent.

Unlike corticosteroids, which have well-documented devastating common side effects with long-term use, as well as limited evidence of efficacy in a maintenance setting, the immunomodulators have been accepted into the medical community as safe, effective long-term treatments in patients with inflammatory bowel disease. Formalized reintroduction trials have been rare; clinical experience has found that many patients who do flare after cessation of therapy are unable to easily regain a lasting remission. The balance of data on safety, efficacy, and decades of experience in the use of these agents currently supports their continued use in a remission maintenance role.

The biological therapies do not boast the same "decades of experience" title, and their high drug costs put more pressure on efforts to limit their long-term use. However, the dramatically rapid relapse rates in every study to date make the likelihood of long-term remission after cessation of therapy highly doubtful. Coupled with the unfortunate lesson learned with infliximab,

whereby an extended hiatus of therapy led to severe infusion-related adverse events and neutralization of the drug by anti-drug antibodies, reintroduction of the same agent will not likely be a realistic option. As there are only a precious few advanced drugs currently available to treat these diseases, it seems treacherous at this point to put patients into a gamble that they are highly likely to lose.

Editor's note (TMB): Clinicians—read carefully. This excellent chapter provides detailed benefit-risk information. If your patient initially responded (60%) or went into remission (40%) on anti-TNF agent; the evidence favoring maintenance therapy with immunomodulators or biologics is further strengthened by the chapter on mucosal healing.

Editor's note added in proof (TMB): Immunomodulator withdrawal from Combination therapy with anti-TNF: At DDW, May 2001, D. Drobne et al. presented an abstract (#279, A70) describing discontinuing IMM therapy from a combination with IFX after > 6 mo therapy and achieving a remission. Loss of response to IFX after discontinuing IMM was predicted by undetectable trough levels of IFX and CRP >5 mg/L during the combination therapy.

Restarting IFX after long drug holiday: F.J. Baert et al. from the same Belgian group reported in an abstract (#280, A70) that restart was successful in 33 of 39 patients but that having undetectable trough levels and ATI (antibodies to IFX) present early after restarting was predictive of no response and/or an infusion reaction.

References

1. O'Donoghue DP, Dawson AM, Powell-Tuck J, Bown RL, Lennard-Jones JE. Double-blind withdrawal trial of azathioprine as maintenance treatment for Crohn's disease. *Lancet.* 1978;2(8097):955–957.

2. Fraser AG, Orchard TR, Jewell DP. The efficacy of azathioprine for the treatment of inflammatory bowel disease: a 30 year review. *Gut.* 2002;50(4):485–489.

3. Bouhnik Y, Lémann M, Mary JY, et al. Long-term follow-up of patients with Crohn's disease treated with azathioprine or 6-mercaptopurine. *Lancet.* 1996;347(8996):215–219.

4. Lémann M, Mary JY, Colombel JF, et al.; Groupe D'Etude Thérapeutique des Affections Inflammatoires du Tube Digestif. A randomized, double-blind, controlled withdrawal trial in Crohn's disease patients in long-term remission on azathioprine. *Gastroenterology.* 2005;128(7):1812–1818.

5. Treton X, Bouhnik Y, Mary JY, et al.; Groupe D'Etude Thérapeutique Des Affections Inflammatoires Du Tube Digestif (GETAID). Azathioprine withdrawal in patients with Crohn's disease maintained on prolonged remission: a high risk of relapse. *Clin Gastroenterol Hepatol.* 2009;7(1):80–85.

6. Vilien M, Dahlerup JF, Munck LK, Nørregaard P, Grønbaek K, Fallingborg J. Randomized controlled azathioprine withdrawal after more than two years treatment in Crohn's disease: increased relapse rate the following year. *Aliment Pharmacol Ther.* 2004;19(11):1147–1152.

7. Pearson DC, May GR, Fick G, Sutherland LR. Azathioprine for maintaining remission of Crohn's disease. *Cochrane Database Syst Rev.* 2000;(2):CD000067.

8. Prefontaine E, Sutherland LR, Macdonald JK, Cepoiu M. Azathioprine or 6-mercaptopurine for maintenance of remission in Crohn's disease. *Cochrane Database Syst Rev 2009*;(1)CD000067.

9. Mackey AC, Green L, Leptak C, Avigan M. Hepatosplenic T cell lymphoma associated with infliximab use in young patients treated for inflammatory bowel disease: update. *J Pediatr Gastroenterol Nutr.* 2009;48(3):386–388.

10. Mackey AC, Green L, Liang LC, Dinndorf P, Avigan M. Hepatosplenic T cell lymphoma associated with infliximab use in young patients treated for inflammatory bowel disease. *J Pediatr Gastroenterol Nutr.* 2007;44(2):265–267.

11. Van Assche G, Van Ranst M, Sciot R, et al. Progressive multifocal leukoencephalopathy after natalizumab therapy for Crohn's disease. *N Engl J Med.* 2005;353(4):362–368.

12. Kleinschmidt-DeMasters BK, Tyler KL. Progressive multifocal leukoencephalopathy complicating treatment with natalizumab and interferon beta-1a for multiple sclerosis. *N Engl J Med.* 2005;353(4):369–374.

13. Van Assche G, Magdelaine-Beuzelin C, D'Haens G, et al. Withdrawal of immunosuppression in Crohn's disease treated with scheduled infliximab maintenance: a randomized trial. *Gastroenterology.* 2008;134(7):1861–1868.

14. Present DH, Meltzer SJ, Krumholz MP, Wolke A, Korelitz BI. 6-Mercaptopurine in the management of inflammatory bowel disease: short- and long-term toxicity. *Ann Intern Med.* 1989;111(8):641–649.

15. Feagan BG, Fedorak RN, Irvine EJ, et al. A comparison of methotrexate with placebo for the maintenance of remission in Crohn's disease. North American Crohn's Study Group Investigators. *N Engl J Med.* 2000;342(22):1627–1632.

16. Rutgeerts P, D'Haens G, Targan S, et al. Efficacy and safety of retreatment with anti-tumor necrosis factor antibody (infliximab) to maintain remission in Crohn's disease. *Gastroenterology.* 1999;117(4):761–769.

17. Targan SR, Hanauer SB, van Deventer SJ, et al. A short-term study of chimeric monoclonal antibody cA2 to tumor necrosis factor alpha for Crohn's disease. Crohn's Disease cA2 Study Group. *N Engl J Med.* 1997;337(15):1029–1035.

18. Hanauer SB, Feagan BG, Lichtenstein GR, et al.; ACCENT I Study Group. Maintenance infliximab for Crohn's disease: the ACCENT I randomised trial. *Lancet.* 2002;359(9317):1541–1549.

19. Sands BE, Anderson FH, Bernstein CN, et al. Infliximab maintenance therapy for fistulizing Crohn's disease. *N Engl J Med.* 2004;350(9):876–885.

20. Sandborn WJ, Hanauer SB, Rutgeerts P, et al. Adalimumab for maintenance treatment of Crohn's disease: results of the CLASSIC II trial. *Gut.* 2007;56(9):1232–1239.

21. Hanauer SB, Sandborn WJ, Rutgeerts P, et al. Human anti-tumor necrosis factor monoclonal antibody (adalimumab) in Crohn's disease: the CLASSIC-I trial. *Gastroenterology.* 2006;130(2):323–333.

22. Colombel JF, Sandborn WJ, Rutgeerts P, et al. Adalimumab for maintenance of clinical response and remission in patients with Crohn's disease: the CHARM trial. *Gastroenterology.* 2007;132(1):52–65.

23. Schreiber S, Khaliq-Kareemi M, Lawrance IC, et al.; PRECISE 2 Study Investigators. Maintenance therapy with certolizumab pegol for Crohn's disease. *N Engl J Med.* 2007;357(3):239–250.

24. Sandborn WJ, Feagan BG, Stoinov S, et al.; PRECISE 1 Study Investigators. Certolizumab pegol for the treatment of Crohn's disease. *N Engl J Med.* 2007;357(3):228–238.

25. Sandborn WJ, Colombel JF, Enns R, et al.; International Efficacy of Natalizumab as Active Crohn's Therapy (ENACT-1) Trial Group; Evaluation of Natalizumab as Continuous Therapy (ENACT-2) Trial Group. Natalizumab induction and maintenance therapy for Crohn's disease. *N Engl J Med.* 2005;353(18):1912–1925.

Antiadhesion Therapies | 112

Sukanya Subramanian, Stephen B. Hanauer, and Joseph B. Kirsner

The prevailing treatment paradigm for IBD uses aminosalicylates, corticosteroids, and immunomodulators as first-line therapies with biologics reserved for refractory patients. The disease location, severity, and responsiveness typically guide therapeutic options.[1] With the inception of biologic therapy, "refractory" inflammatory bowel disease has become more treatable with the potential for disease modification.[2] Nevertheless, even with the introduction of biological therapies directed at TNF-α, failure rates approach 30% to 40%, underscoring an unmet need in long-term management.

As the role of T lymphocytes in disease pathogenesis has been recognized, the mechanisms that govern their margination and extravasation into tissue have elucidiated potential approaches for targeted therapies. Lymphocytes are endowed with the ability to dynamically express cell-surface receptors known as integrins, which allow them to accumulate at sites of inflammation. Although integrins are expressed constitutively by circulating leukocytes with low ligand avidity,[3] under inflammatory duress, expression of these adhesion molecules is upregulated[4] to allow leukocyte arrest, firm adhesion, and diapedesis, and thus, enhancing leukocyte penetration into intestinal tissue, where they perpetuate chronic disease activity. Tissue affinity is determined by the specificity of the integrin expressed. The $\alpha_4\beta_7$-integrin recognizes an adhesion molecule receptor that is heterogeneously but pervasively expressed in human tissue; therefore, natalizumab nonselectively interrupts leukocyte egress. Integrins are believed to have pleiotropic functions[5] beyond the effect on leukocyte trafficking, including interference with lymphocyte activation that may rely on adhesion-dependent cell-signal transduction.[6,7]

NATALIZUMAB

Natalizumab (Tysabri, Elan Pharmaceuticals and Biogen Idec) is a partially humanized monoclonal IgG4 antibody engineered to target the alpha-4 constituent of the integrin heterodimer on leukocytes and interrupt adhesion and diapedesis into tissue. The α_4 integrin exists with either β_1 or β_7 integrin and the pairing enables tissue-specific recognition. Preclinical studies in cotton-top tamarins (new-world monkeys) revealed that α_4 blockade led to attenuation of spontaneous colitis, evidenced by both histological improvement and weight gain.[8] A correlative in vivo pharmacologic effect in humans has been the observation of increased circulating leukocytes as a result of α_4-integrin blockade with natalizumab.[9,10]

Data from patients with multiple sclerosis demonstrated that natalizumab has a half-life of 11 days and drug clearance occurs within 60 days or five elimination half-lives. The pharmacokinetic data in Crohn's disease is limited, however, and the half-life appears shorter, ranging from 4.8 to 6.7 days.[9]

A single dose of 3 mg/kg body weight resulted in saturation of 80% of integrin.[11,12] This level of α_4 integrin saturation accomplishes the desired pharmacodynamic effect.[13]

CLINICAL EFFICACY

Gordon et al. conducted a phase II double-blind, placebo-controlled pilot study in 30 patients with mild to moderately active Crohn's disease.[9] A weight-based single dose of natalizumab (3 mg/kg) was administered with a primary end point of change in the CDAI at 2 weeks. Patients who received natalizumab had a significant reduction in the Crohn's Disease Activity Index (CDAI) compared to baseline; however, there was no difference when compared to placebo. Moreover, though the CDAI remained lower, 50% of patients required rescue therapy at 4 weeks. Although the proportion of patients receiving natalizumab who were in clinical remission was numerically greater (39% vs. 8%, $P = 0.1$). The authors reported no significant differences in inflammatory markers at any stage between treatment groups, and the single dose of natalizumab was well tolerated.

In a larger double-blind, placebo-controlled phase II trial, patients receiving 2 doses of natalizumab, 3 mg/kg, 4 weeks apart had significantly greater response and remission compared to placebo. A higher dose of 6 mg/kg did not augment response rates.[14]

ENACT-1 (Evaluation of Natalizumab As Continuous Therapy) was a randomized, placebo-controlled trial designed to measure the efficacy of natalizumab at inducing clinical response and remission in Crohn's disease.[15] A total of 905 patients with moderate-to-severe Crohn's disease (CDAI 220-450) were randomized in a 4:1 ratio to receive either intravenous natalizumab (300-mg fixed dose) or placebo at 4-week intervals for 2 total doses and were then followed for 12 weeks. The primary end point, induction of clinical response (reduction of CDAI by 70 points from baseline) at week 10, was not statistically different (natalizumab vs. placebo groups: 56% vs. 49%, $P = 0.051$). Of note, the placebo response was strikingly high and not anticipated. The secondary end point of clinical remission (CDAI < 150) at 10 weeks was also not statistically different between the two groups (37% vs. 30%, $P = 0.12$). Although the primary end point was not met, when a more conservative definition of clinical response was applied (100-point reduction of CDAI), the difference in outcomes between natalizumab and placebo treatments became statistically significant due to a relative reduction in placebo responders.

Although natalizumab did not meet statistical criteria for induction, post hoc subgroup analysis revealed clinically important information when patients were stratified according to CRP level, concomitant immunosuppressant use, and prior anti-TNF-α treatment.

Stratification of patients on the basis of CRP level unmasked a significant difference in treatment response, suggesting that active disease based on CRP may distinguish patients who are more likely to respond compared with placebo. In addition, patients receiving concomitant immunomodulators were more likely to respond and achieve clinical remissions with natalizumab at week 10 compared to placebo ($P < 0.05$). Furthermore, patients who had failed previous anti-TNF-α therapy had numerically greater remission rates with natalizumab. However, efficacy was not contingent on prior anti-TNF-α use, as the proportion of responders to natalizumab was equal to that in anti-TNF-α-naïve patients (58% vs. 55%), suggesting that natalizumab may be a viable alternative for induction therapy in nonresponders to anti-TNF therapy.

To further explore the induction benefits of natalizumab for patients with active Crohn's disease, the ENCORE trial was designed to investigate the ability of intravenous natalizumab, 300 mg, every 4 weeks to induce clinical response at week 8 sustained through week 12 ($\geq$ 70 point reduction in CDAI) in patients with moderate-to-severe Crohn's disease with an elevated CRP.[16]

A total of 509 patients were randomized to either natalizumab or placebo. A significant inductive benefit was demonstrated at weeks 8 and 12, with 48% of patients achieving a clinical response in the natalizumab group compared to 32% in the placebo group ($P < 0.001$). This effect was seen at 4 weeks after the initial infusion. Furthermore, clinical remission was achieved by a greater percentage of patients in the natalizumab arm, compared to the placebo arm (26% vs. 16%, $P = 0.002$).

ENACT-2 was an extension of ENACT-1 performed to assess the maintenance benefit of natalizumab.[15,17] At the conclusion of ENACT-1, all responders (CDAI reduction $\geq$ 70) to either natalizumab or placebo were rerandomized to either a dose of natalizumab 300 mg, every 4 weeks, or placebo. The primary end point, sustained response through week 36, was significantly better with monthly natalizumab compared to placebo (61% vs. 28%, $P < 0.001$). Furthermore, natalizumab therapy sustained clinical remission at week 36 compared to placebo (44% vs. 26%, $P = 0.003$). The benefit of natalizumab was consistent at various time points along the course of the clinical trial.

Another important end point from this study was the steroid-sparing potential of natalizumab. A greater proportion of patients who attained remission receiving natalizumab were able to discontinue steroids (45% vs. 22%, $P = 0.01$), a benefit that was durable to week 60 (42% vs. 15%, $P = 0.001$).

An open-label extension study for ENACT-2 was conducted by Panaccione et al. to assess the effect of natalizumab in maintaining remission for one additional year for patients who achieved remission after 15 months enrollment in ENACT 1 and 2.[17] The primary aim was to assess long-term safety and tolerability, and the secondary goal was to evaluate efficacy in maintaining remission. Of the 87 patients who were given an uninterrupted dose of natalizumab at 4-week intervals and in remission at the completion of ENACT-2, 93% of them were in remission after 6 months and 86% at the end of 12 additional months. Of the 11 patients in this cohort who previously failed to respond to infliximab, but achieved remission with natalizumab, 82% (9 of 11) remained in remission with continued natalizumab maintenance.

The impact of natalizumab on the health-related quality of life (HRQoL) was assessed among natalizumab responders from ENACT-1 rerandomized to natalizumab versus placebo in ENACT-2.[18] There was substantial improvement in those who continued to receive natalizumab, and the effect was sustained over a period of 48 weeks after maintenance therapy was initiated.

● IMMUNOGENECITY

Immunogenicity with the use of therapeutic proteins has been an important factor relating to long-term efficacy and side effects related to biologic therapy in Crohn's disease.[19] Potential consequences include hypersensitivity reactions, infusion reactions, and treatment resistance. The ENABLE study conducted by Schreiber et al.[15] assessed the immunogenicity of natalizumab in a cohort of patients from ENACT-1 and ENACT-2. They found that overall immunogenicity was low (36 of 319 patients, 11%) and that the rates of antibody positivity were similar between patients receiving continuous natalizumab (6%) and those with an interrupted regimen (9.9%). Of the patients who received natalizumab continuously, 2 out of 150 patients (1.3%) became newly positive for antibodies. Among all patients who received continuous natalizumab, the overall prevalence of antibody positivity was 6% (9/150). The rate of antibody formation in patients who received natalizumab in ENACT-1 with subsequent placebo in ENACT-2 and then reexposed to natalizumab was 9.9% (14 of 141 patients). Furthermore, 11% of patients developed antibodies with reexposure after a 12-month lapse in natalizumab therapy, compared to 4.4% with a less-than-12-month lapse.

The clinical significance of antibody formation is less clear. Remission rates at 12 months with the background of persistent immunogenicity, though not statistically significant, were somewhat lower in patients who had persistent antibodies (37% vs. 43%). Of the 20 patients who were antibody positive in ENACT-1, 9 developed an acute infusion reaction and only 1 patient experienced a severe reaction characterized by chest pain, dyspnea, and sweating. As has been seen with other biologic agents,[19] concomitant immunosuppressive therapy was associated with a lower rate of antibodies to natalizumab. Furthermore, though the development of immunogenicity does not necessarily translate to a loss of clinical inefficacy, the persistence of antibodies over time may have predictive value for the development of treatment resistance. These findings were similar to the incidence and impact of antibodies to natalizumab in multiple sclerosis clinical trials.[20]

ADOLESCENTS

A phase II single-arm study of three monthly infusions of natalizumab (3 mg/kg) was conducted in 31 adolescent patients with moderate-to-severe Crohn's disease.[21] Concomitant medications included immunomodulator therapy (76%), 5-aminosalicyclic acids (58%), and corticosteroids (37%). Safety and tolerability in adolescent patients were found to be comparable to that seen in adults.[22] Immunogenicity rates were also comparably low (8%). Fifteen patients (39%) experienced adverse events related to infection, though no opportunistic infections were observed. Efficacy as an additional objective of this study was found to be similar to that seen in adult patients. Clinical response defined as a ≥15 point reduction in the pediatric CDAI from baseline and clinical remission defined as a pediatric CDAI ≥10 were 55% and 29% with natalizumab or placebo, respectively, at week 10.

SAFETY AND TOLERABILITY

The overall safety profile of natalizumab has been favorable. In phase III trials, adverse reactions were no different between those receiving natalizumab and placebo; however, sample size was a limitation in detecting extremely rare events.[14,15,23]

Sands et al. evaluated the short-term safety and tolerability of combined natalizumab and infliximab in 79 patients with active Crohn's disease (CDAI ≥ 150). The patients were on infliximab for at least 10 weeks and were randomized to receive either natalizumab or placebo every 4 weeks for a total of 3 infusions.[24] Permissible concurrent medications included stable doses of corticosteroids (equivalent to a dose no more than 25-mg prednisone), 5-aminosalicylic acid compounds, oral antibiotics, and immunomodulators (azathioprine, 6-MP, methotrexate). There were no apparent increases in adverse events with the combination therapies in this small trial.

PROGRESSIVE MULTIFOCAL LEUKOENCEPHALOPATHY

The largest source of trepidation surrounding use of natalizumab has been the occurrence of JC-polyoma-virus-associated progressive multifocal leukoencephalopathy (PML). PML is a demyelinating disorder that manifests with a wide variety and degree of neurological derangements. PML classically presents as a triad of progressive dementia, motor disturbance, and visual deficit.[25] The annual risk of PML with natalizumab therapy in multiple sclerosis is approximately 1 in 1000.[26,27] This opportunistic infection can be rapidly progressive and fatal; moreover, efficacious treatment has been elusive. The relationship to number of infusions, concurrent use of immunomodulators, lack of understanding of the virology, and the paucity of other opportunistic infectious complications has made the association complex.[28] Although causality is clear, the mechanism by which natalizumab interferes with viral regulation remains incompletely understood.[29] JC viremia is believed to be a critical event that precedes clinical PML[30]; however, the feasibility of screening for risk stratification remains to be established.

Plasma exchange (PLEX) has been investigated in multiple-sclerosis patients treated with natalizumab to determine whether this intervention can expedite therapeutic monoclonal antibody clearance.[31] The results of the study showed that PLEX decreased α_4-integrin saturation when natalizumab concentrations are reduced to levels below 1 mcg/ml.[31] Peripheral blood mononuclear cell (PBMC) transmigratory capacity increased to 2.2-fold after PLEX, compared to baseline on natalizumab; however, it is unknown whether this intervention will alter the natural course of PML.

As the α_4-integrin heterodimerizes with either the β_1 or β_7 integrin, neutralization results in a nonspecific blockade of leukocyte homing throughout the body, including the central nervous system (CNS). This lack of specificity and compromised immune surveillance is only one plausible contributor to the development of PML, as increases in other opportunistic infections have not been reported. It is interesting that bacterial infections do not appear more commonly with natalizumab use, potentially due to the absence of α_4-integrins on neutrophils and the lesser impact on neutrophil migration compared with lymphocytes.

The risk of PML has significantly affected patient acceptance of natalizumab therapy for Crohn's disease. In a study conducted by Siegel et al.,[32] Patients were asked to consider trade-offs between specific risk and benefits. Estimates of the likelihood of adverse events were presented as absolute risk rather than relative risk. In a survey of 580 patients, the majority (80%) expressed a preference for natalizumab to obtain a clinically important improvement in disease activity. Not surprisingly, there was greater risk aversion associated with more marginal improvements in disease parameters. Nonetheless, the lowest quantification of risk that patients were willing to endure remained higher than published estimates of serious adverse events at all levels. Nevertheless, there has been a poor, overall acceptance for natalizumab among patients (and physicians) demonstrating more subtle aspects of therapeutic decision making.

FDA GUIDELINES

The risk of PML has limited the FDA approval for natalizumab therapy in Crohn's disease to "monotherapy" without additional immunosuppressive therapy.[27] In addition, patients receiving natalizumab are required to have a neurological evaluation at the time of each infusion (TOUCH program).[33] If patients are unable to discontinue corticosteroid therapy within 6 months of initiating natalizumab, discontinuation of the biologic is recommended.[33]

Current experience with natalizumab has not allowed adequate estimations of embryo/fetal risk from maternal exposure during pregnancy. Of the IgG subclasses, there is preferential placental transport for IgG1 over IgG4 (e.g., natalizumab).[34] Animal studies utilizing 2.3 times the clinical dose of natalizumab used in humans revealed hematological abnormalities, including mild anemia, reduced platelet count, and reduced weight of the liver and thymus as well as increased weight of the spleen in the progeny of treated animals.[27] One series of 23 patients who received natalizumab for Crohn's disease reported 12 live births, 6 elective terminations, and 5 spontaneous abortions.[35] It is unknown whether any adverse outcome was attributable to natalizumab. Natalizumab is classified "Class C" for pregnancy by the FDA in the absence of "adequate and well-controlled studies in pregnant women," with the stipulation that natalizumab "should be used during pregnancy only if the potential benefit justifies the potential risk to the fetus."[27]

SUMMARY

Natalizumab is a recombinant, humanized, monoclonal antibody (IgG4) that antagonizes the α_4 constituent of the $\alpha_4\beta_1$ and $\alpha_4\beta_7$ integrin cell-surface-adhesion molecules on leukocytes and nonspecifically interrupts their egress into tissue, affording a novel mechanistic approach to the treatment of inflammatory bowel disease. Currently available data suggest that it is effective in biologic-naïve patients and, uniquely, in patients failing biologic therapy targeting TNF-α. Natalizumab is generally well tolerated, and the small risk of PML must be balanced against the potential benefits when established therapies are ineffective.

FUTURE APPROACHES TO ANTIADHESION THERAPIES

Recognition of the potential for antiadhesion therapy has led to the development of more specific, $\alpha_4\beta_7$ and β_7 inhibitor, as well as other strategies to treat IBD while avoiding potential affects on viral access and activation in the CNS.[36] Large-scale clinical trials for induction and maintenance of remission in both ulcerative colitis and Crohn's disease are nearing completion with vedolizumab, an anti-$\alpha_4\beta_7$ monoclonal antibody that is a modified version of MLN-002.[37] In preliminary trials in ulcerative colitis there appears to be potential for induction of response and remission in ulcerative colitis.

Clinical development of monoclonal antibodies targeting the β_7 component of integrins as well as MadCam inhibition are also being pursued in early-phase trials[33,36] to further attempt gaining specificity of the gut integrins and avoiding the potential inhibition of immune surveillance in the CNS.

An alternative approach to inhibition of leukocyte adhesion has been studied in both ulcerative colitis and Crohn's disease.[38] Alicaforsen, a human ICAM-1 antisense oligonucleotide, blocks ICAM-1 production by disabling target RNA molecules and blocking the translation of protein. This alters the local inflammatory reaction in the intestinal wall. Early studies with alicaforsen as topical (enema) therapy in ulcerative colitis have been difficult to interpret, though there does appear to be some therapeutic potential that remains to be optimized and formulated in future clinical trials.[39]

CONCLUSIONS

Antiadhesion strategies have had demonstrable benefits in the treatment of Crohn's disease and have demonstrated promise in ulcerative colitis. Natalizumab therapy has been efficacious as an inductive and maintenance treatment for patients with refractory Crohn's disease whether or not they had responded to anti-TNF therapies. However, the acceptance within the GI and patient communities has been hampered by the rare, but devastating, complication of PML. Novel approaches to the targeting of adhesion molecules are currently underway with the hope of harnessing effective and gut-specific inhibition of leukocyte trafficking.

References

1. Lichtenstein GR, Hanauer SB, Sandborn WJ. Management of Crohn's disease in adults. *Am J Gastroenterol.* 2009;104(2):465–483; quiz 464, 484.
2. Vermeire S, van Assche G, Rutgeerts P. Review article: altering the natural history of Crohn's disease—evidence for and against current therapies. *Aliment Pharmacol Ther.* 2007;25(1):3–12.
3. Stewart M, Thiel M, Hogg N. Leukocyte integrins. *Curr Opin Cell Biol.* 1995;7(5):690–696.
4. Stewart M, Hogg N. Regulation of leukocyte integrin function: affinity vs. avidity. *J Cell Biochem.* 1996;61(4):554–561.
5. Clark EA, Brugge JS. Integrins and signal transduction pathways: the road taken. *Science.* 1995;268(5208):233–239.
6. Lobb RR, Hemler ME. The pathophysiologic role of alpha 4 integrins in vivo. *J Clin Invest.* 1994;94(5):1722–1728.
7. Bayless KJ, Meininger GA, Scholtz JM, Davis GE. Osteopontin is a ligand for the alpha4beta1 integrin. *J Cell Sci.* 1998;111 (Pt 9): 1165–1174.
8. Podolsky DK, Lobb R, King N, et al. Attenuation of colitis in the cotton-top tamarin by anti-alpha 4 integrin monoclonal antibody. *J Clin Invest.* 1993;92(1):372–380.
9. Gordon FH, Lai CW, Hamilton MI, et al. A randomized placebo-controlled trial of a humanized monoclonal antibody to alpha4 integrin in active Crohn's disease. *Gastroenterology.* 2001;121(2):268–274.
10. Gordon FH, Amlot PL. The Effect of natalizumab, a humanized monoclonal antibody to the alpha 4 integrin on circulating activated leukocytes in active inflammatory bowel disease (IBD). *Gastroenterology.* 2002;122:A434.
11. Miller DH, Khan OA, Sheremata WA, et al. A controlled trial of natalizumab for relapsing multiple sclerosis. *N Engl J Med.* 2003;348(1):15–23.
12. Sheremata WA, Vollmer TL, Stone LA, Willmer-Hulme AJ, Koller M. A safety and pharmacokinetic study of intravenous natalizumab in patients with MS. *Neurology.* 1999;52(5):1072–1074.
13. Bennet D, Ludden T, Shah J, Floren L, Beckman E. The use of pharmacokinetic (PK) modeling and efficacy data to establish optimal dosing of natalizumab (abstract P130). *Multiple Sclerosis.* 2002;8(suppl): S61.

14. Ghosh S, Goldin E, Gordon FH, et al. Natalizumab for active Crohn's disease. *N Engl J Med.* 2003;348(1):24–32.

15. Sandborn WJ, Colombel JF, Enns R, et al. Natalizumab induction and maintenance therapy for Crohn's disease. *N Engl J Med.* 2005;353(18):1912–1925.

16. Targan SR, Feagan BG, Fedorak RN, et al. Natalizumab for the treatment of active Crohn's disease: results of the ENCORE Trial. *Gastroenterology.* 2007;132:1672–1683.

17. Panaccione R, Colombel J, EnnsR, et al. Natalizumab maintains remission for 2 years in patients with moderately to severely active Crohn's disease and in those with prior infliximab exposure: results from an Open-label Extension Study. *Am J Gastroenterol.* 2006;101:Abstract.

18. Feagan BG, Sandborn WJ, Hass S, Niecko T, White J. Health-related quality of life during natalizumab maintenance therapy for Crohn's disease. *Am J Gastroenterol.* 2007;102(12):2737–2746.

19. Clark M, Colombel JF, Feagan BC, et al. American gastroenterological association consensus development conference on the use of biologics in the treatment of inflammatory bowel disease, June 21–23, 2006. *Gastroenterology.* 2007;133(1):312–339.

20. Calabresi PA, Giovannoni G, Confavreux C, et al. The incidence and significance of anti-natalizumab antibodies: results from AFFIRM and SENTINEL. *Neurology.* 2007;69:1391–1403.

21. Hyams JS, Wilson DC, Thomas A, et al. Natalizumab therapy for moderate to severe Crohn disease in adolescents. *J Pediatr Gastroenterol Nutr.* 2007;44(2):185–191.

22. Grundy J, Pan W-J, Kugathasan S, et al. Pharmacokinetics and pharmacodynamics of natalizumab in a phase 2 study of adolescent patients with Crohn's disease: 147. *J Pediatr Gastroenterol Nutrition.* 2005;41(4):538.

23. Targan SR, Feagan BG, Fedorak RN, et al. Natalizumab for the treatment of active Crohn's disease: results of the ENCORE Trial. *Gastroenterology.* 2007;132(5):1672–1683.

24. Sands BE, Kozarek R, Spainhour J, et al. Safety and tolerability of concurrent natalizumab treatment for patients with Crohn's disease not in remission while receiving infliximab. *Inflamm Bowel Dis.* 2007;13(1):2–11.

25. Major EO, Amemiya K, Tornatore CS, Houff SA, Berger JR. Pathogenesis and molecular biology of progressive multifocal leukoencephalopathy, the JC virus-induced demyelinating disease of the human brain. *Clin Microbiol Rev.* 1992;5(1):49–73.

26. Yousry TA, Major EO, Ryschkewitsch C, et al. Evaluation of patients treated with natalizumab for progressive multifocal leukoencephalopathy. *N Engl J Med.* 2006;354(9):924–933.

27. Tysabri. Package Insert. Biogen Idec and Elan Pharmaceuticals.

28. Tan CS, Koralnik IJ. Progressive multifocal leukoencephalopathy and other disorders caused by JC virus: clinical features and pathogenesis. *Lancet Neurol.* 2010;9(4):425–437.

29. Berger JR. Progressive multifocal leukoencephalopathy and newer biological agents. *Drug Saf.* 2010;33(11):969–983.

30. Van Assche G, Van Ranst M, Sciot R, et al. Progressive multifocal leukoencephalopathy after natalizumab therapy for Crohn's disease. *N Engl J Med.* 2005;353(4):362–368.

31. Khatri BO, Man S, Giovannoni G, et al. Effect of plasma exchange in accelerating natalizumab clearance and restoring leukocyte function. *Neurology.* 2009;72(5):402–409.

32. Johnson FR, Ozdemir S, Mansfield C, et al. Crohn's disease patients' risk-benefit preferences: serious adverse event risks versus treatment efficacy. *Gastroenterology.* 2007;133:769–779.

33. Stefanelli T, Malesci A, De La Rue SA, Danese S. Anti-adhesion molecule therapies in inflammatory bowel disease: touch and go. *Autoimmun Rev.* 2008;7(5):364–369.

34. Garty BZ, Ludomirsky A, Danon YL, Peter JB, Douglas SD. Placental transfer of immunoglobulin G subclasses. *Clin Diagn Lab Immunol.* 1994;1(6):667–669.

35. Bozic C, Belcher G, Kooijmans M, et al. The safety of natalizumab in patients with relapsing multiple sclerosis: an update from TOUCH and TYGRIS. *Neurology.* 2007;68(suppl 3):A111.

36. Bosani M, Ardizzone S, Porro GB. Biologic targeting in the treatment of inflammatory bowel diseases. *Biologics.* 2009;3:77–97.

37. Behm BW, Bickston SJ. Humanized antibody to the alpha4beta7 integrin for induction of remission in ulcerative colitis. *Cochrane Database Syst Rev.* 2009(1): p. CD007571.

38. Barish CF. Alicaforsen therapy in inflammatory bowel disease. *Expert Opin Biol Ther.* 2005;5(10):1387–1391.

39. Miner PB Jr, Wedel MK, Xia S, Baker BF. Safety and efficacy of two dose formulations of alicaforsen enema compared with mesalazine enema for treatment of mild to moderate left-sided ulcerative colitis: a randomized, double-blind, active-controlled trial. *Aliment Pharmacol Ther.* 2006;23(10):1403–1413.

Crohn's Disease in Children and Adolescents | 113

Judith Kelsen, Anna Hunter, and Robert N. Baldassano

This chapter focuses on pediatric approaches to inflammatory bowel disease (IBD) therapy. The indications for use of 5-aminosalicylic acids, antibiotics like metronidazole and ciprofloxacin, and probiotics in the pediatric population are generally similar as in the adult population. The differences in therapy include the use of enteral therapy as primary treatment in children as well as indications for starting biologic and immunomodulatory agents. Those treatment approaches will be discussed here.

⬤ ENTERAL THERAPY

Around 25% of patients with IBD present in childhood, most commonly with evidence of growth retardation. Alarmingly, more than a quarter of these children will suffer permanent growth stunting. One major goal of pediatric medicine is set, therefore, to ensure children reach their optimum height and avoid any nutritional deficit as is commonplace in this severe disease.

The etiology of growth failure in Crohn's disease (CD) is multifactorial. Inflammation is involved with documented elevated proinflammatory cytokines (e.g., interleukin [IL]-1, IL-6, and tumor necrosis factor [TNF]-α) in young patients. Corticosteroids—used to induce remission of CD—target this inflammation but include significant iatrogenic side effects such as osteoporosis and premature closure of bone growth plates exacerbating growth failure. Finally, malabsorption associated with CD causes nutritional height disparities. Together these factors can be quite devastating; 1 in 5 will suffer from a significant reduction in final adult height.

The question then becomes, "how is one to achieve a prompt and steroid-free induction of remission?" Exclusive enteral nutrition (EEN) is a potent and now accepted addition to the armamentarium of Crohn's therapy. In contrast to corticosteroids, EEN does not adversely affect growth.[1] Despite its preferential use in Europe and Canada, EEN still is not widely employed in the United States. Lack of large-scale studies and established effective treatment regimens and poor compliance hinder EEN acceptance in American pediatrics.

Editor's note (TMB): There is a separate chapter on this topic.

Remission Induction

When analyzing the efficacy of IBD treatments, two factors are taken into consideration: induction and maintenance of remission. To date, two Cochrane reviews—one in 2001 and one in 2007—determined that based on available recent studies enteral therapy is not as effective as steroids in induction of remission.[2,3] These Cochrane reviews also showed that there was inadequate data to perform a subgroup analyses by age, disease duration, and disease location. The 2007 review, in particular, found that meta-analysis of six trials including 192 patients treated with enteral nutrition (EN) and 160 treated with steroids yielded a pooled odds ratio (OR) of 0.33 favoring steroid therapy (95% confidence interval [CI] 0.21–0.53). A sensitivity analysis resulted in an increase in the number of participants to 212 in the EN group and 179 in the steroid group but did little to alter the results (OR 0.36; 95% CI 0.23–0.56). Unfortunately, the results of the Cochrane reviews are only as good as the studies that have been performed and evaluated and since that time other studies have increased the amount of data in favor of enteral therapy and also on the components of what makes for successful enteral therapy.

Formula Ingredients

The Cochrane study also looked at comparison of formula ingredients including type of protein and fat content in patients. Of the 10 trials comprising 334 patients examined, there was no reported difference in elemental versus nonelemental formulas. Subgroup analysis comparing elemental versus nonelemental (elemental, semi-elemental, and polymeric) also showed no difference. Further analysis of seven trials including 209 patients treated with EN formulas of differing fat content (low fat < 20 g/1000 kCal versus high fat > 20 g/1000 kCal) demonstrated no statistically significant difference in efficacy (OR 1.13; 95% CI 0.63–2.01). Similarly, the effect of very low fat content (<3 g/1000 kCal) or type of fat (long-chain triglycerides) was investigated, but did not demonstrate a difference in the treatment outcomes of active CD—although a nonsignificant trend was demonstrated favoring very low fat and very low long-chain triglyceride content.

Several Studies Achieved Remission

Multiple studies not included in the Cochrane review have demonstrated that exclusive nutritional therapy, consisting of the administration of enteral formula (polymeric, semi-elemental, or elemental formula) for a period of no less than 6 to 8 weeks, is effective in inducing clinical remission in children with CD. The clinical remission, however, does not always include histologic evidence of remission, with specimens often having signs of inflammation. One prospective study of 14 patients with CD demonstrated that fecal calprotectin levels, an inflammation marker, were reduced after 8 weeks of an exclusive diet of polymeric formula. In addition, almost three-quarters achieved clinical remission by this nutritional modification at 4 weeks of diet modification. Ultimately, 85% of patients were documented to be in clinical remission and had significantly reduced fecal calprotectin levels only 8 weeks into the study.[4]

In a retrospective study, 26 children (15 with a new diagnosis of CD and 12 with long-standing disease) who were exclusively fed a polymeric formula were evaluated. Analysis showed that all newly diagnosed children treated with exclusive enteral therapy achieved remission after 8 weeks of treatment. Four children continued supplementation and remained in remission a year after therapy was initiated.[5] As more evidence, a prospective study with 110 children with Crohn's treated with EEN as a primary therapy boasted a high remission rate, a reduction in inflammatory markers, and significant improvements in patients' weight and body mass index Z-scores. In this study, there was no significant variation in the response to treatment based on disease phenotype.[6] A retrospective study of 37 children treated with enteral therapy with elemental, semi-elemental, and polymeric formulas compared to 10 children who received steroids alone showed similar clinical remission rate after 8 weeks of treatment: 86.5% children receiving nutritional therapy versus 90% treated with corticosteroids. Improvement in mucosal inflammation occurred in 26 out of 37 (64.8%) patients on nutritional therapy and in 4 out of 10 (40%) children on steroids alone ($P < 0.05$). In addition, examination of mucosal healing showed supportive results for nutritional therapy versus steroids (7 vs. 0, $P < 0.005$). The study concluded that enteral therapy was more effective than corticosteroids in improving nutritional status, linear growth recovery, and the duration of clinical remission. Formulary differences were excluded as confounding the results.[7]

Remission Maintenance

Maintenance of remission is a vital component in the evaluation of therapeutic options. Yamamoto et al. conducted a review of studies using EN as primary therapy. The study was designed to evaluate the efficacy of EN for the maintenance of remission in patients with CD who achieved medically or surgically induced remission. Ten studies were included: one randomized controlled trial, three prospective nonrandomized trials, and six retrospective studies. Elemental, semi-elemental, or polymeric diets were used as an oral supplement or a nocturnal tube feeding augmentation to standard diet. Comparing outcomes between patients who received EN and those who did not, the clinical remission rate was significantly higher in those with EN in all seven studies. In two studies, EN showed suppressive effects on endoscopic disease activity. In all four studies investigating impacts of the quantity of enteral formula on clinical remission, higher amounts of enteral formula were associated with higher remission rates: ≥30 kcal/kg ideal body weight/ day (vs. <30 kcal/kg ideal body weight/day), ≥1200 kcal/day (vs. <1200 kcal/day), and ≥1600 kcal/day (vs. <1600 kcal/day). The review concluded that although the evidence level is not high, the available data suggests that EN may be useful for maintaining remission in patients with CD.[8,9]

Certainly, with the known evidence, there exists multiple arguments for using enteral therapy, but how does one use it correctly in the clinical setting? Multiple studies show achievement of disease remission with a 6-to-10-week treatment; however, guidelines for the maintenance therapy are still lacking. European colleagues suggest EEN with an elemental, semi-elemental, or polymeric formula for 4 to 12 weeks for disease remission, followed by a 4-week cycle every 3 to 4 months.

The poor palatability of the formula, however, may result in poor adherence and require the use of nasogastric tube feedings. Also, the minimal percentage of caloric intake from EN required to control disease remains to be determined. Using EN for 1 month every 4 months over a period of 20 months showed a statistically significant benefit on growth compared to use of alternate-day prednisolone. Similar effects were shown by other authors who noted better growth in children treated with EN than steroids within 1 year of study onset.[1]

Exact mechanisms by which enteral therapy works are not completely understood. Studies in mice with induced colitis treated with enteral therapy showed a multitude of changes. It seems that elemental diet reduced the number of colonic bacteria and changed microbial balance within murine intestine. This change led to an increase in acetic and propionic acid levels. Both compounds are short-chain fatty acids believed to have anti-inflammatory properties. Interestingly, TNF-α, IL-6, and amyloid A (markers of inflammation) were reduced in experimental groups, and histopathological analysis of the colonic tissue showed reduction of inflammation.[10]

Finally, in regard to EN mechanism of action, stool analysis of six children with CD treated with exclusive enteral therapy for 8 weeks showed significant changes in intestinal microbiome composition. This alteration in intestinal microbiome balance appeared to partially persist for up to 4 months after discontinuation of treatment. The change in the composition of Bacteroides, for one, was noted to be associated with reduced disease activity and inflammation. Similar animal studies concluded that EEN reduces bacterial diversity and initiates a sustained modulation of all predominant intestinal bacterial groups. EEN may reduce inflammation through modulating intestinal Bacteroides species.[11] EEN alone down regulates proinflammatory cytokines and may partly improve growth by reducing IL-6, a potent inhibitor of insulin growth factor-1 (IGF-1).[12] A dramatic reduction in C-reactive protein, with concomitant increase in IGF-1 and IGFBP-3, was noted within 14 days of commencing EN.[9]

There is limited evidence of the direct benefits of EN on long-term growth; however, almost all the available clinical trials reach a similar conclusion. A meta-analysis showed equal efficacy between EN and corticosteroids and suggested a statistically significant benefit on growth of EN over corticosteroids.

IMMUNOMODULATORY AGENTS

Azathioprine and 6-mercaptopurine (6-MP) are, increasingly, being used in children with CD. In 1990 Verhave et al. demonstrated partial or complete clinical remission in 75% of patients with CD or ulcerative colitis who were treated with azathioprine. In addition, most of the patients who responded to this drug were able to discontinue corticosteroids within 6 months of starting azathioprine.[13,14] Markowitz et al. also demonstrated a significant reduction in steroid use for patients who received 6-MP. He reported that 57% of patients were able to discontinue corticosteroids within 6 months and 80% within 1 year of the initiation of 6-MP.[15] In 2000, Markowitz et al. published the first randomized, placebo-controlled trial evaluating the early use of 6-MP in newly diagnosed pediatric patients with moderate to severe CD. His group found a significantly shorter duration of steroid use and lower cumulative steroid dose at 6, 12, and 18 months among patients who received 6-MP versus placebo. Although remission was initially induced in 89% of both groups, only 9% of patients maintained on 6-MP relapsed whereas 47% of controls relapsed. Long-term remission at 18 months was 89% in the 6-MP group versus 39% in the placebo group.[16]

Given the known side effects of the use of this class of medications including both allergic (pancreatitis, arthralgias, rash, and fever) and nonallergic reactions (leukopenia, thrombocytopenia, infection, hepatitis, and malignancy), safety remains a concern when prescribing this drug to pediatric patients. Kirschner reported that 28% of 95 pediatric patients who received 6-MP or azathioprine had some side effects (most commonly elevated aminotransferase levels) and that cessation of the drug occurred in 18% of patients because of drug hypersensitivity or infection.[17] Other retrospective studies demonstrated mild side effects including leukopenia and elevated aminotransferases in almost 40% of pediatric patients.[13] Immunomodulators are generally well tolerated although the potential for long-term exposure and the possibility of malignancy are a concern.[18] The risks of immunomodulators are contrasted with the benefits of steroid sparing in vulnerable pediatric patients.[19]

Although the Markowitz study recommended the early use of 6-MP or azathioprine for all newly diagnosed pediatric patients with moderate to severe CD, clearer guidelines for selected use have not been reported. In a study by Jacobstein et al. it was found that patients with lower serum albumin at diagnosis (3.1 g/dL vs. 3.75 g/dL) and higher Pediatric Crohn's Disease Activity Index (PCDAI) at diagnosis (40 vs. 24) were significantly more likely to be started on immunomodulators. In addition, all patients with serum albumin 2.8 g/dL or less were placed on immunomodulators within 6 months of diagnosis versus only 45% of patients with serum albumin of 2.9 g/dL or greater.[20]

Grossman et al. found that in patients younger than 5 years, higher doses are required in order to induce and maintain remission. These patients often required 3 mg/kg or greater.[21]

Methotrexate

Limited studies exist evaluating the use of methotrexate in pediatric IBD. In the only published full study to date assessing clinical outcomes with subcutaneous methotrexate, Mack et al. established clinical efficacy with this medication. In a study of 14 patients with steroid-dependent CD who failed or did not tolerate 6-MP, 9 (64%) demonstrated improvement within 4 weeks of initiation of therapy.[22]

Side effects including gastrointestinal problems (nausea, anorexia, and diarrhea), headaches, dizziness, fatigue, and mood changes have been reported. In addition, leukopenia, thrombocytopenia, pulmonary toxicity, and opportunistic infections are also possible. Hepatotoxicity, although still a concern, is less common than once thought.[13] Recent data in pediatrics suggests that oral methotrexate may be better tolerated and has similar bioavailability to the subcutaneous form.[23]

BIOLOGIC THERAPY: ANTI-TNF ANTIBODY

Treatment with anti-TNFα antibody, infliximab, has greatly changed the therapeutic approach in both adult and pediatric CD. Several anti-TNFα therapies, in addition to infliximab, have been approved for the use of moderate to severe CD and ulcerative colitis. These include adalimumab and certolizumab. Infliximab is thus far the only one of the medications approved for the use of medical refractory CD in pediatrics. Infliximab is a chimeric monoclonal IgG-1 TNFα antibody. Its composition is 75% a human constant, and 25% is composed of a murine variable region.[24] TNFα is a proinflammatory cytokine. Evidence has demonstrated that there is increased number of TNF-producing cells in the lamina propria of patients with CD.[25] Infliximab is an effective therapy through several mechanisms. It neutralizes TNF, blocks leukocyte migration, and induces apoptosis of T lymphocytes and monocytes.[26] It is administered intravenously with three 5 mg/kg doses to comprise the induction schedule at weeks 0, 2, and 6. It is then administered as maintenance therapy every 8 to 12 weeks. The second agent, adalimumab, is a humanized IgG-4 anti-TNFα antibody. It is administered subcutaneously every other week. In adults, the first two doses are loading doses of 160 and 80 mg, respectively, followed by a maintenance dose of 40 mg. Certolizumab is a humanized PEGylated Fab[1] fragment of a monoclonal anti-TNFα antibody. It is administered subcutaneously once a month, at a dose of 400 mg in adults.

Infliximab was first approved for the treatment of adults with CD in 1998 and for pediatrics in 2006. It was approved for the use of ulcerative colitis in adults in 2005. Adalimumab was approved for adults with CD in 2007 and certolizumab was approved for CD in 2008. Natalizumab is a humanized monoclonal antibody against the cellular adhesion molecule α4-integrin. It was approved in 2008 for the treatment of adult CD in the United States, but is being monitored closely because of potential progressive multifocal leukoencephalopathy.

Infliximab

The first pediatric trial was completed in 1998, in an open-label multicenter trial. Twenty-one patients were divided into three groups and received infliximab at three doses—1, 5, and 10 mg/kg per dose as a single infusion.[27] Response was defined as improvement in the PCDAI of equal or more than 10 points. Clinical remission was defined as PCDAI of less than 10. All patients demonstrated approximately 50% improvement in

PCDAI by week 2. All patients achieved clinical response, and 10 children achieved clinical remission.[27-29] The REACH study (Randomized, multicentered, open-label study to evaluate the safety and efficacy of anti-TNF alpha chimeric monoclonal antibody in pediatric subjects with moderate to severe CD) evaluated the safety and efficacy of infliximab in pediatric CD, which was published in 2007.[27] This study evaluated 112 patients, ranging in age from 6 to 17 years of age with median disease duration of 1. 6 years, with moderate to severe CD (defined by PCDAI > 30). Patients were required to be on concurrent immunomodulator therapy. All patients received three induction doses at weeks 0, 2, and 6 of 5 mg/kg per dose. Patients who responded were then randomized at week 10 to receive infliximab every 8 weeks or every 12 weeks for a total of 46 weeks. Patients who lost response to 5 mg/kg every 8 or 12 weeks were allowed to cross over to receive 10 mg/kg, and patients who lost response in the every-12-week group were crossed over to 5 or 10 mg/kg dose every 8 weeks depending on when they lost response (before or after the 8 weeks). Patients were clinically followed through week 54. The primary end point was clinical response at week 10, defined by decrease in PCDAI score from baseline by 15 points or more, and total PCDAI of 30 points or less. The results of the trial demonstrated an overall response rate of 88% and remission rate of 59% at week 10. At week 54, a statistically higher proportion of patients receiving infliximab every 8 weeks achieved clinical response and clinical remission of 63.5% and 56%, respectively. This is in contrast to the every-12-week group who achieved 33% response and 23.5% remission. Adverse events were comparable in both groups.

Ulcerative Colitis and Infliximab

In pediatric ulcerative colitis, initial reports included two small case series with a total of 17 patients of which 14 responded including all five patients with fulminant colitis.[30,31] Subsequently, a later study including 27 pediatric patients was published and confirmed these results. Two further studies were published; the first study included 40 patients and up to 36 months of follow-up. The second trial included 22 patients and demonstrated efficacy in steroid-resistant or steroid-dependent pediatric ulcerative colitis.

Adalimumab in CD

A recent study, Retrospective Evaluation of the Safety and Effect of Adalimumab Therapy (RESEAT), was published that evaluated the pediatric experience with adalimumab. It included 115 patients from 12 centers. Patients had received at least one dose and were followed up for 12 months. Clinical remission and response was based on the PCDAI as well as the physician global assessment (PGA). Response was defined as decrease of the PGA from moderate/severe to mild/inactive, or from mild to inactive. Remission was defined as a PGA of inactive. Response in the PCDAI was defined when a PCDAI > 30 decreased to ≥15. Remission was defined as a PCDAI of ≤10. Ninety-five percent of patients had prior infliximab exposure. Majority of patients discontinued infliximab secondary to infusion reactions, loss of response, or preference for subcutaneous injections. All patients received adalimumab on an every-other-week schedule. The first

two doses were considered induction doses. Nineteen percent of patients received 160 mg followed by 80 mg as the induction dose. Forty-one percent of patients received induction doses of 80 mg followed 2 weeks later by 40 mg. Seventeen percent patients received 40 mg for both induction doses. In regard to maintenance, 85% of patients continued on 40 mg every other week, whereas 12% were initiated on 40 mg weekly. Five percent received 80 mg weekly, and 4% received 20 mg weekly. During the course of the trial period, 25% of patients had the dose increased, 93% of these patients achieved this escalation through weekly scheduling of the drug administration. The remaining two patients were already receiving weekly 40-mg injections, and therefore increased to 80 mg weekly. Results demonstrated that within 3 months of initiation of therapy mean PCDAI decreased 63% and percentage of patients with inactive or mild disease increased from 14% to 82%. These improvements were sustained at 6 and 12 month follow-ups.

There are currently no reports on the use of certolizumab in pediatric IBD, but a large prospective trial is ongoing.

There is only one published trial of natalizumab in pediatric CD, and this was in 31 adolescents who received three intravenous 3 mg/kg infusions. Clinical response was defined by decrease in baseline PCDAI by 15 points and remission was defined as PCDAI ≤ 10. This was greatest seen in week 10, with response of 55% and remission of 29%. However, this medication has been limited in pediatrics due to the concern of the adverse effect of progressive multifocal leukoencephalopathy.

Growth Rate Improvement

Growth failure is a significant challenge in pediatric IBD. Several studies, including REACH, have demonstrated the positive effect of infliximab on growth and bone strength on patients with CD. This effect can be seen as early as 6 months after initiating treatment. The REACH trial evaluated the effect of linear growth prospectively. One subgroup of 38 patients with at least a delay of 1 year in bone age (measured by bone x-ray) at the start of the trial demonstrated an improvement in mean height Z score from −1.5 to +0.3 from week 0 to week 30 and to 0.5 at week 54. This benefit was greater in those patients receiving infliximab on an every-8-week schedule.[32]

Safety

The three main categories of concern in regard to infliximab include infusion reactions, infectious complications, and the risk of malignancy. Infusion reactions are due to the formation of antibodies to the murine portion of the drug. The antibodies are associated with acute infusion reactions, loss of response, and delayed hypersensitivity reactions.[33] The largest pediatric series describing infliximab use in the pediatric population included six centers in which 243 patients received 1652 infusion.[20] Similar to the adult data, there was a 3.6% rate of infusion reactions in 16.5% of patients seen. Acute infusion reactions include shortness of breath, urticaria, palpitations, headache, flushing, and hypotension. Pretreatment with antipyretics, corticosteroids, or antihistamines did not prevent the occurrence of infusion reactions. However, premedication did prevent further reactions once an infusion reaction took place. Although infusion reactions are not indications to stop therapy, often treatment is changed to adalimumab. Delayed infusion reactions, or serum sickness, occur 4 to 9 days after an infusion and are characterized by arthralgias, skin rash, myalgias, fever, and leukocytosis. It is a rare reaction, occurring in approximately 0% to 3% of the patients who receive infliximab. These patients require aggressive treatment with 5 days of oral corticosteroids administered before infliximab infusions for 2 to 3 days. However, most patients benefit from changing to another anti-TNF.[33–38] Recent studies in pediatrics have focused on the role that human antichimeric antibodies (HACA otherwise known as antibodies to infliximab or ATI) play in infusion reactions and efficacy of the medication. Miele et al. evaluated the role that HACA plays in infusion reactions and found that they occurred in higher proportions in patients who were HACA positive than those who were HACA negative. In addition, they found that patients with HACA levels above 8.0 µg/mL were more likely to have infusion reactions, and that concomitant immunomodulator use was associated with a lower risk of developing HACA.[34]

There have been reports of infectious complications with the use of infliximab as well as other anti-TNFα therapies. In the largest pediatric infliximab trial, the rate of infections was 3.9% and consisted mainly of upper respiratory infections. There have been more serious infections documented as well, such as pneumonia, herpes zoster, and abscesses.[39] All patients are screened for tuberculosis prior to starting therapy.

The most significant concern that exists with the anti-TNF therapy, and for all therapy that is used for IBD today, is the risk of malignancy. Currently, the Food and Drug Administration has issued a drug warning label for infliximab and Humira due to this risk. A meta-analysis of the nine trials including 3493 patients who received either infliximab or adalimumab showed pooled OR for malignancy of 3.3.[40] Of 26 malignancies, 10 were lymphomas. This analysis demonstrated that malignancies tended to occur in those patients who were treated with higher doses. However the data is conflicting. It has been difficult to establish the malignancy risk of these agents and the inherent risk of cancer in patients with IBD as well as the risk of dual therapy with immunomodulators. Rare cases of hepatosplenic T-cell lymphoma have been reported; all of the cases occurred in patients on concomitant treatment with 6-MP or azathioprine.

Editor's note (TMB): There is a chapter on the effect of hepatosplenic T-cell lymphoma on decision making in young patients.

Combination Therapy

The role of early top-down infliximab or immunomodulators in steroid-naïve children with CD[41] or infliximab monotherapy in children with CD exposed to steroids[42] needs to be evaluated in light of the recent adult trials showing treatment efficacy and a reduced need for steroids in patients taking these agents.

There has been recent evidence in the adult population that early aggressive intervention yields better results than the traditional "step-up" approach. A 2-year multicenter prospective trial of 133 patients were randomized to a top-down treatment in which they received three infliximab treatments and azathioprine, or traditional corticosteroids followed by an immunomodulator or infliximab therapy.[41] The conclusion of the study was that early treatment with infliximab and azathioprine was more effective than conventional therapy for induction of therapy, as well as for decreased use of steroids. A second adult trial, SONIC (Study of Patients with Crohn's Disease Naïve to Immunomodulators and Biologic Therapy) trial, compared infliximab alone, infliximab plus azathioprine, and azathioprine alone in adult patients with CD.[29] The study concluded that combination therapy with infliximab and azathioprine together was more effective than either therapy used alone. It also demonstrated that infliximab as monotherapy was superior to azathioprine when used as monotherapy.

Editor's note (TMB): The REACH study in pediatric patients with recent onset also included immunomodulator therapy at the outset.

In pediatrics, it is critical that a long-term prospective trial is conducted in order to assess the safety and efficacy of the top-down approach, as well as monotherapy versus dual therapy treatments. Early use of biologic therapy as monotherapy may decrease the risk of hepatosplenic T-cell lymphoma, which, thus far, has only been reported in patients treated with dual therapy or with azathioprine alone. In addition, the use of anti-TNF therapy has demonstrated improvement in bone health strength as well as growth. As the fields of genomics, metagenomics, and the microbiome expand, it is our hope that the goal of patient-targeted therapy will become more realistic.

References

1. Heuschkel R, Salvestrini C, Beattie RM, Hildebrand H, Walters T, Griffiths A. Guidelines for the management of growth failure in childhood inflammatory bowel disease. *Inflamm Bowel Dis.* 2008;14(6):839–849.

2. Zachos M, Tondeur M, Griffiths AM. Enteral nutritional therapy for inducing remission of Crohn's disease. *Cochrane Database Syst Rev.* 2001;(3):CD000542.

3. Zachos M, Tondeur M, Griffiths AM. Enteral nutritional therapy for induction of remission in Crohn's disease. *Cochrane Database Syst Rev.* 2007;(1):CD000542.

4. Navas López VM, Blasco Alonso J, Sierra Salinas C, Barco Gálvez A, Vicioso Recio MI. Efficacy of exclusive enteral feeding as primary therapy for paediatric Crohn's disease. *An Pediatr (Barc).* 2008;69(6):506–514.

5. Day AS, Whitten KE, Lemberg DA, et al. Exclusive enteral feeding as primary therapy for Crohn's disease in Australian children and adolescents: a feasible and effective approach. *J Gastroenterol Hepatol.* 2006;21(10):1609–1614.

6. Buchanan E, Gaunt WW, Cardigan T, Garrick V, McGrogan P, Russell RK. The use of exclusive enteral nutrition for induction of remission in children with Crohn's disease demonstrates that disease phenotype does not influence clinical remission. *Aliment Pharmacol Ther.* 2009;30(5):501–507.

7. Berni Canani R, Terrin G, Borrelli O, et al. Short- and long-term therapeutic efficacy of nutritional therapy and corticosteroids in paediatric Crohn's disease. *Dig Liver Dis.* 2006;38(6):381–387.

8. Yamamoto T, Nakahigashi M, Umegae S, Matsumoto K. Enteral nutrition for the maintenance of remission in Crohn's disease: a systematic review. *Eur J Gastroenterol Hepatol.* 2010;22(1):1–8.

9. Fell JM, Paintin M, Arnaud-Battandier F, et al. Mucosal healing and a fall in mucosal pro-inflammatory cytokine mRNA induced

by a specific oral polymeric diet in paediatric Crohn's disease. *Aliment Pharmacol Ther.* 2000;14(3):281–289.

10. Kajiura T, Takeda T, Sakata S, et al. Change of intestinal microbiota with elemental diet and its impact on therapeutic effects in a murine model of chronic colitis. *Dig Dis Sci.* 2009;54(9):1892–1900.

11. Leach ST, Mitchell HM, Eng WR, Zhang L, Day AS. Sustained modulation of intestinal bacteria by exclusive enteral nutrition used to treat children with Crohn's disease. *Aliment Pharmacol Ther.* 2008;28(6):724–733.

12. Bannerjee K, Camacho-Hübner C, Babinska K, et al. Anti-inflammatory and growth-stimulating effects precede nutritional restitution during enteral feeding in Crohn disease. *J Pediatr Gastroenterol Nutr.* 2004;38(3):270–275.

13. Escher JC, Taminiau JA, Nieuwenhuis EE, Büller HA, Grand RJ. Treatment of inflammatory bowel disease in childhood: best available evidence. *Inflamm Bowel Dis.* 2003;9(1):34–58.

14. Verhave M, Winter HS, Grand RJ. Azathioprine in the treatment of children with inflammatory bowel disease. *J Pediatr.* 1990;117(5):809–814.

15. Markowitz J, Rosa J, Grancher K, Aiges H, Daum F. Long-term 6-mercaptopurine treatment in adolescents with Crohn's disease. *Gastroenterology.* 1990;99(5):1347–1351.

16. Markowitz J, Grancher K, Kohn N, Lesser M, Daum F. A multicenter trial of 6-mercaptopurine and prednisone in children with newly diagnosed Crohn's disease. *Gastroenterology.* 2000;119(4):895–902.

17. Kirschner BS. Safety of azathioprine and 6-mercaptopurine in pediatric patients with inflammatory bowel disease. *Gastroenterology.* 1998;115(4):813–821.

18. Sokol H, Beaugerie L. Inflammatory bowel disease and lymphoproliferative disorders: the dust is starting to settle. *Gut.* 2009;58(10):1427–1436.

19. Griffiths AM. Specificities of inflammatory bowel disease in childhood. *Best Pract Res Clin Gastroenterol.* 2004;18(3):509–523.

20. Jacobstein DA, Markowitz JE, Kirschner BS, et al. Premedication and infusion reactions with infliximab: results from a pediatric inflammatory bowel disease consortium. *Inflamm Bowel Dis.* 2005;11(5):442–446.

21. Grossman AB, Noble AJ, Mamula P, Baldassano RN. Increased dosing requirements for 6-mercaptopurine and azathioprine in inflammatory bowel disease patients six years and younger. *Inflamm Bowel Dis.* 2008;14(6):750–755.

22. Mack DR, Young R, Kaufman SS, Ramey L, Vanderhoof JA. Methotrexate in patients with Crohn's disease after 6-mercaptopurine. *J Pediatr.* 1998;132(5):830–835.

23. Stephens MC, Baldassano RN, York A, et al. The bioavailability of oral methotrexate in children with inflammatory bowel disease. *J Pediatr Gastroenterol Nutr.* 2005;40(4):445–449.

24. Rutgeerts P, Van Assche G, Vermeire S. Review article: Infliximab therapy for inflammatory bowel disease–seven years on. *Aliment Pharmacol Ther.* 2006;23(4):451–463.

25. Breese EJ, Michie CA, Nicholls SW, et al. Tumor necrosis factor alpha-producing cells in the intestinal mucosa of children with inflammatory bowel disease. *Gastroenterology.* 1994;106(6):1455–1466.

26. Van den Brande JM, Braat H, van den Brink GR, et al. Infliximab but not etanercept induces apoptosis in lamina propria T-lymphocytes from patients with Crohn's disease. *Gastroenterology.* 2003;124(7):1774–1785.

27. Baldassano R, Braegger CP, Escher JC, et al. Infliximab (REMICADE) therapy in the treatment of pediatric Crohn's disease. *Am J Gastroenterol.* 2003;98(4):833–838.

28. Baldassano RN. Surpassing conventional therapies: the role of biologic therapy. *J Pediatr Gastroenterol Nutr.* 2001;33(suppl 1):S19–S26.

29. Stephens MC, Shepanski MA, Mamula P, Markowitz JE, Brown KA, Baldassano RN. Safety and steroid-sparing experience using infliximab for Crohn's disease at a pediatric inflammatory bowel disease center. *Am J Gastroenterol.* 2003;98(1):104–111.

30. Mamula P, Markowitz JE, Brown KA, Hurd LB, Piccoli DA, Baldassano RN. Infliximab as a novel therapy for pediatric ulcerative colitis. *J Pediatr Gastroenterol Nutr.* 2002;34(3):307–311.

31. Mamula P, Markowitz JE, Cohen LJ, von Allmen D, Baldassano RN. Infliximab in pediatric ulcerative colitis: two-year follow-up. *J Pediatr Gastroenterol Nutr.* 2004;38(3):298–301.

32. Thayu M, Leonard MB, Hyams JS, et al.; Reach Study Group. Improvement in biomarkers of bone formation during infliximab therapy in pediatric Crohn's disease: results of the REACH study. *Clin Gastroenterol Hepatol.* 2008;6(12):1378–1384.

33. Cheifetz A, Smedley M, Martin S, et al. The incidence and management of infusion reactions to infliximab: a large center experience. *Am J Gastroenterol.* 2003;98(6):1315–1324.

34. Miele E, Markowitz JE, Mamula P, Baldassano RN. Human anti-chimeric antibody in children and young adults with inflammatory bowel disease receiving infliximab. *J Pediatr Gastroenterol Nutr.* 2004;38(5):502–508.

35. Vermeire S, Noman M, Van Assche G, Baert F, D'Haens G, Rutgeerts P. Effectiveness of concomitant immunosuppressive therapy in suppressing the formation of antibodies to infliximab in Crohn's disease. *Gut.* 2007;56(9):1226–1231.

36. Vermeire S, Noman M, Van Assche G, et al. Autoimmunity associated with anti-tumor necrosis factor alpha treatment in Crohn's disease: a prospective cohort study. *Gastroenterology.* 2003;125(1):32–39.

37. Crandall WV, Mackner LM. Infusion reactions to infliximab in children and adolescents: frequency, outcome and a predictive model. *Aliment Pharmacol Ther.* 2003;17(1):75–84.

38. Colombel JF, Loftus EV Jr, Tremaine WJ, et al. The safety profile of infliximab in patients with Crohn's disease: the Mayo clinic experience in 500 patients. *Gastroenterology.* 2004;126(1):19–31.

39. Hyams J, Crandall W, Kugathasan S, et al.; REACH Study Group. Induction and maintenance infliximab therapy for the treatment of moderate-to-severe Crohn's disease in children. *Gastroenterology.* 2007;132(3):863–873; quiz 1165.

40. Bongartz T, Sutton AJ, Sweeting MJ, Buchan I, Matteson EL, Montori V. Anti-TNF antibody therapy in rheumatoid arthritis and the risk of serious infections and malignancies: systematic review and meta-analysis of rare harmful effects in randomized controlled trials. *JAMA.* 2006;295(19):2275–2285.

41. D'Haens G, Baert F, van Assche G, et al.; Belgian Inflammatory Bowel Disease Research Group; North-Holland Gut Club. Early combined immunosuppression or conventional management in patients with newly diagnosed Crohn's disease: an open randomised trial. *Lancet.* 2008;371(9613):660–667.

42. Colombel JF, Sandborn WJ, Reinisch W, et al. Infliximab, azathioprine, or combination therapy for Crohn's disease. *N Engl J Med.* 2010;362(15):1383 -1395.

Influence of Hepatosplenic Lymphoma on Management Decisions

114

Jeffrey S. Hyams

The use of immunomodulators and biologic therapy has become standard-of-care in the treatment of inflammatory bowel disease (IBD) and has been associated with improved outcomes and better quality of life. These therapies have also been associated with complications including increased susceptibility to opportunistic infection and certain malignancies. Potential adverse events associated with biologic therapy for IBD reached a new level of concern in May 2006 with the initial pediatric approval of infliximab by the Food and Drug Administration and the subsequent black box warning that appeared in August 2006 concerning hepatosplenic T-cell lymphoma (HSTCL). HSTCL was to most gastroenterologists a totally unknown entity. The gastroenterology community soon learned that HSTCL was a very rare and aggressive non-Hodgkin's lymphoma (NHL) that primarily targeted young males and was almost uniformly fatal. Suddenly, and particularly for pediatric gastroenterologists, there was a heightened concern that the treatment of IBD could prove fatal. This chain of events caused a reappraisal of treatment modalities and for this practitioner influenced the way in which I use biologic therapy and immunomodulators. An understanding of the pathobiology and epidemiology of HSTCL is required to appreciate the background in which management decisions are now made.

HSTCL—GENERAL CONSIDERATIONS

In 1981 a report appeared describing three patients with an aggressive and fatal lymphoma that was termed erythrophago-cytic Tγ lymphoma.[1] Almost 10 years later, the name hepatosplenic γδ T-cell lymphoma was proposed because subsequent cases had all expressed the γδ T-cell receptor.[2] Additional clinical data revealed that some HSTCL expressed the αβ T-cell receptor[3] and it became clear that HSTCL can express either T-cell receptor. In 2001, the World Health Organization classified HSTCL as a distinct disorder under the classification of peripheral (extranodal) T-cell lymphomas.

The pathobiology of HSTCL is poorly understood. γδ T cells become activated after antigenic stimulation and, through cytotoxic enzymes, kill microorganisms or infected cells. γδ T cells are found in the splenic red pulp and in mucosal membranes such as the gastrointestinal tract or respiratory system and are felt to be part of the innate immune system.[4] Commonly, subjects with HSTCL have a history of chronic antigenic stimulation in the setting of immunosuppression; it has been postulated that primary or acquired immunodeficiency can predispose to HSTCL.[5] A defect in immunosurveillance may predispose to proliferation of cells undergoing malignant transformation following viral infection, particularly Epstein-Barr virus (EBV). However, as noted earlier, EBV infection is rare in HSTCL. It is more likely that exposure to antimetabolites such as azathioprine or 6-mercaptopurine cause DNA damage leading to defects in control of cellular proliferation or apoptosis resulting in malignant transformation. The relevance of this latter hypothesis to IBD is obvious.

The literature on HSTCL is modest and only about 200 cases have been described. The two largest series combined describe 66 patients.[5,6] About one-third of patients in the literature had previous organ transplantation or received immune-modifying agents for other indications. Though HSTCL has been described from infancy up to 80 years of age, the median age has been 32 years, and 70% of subjects are male. Table 114.1 shows the most common clinical and laboratory findings. It must be emphasized that these patients lack adenopathy and more commonly present with fever, weight loss, hepatosplenomegaly, and abdominal pain. The disease is always disseminated at diagnosis with involvement of liver, spleen, and bone marrow. Serum aminotransferases are commonly elevated and an erroneous diagnosis of hepatitis can be made; liver biopsy may be misleading and has suggested autoimmune hepatitis.[7]

Diagnosis

HSTCL is not an immediately easy diagnosis as malignant cells appear similar to normal activated T cells; immunohistochemistry

TABLE 114.1 Presenting Features of Hepatosplenic T-Cell Lymphoma[a]

Feature	% of Actual Cases
Splenomegaly	98
Hepatomegaly	77
Fever, weight loss	70
Jaundice	29
Thrombocytopenia	89
Anemia	80
Elevated LDH	59
Leukopenia	50
Elevated aminotransferases	40

[a]Adapted from Belhadj et al.[5] and Weidmann.[6]
LDH, lactate dehydrogenase.

and flow cytometry are mandatory for the correct diagnosis. Common surface antigen expression is TdT (−), CD2+, CD3+, CD4−, CD5−, CD7−, occasionally CD16+, rarely CD8+ and CD56±. Evidence of EBV infection is usually absent. The cytotoxic proteins granzyme and perforin are negative and T-cell intracellular antigen-1 is positive. This pattern distinguishes HSTCL from other γδ T-cell NHL, which express granzyme and perforin.[8] Cytogenetic abnormalities such as trisomy 8 and isochrome 7q are common. Erythrophagocytosis in the bone marrow can be prominent.

● WHAT IS THE RELATIONSHIP OF HSTCL AND IBD?

To put the rarity of HSTCL in perspective, the incidence of NHL in subjects 10 to 19 years of age is approximately 20/1,000,000 (1 in 50,000) subjects per year, slightly higher for people in their 20s, and about 80/1,000,000 for people in their late 30s.[9] Peripheral T-cell lymphomas make up about 10% to 15% of all NHL, and HSTCL represents about 5% of peripheral T-cell lymphomas (i.e., HSTCL represents less than 1% of NHL).[10] Thus, one would presume an annual incidence of HSTCL in adolescents of 1/5,000,000 subjects. Given that there are likely 50,000 to 100,000 pediatric patients with IBD in the United States, we would expect one case of HSTCL every 50 to 100 years. To date there have been 40 reported cases worldwide of HSTCL in subjects with IBD (see following section). Several cases have appeared in the medical literature[7,11–16,16a] and the rest have been identified by reports from the pharmaceutical industry. Seven of these cases have been in patients less than 20 years of age.

Thiopurine Use

The common thread for all subjects with IBD who have developed HSTCL has been treatment with a thiopurine. As of January 2011 there have been 16 reports of subjects treated with thiopurines only and 24 reports of subjects who have been treated with infliximab and a thiopurine who have developed

HSTCL[8,9,11–16,16a] (data on file, Centocor, Horsham, Pennsylvania). For this latter group the age range was 12 to 40 years (mean age 22 years) at the time of diagnosis, and all except one was male. The mean number of infliximab infusions was 10 (range 1–24) and five patients had 3 or less infusions. There have been two cases of HSTCL in IBD patients receiving adalimumab, both of whom previously also received infliximab and a thiopurine. There have been *no cases* of HSTCL developing in IBD patients treated with an anti-tumor necrosis factor (TNF) agent without previous thiopurine exposure, in IBD patients treated with an anti-TNF agent and methotrexate, or in IBD patients treated with methotrexate alone.

Possible Contributing Factors to HSTCL in IBD Patients

It is important to speculate why there has been what appears to be a markedly increased recognition of HSTCL in the IBD population over the past several years. First, it is possible that this malignancy has previously occurred but has not been recognized as HSTCL because special expertise is required for identification. Previous cases may have been called T-cell NHL and not further classified as HSTCL. Second, the past decade has witnessed a marked increase in the use of thiopurines and the advent of biologic therapy with anti-TNF agents. As noted earlier, thiopurines are known to cause DNA damage, and azathioprine has been classified as a human carcinogen.[17] Though studies are conflicting, recent evidence suggests an increased association of lymphoma (not HSTCL) with thiopurine use.[18]

Editor's note (TMB): There is a separate chapter on lymphoma risk from the French Consortium.

Ionizing radiation is also a cause of DNA damage, and the frequency of computed tomography scan examinations and their attendant radiation exposure has dramatically increased in the pediatric population over the past decade.[19] Recent literature has emphasized the potential increased likelihood of malignancy following exposure to ionizing radiation from diagnostic imaging studies, as well as the particular sensitivity of pediatric patients.[20–23]

Editor's note (TMB): There is a separate chapter on risks of medication.

Immune surveillance is impaired in the presence of *thiopurines* as well as with treatment with anti-TNF agents. Though it has been controversial as to whether Crohn's disease itself (regardless of therapy) may be associated with an increased likelihood of lymphoma, the association of chronic inflammation and autoimmune disorders (e.g., rheumatoid arthritis) with lymphoma has long been known.[24] However, in the latter situations, lymphoma development has more commonly been of the B-cell variety (an excellent review of the presumed pathogenesis of lymphomas has recently been published[25]). Given that Crohn's disease is a condition in which chronic inflammation is present in a mucosal surface (site of γδ T cells), diagnostic studies with ionizing radiation are common, thiopurines that can cause chromosomal damage are frequently used, and immune-modifying drugs are common, it would appear to be the "perfect storm" for the development of malignancy.

● HSTCL INFLUENCE ON THERAPEUTIC DECISIONS

The recognition of HSTCL has greatly impacted therapeutic and diagnostic decision making in young patients with IBD. The concept of benefit versus risk has become much more real with HSTCL. I will summarize the therapeutic issues in light of HSTCL.

Choice of Immunomodulator

Given that HSTCL has only been described in IBD patients previously treated with thiopurines, many pediatric IBD physicians are now questioning whether 6-mercaptopurine/azathioprine or methotrexate should be the immunomodulator of choice for children and adolescents requiring an immunomodulator. Given that up to 80% of children newly diagnosed with Crohn's disease and 50% of those with ulcerative colitis receive an immunomodulator within 1 to 2 years of diagnosis,[26] this question is of clear and present relevance. Thiopurines have been used extensively in children with IBD and have definitively been shown to maintain remission and spare corticosteroid therapy.[26,27] The availability of TPMT testing (thiopurine methyltransferase) prior to initiation of thiopurine therapy has provided an additional measure of safety by avoiding exposure of TPMT deficient homozygotes. Monitoring 6-thioguanine levels has been shown by some to help guide actual dosing in those treated with thiopurines.[28] Though *methotrexate* has been used for some time, widespread experience with it in IBD is less than with thiopurines, and though it has been shown to be useful in Crohn's disease in both adults and children,[29,30] its utility in ulcerative colitis has not been proven. I have seen a real shift toward increased use of methotrexate as the primary immunomodulator in children with Crohn's disease, though there are no data comparing thiopurines to methotrexate in either adult or pediatric patients.

Use of Concomitant Immunomodulators with an Anti-TNF Agent

At present, the vast majority of pediatric patients starting a biologic agent have failed thiopurine therapy, or are starting a thiopurine and biologic agent together in the setting of corticosteroid-refractory or -dependent disease. Given the apparent strong signal of an increased number of cases of HSTCL in patients with a history of treatment with both a thiopurine and an anti-TNF agent, there are several considerations that are required.

The first question is whether concomitant immunomodulator therapy increases the effectiveness of an anti-TNF agent. There are studies of all the anti-TNF agents (infliximab, adalimumab, and certolizumab) used in a maintenance fashion that show that concomitant therapy with an immunomodulator was not associated with greater efficacy at the primary end points for the studies.[31–33] It needs to be pointed out, however, that these studies were generally with patients who had been on chronic immunomodulator therapy that had failed to control disease when the biologic agent was started. Withdrawal of immunomodulators in subjects on chronic maintenance therapy with infliximab was associated with similar outcomes compared to when immunomodulatory therapy was continued.[34]

In contrast, the recent SONIC study, which examined adults with Crohn's disease who were both immunomodulator and biologic therapy naïve, demonstrated that the coadministration of azathioprine and infliximab was superior to either azathioprine alone or infliximab alone in inducing clinical remission and mucosal healing at 26 weeks.[35] Subgroup analysis of only those patients with endoscopic evidence of active disease and an elevated C-reactive protein (CRP) at the start of the study did not show a significant difference in efficacy between the infliximab-alone group and the infliximab/azathioprine group. The SONIC data are now out to 50 weeks, and further long-term analysis at 2 years will be needed to help further distinguish whether potential added efficacy outweighs the risk of concomitant therapy.

If there is no apparent increase in efficacy by continuing an immunomodulator that has failed in achieving success at the time a biologic agent is started, is there any reason to continue it? The one potentially important observation in this regard is that infliximab levels are higher and CRP levels are lower in those who continue dual therapy than in those on the biologic agent alone.[36,37]

Given the information provided earlier, I stop the thiopurine when a biologic agent is begun largely because of no evidence of added efficacy and the specter of HSTCL in the setting of dual therapy. My feeling is that one is adding risk and not benefit by giving dual therapy. Other pediatric gastroenterologists will continue the thiopurine through the first few months of infliximab therapy until a maintenance schedule is established. There are no data on comparable safety between the two approaches. For patients receiving methotrexate as their immunomodulator, the approach is also less than clear. The recent COMMIT trial suggests that methotrexate plus infliximab is no better than infliximab alone.[38] However, some gastroenterologists will continue methotrexate at low dose (7.5 mg weekly) to decrease antibody formation and perhaps extend half-life of the infliximab.

Another unresolved clinical situation is whether dual therapy with an immunomodulator and an anti-TNF agent can be used as a bridge to long-term thiopurine use alone. In other words, in a corticosteroid-refractory or -dependent patient in whom the clinician does not have several months to wait for a thiopurine to become effective, should one use an anti-TNF agent for a brief period to allow corticosteroid withdrawal and clinical improvement while the thiopurine is becoming effective? Whether such a brief coexposure adds significant risk to a patient is not clear.

Much of the decision making also hinges on the perspective of the clinician toward long-term biologic therapy. If the intent at the start of anti-TNF therapy is to continue it indefinitely then there would appear to be little reason to use an immunomodulator concomitantly. The likelihood of antibody development to infliximab, for example, with scheduled maintenance therapy is not significantly different with or without a concomitant immunomodulator. If the intent is to use infliximab episodically then a concomitant immunomodulator does decrease antibody formation. In this latter situation, however, one could switch to either adalimumab or certolizumab if necessary.

Editor's note (TMB): The chapter on "Balancing Benefits and Risks of Biologic Therapy" presents some other aspects of this dilemma.

Therapy of HSTCL

At present there are no predictive tests to identify those individuals more likely to develop HSTCL or to make a diagnosis before the disease becomes disseminated. Once a diagnosis of HSTCL is established, the prognosis is generally grim.[5,6] Aggressive chemotherapeutic regimens, antilymphocyte antibodies, and stem cell transplantation have been used with success in rare patients.[39–41]

References

1. Kadin ME, Kamoun M, Lamberg J. Erythrophagocytic T gamma lymphoma: a clinicopathologic entity resembling malignant histiocytosis. *N Engl J Med.* 1981;304(11):648–653.

2. Farcet JP, Gaulard P, Marolleau JP, et al. Hepatosplenic T-cell lymphoma: sinusal/sinusoidal localization of malignant cells expressing the T-cell receptor gamma delta. *Blood.* 1990;75(11):2213–2219.

3. Macon WR, Levy NB, Kurtin PJ, et al. Hepatosplenic alphabeta T-cell lymphomas: a report of 14 cases and comparison with hepatosplenic gammadelta T-cell lymphomas. *Am J Surg Pathol.* 2001;25(3):285–296.

4. Vega F, Medeiros LJ, Gaulard P. Hepatosplenic and other gammadelta T-cell lymphomas. *Am J Clin Pathol.* 2007;127(6):869–880.

5. Belhadj K, Reyes F, Farcet JP, et al. Hepatosplenic gammadelta T-cell lymphoma is a rare clinicopathologic entity with poor outcome: report on a series of 21 patients. *Blood.* 2003;102(13):4261–4269.

6. Weidmann E. Hepatosplenic T cell lymphoma. A review on 45 cases since the first report describing the disease as a distinct lymphoma entity in 1990. *Leukemia.* 2000;14(6):991–997.

7. Thayu M, Markowitz JE, Mamula P, Russo PA, Muinos WI, Baldassano RN. Hepatosplenic T-cell lymphoma in an adolescent patient after immunomodulator and biologic therapy for Crohn disease. *J Pediatr Gastroenterol Nutr.* 2005;40(2):220–222.

8. Cooke CB, Krenacs L, Stetler-Stevenson M, et al. Hepatosplenic T-cell lymphoma: a distinct clinicopathologic entity of cytotoxic gamma delta T-cell origin. *Blood.* 1996;88(11):4265–4274.

9. Surveillance Epidemiology and End Results (SEER). Cancer Statistics Review, 1975–2006. Bethesda, MD: National Cancer Institute. http://seer.cancer.gov

10. Jaffe E, Harris NL, Stein H, et al. *World Health Organization Classification of Tumors/Pathology and Genetics of Tumors of Haematopoietic and Lymphoid Tissues.* Lyon, France: International Agency for Research Press; 2001.

11. Navarro JT, Ribera JM, Mate JL, et al. Hepatosplenic T-gammadelta lymphoma in a patient with Crohn's disease treated with azathioprine. *Leuk Lymphoma.* 2003;44(3):531–533.

12. Drini M, Prichard PJ, Brown GJ, Macrae FA. Hepatosplenic T-cell lymphoma following infliximab therapy for Crohn's disease. *Med J Aust.* 2008;189(8):464–465.

13. Zeidan A, Sham R, Shapiro J, Baratta A, Kouides P. Hepatosplenic T-cell lymphoma in a patient with Crohn's disease who received infliximab therapy. *Leuk Lymphoma.* 2007;48(7):1410–1413.

14. Mackey AC, Green L, Liang LC, Dinndorf P, Avigan M. Hepatosplenic T cell lymphoma associated with infliximab use in young patients treated for inflammatory bowel disease. *J Pediatr Gastroenterol Nutr.* 2007;44(2):265–267.

15. Mittal S, Milner BJ, Johnston PW, Culligan DJ. A case of hepatosplenic gamma-delta T-cell lymphoma with a transient response to fludarabine and alemtuzumab. *Eur J Haematol.* 2006;76(6):531–534.

16. Rosh JR, Gross T, Mamula P, Griffiths A, Hyams J. Hepatosplenic T-cell lymphoma in adolescents and young adults with Crohn's disease: a cautionary tale? *Inflamm Bowel Dis.* 2007;13(8):1024–1030.

16a. Kotlyar D, Blonski W, Diamond RH, et al. A systematic review of factors that contribute to hepatosplenic lymphoma in patients with inflammatory bowel diseases. *Clin Gastroenterol Hepatol.* 2011;9:36 -41.

17. Karran P. Thiopurines, DNA repair and therapy-related cancer. *Brit Med Bull.* 2007;1–18.

18. Kandiel A, Fraser AG, Korelitz BI, Brensinger C, Lewis JD. Increased risk of lymphoma among inflammatory bowel disease patients treated with azathioprine and 6-mercaptopurine. *Gut.* 2005;54(8):1121–1125.

19. Brody AS, Frush DP, Huda W, Brent RL; American Academy of Pediatrics Section on Radiology. Radiation risk to children from computed tomography. *Pediatrics.* 2007;120(3):677–682.

20. Brenner DJ, Hall EJ. Computed tomography—an increasing source of radiation exposure. *N Engl J Med.* 2007;357(22):2277–2284.

21. Brenner DJ, Sachs RK. Estimating radiation-induced cancer risks at very low doses: rationale for using a linear no-threshold approach. *Radiat Environ Biophys.* 2006;44(4):253–256.

22. Mazrani W, McHugh K, Marsden PJ. The radiation burden of radiological investigations. *Arch Dis Child.* 2007;92(12):1127–1131.

23. Kleinerman RA. Cancer risks following diagnostic and therapeutic radiation exposure in children. *Pediatr Radiol.* 2006;36(suppl 2):121–125.

24. Baecklund E, Iliadou A, Askling J, et al. Association of chronic inflammation, not its treatment, with increased lymphoma risk in rheumatoid arthritis. *Arthritis Rheum.* 2006;54(3):692–701.

25. Blinder V, Fisher SG; Lymphoma Research Foundation, New York. The role of environmental factors in the etiology of lymphoma. *Cancer Invest.* 2008;26(3):306–316.

26. Punati J, Markowitz J, Lerer T, et al.; Pediatric IBD Collaborative Research Group. Effect of early immunomodulator use in moderate to severe pediatric Crohn disease. *Inflamm Bowel Dis.* 2008;14(7):949–954.

27. Markowitz J, Grancher K, Kohn N, Lesser M, Daum F. A multicenter trial of 6-mercaptopurine and prednisone in children with newly diagnosed Crohn's disease. *Gastroenterology.* 2000;119(4):895–902.

28. Dubinsky MC, Lamothe S, Yang HY, et al. Pharmacogenomics and metabolite measurement for 6-mercaptopurine therapy in inflammatory bowel disease. *Gastroenterology.* 2000;118(4):705–713.

29. Feagan BG, Rochon J, Fedorak RN, et al. Methotrexate for the treatment of Crohn's disease. The North American Crohn's Study Group Investigators. *N Engl J Med.* 1995;332(5):292–297.

30. Turner D, Grossman AB, Rosh J, et al. Methotrexate following unsuccessful thiopurine therapy in pediatric Crohn's disease. *Am J Gastroenterol.* 2007;102(12):2804–2812; quiz 2803, 2813.

31. Hanauer SB, Feagan BG, Lichtenstein GR, et al.; ACCENT I Study Group. Maintenance infliximab for Crohn's disease: the ACCENT I randomised trial. *Lancet.* 2002;359(9317):1541–1549.

32. Colombel JF, Sandborn WJ, Rutgeerts P, et al. Adalimumab for maintenance of clinical response and remission in patients with Crohn's disease: the CHARM trial. *Gastroenterology.* 2007;132(1):52–65.

33. Schreiber S, Khaliq-Kareemi M, Lawrance IC, et al.; PRECISE 2 Study Investigators. Maintenance therapy with certolizumab pegol for Crohn's disease. *N Engl J Med.* 2007;357(3):239–250.

34. Van Assche G, Magdelaine-Beuzelin C, D'Haens G, et al. Withdrawal of immunosuppression in Crohn's disease treated

with scheduled infliximab maintenance: a randomized trial. *Gastroenterology.* 2008;134(7):1861–1868.

35. Colombel JC, Sandborn WJ, Reinisch W, et al. Infliximab, azathioprine, or combination therapy for Crohn's disease. *N Engl J Med.* 2010;362:1383–1395.

36. Rutgeerts P, Feagan BG, Lichtenstein GR, et al. Comparison of scheduled and episodic treatment strategies of infliximab in Crohn's disease. *Gastroenterology.* 2004;126(2):402–413.

37. Van Assche G, Vermeire S, Rutgeerts P. Optimizing treatment of inflammatory bowel diseases with biologic agents. *Curr Gastroenterol Rep.* 2008;10(6):591–596.

38. Feagan B, McDonald J, Panaccione R, et al. A randomized trial of methotrexate in combination with infliximab for the treatment of Crohn's disease. *Gastroenterology.* 2008;135:294

39. Moleti ML, Testi AM, Giona F, et al. Gamma-delta hepatosplenic T-cell lymphoma. Description of a case with immunophenotypic and molecular follow-up successfully treated with chemotherapy alone. *Leuk Lymphoma.* 2006;47(2):333–336.

40. Otrock ZK, Hatoum HA, Salem ZM, et al. Long-term remission in a patient with hepatosplenic gammadelta T cell lymphoma treated with bortezomib and high-dose CHOP-like chemotherapy followed by autologous peripheral stem cell transplantation. *Ann Hematol.* 2008;87(12):1023–1024.

41. Konuma T, Ooi J, Takahashi S, et al. Allogeneic stem cell transplantation for hepatosplenic gammadelta T-cell lymphoma. *Leuk Lymphoma.* 2007;48(3):630–632.

Balancing Benefits and Risks of Biologic Therapy | 115

Corey A. Siegel

The past decade has brought significant changes in the available treatment options for patients with inflammatory bowel disease (IBD). Until the antitumor necrosis factor (anti-TNF) agent infliximab became available in 1998, we were limited to 5-aminosalicylate drugs, corticosteroids, and immunomodulators, including 6-mercaptopurine (6-MP), azathioprine, and methotrexate. The successful early trials of infliximab for Crohn's disease led to larger and longer-term induction and maintenance studies for both luminal and perianal disease.[1,2] Other anti-TNF drugs followed with similar results, and in addition to infliximab, adalimumab and certolizumab pegol form this important drug class for the treatment of Crohn's disease.[3,4] Infliximab is also approved by the Food and Drug Association (FDA) for ulcerative colitis, but the majority of data available regarding the use of anti-TNF agents are for Crohn's disease. The newest medication available for the treatment of Crohn's disease is natalizumab, an alpha-4 integrin molecule, which presents a new treatment option for patients who have not responded (or lost response) to anti-TNF agents.

A rapidly growing body of research has focused on optimizing the use of these medications to further enhance the treatment response. Anti-TNF agents were first used only after the failure of standard therapies and for our sickest patients. However, evidence that using these medications earlier in the course of Crohn's disease can increase remission rates and avoid the use of corticosteroids has started a shift in the treatment paradigm.[5] Previously, we waited for proof (e.g., failure of immunomodulators, complications of disease, multiple surgeries) that these medications were required. When they were initiated patients and physicians had little question that they were justified. Now, with the D'Haens "top-down" results we have some evidence that we can do better by anticipating future problems and treating patients before complications develop.[5]

● KNOWN BENEFITS AND RISKS OF BIOLOGIC THERAPY

Data and opinions are accumulating to support the idea of the early use of biologic therapy. Because these medications are associated with severe (albeit rare) life-threatening side effects, trade-offs need to be understood and accepted by patients before proceeding with this treatment approach. This chapter aims to describe the known benefits and risks of biologic therapy and to explore the trade-offs that patients need to understand in order to be more involved in medical decisions and receive care that fits with their personal preferences.

Benefits of Treatment

Infliximab, adalimumab, and certolizumab pegol have had similar response and remission rates in the pivotal clinical trials. There are differences in study design, patient population, and endpoints, but overall it is difficult to distinguish a meaningful difference in efficacy between the three anti-TNF agents. When reviewing expected benefit of anti-TNF therapy with patients, I separate the chance of initial response and the likelihood of maintaining that response over the period of 1 year. From results of the three maintenance studies with a similar design (open-label induction followed by randomization of responders to treatment or placebo) patients can expect a response rate of approximately 60%. Of the responders, about 34% of patients in the active treatment arm maintain clinical remission at 1 year compared to 13% in the placebo arms. Fig. 115.1 displays this summary information in a format that can be reviewed with patients. The steroid-free remission rates at 1 year are a little bit lower, with 29% of treated patients in remission and off steroids versus 7% in the placebo groups.

The ENACT 1 and 2 studies for natalizumab had a similar design to the above-described anti-TNF randomized controlled trials.[6] Similar to the anti-TNFs, almost 60% of patients show an initial response to natalizumab. In ENACT 2, 55% of the intention-to-treat population maintained a clinical remission at the end of 15 months. Because natalizumab is currently approved only for patients who have previously received an anti-TNF agent, Fig. 115.2 reports the 15-month remission rate in the anti-TNF failure population.

Although results of the randomized controlled trials of the biologic agents are similar, remission rates in clinical practice

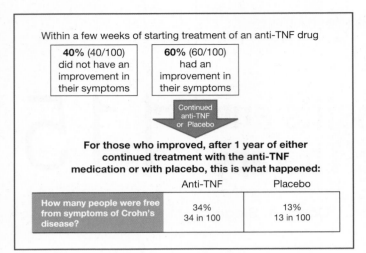

FIGURE 115.1 • Estimate of initial response and remission rate to anti-TNF treatment from randomized controlled trials. Results based on weighted average from ACCENT1, CHARM, and Precise 2 (only response rate since trial ended at 6 months).[1,3,4]

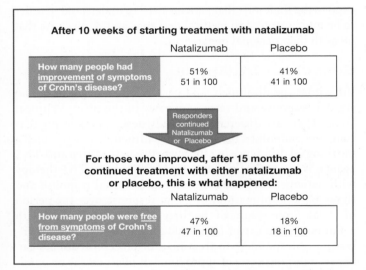

FIGURE 115.2 • Results from the ENACT 1 and 2 trials for patients who previously failed anti-TNF therapy. The week 10 rate of improvement refers to a drop in the Crohn's disease activity index of 70 points. Anti-TNF failure is defined as: (1) no response to initial treatment, or (2) lost response with continued treatment, or (3) discontinuation due to adverse event, or (4) discontinuation due to infusion reaction.[6]

may be higher. Rigid clinical trial design typically prohibits measures that might improve response rates (e.g., more frequent or higher anti-TNF doses), and patients included in clinical trials are not always representative of the general population of those with Crohn's disease. Therefore, trial results are a good starting point for discussions of expected treatment benefit, but individual patients likely have a higher (or lower) chance of response on the basis of their personal characteristics. An area of uncertainty is the durability of anti-TNF treatment.

Observational studies have shown that the majority of patients who are in remission after 1 year of treatment continue to stay in remission, but true long-term placebo-controlled withdrawal studies are lacking.

Risks of Crohn's Disease

The treatment of Crohn's disease aims to improve symptoms and to prevent complications. Overall, the goal is to improve quality of life. Poorly treated Crohn's disease leads to a similar quality of life as those with severe angina, and patients may have frequent hospitalizations, loss of time from work and family, and excessive healthcare costs. Although surgery can be used as a successful treatment modality for Crohn's disease, changing the natural history of disease and preventing surgeries is an important goal of therapy. As reported by Dr. Munkholm in 1993, 40% of patients with Crohn's disease have surgery after their first year of disease, 50% have surgery by 5 years, and 80% undergo at least one surgery after 20 years of disease.[7] Unfortunately, these rates have not changed significantly over the past 25 years.[8] Patients often ask about the risk of dying from Crohn's disease. Although a large population-based cohort study showed a statistically significantly elevated standardized mortality ratio of 1.4 (95% confidence interval [CI] = 1.2–1.6), in absolute terms this translates to approximately 57 deaths per 10,000 patient-years in patients with IBD versus 50 deaths per 10,000 patient-years in the general population.[9] The increased deaths came predominantly as a result of infections, respiratory disease, and digestive disease other than IBD. An evaluation of a large database from the United Kingdom agreed that Crohn's disease was associated with an increased mortality and that it was those patients with more severe disease (HR = 2.44, 95% CI = 1.84–3.25) or using prednisone (HR = 2.48, 95% CI = 1.85–3.31) who were at the highest risk. Therefore, effective treatment of Crohn's disease does not only result in symptomatic control but, presumably, a mortality benefit.

Risks of Biologic Treatment

Biologic therapies bear a risk of side-effects that need to be considered before initiating one of these medications (Table 115.1). Some are common, but typically mild and self-limited, such as infusion reactions, headaches, or nonserious infections. Others are serious, may be life-threatening, but fortunately are very rare. Table 115.2 shows the frequency of common events seen in the major RCTs. It is important to note that patient populations and trial duration are different across studies, as are definitions of adverse events. Overall, rates are similar and it is difficult to detect meaningful safety differences between these agents.

Serious Events

The serious events should be considered more heavily in medical decision making. These risks need to be weighed carefully for individual patients against the expected benefit of treatment. There are a number of reported side effects that are difficult to quantify accurate incidence rates for, due to paucity of data. For example, early clinical trials of the anti-TNF agent lenercept for the treatment of multiple sclerosis (MS) led to a higher rate of exacerbations in the treatment group, and since, demyelinating

TABLE 115.1 Side-Effects Associated with Anti-TNF Agents

Common but Minor

Hypersensitivity reactions

    Infusion reactions (IV delivery)

    Injection site reactions (SQ delivery)

    Serum sickness/delayed hypersensitivity

Immunogenicity (antibodies to drug)*

Headache

Rash

Infections

    URI, bronchitis, UTI

Rare but Serious

Infections

    Pneumonia, septic arthritis

    Prosthetic and postsurgical infections,

    Erysipelas, cellulitis, diverticulitis,

    Pyelonephritis

    Tuberculosis and opportunistic infections

    Coccidiomycosis, histoplasmosis,

    Pneumocytosis, nocardiosis, cytomegalovirus

    Hepatitis B reactivation

Demyelinating disorders

Autoantibodies

    Lupus

Pancytopenia/aplastic anemia

Heart failure

Hepatotoxicity

    Acute liver failure

    Hepatitis/jaundice

Malignancy

    Lymphoma (NHL, HSTCL)

    Solid tumors

    Nonmelanoma skin cancers

This is a compilation taken from the package inserts for infliximab, adalimumab, and certolizumab. Some adverse events may have not been reported with all medications.
*Undetermined clinical significance.
TNF, tumor necrosis factor; IV, intravenous; SQ, subcutaneous; URI, upper respiratory infection; UTI, urinary tract infection; NHL, non-Hodgkin's lymphoma; HSTCL, hepatosplenic T-cell lymphoma. Adapted from Siegel CA. Risks of biologic therapy for inflammatory bowel disease. In: Bernstein CN, ed. *IBD Yearbook*, Vol. 6. London: Remedica; 2009.

TABLE 115.2 Adverse Events Seen with Biologic Agents in Clinical Trials ≥ 12 Weeks Duration

	ACCENT I[1]	CHARM[3]	PRECISE 2[4]	ENACT[6]
Agent	IFX	ADA	CZP	NAT
Subjects^	385	517	216	214
Follow-up (weeks)	54	56	26	60
Discontinued due to adverse event (%)	12	6	8	14
Infusion/injection site reaction (%)	21	5	3	7
Infections* (%)	30	45	6	62
Serious infections (%)	4	3	3	3

^Included only patients who received active treatment for the entire follow-up period.
*Not serious, but may have required antibiotics.
IFX, infliximab; ADA, adalimumab; CZP, certolizumab pegol; NAT, natalizumab.
Adapted from Siegel CA. Risks of biologic therapy for inflammatory bowel disease. In: Bernstein CN, ed. *IBD Yearbook*, Vol. 6. London: Remedica; 2009.

disease has been reported with all three of the anti-TNFs approved for Crohn's disease. Similarly, infliximab was studied for the treatment of congestive heart failure (CHF) but led to a higher rate of CHF exacerbations in a dose-dependent fashion. Other reported events associated with anti-TNF use include autoimmunity (e.g., lupus), hepatitis and hepatic failure, pancytopenia, alveolar hemorrhage, and psoriasiform eruptions.

Serious Infections

The adverse events that have received the most attention by patients and physicians are serious infections and malignancy. In the large prospective TREAT registry the risk of serious infections was elevated in patients receiving anti-TNF therapy, but in the multivariate analysis it only appeared to be the patients who were receiving corticosteroids (HR = 2.0, 95% CI = 1.4–2.9) or narcotics (HR = 2.7, 95% CI = 1.9–4.0) that were at risk.[10] A case-control study from the Mayo clinic corroborated the concern that the combination of medications leads to a higher rate of infections as they showed an odds ratio of 2.9 (95% CI = 1.5–5.3) for developing an opportunistic infection on one medication, which increased to 14.5 (95% CI = 4.9–43) if patient is given a combination of prednisone with 6-MP/aza-thioprine, or infliximab.[11] Mortality related to sepsis in patients taking infliximab has been reported as 4/1000 patient-years in one systematic review and up to 1/100 exposed patients at the Mayo clinic.[12,13] However, the average age of the patients who died was about 60 years; many had comorbidities, and most had long-standing disease and were on concomitant medications. A majority of patients treated with infliximab do not fit into this high-risk group but some do. We can feel reassured that typical patients who are candidates for anti-TNF therapy are at lower risk, but we still need to consider the possibility of severe, life-threatening infections in all patients.

Opportunistic Infections

The risks of respiratory infections, including tuberculosis (TB) and histoplasmosis, should also be discussed with patients. In a large study in the United States that addressed patients with rheumatoid arthritis taking infliximab, the risk of developing TB was approximately 5 per 10,000 patient-years of exposure (compared to about 0.6 per 10,000 patient-years in the general population).[14] Of the four patients who developed TB in this study, three had a positive tuberculin skin test (TST) prior to initiating infliximab, and the fourth had a suspected history of prior TB. Interestingly, all were women and their average age was 61 years. A history of TB exposure should be carefully taken, along with screening using either a TST ($\pm$ CXR) or serologic assay for TB such as QuantiFERON Gold. Invasive fungal infections such as histoplasmosis, coccidiomycosis, and blastomycosis have also been reported and were the focus of a new black-box warning for anti-TNF agents in September 2006. These infections are predominantly a problem in endemic regions (Midwest/Ohio and Mississippi river valleys for blastomycosis/histoplasmosis, Southwest for coccidiomycosis), but obtaining a travel history and prior location of residence is important.

Malignancy

The risk of malignancy associated with anti-TNF treatment is of significant concern to patients and providers. There has been no clear association with solid tumors other than nonmelanoma skin cancer that probably occurs at a higher rate (as they do with immunomodulators). However, there does appear to be an increased risk of non-Hodgkin's lymphoma (NHL). In a meta-analysis including almost 9000 patients and more than 20,000 patient-years, the rate of NHL in patients receiving combination therapy with anti-TNF and immunomodulators was 6.1 per 10,000 patient-years.[15] Compared to the general population (based on the Surveillance, Epidemiology and End Results registry), which showed an overall rate of NHL prevalence at 2.1 per 10,000 patient-years, this is a significantly elevated standardized incidence ratio (SIR) of 3.23 (95% CI = 1.5–6.9). Compared to a population of patients receiving immunomodulators alone, the SIR is 1.7 (95% CI = 0.5–7.1), but this is not statistically significant. A conclusion from these data and others is that both immunomodulators and the combination of immunomodulators and anti-TNF therapy lead to a slight increase in risk of NHL. We do not have enough data on anti-TNF monotherapy to determine whether this class of drug used on its own increases the NHL risk. I suspect that it does, to about the same magnitude as immunomodulator monotherapy.

Editor's note (TMB): There is a separate chapter on lymphoma in IBD.

Hepatosplenic T-cell Lymphoma (HSTCL) is another form of NHL that was only recently described in association with IBD therapy and, unfortunately, is almost universally fatal. Previously, 16 cases had been described in patients receiving immunomodulator monotherapy. As of early 2011, 24 cases of HSTCL had been reported in patients receiving infliximab or adalimumab in combination with an immunomodulator (6-MP/azathioprine; Data on file, Centocor, Inc., February 2011). The average age of the patients with HSTCL was 27 at the time of diagnosis with a range of 12to 58 years. They had received from 1 to 24 doses of anti-TNF, and the majority had more than three infusions. Interestingly, 22 of the 24 patients were men. As we do not have the ability to determine the denominator of patients in the at-risk age/gender group who have received anti-TNF therapy, calculating an accurate rate is difficult, but we can try to make an estimate. More than 1 million patients have been treated worldwide with infliximab (for all indications) of which more than 300,000 have Crohn's disease. Assuming that at least half of these Crohn's patients are between the ages of 12 and 58 and half are men, then somewhere in the range of 75,000 young men may have been exposed to infliximab. Therefore, a conservative estimate is 15 male cases out of 75,000 patients, which translates to 2 patients per 10,000 exposed. The rate is probably lower because the denominator of patient-years is likely higher, but it is fairly safe to say that the rate is not higher than 2 per 10,000.

Editor's note (TMB): There is a separate chapter on risk and benefit considerations in teenaged patients.

Progressive Multifacet Leukoencephalopathy

The biggest safety concern regarding natalizumab is the association with progressive multifocal leukoencephalopathy (PML). PML is a neurodegenerative disease resulting from JC-virus infection. In 2005 natalizumab was withdrawn from the market for the treatment of MS, and Crohn's disease studies were halted based on the report of PML in three patients (one with Crohn's disease, two with MS). Since then, a number of additional patients have been identified (Data on file, Elan Pharmaceuticals, March 2011). As of March 2011 there have been over 100 confirmed cases of PML in patients receiving natalizumab. All of these patients except one were receiving treatment for MS. All patients received at least one year of therapy before symptoms of PML were identified. PML is a concerning disease and has a high rate of death or significant disability. Outcomes have been variable in these reported patients. By early 2011, approximately 80,000 patients have been treated with natalizumab worldwide. The estimated incidence is about 1 per 1000 treated patients. This estimation is slightly higher than the 6 per 10,000 rate of NHL associated with anti-TNF therapy. The threshold of risk patients or their physicians will accept is variable (see "Patient Perceptions and Risk Thresholds" section), but this very small chance of developing PML will have to be weighed against the relatively high response rate, even in patients who have failed anti-TNF therapy. Despite the expected benefits and rarity of PML, patients and physicians are still hesitant to accept this treatment. A successful strategy that I have used in talking with patients is to suggest that they take natalizumab for 12 weeks and then we will assess for a response. I reassure them that no cases of PML have been reported before 1 year of therapy. Then, if they are responding, patients typically perceive the benefit-risk balance more in favor of benefit and want to continue treatment because they now have proof that the drug is working. If they are not better—clearly the medication is stopped. With this strategy, all of the patients I have treated with natalizumab who have responded chose to continue with long-term maintenance, despite significant hesitations they had before initiating therapy.

Treatment Strategies to Optimize the Trade-Offs of Benefits and Risks

The trade-off of benefits versus risks needs to be determined on an individual-patient basis. Patients who are at most risk from their disease will benefit the most from effective treatment. In contrast, a patient with mild disease who is in a high-risk group for an adverse event (e.g., elderly on concomitant medications or young men) will have a less favorable benefit-risk ratio. In addition, patients will have varying thresholds of how much risk of treatment they are willing to tolerate and how much treatment benefit they will demand in order to accept that stated risk.

A decision analysis was performed exploring the benefits versus the risks of therapy for Crohn's disease patients treated with infliximab.[13] In the hypothetical clinical trial constructed for the decision analysis, 100,000 patients received infliximab and 100,000 patients received "standard therapy," defined as continued 5-aminosalicylate (5-ASA), corticosteroid, or immunomodulator therapy. In the infliximab group more than 12,000 more patients achieved clinical remission and more than 4000 patients avoided surgery. This was at the expense of 142 more lymphomas in the infliximab group, and 271 more deaths in the infliximab group, mostly attributable to sepsis. Despite the increased rate of lymphoma and death, overall there was a benefit in quality of life for the infliximab group (0.02 more quality-of-life-adjusted years [QALYs] for infliximab-treated patients) based on its substantial clinical benefit. The original analysis was performed with a lymphoma rate of 2 per 1000 patient-years, which is higher than the recent estimate of 6 per 10,000 patient-years. When running the analysis again with this updated lymphoma rate, there are fewer lymphomas in the infliximab-treated patients, but the mortality is still higher than standard therapy as most of the deaths are relate to sepsis, not lymphoma. The QALYs did not change. This analysis not only reaffirms the treatment benefit afforded by anti-TNF therapy but also reminds us that there is a cost and proper patient selection to optimize the benefit-risk balance is critical.

Benefits of Early Therapy

The ratio could be maximized by either increasing the benefit or decreasing the risk. Recent studies exploring treatment strategies have shown that we can increase the treatment response to infliximab higher than what had been seen in the RCTs reported previously. First, D'Haens and colleagues showed that early treatment (within 2 years of Crohn's disease diagnosis) with combination immunomodulator and anti-TNF therapy was superior to standard therapy. Standard therapy included sequential treatment with corticosteroids followed by azathioprine, and then anti-TNFs only, if they were unable to taper off corticosteroids despite azathioprine. In the early combination group 62% achieved steroid-free remission at the end of 1 year compared to 42% in the standard therapy group. There were slightly more serious adverse events in the early combination group (31% vs. 25%), but this was not statistically significant. Despite the methodological limitations of this open-label study,

an important message is that initiation of biologics earlier in the course of disease may enhance efficacy of treatment.

Another important question is the necessity of using anti-TNF therapy in combination with immunomodulators, as opposed to anti-TNF therapy used on its own. There were two recent RCTs addressing this question, but they had important differences in study design. The COMMIT study randomized patients to infliximab monotherapy or infliximab with methotrexate.[16] Results showed no difference between these treatment groups. The SONIC study randomized patients to azathioprine monotherapy, infliximab monotherapy, or combination therapy.[17] Here, results showed a statistically significant improvement in remission rates for combination therapy without a difference in serious adverse events. COMMIT included patients who had Crohn's disease for an average of 10 years, 25% had previously been exposed to 6-MP or azathioprine, and all patients were induced into remission with corticosteroids. SONIC included patients who had Crohn's disease for an average of 2 years, all were naïve to immunomodulators, and less than one third of patients were concomitantly on corticosteroids. These two patient populations are different, which may be important in deciding which patients deserve combination therapy. My belief is that these SONIC results lead us to favor combination therapy in patients with recent-onset disease, as we can increase their benefit of response, without significantly increasing risk. Exceptions are young men (who are the most at risk for HSTCL) and those older than 60 (who are at most risk from life-threatening infections). In these groups, consideration of personal disease characteristics associated with more debilitating disease (i.e., extent of disease, prior surgery, perianal involvement) should guide the decision.

Patient Perceptions and Risk Thresholds

Patients receive information about medical treatments from a variety of resources. Although most are well intentioned, much of the data communicated are unfortunately inaccurate and misleading. A survey of patients' perceptions of benefits and risks of biologic therapy confirmed this concern.[18] The majority of patients believed that infliximab would lead to remission of Crohn's disease over 50% of the time at 1 year, and almost 20% of patients expected a 70% 1-year remission rate. More than one third of patients responded that infliximab carried no increased risk of lymphoma, and when presented a scenario of a "new" drug for Crohn's disease that carried risks mirroring those of infliximab, 64% of patients responded that they would not take the medication, despite its described benefits. These results should raise awareness that patients oftentimes have misinformation and need help in understanding the expected benefits of treatment and the risks of therapy and of their disease.

Patients are willing to accept the risk of serious treatment side effects to varying degrees. This was quantified for patients with Crohn's disease.[19] In a large online survey of nearly 600 patients, using the technique of conjoint analysis, patients' thresholds of how much risk they were willing to accept for death due to sepsis, lymphoma, or PML were calculated. A few interesting patterns were revealed. First, despite the outcome of death, patients were more concerned about PML than the other adverse outcomes. Next, patients were willing to accept a higher risk when the treatment benefit was more robust. In addition, in general, the amount of risk patients were willing to take was higher than the risks that have been noted in the literature. These data suggest that patients are willing to accept the risk of sepsis, lymphoma, and PML, but only if they can expect a meaningful response to therapy. In a separate study using the same survey, parents of patients with Crohn's disease were also questioned.[20] Parents were willing to take higher risks for their children than the adult patients were for themselves, but only if the child had severely active disease. Conversely, if the children had less severe disease, parents were risk averse and were willing to accept a much lower magnitude of risk than the adult patients were. The study was also performed with gastroenterologists.[21] The physicians included in this study were also willing to accept a risk of sepsis, lymphoma, or PML at rates higher than that already reported and, in some cases, higher than patients. Taken together, these data teach us that patients, parents, and physicians are willing to accept the risks of the rare but serious side effects associated with biologic therapy. However, it is the job of physicians to determine when the expected treatment benefit is high enough to expose our patients to these risks.

● CONCLUSIONS

Biologic therapy has changed the lives of many of our patients by offering substantial clinical improvement when other medications have failed. These medications are not without risk, but the chance of serious adverse events are very small, and in most patients, the treatment benefits will outweigh these risks. Current research is focusing on predicting individuals' disease course and treatment response that will help both physicians and patients in making decisions regarding the appropriate timing for biologic therapy. In addition to personalizing treatment choices, it is critical to allow patients to clearly understand the benefits and risks of therapy. Thus, we should not only have our goal as prescribing the most appropriate medical therapy on the basis of best available evidence but also on helping our patients make treatment choices that fit with their personal preferences.

References

1. Hanauer SB, Feagan BG, Lichtenstein GR, et al.; ACCENT I Study Group. Maintenance infliximab for Crohn's disease: the ACCENT I randomised trial. *Lancet*. 2002;359(9317):1541–1549.

2. Sands BE, Anderson FH, Bernstein CN, et al. Infliximab maintenance therapy for fistulizing Crohn's disease. *N Engl J Med*. 2004;350(9):876–885.

3. Colombel JF, Sandborn WJ, Rutgeerts P, et al. Adalimumab for maintenance of clinical response and remission in patients with Crohn's disease: the CHARM trial. *Gastroenterology*. 2007;132(1):52–65.

4. Schreiber S, Khaliq-Kareemi M, Lawrance IC, et al.. Maintenance therapy with certolizumab pegol for Crohn's disease. *N Engl J Med*. 2007;357(3):239–250.

5. D'Haens G, Baert F, van Assche G, et al. Early combined immunosuppression or conventional management in patients with newly diagnosed Crohn's disease: an open randomised trial. *Lancet*. 2008;371(9613):660–667.

6. Sandborn WJ, Colombel JF, Enns R, et al. Natalizumab induction and maintenance therapy for Crohn's disease. *N Engl J Med*. 2005;353(18):1912–1925.

7. Munkholm P, Langholz E, Davidsen M, Binder V. Intestinal cancer risk and mortality in patients with Crohn's disease. *Gastroenterology*. 1993;105(6):1716–1723.

8. Cosnes J, Nion-Larmurier I, Beaugerie L, Afchain P, Tiret E, Gendre JP. Impact of the increasing use of immunosuppressants in Crohn's disease on the need for intestinal surgery. *Gut*. 2005;54(2):237–241.

9. Hutfless SM, Weng X, Liu L, Allison J, Herrinton LJ. Mortality by medication use among patients with inflammatory bowel disease, 1996–2003. *Gastroenterology*. 2007;133(6):1779–1786.

10. Lichtenstein GR, Feagan BG, Cohen RD, et al. Serious infections and mortality in association with therapies for Crohn's disease: TREAT registry. *Clin Gastroenterol Hepatol*. 2006;4(5):621–630.

11. Toruner M, Loftus EV Jr, Harmsen WS, et al. Risk factors for opportunistic infections in patients with inflammatory bowel disease. *Gastroenterology*. 2008;134(4):929–936.

12. Colombel JF, Loftus EV Jr, Tremaine WJ, et al. The safety profile of infliximab in patients with Crohn's disease: the Mayo clinic experience in 500 patients. *Gastroenterology*. 2004;126(1):19–31.

13. Siegel CA, Hur C, Korzenik JR, Gazelle GS, Sands BE. Risks and benefits of infliximab for the treatment of Crohn's disease. *Clin Gastroenterol Hepatol*. 2006;4(8):1017–24; quiz 976.

14. Wolfe F, Michaud K, Anderson J, Urbansky K. Tuberculosis infection in patients with rheumatoid arthritis and the effect of infliximab therapy. *Arthritis Rheum*. 2004;50(2):372–379.

15. Siegel CA, Marden SM, Persing SM, Larson RJ, Sands BE. Risk of lymphoma associated with combination anti-tumor necrosis factor and immunomodulator therapy for the treatment of Crohn's disease: a meta-analysis. *Clin Gastroenterol Hepatol*. 2009;7(8):874–881.

16. Feagan BG, McDonald J, Ponich T, et al. Combination of maintenance methotrexate-infliximab trial (COMMIT). Presented at: Digestive Disease Week; May, 2008. Abstract 682C.

17. Colombel JF, Sandborn WJ, Reinish W, et al. Infliximab, azathioprine, or combination therapy for Crohn's disease. *N Engl J Med*. 2010;362:1383–1395.

18. Siegel CA, Levy LC, Mackenzie TA, Sands BE. Patient perceptions of the risks and benefits of infliximab for the treatment of inflammatory bowel disease. *Inflamm Bowel Dis*. 2008;14(1):1–6.

19. Johnson FR, Ozdemir S, Mansfield C, et al. Crohn's disease patients' risk-benefit preferences: serious adverse event risks versus treatment efficacy. *Gastroenterology*. 2007;133(3):769–779.

20. Johnson FR, Ozdemir S, Mansfield C, Hass S, Siegel CA, Sands BE. Are adult patients more tolerant of treatment risks than parents of juvenile patients? *Risk Anal*. 2009;29(1):121–136.

21. Sands BE, Siegel CA, Johnson FR, Ozdemir S, Hass S, Miller DW. Gastroenterologists' tolerance for Crohn's disease treatment risks. Presented at the United European Gastroenterology Week, Paris, October, 2007.

Medical Treatment Options for Perianal Crohn's Disease | 116

Sara N. Horst and David A. Schwartz

The development of perianal Crohn's disease can, significantly, negatively impact a patient's quality of life. Typically, patients will present with perianal pain or drainage. Unfortunately, the disease process will frequently lead to incontinence and/or the need for proctectomy. Over the last decade, the treatment of this dreaded manifestation of Crohn's disease has improved. The concept of a multimodality approach to this problem using both medical and surgical therapy has largely become the standard of care. Surgical therapy for perianal Crohn's disease will be covered in a separate chapter. However, it is important to note that medical therapy seems to be much more effective if a surgeon has first established drainage of all abscesses present and has placed setons in any complex fistulas that are present. The focus of this chapter will be the medical treatment options for patients with fistulizing perianal Crohn's disease.

EPIDEMIOLOGY

Fistulas are common in Crohn's disease. The cumulative frequency of perianal fistulous disease ranges from 17% to 43% in reports from referral centers. Population cohort studies from Europe and the United States have shown similar rates of perianal fistulas in patients with Crohn's disease, at 23% and 21%, respectively.[1,2] Another population-based retrospective study of patients with Crohn's disease in the Canadian province of Manitoba found that perianal fistulas alone were reported in 9.9% to 14.0% of patients, and both luminal and perianal disease was reported in 3.3% to 7.7%.[3] In the cohort from Olmsted County, Minnesota, the cumulative risk for developing a perianal fistula among patients with Crohn's disease diagnosed between 1970 and 1993 was 21% after 10 years and 26% after 20 years. An evaluation of fistulizing disease by type showed 54% fistulas originated in the perianal region.[2]

Perianal Crohn's disease often occurs at, or around, the time of diagnosis. In a Swedish cohort study, 25% with fistulizing disease had anal fistula more than 6 months prior to when they were diagnosed with Crohn's disease; another 46% developed fistula within 6 months of diagnosis.[1]

The risk of developing perianal fistulas increases as the luminal manifestation of the disease decreases. Crohn's patients with rectal inflammation have the highest risk of developing perianal Crohn's disease, and those with ileal disease have the lowest risk. In the Swedish cohort study, 90% patients with perianal fistula had colitis and rectal disease, compared with 41% with colon disease and rectal sparing, and only 12% with isolated small bowel disease.[1]

Fistulas in patients with Crohn's disease tend to be chronic and relapsing. In Olmstead County, the recurrence rate was estimated to be 34%. In this study, the mean time to fistula closure was 14 weeks, and mean time to recurrence was 2.8 years. In total, 82% of these patients ultimately required surgery (21% required proctectomy).[2]

ANATOMY AND CLASSIFICATION

It is important to understand the anatomy of the anal canal in order to define fistulizing disease. The anal canal comprises

- internal anal sphincter: continuation of circular smooth muscle from rectum
- external anal sphincter: downward extension of skeletal muscle from puborectalis

The intersphincteric space lies in between the two sphincters. The dentate line marks the point of transition from transitional and columnar epithelium of rectum to squamous epithelium of anus and is usually in the middle portion of internal anal sphincter. Anal crypts, which contain anal glands at the base, are present at the dentate line. These can sometimes penetrate into intersphincteric space and can be a source of fistula (**Fig. 116.1**).

Classification schemes for perianal fistulas are extremely important as it facilitates communication between clinicians and surgeons and helps to identify patients who would benefit from surgical intervention. The two most commonly used classification systems are the Parks classification and the simple/complex scheme.

The Parks classification scheme is the most anatomically accurate. It involves five types of perianal fistulas, using the external sphincter as central point of reference and these include intersphincteric, transphincteric, suprasphincteric,

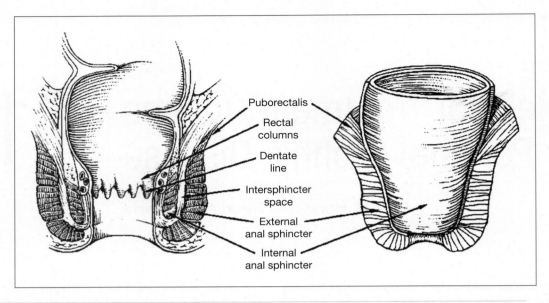

FIGURE 116.1 • Schematic diagram of the perianal region. Reproduced with permission from Sandborn et al.[4]

extrasphincteric, and superficial. Branching or horseshoeing and the location are noted. However, this classification does not include factors such as abscess presence or fistulous connection to other structures such as bladder or vagina, which are important in determining the appropriate therapies.

In 2003, an AGA technical review was published and proposed a more clinically relevant approach to classifying fistulas. A simple fistula is defined as a low, single external opening and is superficial, intersphincteric, or low transphincteric, and there is no evidence of abscess, rectovaginal fistula, or anorectal stricture. A complex fistula is defined as a high transphincteric, extrasphincteric, or suprasphincteric fistula with multiple external openings, and it may have horseshoeing or perianal abscesses and/or rectovaginal fistulas. These fistulas may have strictures and active rectal inflammation. This is clinically important as several studies have shown better outcomes for simple fistulas.[4]

● MEDICAL THERAPIES

The natural history of Crohn's perianal fistulas may be changing as immunosuppressive and anti-tumor necrosis factor (TNF) medications have emerged as effective medical treatments for these patients. A summary of the potential medical treatments options will be outlined in the following sections.

Antibiotics

Antibiotics are the most commonly used treatment for perianal Crohn's disease. They are used for both their activity in perianal sepsis and for their anti-inflammatory properties. The most common antibiotics used are metronidazole at doses of 750 to 1000 mg/day or ciprofloxacin at 1000 to 1500 mg/day for up to 2 to 4 months. Adverse events commonly associated with metronidazole include metallic taste, glossitis, nausea, and a distal peripheral sensory neuropathy. Adverse events

with ciprofloxacin occur less commonly but include headache, nausea, diarrhea, and rash.

There have been multiple case reports regarding the benefit of metronidazole in patients with perianal Crohn's disease.[4] One of the larger studies was an open-label study of metronidazole at 20 mg/kg/day in 21 consecutive patients with Crohn's disease and perianal fistulas. All patients had a clinical response defined as a decrease in pain and tenderness. Fistula closure occurred in 83% of patients. Clinical improvement was noted after 6 to 8 weeks of therapy.[5] Given the high rate of adverse events with metronidazole, physicians began using ciprofloxacin in the 1980s. Similar to metronidazole, recurrence is common after discontinuation of therapy.[4]

Recently, a randomized, double-blinded, placebo-controlled study evaluated ciprofloxacin or metronidazole for the treatment of perianal fistulas in patients with Crohn's disease. Twenty-five patients were randomized to ciprofloxacin 500 mg (10 patients), metronidazole 500 mg (7 patients), or placebo (8 patients) twice daily for 10 weeks. Response (≥50% reduction in the number of draining fistulas) at week 10 was seen in 4 patients (40%) treated with ciprofloxacin, 1 patient (14.3%) treated with metronidazole, and 1 patient (12.5%) with placebo. One patient ($P = 0.43$) from both the ciprofloxacin and placebo, and 5 (71.4%; $P < 0.02$) treated with metronidazole dropped out of the study. This small study suggested that remission and response occurred more often in patients treated with ciprofloxacin, but the differences were not significant.[6]

Antibiotics may also be beneficial in bridging to immunosuppressive therapy. A prospective open-label trial of 52 patients was done. Patients were divided into three groups: antibiotics only, addition of azathioprine (AZA; 2–2.5 mg/kg/day) after 8 weeks, and antibiotics added to those already on AZA at onset of the study. At week 8, 50% of patients had responded to antibiotic therapy and there was no statistical difference between those who were on concomitant immunosuppressive therapy at onset and those who were not (41% vs. 54%). However, at week 20, those who were maintained on AZA were more likely to maintain their response after the antibiotics were discontinued (48% vs. 15% $P = 0.03$).[7]

Azathioprine and 6-Mercaptopurine

The use of AZA and 6-mercaptopurine (6-MP), in current clinical practice, is based on a meta-analysis of five controlled trials in which fistula closure was a secondary end point and uncontrolled case series in adults and children. No prospective trials exist to date evaluating these medications with fistula closure as primary end point.[8] A total of 70 patients were included in the meta-analysis analyzing studies where fistula closure was a secondary end point. This analysis found that 22 of 42 (54%) patients with perianal Crohn's disease who received AZA/6-MP responded versus only 6 of 29 (21%) patients who received placebo (odds ratio = 4.44). Caution should be taken as the primary goal of these studies was to treat active inflammatory Crohn's disease and was not designed primarily to look at the effect on perianal fistulas. In fact, only one of the studies stratified the patients for the presence of fistulas at randomization.

It is important to optimize the dose of these medications to achieve maximal effect. Doses of 2.0 to 2.5 mg/kg/day of AZA and 1.0 to 1.5 mg/kg/day of 6-MP have been shown to be the most efficacious. Adverse events including leukopenia, allergic reactions, infections, pancreatitis, and drug-induced hepatitis are reported to occur in 9% to 15% of patients receiving these medications for inflammatory bowel disease. Patient's leukocyte count and liver transaminase levels should be monitored throughout treatment.[4]

Cyclosporine

Multiple small uncontrolled case series have reported use of intravenous cyclosporine to treat fistulizing disease. Medication is administered via intravenous continuous infusion (secondary to poor oral bioavailability) at a dose of 4 mg/kg/day. Clinical improvement occurs rapidly, usually within 1 to 2 weeks. The overall initial response rate was 83% in these case series. When these patients were converted to oral cyclosporine, relapses tended to occur.[4] Clinicians have used intravenous infusion as the initial "rescue therapy," and oral cyclosporine as "bridge therapy" while other treatments are initiated such as AZA/6-MP. Adverse events in patients treated with cyclosporine include renal insufficiency, hirsutism, hypertension, paresthesias, headaches, seizures, tremor, gingival hyperplasia, hepatotoxicity, and increased incidence of infection.[6]

Tacrolimus

Tacrolimus has been reported for use in patients with refractory fistulizing Crohn's disease. In one placebo-controlled trial, 48 patients were randomized to tacrolimus standard dose 0.2 mg/kg/day versus placebo for 10 weeks. In the tacrolimus group, 43% had fistula improvement (closure of ≥50% fistulas for >4 weeks) compared with 8% placebo patients ($P = 0.004$). However, complete fistula closure was only achieved in 10% of the patients who received tacrolimus. Fistula closure in the treatment group was not improved with concomitant immunosuppressive therapy with AZA/6-MP (38% closure with therapy vs. 50% without). Number of adverse events was higher in the treatment group (5.2 vs. 3.9; $P = 0.009$) including headache, insomnia, elevated creatinine, paresthesias, and tremor. Of 15 patients in the treatment arm who had been treated with infliximab in the past, 7 (47%) improved with treatment.[9] Therefore, in patients who have failed infliximab treatment, this may offer an alternative therapy to colectomy.

Some authors have suggested that longer courses of treatment (>6 months) may improve fistula healing rates with tacrolimus. One small prospective, open-label study was conducted, in which 10 patients who had fistulas (4 were perianal) previously and were unsuccessfully treated with all conventional therapy (i.e., antibiotics, azathioprine, or 6-MP and infliximab) were treated with oral long-term tacrolimus (0.05 mg/kg every 12 hours) and followed for 6 to 24 months. These patients were evaluated for response or remission with the perianal Crohn's Disease Activity Index and magnetic resonance imaging (MRI)-based scores. Four patients had a partial clinical response and five patients a complete clinical response. The use of tacrolimus requires regular monitoring of renal function and drug levels.[6]

Methotrexate

Methotrexate is generally used as third-line agent for patients with luminal Crohn's who are intolerant to AZA or 6-MP, and it has been used similarly for patients with perianal Crohn's disease. A few uncontrolled studies have evaluated the use of methotrexate in fistulizing Crohn's disease. In one retrospective case series of 16 Crohn's disease patients with perianal fistulas, 4 (25%) had complete closure and 5 (31%) had partial closure.[10] Further studies are needed prior to methotrexate use being recommended for fistulizing Crohn's disease.

Anti-TNFα Antibodies

Infliximab

Infliximab was the first drug in this class. It is a murine/human chimeric monoclonal antibody directed toward soluble and membrane-bound TNFα. There have been two randomized double-blinded, placebo-controlled trials demonstrating infliximab's efficacy for fistulizing Crohn's disease. The first study evaluated infliximab induction therapy, and included 94 patients with perianal or abdominal fistulas and were randomized to control group or to receive 5 mg/kg or 10 mg/kg of infliximab at weeks 0, 2, and 6. The primary end point was ≥ 50% reduction in the number of draining fistulas, and the secondary end point was fistula closure. Sixty-eight percent of patients in the 5-mg/kg group and 56% of patients in the 10-mg/kg group versus 26% controls reached the primary end point. Fifty-five percent of the 5-mg/kg group and 38% of the 10-mg/kg group vs. 13% of control group reached the secondary end point. The median length of time to fistula closure was 3 months.[11]

The ACCENT II trial evaluated infliximab maintenance therapy. Time to loss of response was the primary end point. Three hundred and six patients were enrolled and received 5 mg/kg infliximab at week 0, 2, and 6. Of those patients, 195 (64%) demonstrated response to therapy at weeks 10 and 14.

At week 14, responders were then randomized to infliximab 5 mg/kg or placebo every 8 weeks until week 54. Time to loss of response was 40 weeks versus 14 weeks in the infliximab maintenance group versus placebo group, respectively. Thirty-six percent of patients in the infliximab group maintained cessation of drainage at week 54 compared to 19% of the placebo group (*P* = 0.009).[12] A secondary analysis of the results of the ACCENT II trial by Lichtenstein et al. showed that infliximab maintenance resulted in significantly fewer hospitalizations, number of surgeries, and mean number of hospital days.[13]

Doses proven to be efficacious in clinical trials include induction therapy with 5 mg/kg at week 0, 2, and 6, and maintenance therapy of 5 mg/kg every 8 weeks. Doses may be escalated to 10 mg/kg per dose or the dosing frequency shortened if loss of response is seen at the lower dose. Adverse events observed in patients treated with infliximab include infusion reactions, an increased rate of infections including tuberculosis and other opportunistic infections, delayed hypersensitivity reactions, formations of antibodies to infliximab, formation of double-stranded DNA antibodies, and, in rare cases, drug-induced lupus. All patients should have a purified protein derivative (PPD) placed and hepatitis B status checked prior to initiation of any anti-TNF antibody.

Adalimumab

Adalimumab is a fully humanized monoclonal antibody to TNF. Multiple trials and case reports have been published regarding the use of adalimumab in Crohn's disease. The efficacy of adalimumab for fistulizing Crohn's disease was evaluated as a major secondary end point of the CHARM trial. Among the randomized responders to the two open-label doses of adalimumab, maintenance adalimumab resulted in complete fistula closure at week 56 in 39% of patients compared to 13% of patients on placebo who had only received induction adalimumab (*P* = 0.043). At long-term follow-up, of all patients with healed fistulas at week 56 (both adalimumab and placebo groups), 90% (28 of 31) maintained healing following 1 year of open-label adalimumab therapy. Of the adalimumab-treated patients with fistulas at baseline, approximately 60% (23 of 37) had maintained fistula healing after 2 years of therapy. There were significant decreases in the mean number of draining fistulas per day among adalimumab-treated patients compared with placebo-treated patients during the double-blind treatment period. For all randomized patients, the mean number of draining fistulas per day was 1.34 for placebo compared with a mean of 0.88 for the combined adalimumab groups (*P* = 0.002).[14] In clinical trials, adverse events attributed to adalimumab are similar to infliximab. Patients start at 160 mg given subcutaneously. This is followed by 80 mg at week 2 and then 40 mg every other week. Dose can be escalated to 40 mg weekly if there is a partial response, or loss of response, with every other week dosing. As with infliximab, patients should have a PPD placed and hepatitis B status checked prior to initiation of therapy.

Other Biologic Therapies Approved for Crohn's Disease

Currently, there is no data to support use of certolizumab and natalizumab in patients with fistulizing Crohn's disease.

Miscellaneous Nonsurgical Therapies

Therapies including elemental diets, total parenteral nutrition, mycophenolate mofetil, thalidomide, granulocyte colony-stimulating factor, and hyperbaric oxygen have been reported in uncontrolled case series and case reports as being effective in the treatment of perianal Crohn's disease. However, no controlled trials exist.[4]

● TREATMENT ALGORITHM FOR PERIANAL FISTULAS

The goal of therapy is to achieve complete fistula closure and avoid some of the frequent complications that negatively affect a patient's quality of life. One can best achieve this by employing a "top-down" medical approach to patients with perianal Crohn's disease. It is important to stress again that the best outcomes are achieved when combination medical and surgical therapy are used together. The surgical options for these patients are beyond the scope of this chapter and are reviewed in a chapter 32.

A straight-forward way to approach these patients is to begin by assessing their luminal disease with a flexible sigmoidoscopy or colonoscopy. This is done mainly to assess the amount of inflammation present in the rectum. Next, the perianal disease is mapped out with either a pelvic MRI or a rectal endoscopic ultrasound (EUS). Digital rectal examination can be inaccurate; imaging to further delineate fistula type and extent is therefore necessary. Imaging modalities such as EUS and MRI can provide the virtual roadmap for therapy and is recommended with exam under anesthesia (EUA) for a comprehensive evaluation of extent of perianal disease (see Chapter 32 for further discussion). This helps one determine if any abscess exists and the type of fistulas that are present. Once this is done, one should be able to divide patients into categories based on the type of fistula (simple vs. complex), degree of rectal inflammation present, and the severity of symptoms.

The medical treatment strategies for the different fistulas are outlined as follows.

Simple Perianal Fistulas

The treatment goal for simple fistulas should be complete fistula closure. Potential treatment options include antibiotics, AZA/6-MP, infliximab, and fistulotomy[4] (**Fig. 116.2**). Often, these fistulas do well with isolated medical therapy alone.

Antibiotics—Antibiotics are used widely in the treatment of simple fistulas and have been recommended in practice guidelines and treatment algorithms.

Immunosuppressive agents—AZA/6-MP can be used to treat simple fistulas and are recommended in treatment guidelines. However, this treatment strategy has not been evaluated in a randomized placebo-controlled trial. These agents are slow acting and may be more useful in maintaining fistula closure than in inducing fistula closure. One trial has shown that immunomodulators are useful in maintaining fistula closure when antibiotics were used to induce fistula closure.[7]

Anti-TNF Therapy—Placebo-controlled trials have shown that infliximab and adalimumab are effective in reducing the

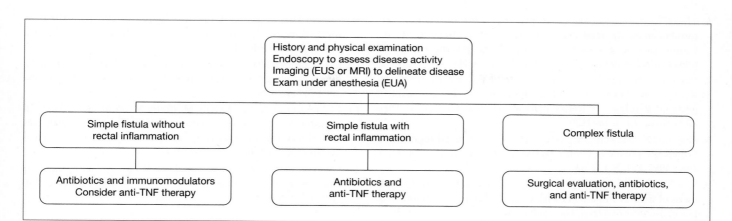

FIGURE 116.2 • Current treatment algorithm for managing patients with perianal fistulas in Crohn's disease.

number of draining fistulas and maintenance of that reduction. Concomitant immunosuppressive therapy may be useful, but further studies need to evaluate this treatment strategy.

Recommendations—Although there is no good prospective data (level 1 evidence) to make clear recommendations about whether antibiotics, immunosuppression with AZA/6-MP, or anti-TNF antibodies or a combination of these treatments are the preferred strategy for treating simple Crohn's perianal fistulas, in general, one should have a low threshold to begin anti-TNF therapy in these patients in order to prevent the progression of a simple fistula into a complex one. In addition, if a patient has a simple fistula with active proctitis, it is important to address the rectal inflammation in order to improve the chance of healing, particularly if surgical therapy is to be considered. In this situation, strong consideration should be taken of anti-TNF treatment to help improve the proctitis and close the fistula.

Complex Perianal Fistulas

The treatment goals for complex fistula are slightly different than with simple fistulas and usually involve trying to achieve cessation of drainage without true fistula closure. Potential treatments include antibiotics, AZA/6-MP, infliximab and adalimumab, and surgery (placement of noncutting setons, endorectal advancement flaps, repair of rectovaginal fistulas, fecal diversion, and proctectomy). Tacrolimus and cyclosporine are reserved for those patients who are refractory or intolerant to anti-TNF therapy.

Antibiotics—Antibiotics are widely used in complex fistula treatment. Relapse rates are high after antibiotic treatment is discontinued so antibiotics should likely be used in combination with other medical or surgical therapies.

Immunosuppressive agents—Immunosuppression with AZA/6-MP has been recommended for use in complex fistulas, but, as in simple fistulizing disease, no placebo-controlled trials exist regarding this treatment strategy and these medications are slow acting. Therefore, they are likely more useful in maintaining fistula closure as in simple fistulas.

Anti-TNF therapy—As mentioned previously, infliximab has been shown in placebo-controlled trials to reduce the number of draining fistulas and maintain fistula closure. Trials

have shown, as a secondary end point, that adalimumab has improved the fistula closure rate.

Other medical options—Tacrolimus and cyclosporine can rarely be used in some patients that fail all other medical and surgical therapies.

CONCLUSION

Perianal disease is a common manifestation of Crohn's disease and can be associated with significant morbidity, including need for proctectomy. Treatment should begin with assessing the type and extent of fistulizing process and any associated abscess with imaging techniques such as EUS and MRI to be used in conjunction with surgical evaluation. Medical and surgical combined treatment strategies have been shown to lead to improved outcomes and will be needed in most patients. A minority of patients with simple fistulas may achieve cure with either medical therapy or surgical treatment alone. The remainder of patients will likely require control of fistula drainage with noncutting setons and then the initiation of medical therapy that includes antibiotics, AZA/6-MP, and anti-TNF therapies with infliximab or adalimumab. Tacrolimus and cyclosporine can be considered in rare patients with refractory disease who have failed other multimodality therapies.

References

1. Hellers G, Bergstrand O, Ewerth S, Holmström B. Occurrence and outcome after primary treatment of anal fistulae in Crohn's disease. *Gut.* 1980;21(6):525–527.
2. Schwartz DA, Loftus EV Jr, Tremaine WJ, et al. The natural history of fistulizing Crohn's disease in Olmsted County, Minnesota. *Gastroenterology.* 2002;122(4):875–880.
3. Tang LY, Rawsthorne P, Bernstein CN. Are perineal and luminal fistulas associated in Crohn's disease? A population-based study. *Clin Gastroenterol Hepatol.* 2006;4(9):1130–1134.
4. Sandborn WJ, Fazio VW, Feagan BG, Hanauer SB; American Gastroenterological Association Clinical Practice Committee. AGA technical review on perianal Crohn's disease. *Gastroenterology.* 2003;125(5):1508–1530.
5. Bernstein LH, Frank MS, Brandt LJ, Boley SJ. Healing of perineal Crohn's disease with metronidazole. *Gastroenterology.* 1980;79(2):357–365.

6. Thia KT, Mahadevan U, Feagan BG, et al. **Ciprofloxacin or metronidazole for the treatment of perianal fistulas in patients with Crohn's disease: a randomized, double-blind, placebo-controlled pilot study.** *Inflamm Bowel Dis.* 2009;15(1):17–24.

7. Dejaco C, Harrer M, Waldhoer T, Miehsler W, Vogelsang H, Reinisch W. **Antibiotics and azathioprine for the treatment of perianal fistulas in Crohn's disease.** *Aliment Pharmacol Ther.* 2003;18(11–12):1113–1120.

8. Pearson DC, May GR, Fick GH, Sutherland LR. **Azathioprine and 6-mercaptopurine in Crohn disease. A meta-analysis.** *Ann Intern Med.* 1995;123(2):132–142.

9. Sandborn WJ, Present DH, Isaacs KL, et al. **Tacrolimus for the treatment of fistulas in patients with Crohn's disease: a randomized, placebo-controlled trial.** *Gastroenterology.* 2003;125(2):380–388.

10. Mahadevan U, Marion JF, Present DH. **Fistula response to methotrexate in Crohn's disease: a case series.** *Aliment Pharmacol Ther.* 2003;18(10):1003–1008.

11. Present DH, Rutgeerts P, Targan S, et al. **Infliximab for the treatment of fistulas in patients with Crohn's disease.** *N Engl J Med.* 1999;340(18):1398–1405.

12. Sands BE, Anderson FH, Bernstein CN, et al. **Infliximab maintenance therapy for fistulizing Crohn's disease.** *N Engl J Med.* 2004;350(9):876–885.

13. Lichtenstein GR, Yan S, Bala M, Blank M, Sands BE. **Infliximab maintenance treatment reduces hospitalizations, surgeries, and procedures in fistulizing Crohn's disease.** *Gastroenterology.* 2005;128(4):862–869.

14. Colombel JF, Schwartz DA, Sandborn WJ, et al. **Adalimumab for the treatment of fistulas in patients with Crohn's disease.** *Gut.* 2009;58(7):940–948.

Evidence-Based Integrative Therapy in IBD

117

Joyce M. Koh, Laura K. Turnbull, John O. Clarke, and
Gerard E. Mullin

Botanicals; food-based supplements, including prebiotics and probiotics; and acupuncture are considered to be "complementary and alternative medicine" (CAM) modalities but have been used for millennia to treat a myriad of ailments. The efficacy and safety of many CAM therapies are unknown; however, their vast usage is such that they cannot be ignored. A recent CDC survey showed that almost 4 out of 10 American adults utilize CAM.[1] CAM use may be higher in inflammatory bowel disease (IBD) due to the chronicity of the disease.[2] The utilization of CAM, commonly accepted to be 50% in patients with IBD, has been well studied (Table 117.1).[1–3]

Integrative medicine combines conventional medical practice with CAM approaches that are safe and effective. The Institute of Medicine regards integrative medicine to be a crucial issue and considers it as an approach to patient care that may yield better outcomes. It is an approach to medicine that "takes into account biological, psychological, social, and spiritual aspects of individual's lives."[3]

Many CAM therapies await further research to illustrate their mechanisms of action, efficacy, and safety. Nevertheless, this chapter aims to review selected aspects of integrative therapy by briefly alluding to proposed mechanisms of action, benefits, as well as indications. Because there are so many modalities currently in use and a wide variety of supplements employed, we will be selective in our discussion. It is our goal to provide familiarization with this very crucial area of medical practice, particularly because CAM therapies are continually expanding and increasing numbers of our patients are utilizing them.

Editor's note (TMB): There is an additional chapter on CAM approaches in the behavioral modification section of this volume.

DIET THERAPY IN IBD

The use of diet and dietary supplements to control inflammation and facilitate healing is an area of great interest and promise in integrative medicine. Diet is thought to play an important role in the immunopathogenesis and treatment of IBD. We offer a brief review of current evidence for dietary constituents as risk factors for development of IBD. We also outline the efficacies of dietary therapies and supplements in IBD.

Evidence from a variety of investigators supports the notion that diet plays a role in disease development. Overall, it appears that overconsumption of a Westernized diet consisting of high contents of monounsaturated fats, saturated fats, omega-6 fatty acids, as well as large amounts of refined sugars, is a risk factor for both ulcerative colitis (UC) and Crohn's disease (CD).[4] Furthermore, increased refined sugar intake and high overall carbohydrate intake precedes the development of CD (Tables 117.2 and 117.3).[5] Transfats can be proinflammatory in nature.[6] Increased consumption of chemically modified fats (i.e., those found in margarine) may be involved in the etiology of UC.[7] There is an inverse association between dietary intake of vegetables, fruits, fish, fiber, and omega-3 fatty acids and the subsequent development of CD in children.[8]

Similar to the aforementioned study conducted in the United States, studies in Japan whose diet is becoming more Westernized with fast-foods are showing the same trends. For example, the rise in CD in Japan is associated with an increased total intake of animal fat and an increased ratio of omega-6 to omega-3 fats.[9] More recently, investigators from the United Kingdom reported that individuals consuming higher amounts of omega-6 fatty acids from red meat were also at increased risk for UC.[10] Taken together, these data suggest that animal protein-rich diets with a high content of refined sugars appear to place individuals more at risk, whereas plant-based proteins with higher omega-3 fats may be protective.

DIETARY SUPPLEMENTS IN IBD

There are innumerable nutraceutical supplements in use by IBD patients. All patients should be carefully asked about their use of supplements, probiotics, and foods/diets. Both patients and providers often view these treatments as "natural supplements"; therefore patients may not recognize the importance of sharing this information with their provider. Certainly the more familiar and

TABLE 117.1 Utilization of Complementary and Alternative Medicine in Inflammatory Bowel Disease

Does it work?			
CAM	Satisfied	Unsatisfied	No Change
Probiotics	57%	14%	16%
Acupuncture	49%	21%	20%
Boswellia extract	44%	12%	27%
Homeopathy	9%	24%	35%
Who is using it?			
21–68% of IBD pts in USA, F>M, CD>UC			
Why are they using it?			
Better control of disease	64%		
Good for stress	63%		
Which forms of CAM are being used?			
Homeopathy	52–55%		
Diet change and supplements	22–45%		
Probiotics	43%		

The use of complementary and alternative medicine (CAM) in patients with inflammatory bowel disease has been well studied. The usage of CAM varies from 21% to 68% but is commonly accepted to be 50% in patients with inflammatory bowel disease (IBD).[1–3] Table provided courtesy of G. Mullin.

accepting healthcare providers are with these nonallopathic treatments, the more likely patients are to disclose this information.

Essential Fatty Acids

Essential fatty acids (EFAs) are dietary constituents that cannot be synthesized endogenously and must be obtained via the diet for optimal health. Omega-3 EFAs are found in a wide variety of foods including flax seeds, eggs of hens on a diet rich in flaxseed, walnuts, cultivated plants, hemp seeds, and fish (deep-water fatty fish such as mackerel, herring, sardines, and wild-caught salmon). Fish oil can be administered as either raw fish oil or as an enteric-coated capsule. A dose of up to 3 g per day of eicosapentaenoic acid (EPA) plus docosahexaenoic acid (DHA) has been determined to be safe for general consumption.

Omega-3 EFAs appear to work through many mechanisms (Fig. 117.1). The net result is an inhibition of both the cyclooxygenase (COX) pathway (primarily COX-2) and the 5-lipoxygenase pathway, the key pathways in the inflammatory cascade. One of the many results is decreased production of proinflammatory leukotriene B_4. Omega-3 EFA regulates transcription factors such as peroxisome proliferator–activated receptors, with resultant downregulation of inflammatory processes. They also inhibit NF-kB and decrease the release of the proinflammatory cytokines IL-1β and TNF-α.[11,12]

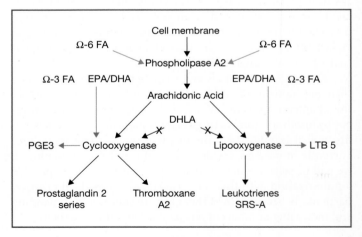

FIGURE 117.1 • Omega-3 (ω-3) modulation of the arachidonic acid cascade. ω-6 Fatty acids appear to promote the production of phospholipase A2 (PLP A2) and arachidonic acid (AA) and production of noxious proinflammatory eicosanoids such as prostaglandin-2 series (PGE2), leukotrienes (LTB) such as slow reactive releasing substance (SRS-A), and thromboxane A2 (TXA2). ω-3 Fatty acids, in contrast, downregulate production of proinflammatory eicosanoids by competitive inhibition of the enzymes cyclooxygenase-2 (COX-2) and 5′-Lipooxygenase (5′LPO) for AA, thus leading to preferential production of the prostaglandin-3 series (PGE3) and leukotriene-5 series (LTB5). Figure provided courtesy of G. Mullin.

TABLE 117.2 Carbohydrate: Observational Studies Investigating Consumption of Sugar-Containing Foods

Reference	Country	Subjects (n)	Controls (n)	Length of Time Postdiagnosis (Years)	Diet Investigated	Method	Significant Associations
Martini et al. (1976)	Germany	63 CD	63	Mean 4.5	Predisease	Postal questionnaire	CD consumed more sweets and pastries a week
Katschinski et al. (1988)	UK	104 CD	153 GP register	NP	Current and changes in past 10 yrs	Postal questionnaire 6 questions	CD associated with higher intake of confectionery
Epidemiology Group of the Research Committee of IBD in Japan (1994)	Japan	101 UC	143	Within 3	NP	Self-administered questionnaire	No difference in intake of soft drinks
Russel et al. (1998)	The Netherlands	290 CD	616 population controls	Within 5	Pre-symptoms	Questionnaire	Association between CD and cola drinks, chewing gum and chocolate
		398 UC					Association between UC and cola drinks and chocolate
							Decreased risk in both with high intake of citrus fruits

The intake of confectionery, preserves, biscuits, and cakes 1 to 3 years prior to the onset of the disease was found to be significantly higher compared with controls who had been instructed to record current diet. As indicated previously, comparison between current diet and recall of a diet from 1 to 3 years earlier may be problematic. Nevertheless, other studies support this association with sweet foods.
Reproduced with permission from Chapman-Kiddell et al.[55]

Biochemical studies indicate that 25% of patients with IBD show evidence of EFA deficiency.[13] Numerous studies have evaluated the effects of fish oil on IBD. Enteral fish oil supplements led to improvement in IBD in animal models,[14,15] and these findings were corroborated in small clinical trials.[16–18] A variety of studies have been performed exploring the roles of ω-3 EFA in the treatment of UC, but the methodology and endpoints have varied. Using clinical scores as an outcome, three of five studies showed significant clinical improvement in the fish oil arm.[19–21]

Utilizing endoscopic endpoints, three of three studies showed statistically significant improvement in the study group that received fish oil supplementation.[30–32] With endpoint of histologic improvement, only one[32] of three[28,30,31] studies reported significant improvement in the fish oil–treated arm.[27] However, data pertaining to steroid requirements suggest that ω-3 EFAs may reduce the need for or dose of corticosteroids among patients with IBD.

The Cochrane Collaboration recently composed a report concluding that an enteric-coated omega-3 EFA supplement reduced the 1-year relapse rate by half with an absolute risk reduction of 31% and a number needed to treat (NNT) of only 3. Two randomized, double-blind, placebo-controlled studies (Epanova Program in Crohn's Study 1 and 2 [EPIC-1] and [EPIC-2]) were conducted between January 2003 and February 2007 at 98 centers in Canada, Europe, Israel, and the United States. The goal of these studies was to determine whether omega-3 fatty acids could sustain remission once it is achieved in CD. Clinical relapse was defined by a CDAI score of 150 points or greater, an increase of more than 70 points from the baseline CDAI value, or initiation of treatment for active CD. In both EPIC-1 and EPIC-2, there were no significant differences in the CD relapse rate for placebo versus fish oils (Fig. 117.2).

Recently, a randomized, placebo-controlled trial by Seidner et al. evaluated an oral supplement enriched with fish oil on disease activity and medication use in patients with mild-to-

TABLE 117.3 Carbohydrate: Observational Studies Investigating Intake of Sugar-Containing Foods and Added Sugar Consumption

Reference	Country	Subjects n	Controls n	Length of Time Postdiagnosis (Years) Mean ± Standard Deviation	Diet Investigated	Method	Significant Associations
Mayberry et al. (1978)	UK	100 CD	100 # Clinic patients and relatives	8.9 ± 7.2	Current	Questionnaire	CD patients added more sugar to tea, coffee, cereals and drinks than controls
Mayberry et al. (1980)	UK	120 CD	# Clinic patients and relatives 100 UC	CD 10.1 ± 7.2	Current and pre-symptoms	Postal questionnaire	CD patients used more sugar
				UC 8.7 ± 7.6			Larger percentage CD added sugar to beverages and cereals currently and pre-symptoms
Silkoff et al. (1980)	Israel	27 CD	27 # Clinic	NP	Previous week and at onset of symptoms	Questionnaire	CD patients consumed more total sugars both at onset and during the previous week
Mayberry et al. (1981)	UK	32 CD	32 # Clinic patients or relatives	Within 1	Current and pre-symptoms	Postal questionnaire	Intake added and total sugar greater in CD both current consumption and prior to symptoms
Katschinski et al. (1988)	UK	104 CD	153 GP register	Up to 10	Current and changes in past 10 yrs	6 question postal questionnaire	RR CD in smokers not related to added sugar. RR CD in nonsmokers increased with increasing sugar intake.

Several studies used questionnaires specific to the intake of added sugar and sugar-containing foods (Table 117.3). Investigators found that significantly more number of CD patients than controls added sugar to beverages and cereals, with later studies by the same researchers confirming a higher sugar intake in CD patients at and prior to symptom onset. The influence of disease activity or treatment on current diet was not considered. These early studies focused on individual foods, and the results do not necessarily reflect total sugar intake. Nor did they adjust for energy to ensure that any association between sugar intake and IBD was independent of total energy intake.
Reproduced with permission from Chapman-Kiddell et al.[55]
CD, Crohn's disease; UC, ulcerative colitis; RR, relative risk; NP, not provided.

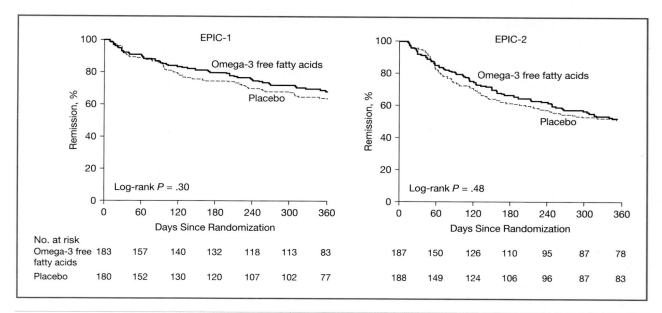

FIGURE 117.2 • Kaplan–Meier estimates of the time to relapse in the omega-3 free fatty acids and placebo groups for EPIC-1 and EPIC-2. This shows the proportion of patients that remained in remission over time. No significant differences were observed between the two treatment groups in either trial. In EPIC-1, 54 patients treated with omega-3 free fatty acids and 62 patients treated with placebo experienced a clinical relapse. The proportion of patients assigned to receive omega-3 free fatty acids who experienced a relapse within 360 days was estimated to be 31.6%, compared with 35.7% for those who received placebo (HR = 0.82; 95% CI = 0.57–1.19, P = 0.30). In EPIC-2, 84 patients treated with omega-3 free fatty acids and 94 patients treated with placebo experienced a clinical relapse. The proportion of patients assigned to receive omega-3 free fatty acids who experienced a relapse within 360 days was estimated to be 47.8%, compared with 48.8% of those who received placebo (HR = 0.90, 95% CI = 0.67–1.21, P = 0.48). Reproduced with permission from Feagan BG, Sandborn WJ, Mittmann U, et al. Omega-3 free fatty acids for the maintenance of controlled trials remission in Crohn disease: The EPIC randomized controlled trials. *JAMA*. 2008;299(14):1690–1697.

moderate UC.[22] Clinical and histologic parameters, as well as medication usage, were assessed over 6 months in the 86 patients who completed the study. Both groups (oral supplement and placebo) showed similar improvement in clinical and histologic indices. However, the treatment group required less prednisone to control clinical symptoms when compared to the placebo group.

In summary; despite animal models and scattered clinical studies; it is unclear as to whether fish oil supplements can maintain remission of IBD. Well-designed clinical trials are required to explore whether nutraceutical supplements can be used in conjunction with conventional therapies to optimize treatment of IBD.

Folate

Multiple nutritional deficiencies are known to be problematic in IBD (Table 117.4). Folic acid and vitamin D are two of the most common ones. Folic acid, a member of the B-complex family, is involved in many important body processes, including DNA synthesis. Thus, folic acid has been studied for its ability to circumvent dysplasia as a consequence of long-standing IBD, with disappointing results (Table 117.3).

The majority of IBD patients are deficient in folic acid.[23] Low folate levels in IBD may be caused by medications (i.e., sulfasalazine) that impair folic acid transport and malabsorption from loss of surface area due to underlying disease or surgery.[24]

Hyperhomocysteinemia, a known inducer of a hypercoagulable state seen in 26.5% of patients with IBD as compared to only 3.3% of controls,[25] is associated with a low serum folate level and can predispose to the development of deep venous thromboses. There currently is no evidence to supplement IBD patients with folate unless they have a folate deficiency.

Vitamin D

Vitamin D is now widely recognized as a regulator of the immune system (Fig. 117.3). Deficiency of vitamin D may also be a risk factor for IBD.[26,38] The incidence of IBD is higher at northern latitudes, and relapses occur more commonly in autumn and winter months when levels of sunlight are low. Reduced blood levels of 25-OH cholecalciferol, the major vitamin D metabolite, are common in patients with CD and are related to malnutrition and lack of sun exposure.[27,28] Administration of vitamin D (1000 IU per day for 1 year) prevented bone loss in patients with active CD.[29] The major causes of bone loss in IBD, however, are the effects of inflammatory cytokines and glucocorticoid therapy,[30] not vitamin D status.

Editor's note (TMB): There are two separate chapters, one in volume 1, and one in volume 2 on bone health in IBD.

Probiotics in IBD

Probiotics, consistently listed as one of the top nutritional supplements used by patients with IBD, may have many beneficial effects (Fig. 117.4). Of these, modulation of the intestinal

TABLE 117.4 Vitamin and Mineral Deficiencies in IBD

Deficiency	CD (%)	UC (%)	Treatment
Vitamin B12	48	5	1000 µg/day × 7 days then q month
Folate	67	30–40	1 mg/day
Vitamin A	11	Unknown	5,000–25,000 IU/day
Vitamin D	75	35	5,000–25,000 IU/day
Calcium	13	Unknown	1,000–1,200 mg/day
Potassium	5–20	Unknown	Variable
Iron	39	81	Fe Gluconate 300 mg TID
Zinc	50	Unknown	Zn Sulfate 220 mg daily or BID

This table illustrates the frequency of vitamin and mineral insufficiencies in patients with IBD. Of note, patients with Crohn's disease are vulnerable to vitamin B12, folate, zinc, and vitamin D deficiency due to their small-bowel disease and malabsorption of fat and diminished surface area for absorption due to damage to the surface epithelium. Thus, all patients with IBD should be screened annually for vitamins and minerals as shown here to avoid deficiencies of the micronutrients.

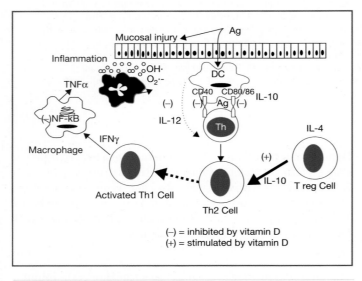

FIGURE 117.3 • Immunomodulatory role of vitamin D in inflammatory bowel disease. In Crohn's disease, bacterial antigens drive antigen-presenting cells (DCs) to produce cytokines such as interleukin-12 (IL-12) to drive a T-helper 1 (Th1) proinflammatory response to induce macrophages that produce TNFα and neutrophil chemoattractive agents that ultimately result in the production of noxious agents and tissue injury. The damaged intestinal tissue is more permeable to antigens that drive the vicious cycle of antigen presentation, local immune activation, and tissue injury. Antiinflammatory cytokines such as interleukin-10 (IL-10), made by regulatory T cells (T regs), antagonize Th1 proinflammatory processes by stimulating T-helper-2 function. Vitamin D antagonizes Th1 proinflammatory responses by interfering with antigen presentation and Th1 activation, upregulating Th2 cytokines and downregulating NF-kB in macrophages. Figure provided by courtesy of G. Mullin.

immune response is a key to effective treatment of IBD. There are many preparations available. We will briefly summarize the data for the use of probiotics in IBD in the context of "alternative therapies" because it is covered elsewhere in other chapters. Unfortunately, the quality of studies utilizing probiotics in UC and CD makes it difficult to make a recommendation for or against their use. Thus far, there are more data showing benefit in UC than in CD (Table 117.5). Nevertheless, the absence of data should not necessarily rule out the use of therapy.

VSL-3 is a well-studied probiotic preparation that is available in the United States. Each dose contains 450 billion live bacteria per packet. The bacteria included are *Bifidobacterium breve, Bifidobacterium longum, Bifidobacterium infantis, Lactobacillus acidophilus, Lactobacillus plantarum, Lactobacillus paracasei, Lactobacillus bulgaricus,* and *Streptococcus thermophilus*.[31] A well-designed clinical trial was able to show that VSL-3 used along with 5-ASA for induction of remission in UC led to remission faster than when 5-ASA was used alone.[32] It seems that VSL-3 is also useful in preventing relapse, specifically of pouchitis.[33]

Editor's note (TMB): There are chapters on probiotic use in UC and in CD elsewhere in this set of volumes.

Saccharomyces boulardii is a plant-derived yeast that may be of benefit in both UC and CD. An uncontrolled pilot study showed benefit in inducing remission of active UC when *S. boulardii* was added to mesalamine. A controlled trial found benefit for reducing frequency of diarrhea in patients with stable, active CD.[34] In addition, *S. boulardii* with mesalamine resulted in fewer relapses in comparison to just mesalamine therapy in patients with CD.

Although probiotics are termed "beneficial organisms," there are reports of fungemia and bacteremia in critically ill or immunocompromised patients.[35] Therefore, their use should be limited in such settings and always under supervision.[36]

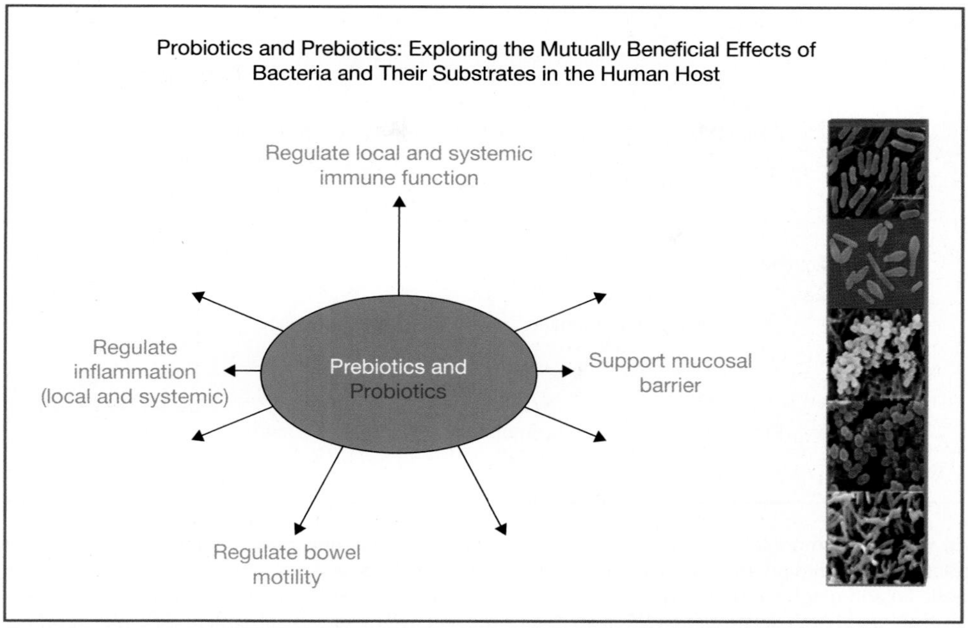

FIGURE 117.4 • Mechanisms of action of probiotics in inflammatory bowel disease. Prevent GI infections: probiotics have been shown to antagonize adherence of *H. pylori*, prevent systemic infections, regulate immune function, regulate metabolic pathways; hepatic: glucose control, reduce serum cholesterol, correct hepatic encephalopathy, enhance nutrient utilization and metabolism, vitamin synthesis, decrease lactose intolerance, enhance mineral absorption, bowel motility disorders, regulate appetite (Leptin, Ghrelin), prevent inflammatory and malignant GI and other epithelial based tissues. Probiotics also prevent clonal expansion of pathogens interference with mucosal binding of pathogen maintain barrier function, maintains short-chain fatty acid levels (SCFAs: primary fuel for colonocyte), modulates the immune response, enhances macrophage function, and enhances intestinal motility. The effects of these colonic foods are largely mediated by their interaction with the microflora, now considered a vital organ in regulating epithelial-cell development, instructing innate immunity and providing nourishment. Figure provided courtesy of G. Mullin.

TABLE 117.5 Probiotic Clinical Trials in Ulcerative Colitis

Author	Year	Probiotic	Result
Kruis	1997	*E. coli* Nissle1917	Equal to mesalamine
Venturi	1999	*E. coli* Nissle 1917	Equal to mesalamine
Rembacken	1999	*E. coli* Nissle 1917	Equal to mesalamine
Gustlandi	2003	*S. boulardii*	Equal to mesalamine
Ishikawa	2003	Bifidobacterium milk	Superior to placebo
Borody	2003	Stool enema	Improved
Kruis	2004	*E. coli* Nissle 1917	Superior to conventional medications
Kato	2004	Bifidobacteria milk	Sup to placebo
Furrie	2005	Bifidobacteria + Fiber	Improved

Nine clinical trials were performed to determine the potential benefit of probiotics on the course of ulcerative colitis. Four trials showed that probiotics had equal efficacy to mesalamine. All other trials showed that probiotics were superior to conventional medications, superior to placebo or overall improved. Overall, the results of these studies appear to favor use of probiotics for ulcerative colitis.[56-63] Table provided courtesy of G. Mullin.

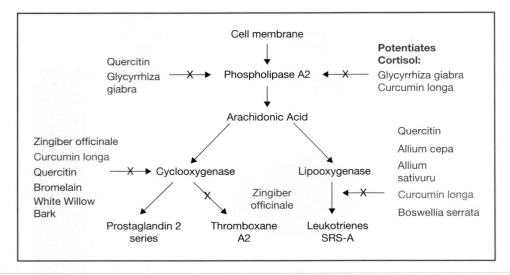

FIGURE 117.5 • Botanical modulation of arachidonic acid cascade. Polyphenols have a number of different mechanisms for downregulating inflammation and modulating immunity. A number of botanicals, including polyphenols (curcumin, boswelia, quericitin and ginger), interfere with the production of noxious proinflammatory eicosanoids such as prostaglandin-2 series (PGE2), leukotrienes (LTB) such as slow reactive releasing substance (SRS-A), thromboxane A2 (TXA2) via inhibition of the enzymes cyclooxygenase-2 (COX-2), and 5'-Lipooxygenase (5'LPO). Figure provided courtesy of G. Mullin.

Prebiotics in IBD

Prebiotics are probably less well known and, therefore, utilized less compared to probiotics. They are nondigestible dietary carbohydrates. Examples include bran, psyllium husk, resistant (high amylose) starch, inulin, lactulose, and oligosaccharides consisting of short-chain complexes of sucrose, galactose, fructose, glucose, maltose, or xylose. Prebiotics preferentially encourage growth and modify activity of beneficial intestinal bacteria. Bacterial fermentation of prebiotics yields short-chain fatty acids such as butyrate, which may be antiinflammatory and may reduce intestinal permeability.[37] Unblinded study of germinated barley foodstuff has shown an increased remission rate in UC patients, over 12 months.[38] Other prebiotics that have shown promise in placebo-controlled trials include wheatgrass juice[39] and inulin.

Botanicals in IBD

In traditional Chinese medicine and Ayurveda, herbal extracts are the mainstay of treatment for IBD and appear to be effective when used by trained practitioners. Polyphenols, found in food substances produced from plants, are believed to play a biologically active role and have been shown to be potentially immune modulating (Fig. 117.5).[40] There is clinical evidence in humans for use of two polyphenols in IBD, curcumin and boswellia.[41]

Curcumin

Turmeric, the major spice in curry, is made from the herb *Curcuma longa* and has been used in Ayurvedic medicine since ancient times. The major chemical constituents of turmeric are curcuminoids, the most prominent of which is curcumin. Recently, studies have demonstrated that curcumin is an inhibitor of NF-kB and leads to downstream regulation and inhibition of proinflammatory genes and cytokines.[42] Administration of curcumin has also been reported to modulate a host of other cytokines and signaling pathways.[43]

Seven studies involving curcumin administration to animal colitis models showed clinical and histopathological improvement and, where measured, decreased inflammatory cytokine production.[44] In a pilot study involving open-label administration of curcumin preparation to five patients with UC and five patients with CD, 9 out of 10 patients reported improvement at the conclusion of the 2-month study. Four of the five patients with UC were able to decrease or eliminate their medications.[45] In a larger, randomized, double-blind multicenter trial involving 89 patients with quiescent UC, administration of 1 g of curcumin twice daily resulted in both clinical improvement and a statistically significant decrease in the rate of relapse.[46] Given its excellent safety profile as well as the results discussed previously, curcumin is poised to have a prominent role in the future management of IBD.

Editor's note (TMB): Curcumin has also been shown to decrease polyp growth in Familial polyposis (Giardiello, et al).

Boswellia

The Ayurvedic herb, *Boswellia serrata* (Indian frankincense), inhibits leukotriene biosynthesis by noncompetitive inhibition of 5-lipoxygenase.[47] During a small 6-week trial, 350 mg 3 times a day of boswellia gum resin was as effective as sulfasalazine (1000 mg 3 times a day) in reducing symptoms or laboratory abnormalities of patients with active UC.[48] In a randomized, double-blind study from Germany, a proprietary boswellia extract (H15) was found to be as effective as mesalamine in improving symptoms of active CD.[49]

● ACUPUNCTURE

Acupuncture and moxibustion (using herbs in acupuncture points through burning or needling) are commonly used in traditional

Chinese medicine for treatment of UC. Mechanisms by which acupuncture and moxibustion modulate the immune system are not entirely clear. Studies from the Chinese and Western literature suggest that they may regulate gastrointestinal motor activity and secretion through opioid and other neural pathways.[50]

Uncontrolled studies from China as well as those comparing these modalities against standard Western treatments claim excellent results; however, rates of response to Western treatments seem smaller than would be expected.[51,52] In the Western literature, a randomized controlled study of acupuncture and moxibustion as treatment for active CD showed no significant difference in CDAI score and quality of life between the treatment group and the placebo group undergoing sham acupuncture.[53] These results were echoed in a study of UC patients with similar design.[54] In general, the data for acupuncture in IBD has not been convincing.

● CONCLUSION

Integrative medicine is an exciting, dynamic field that holds much promise. Familiarity with these modalities and continued investigations allow us to offer possibly superior treatments or treatments that may help spare or decrease the use of toxic conventional therapies. In the interim, just as with conventional medicine, integrative medicine is best practiced with continued open communication between patients and providers in an attempt to render the best care possible.

References

1. Barnes PM, Bloom B, Nahin R. CDC National Health Statistics Report #12. Complementary and Alternative Medicine Use Among Adults and Children: United States, 2007. December 2008.

2. Langhorst J, Anthonisen IB, Steder-Neukamm U, et al. Amount of systemic steroid medication is a strong predictor for the use of complementary and alternative medicine in patients with inflammatory bowel disease. Results From a German National Survey. *Inflamm Bowel Dis.* 2005;11(3):287–295.

3. www.iom.edu/?id=59924

4. Persson PG, Ahlbom A, Hellers G. Diet and inflammatory bowel disease: a case-control study. *Epidemiology.* 1992;3(1):47–52.

5. Reif S, Klein I, Lubin F, Farbstein M, Hallak A, Gilat T. Pre-illness dietary factors in inflammatory bowel disease. *Gut.* 1997;40(6):754–760.

6. Mozaffarian D, Aro A, Willett WC. Health effects of trans-fatty acids: experimental and observational evidence. *Eur J Clin Nutr.* 2009;63(suppl 2):S5–21.

7. Dietary and other risk factors of ulcerative colitis. A case-control study in japan. Epidemiology group of the research committee of inflammatory bowel disease in japan. *J Clin Gastroenterol.* 1994;19:166–171

8. Amre DK, D'Souza S, Morgan K, et al. Imbalances in dietary consumption of fatty acids, vegetables, and fruits are associated with risk for crohn's disease in children. *Am J Gastroenterol.* 2007;102(9):2016–2025.

9. Shoda R, Matsueda K, Yamato S, Umeda N. Epidemiologic analysis of Crohn disease in Japan: increased dietary intake of n-6 polyunsaturated fatty acids and animal protein relates to the increased incidence of Crohn disease in Japan. *Am J Clin Nutr.* 1996;63(5):741–745.

10. Hart AR. Linolenic acid, a dietary polyunsaturated fatty acid, and the aetiology of ulcerative colitis-A European Prospective Cohort Study. *Gut.* 2009 July 23. [Epub ahead of print]

11. Goldberg RJ, Katz J. A meta-analysis of the analgesic effects of omega-3 polyunsaturated fatty acid supplementation for inflammatory joint pain. *Pain.* 2007;129(1–2):210–223.

12. Nieto N. Ethanol and fish oil induce NFkappaB transactivation of the collagen alpha2(I) promoter through lipid peroxidation-driven activation of the PKC-PI3K-Akt pathway. *Hepatology.* 2007;45(6):1433–1445.

13. Siguel EN, Lerman RH. Prevalence of essential fatty acid deficiency in patients with chronic gastrointestinal disorders. *Metab Clin Exp.* 1996;45(1):12–23.

14. Vilaseca J, Salas A, Guarner F, Rodríguez R, Martínez M, Malagelada JR. Dietary fish oil reduces progression of chronic inflammatory lesions in a rat model of granulomatous colitis. *Gut.* 1990;31(5):539–544.

15. Empey LR, Jewell LD, Garg ML, Thomson AB, Clandinin MT, Fedorak RN. Fish oil-enriched diet is mucosal protective against acetic acid-induced colitis in rats. *Can J Physiol Pharmacol.* 1991;69(4):480–487.

16. Lorenz R, Weber PC, Szimnau P, Heldwein W, Strasser T, Loeschke K. Supplementation with n-3 fatty acids from fish oil in chronic inflammatory bowel disease–a randomized, placebo-controlled, double-blind cross-over trial. *J Intern Med Suppl.* 1989;731:225–232.

17. Hillier K, Jewell R, Dorrell L, Smith CL. Incorporation of fatty acids from fish oil and olive oil into colonic mucosal lipids and effects upon eicosanoid synthesis in inflammatory bowel disease. *Gut.* 1991;32(10):1151–1155.

18. Salomon P, Kornbluth AA, Janowitz HD. Treatment of ulcerative colitis with fish oil n–3-omega-fatty acid: an open trial. *J Clin Gastroenterol.* 1990;12(2):157–161.

19. Aslan A, Triadafilopoulos G. Fish oil fatty acid supplementation in active ulcerative colitis: a double-blind, placebo-controlled, cross-over study. *Am J Gastroenterol.* 1992;87(4):432–437.

20. Loeschke K, Ueberschaer B, Pietsch A, et al. n-3 fatty acids only delay early relapse of ulcerative colitis in remission. *Dig Dis Sci.* 1996;41(10):2087–2094.

21. Varghese T, Coomansingh D. Clinical response of ulcerative colitis with dietary omega-3 fatty acids: a double-blind randomized study. *Br J Surg.* 2000;87:AB73.

22. Seidner DL, Lashner BA, Brzezinski A, et al. An oral supplement enriched with fish oil, soluble fiber, and antioxidants for corticosteroid sparing in ulcerative colitis: a randomized, controlled trial. *Clin Gastroenterol Hepatol.* 2005;3(4):358–369.

23. Goh J, O'Morain CA. Review article: nutrition and adult inflammatory bowel disease. *Aliment Pharmacol Ther.* 2003;17(3):307–320.

24. Mason JB. Folate, colitis, dysplasia, and cancer. *Nutr Rev.* 1989;47(10):314–317.

25. Papa A, De Stefano V, Danese S, et al. Hyperhomocysteinemia and prevalence of polymorphisms of homocysteine metabolism-related enzymes in patients with inflammatory bowel disease. *Am J Gastroenterol.* 2001;96(9):2677–2682.

26. Lim WC, Hanauer SB, Li YC. Mechanisms of disease: vitamin D and inflammatory bowel disease. *Nat Clin Pract Gastroenterol Hepatol.* 2005;2(7):308–315.

27. Harries AD, Brown R, Heatley RV, Williams LA, Woodhead S, Rhodes J. Vitamin D status in Crohn's disease: association with nutrition and disease activity. *Gut.* 1985;26(11):1197–1203.

28. Vogelsang H, Ferenci P, Woloszczuk W, et al. Bone disease in vitamin D-deficient patients with Crohn's disease. *Dig Dis Sci.* 1989;34(7):1094–1099.

29. Vogelsang H, Ferenci P, Resch H, Kiss A, Gangl A. Prevention of bone mineral loss in patients with Crohn's disease by long-term oral vitamin D supplementation. *Eur J Gastroenterol Hepatol.* 1995;7(7):609–614.

30. Trebble TM, Wootton SA, Stroud MA, et al. Laboratory markers predict bone loss in Crohn's disease: relationship to blood mononuclear cell function and nutritional status. *Aliment Pharmacol Ther.* 2004;19(10):1063–1071.

31. http://www.vsl3.com/healthcare.asp

32. Tursi A, Brandimarte G, Giorgetti GM, Forti G, Modeo ME, Gigliobianco A. Low-dose balsalazide plus a high-potency probiotic preparation is more effective than balsalazide alone or mesalazine in the treatment of acute mild-to-moderate ulcerative colitis. *Med Sci Monit.* 2004;10(11):PI126–131.

33. Mimura T, Rizzello F, Helwig U, et al. Once daily high dose probiotic therapy (VSL#3) for maintaining remission in recurrent or refractory pouchitis. *Gut.* 2004;53(1):108–114.

34. Guslandi M, Mezzi G, Sorghi M, Testoni PA. Saccharomyces boulardii in maintenance treatment of Crohn's disease. *Dig Dis Sci.* 2000;45(7):1462–1464.

35. Singhi SC, Baranwal A. Probiotic use in the critically ill. *Indian J Pediatr.* 2008;75(6):621–627.

36. Snydman DR. The safety of probiotics. *Clin Infect Dis.* 2008;46(suppl 2):S104–11; discussion S144.

37. Kinoshita M, Suzuki Y, Saito Y. Butyrate reduces colonic paracellular permeability by enhancing PPARgamma activation. *Biochem Biophys Res Commun.* 2002;293(2):827–831.

38. Hanai H, Kanauchi O, Mitsuyama K, et al. Germinated barley foodstuff prolongs remission in patients with ulcerative colitis. *Int J Mol Med.* 2004;13(5):643–647.

39. Ben-Arye E, Goldin E, Wengrower D, Stamper A, Kohn R, Berry E. Wheat grass juice in the treatment of active distal ulcerative colitis: a randomized double-blind placebo-controlled trial. *Scand J Gastroenterol.* 2002;37(4):444–449.

40. Shapiro H, Singer P, Halpern Z, Bruck R. Polyphenols in the treatment of inflammatory bowel disease and acute pancreatitis. *Gut.* 2007;56(3):426–435.

41. Mazzon E, Muià C, Paola RD, et al. Green tea polyphenol extract attenuates colon injury induced by experimental colitis. *Free Radic Res.* 2005;39(9):1017–1025.

42. Jobin C, Bradham CA, Russo MP, et al. Curcumin blocks cytokine-mediated NF-kappa B activation and proinflammatory gene expression by inhibiting inhibitory factor I-kappa B kinase activity. *J Immunol.* 1999;163(6):3474–3483.

43. Duvoix A, Blasius R, Delhalle S, et al. Chemopreventive and therapeutic effects of curcumin. *Cancer Lett.* 2005;223(2):181–190.

44. Sugimoto K, Hanai H, Tozawa K, et al. Curcumin prevents and ameliorates trinitrobenzene sulfonic acid-induced colitis in mice. *Gastroenterology.* 2002;123(6):1912–1922.

45. Holt PR, Katz S, Kirshoff R. Curcumin therapy in inflammatory bowel disease: a pilot study. *Dig Dis Sci.* 2005;50(11):2191–2193.

46. Hanai H, Iida T, Takeuchi K, et al. Curcumin maintenance therapy for ulcerative colitis: randomized, multicenter, double-blind, placebo-controlled trial. *Clin Gastroenterol Hepatol.* 2006;4(12):1502–1506.

47. Hammon HP. Boswellic acids (components of frankincense) as the active principle in treatment of chronic inflammatory diseases. *Wien Med Wochenschr.* 2002;152(15–16):373–378.

48. Gupta I, Parihar A, Malhotra P, et al. Effects of gum resin of Boswellia serrata in patients with chronic colitis. *Planta Med.* 2001;67(5):391–395.

49. Gerhardt H, Seifert F, Buvari P, Vogelsang H, Repges R. [Therapy of active Crohn disease with Boswellia serrata extract H 15]. *Z Gastroenterol.* 2001;39(1):11–17.

50. Li Y, Tougas G, Chiverton SG, Hunt RH. The effect of acupuncture on gastrointestinal function and disorders. *Am J Gastroenterol.* 1992;87(10):1372–1381.

51. Chen YC, Chen FP, Chen TJ, Chou LF, Hwang SJ. Patterns of traditional Chinese medicine use in patients with inflammatory bowel disease: a population study in Taiwan. *Hepatogastroenterology.* 2008;55(82–83):467–470.

52. Schneider A, Streitberger K, Joos S. Acupuncture treatment in gastrointestinal diseases: a systematic review. *World J Gastroenterol.* 2007;13(25):3417–3424.

53. Joos S, Brinkhaus B, Maluche C, et al. Acupuncture and moxibustion in the treatment of active Crohn's disease: a randomized controlled study. *Digestion.* 2004;69(3):131–139.

54. Joos S, Wildau N, Kohnen R, et al. Acupuncture and moxibustion in the treatment of ulcerative colitis: a randomized controlled study. *Scand J Gastroenterol.* 2006;41(9):1056–1063.

55. Chapman-Kiddell CA, Davies PS, Gillen L, Radford-Smith GL. Role of diet in the development of inflammatory bowel disease. *Inflamm Bowel Dis.* 2010;16(1):137–151.

56. Kruis W, Fric P, Pokrotnieks J, et al. Maintaining remission of ulcerative colitis with the probiotic *Escherichia coli* Nissle 1917 is as effective as with standard mesalazine. *Gut.* 2004; 53(11):1617–1623.

57. Ishikawa H, Akedo I, Umesaki Y, Tanaka R, Imaoka A, Otani T. Randomized controlled trial of the effect of bifidobacteria-fermented milk on ulcerative colitis. *J Am Coll Nutr.* 2003; 22(1):56–63.

58. Kato K, Mizuno S, Umesaki Y, et al. Randomized placebo-controlled trial assessing the effect of bifidobacteria-fermented milk on active ulcerative colitis. *Aliment Pharmacol Ther.* 2004;20(10):1133–1141.

59. Borody TJ, Warren EF, Leis S, Surace R, Ashman O. Treatment of ulcerative colitis using fecal bacteriotherapy. *J Clin Gastroenterol.* 2003;37(1):42–47.

60. Furrie E, Macfarlane S, Kennedy A, et al. Synbiotic therapy (Bifidobacterium longum/Synergy 1) initiates resolution of inflammation in patients with active ulcerative colitis: a randomised controlled pilot trial. *Gut.* 2005;54(2):242–249.

61. Kruis W, Schutz E, Fric P, Fixa B, Judmaier G, Stolte M. Double-blind comparison of an oral *Escherichia coli* preparation and mesalazine in maintaining remission of ulcerative colitis. *Aliment Pharmacol Ther.* 1997;11(5):853–858.

62. Rembacken BJ, Snelling AM, Hawkey PM, Chalmers DM, Axon AT. Non-pathogenic *Escherichia coli* versus mesalazine for the treatment of ulcerative colitis: a randomised trial. *Lancet.* 1999;354(9179):635–639.

63. Guslandi M, Mezzi G, Sorghi M, Testoni PA. *Saccharomyces boulardii* in maintenance treatment of Crohn's disease. *Dig Dis Sci.* 2000;45(7):1462–1464.

Stem-Cell Transplantation for Refractory Crohn's Disease | 118

Robert M. Craig and Richard K. Burt

● INTRODUCTION

Crohn's disease (CD) is a chronic, immunologically mediated illness and of unknown etiology but probably induced by an exposure to intestinal bacteria or their component antigens leading to an excessive Th1-mediated chronic inflammation of the gastrointestinal tract in patients with genetic susceptibility.[1,2] The etiology of CD is unknown, but its pathophysiology is related to immune dysregulation or autoimmunity. Recently genetic modifications have been identified in the production of CARD/NOD2 proteins in some patients with CD,[3-8] especially those with ileal involvement and strictures. These proteins function as gatekeepers and can control access to various antigens from the gastrointestinal tract, performing roles in the innate immune system. Presumably genetic defects in this system allow easier access to putative antigens responsible for generating the inflammatory processes seen in CD. In addition, other susceptibility genes have been described in CD, though they are less common and less well characterized.[9] The antigen or antigens involved in the ensuing process are probably derived from gut bacteria, which function as the trigger mechanism, enlisting the acquired immune system with predominantly TH1 lymphocyte reactivity.

Regardless of the precise pathophysiology of CD, abnormal lymphocyte responsiveness is critically involved. Much of the therapy for CD involves opposing lymphocyte reactivity or its cytokine products, including corticosteroids, immunosuppressives, and anti-TNF-alpha. However, the treatment is often unsuccessful in controlling many patients' disease, and some are ravaged with severe illness in spite of all known therapy. Regardless of the therapy employed, many patients remain very sick in spite of therapy, after all therapeutic options have been exhausted.[10-19] Although not well characterized, a distinct excessive mortality from CD exists in this group of patients.[20-27] In addition, patients with severe, refractory disease suffer from an inability to eat, frequent nausea, vomiting, diarrhea, malnutrition, growth retardation in children, fistulae, abdominal pain, multiple surgeries, extraintestinal symptoms, iatrogenic addiction to narcotics, and toxicities of therapy.

A more drastic, therapeutic approach has been proposed for these patients who are refractory to standard treatment: bone marrow ablation with stem-cell rescue. Herein we describe the early experience of bone marrow transplantation for malignant disease in patients with incidental CD, the distinction between allogeneic and autologous hematopoietic stem cell transplantation (HSCT), the difference between hematoablation for malignant disease and immune ablation for autoimmune disease, MSC transplantation, and the experience of us and others of autologous HSCT with immune ablation for refractory CD.

● EARLY EXPERIENCE OF ALLOGENEIC BONE MARROW TRANSPLANTATION WITH INCIDENTAL CD

The rationale for immune ablation and HSCT derived from the concept that a more radical immune ablation with stem-cell rescue might promote remission in these patients. This was supported by reports of bone marrow or allogeneic HSC transplantation for malignant disease in patients with incidental CD, who went into remission.[28-32] These patients underwent hematoablation therapy, which is more rigorous than immune ablative therapy, and carries a higher mortality and risk of complications. In addition, allogeneic transplantation was used rather than autologous, which has the advantage of supplying the patient with a completely new immune system, but carries the risk of graft-versus-host disease (GVHD). Two transplant-related deaths were reported, perhaps related to the more rigorous, hematoablative chemotherapy. Eleven of the reported patients had a sustained remission, suggesting that there is a role for immune ablation and HSCT in patients with CD who have failed conventional therapy.

● RISK VERSUS BENEFIT OF IMMUNE ABLATION AND HSCT

In order to assess risks versus benefits in any new therapy for CD, it is necessary to compare the anticipated mortality for the new therapy to the intrinsic mortality from severe CD and its therapy. Although data are varied, most studies show increased mortality from CD above expected mortality rates for given populations.[20–27] For example, a recent European study showed a mortality rate nearly twice as high as expected over 10 years.[27]

The mortality experience with immune ablation and HSCT in autoimmune diseases at our medical center is about 1.6% (3 patients out of approximately 180), due to the procedure, which is clearly an acceptable mortality rate.[33,34] Our low mortality rate probably derives from our extensive experience with this procedure and our use of immune ablation rather than myeloablative chemotherapy. However, autologous HSCT is not expected to alter a genetic tendency to develop CD, making the risk of disease recurrence higher than after allogeneic HSCT, in which a recipient's immune and hematologic system is replaced with a genetically non–disease-prone donor.

● MESENCHYMAL STEM-CELL THERAPY

Mesenchymal stem cells (MSCs), originally identified as the cells adhering to plastic flasks from bone marrow aspirates, are obtained from adipose tissue or bone marrow[35,36]. Preliminary reports of their use in refractory GVHD suggest a salutary role, supporting their having an immunomodulatory effect.[37] In autoimmune diseases, it is uncertain whether the beneficial effects of immune ablation and stem-cell transplantation are solely due to the immune ablation and whether the infusion of the stem cells merely shortens the time of bone marrow hypoplasia and does not have a fundamental role in immune suppression. However, recent studies in a murine model of inflammatory bowel disease suggest that the infusion of stem cells have a primary role in correcting attendant microcirculatory abnormalities.[38] In humans, however, it remains controversial whether the HSC or MSC has a beneficial role by itself, promoting healthy small-bowel tissue as the stem cells home to diseased areas. Controlled studies are in process testing this hypothesis.

● AUTOLOGOUS HSCT PROCEDURE

Candidates for HSCT should have clinical and histological evidence of CD, be less than 60 years old, and have failed conventional therapy, including infliximab or other TNF-alpha antibody, corticosteroids, 5-ASA products, antibiotics, and azathioprine or 6-mercaptopurine.[39] Each patient should have a persistent Crohn's Disease Activity Index (CDAI) of 225 to 400 or a severity index (CSI, Table 118.1) of 17 or greater.[21] Patients with significant heart disease, liver disease unrelated to CD, hematologic disease, active infection, toxic megacolon, or intestinal perforation should be excluded.

HSC Harvest

Peripheral blood stem cells are mobilized with cyclophosphamide followed by granulocyte colony-stimulating factor (G-CSF). After the WBC rebounds, leukaphereses is continued daily until an enriched target CD34$^+$ cell count (2.0×10^6/kg) is achieved. T-cell depletion is performed by enrichment of CD34$^+$ cells using immunoselection techniques. The HSC graft is cryopreserved until the date of transplantation (reinfusion).

TABLE 118.1 Crohn's Severity Index (CSI)	
Feature	Score
Diarrhea	
3–10/day	1
>10/day	2
Pain Intermittent cramping	1
Steady, mild to moderate	2
Steady, severe	3
Chronic opiate use for pain	2
Well-being	
Fair	1
Poor	2
Terrible	3
Corticosteroid use	2
Immunosuppressives use	2
5-ASA or antibiotic use	1
TPN use	3
Enteropathic arthritis/arthralgias	1
Hepatobiliary complication	2
Perianal fistula or abscess	2
Entero-entero fistula	2
Entero-vaginal fistula	2
Entero-vesical fistula	2
Entero-cutaneous fistula	2
Perianal fissure, anal pain	1
Vulvar inflammation	1
Intestinal obstruction	2
Abdominal mass	2
Erythema nodosum	1
Pyoderma gangrenosa	2
Aphthous stomatitis	1
Iritis	2
Fever > 1 week	2
Weight loss	
10% of usual	1
20% of usual	2
Hematocrit	
1–5 less than normal	1
5 or more less than normal	2

Continued

TABLE 118.1 *Continued*

Feature	Score
Serum albumin	
2.5–3.5	1
<2.5	2
CRP abnormality	1
ESR > 20	1
Colonoscopic abnormality	
Mild	1
Moderate	2
Severe	3
Small bowel radiographic inflammation	
Mild	1
Moderate	2
Severe	3
Upper GI endoscopy abnormality	
Mild	1
Moderate, severe	2, 3

From Oyama et al.[39]

Conditioning Regimen

The conditioning regimen consists of cyclophosphamide 50 mg/kg/day and antithymocyte globulin (ATG) for the 4 days prior to HSC infusion. Mesna is administered along with the cyclophosphamide to prevent hemorrhagic cystitis, and methylprednisolone, 1.0 g/day, is administered prior to each dose of ATG to prevent infusion reactions. G-CSF, 5 mcg/kg/day, is started on the day of reinfusion and continued until the absolute neutrophil count (ANC) reaches 500/μl .

Supportive Care

Patients are treated on a high-efficiency-particulate-air-filtered medical floor. A low microbial diet, oral ciprofloxacin 500 mg twice daily, fluconazole 400 mg once daily, metronidazole 500 mg 3 times daily, valacyclovir 500 mg 3 times daily, and aerosolized pentamidine, 300 mg upon admission, are administered. When the neutrophil count drops to less than 500/mcl the ciprofloxacin is discontinued and intravenous piperacillin/tazobactam, 3.375 g every 4 hours, is started. Metronidazole and piperacillin/tazobactam are stopped upon neutrophil recovery. Valacyclovir 500 mg twice daily and fluconazole 400 mg once daily are continued for 12 and 6 months post-HSCT, respectively. Trimethoprim/sulfamethoxazole double strength (160 mg/800 mg) 3 times weekly is started upon hematopoietic engraftment and continued for 6 months post-HSCT. Hemoglobin levels and platelet counts are maintained above

8 g/dL and 20,000/mcl, respectively, with leukoreduced, irradiated, and cytomegalovirus-safe blood transfusions. All immunosuppressive and disease-modifying agents are discontinued upon the stem-cell mobilization except systemic corticosteroids that are tapered as outpatients.

● RESULTS, AUTOLOGOUS HSCT, AND IMMUNE ABLATION

Four case reports of patients who received an autologous HSCT for cancer showed prolonged remissions of their incidental CD.[40–43] These case studies gave impetus to the largest reported series of immune ablation and HSCT as primary therapy for CD, which included 21 Caucasian patients, 10 women, and 11 men, aged between 15 and 42 years[39,44] (Table 118.2, Figs. 118.1–118.5). Five patients had significant pre-HSCT complications from standard immunosuppressive therapies, including hepatotoxicity, fever, pancreatitis, and pancytopenia. The durations post-HSCT are 6 years for 1 patient, 5 years for 7 patients, 4 years for 3 patients, 3 years for 6 patients, 2 years for 2 patients, and 1 year for 2 patients. A total of 20 patients are surviving. One died of an accidental death 3.5 years posttransplant, also included in the 3-year duration listing above, following which a postmortem examination revealed no evidence of CD.

Neutrophil and platelet engraftment occurred in 8 to 11 days following HSC infusion. Platelet and red blood cell transfusions were regularly employed during the pancytopenic phase. Hospital discharge occurred in 10 to 17 days. Engraftment was prompt and complete, and no one developed late cytopenias.

Besides fever that was either neutropenic or disease related, the procedure was well tolerated without a documented early or late infection. One patient (patient T) had a central-line infection following discharge. Two patients with CD-related fever prior to HSCT continued to have peritransplant fever for 7 and 14 days, respectively, which resolved following the neutrophil engraftment. No CMV reactivation, infection, or disease occurred after the HSCT.

Follow-up evaluations have been available for all 21 patients. The CDAI and CSI had a rapid and dramatic post-HSCT improvement ($P < 0.001$ for each time interval compared to baseline), unless a relapse ensued. Note that some of the patients accessed more recently initially had a lower CDAI, as they met the CSI, but not the CDAI, criterion. The improvements in the sedimentation rate and CRP are less apparent. Figs. 118.1 to 118.4 describe each individual data point, and P values are included in the figure legends. In addition, the diarrhea and abdominal pain usually stopped prior to hospital discharge. All patients eventually came off all immunosuppressive therapies post-HSCT. Karnofsky performance scale, quality-of-life scores, lassitude, appetite, and oral intake improved in most patients, either immediately or gradually post HSCT, unless intestinal obstruction occurred or the patient had a relapse (see the following). The quality-of-life scores were not quantified, as they were predominantly subjective indices, and, for the most part, their findings were included in both the CDAI and CSI.

Endoscopic response was included as part of the CSI, where colonoscopic severity of illness was graded 0 to 3 (0 = normal, 1 = mild disease, 2 = moderate disease, and 3 = severe disease).

TABLE 118.2 Patient Demographics Pre-HSCT

Subj	CDAI	Age/Sex	CSI	Disease Duration (Years)	Disease Location	Surgery	Smoker	ASCA Pre		ASCA post	
								IgA	IgG	IgA	IgG
A.	305	21 F	32	10	SB and Colon	Sig Rsx	No	ND	ND	90	40
						SB Rsx					
B.	271	16 M	33	7	Colon	None	No	66	86	41	79
C.	277	38 F	30	20	SB and Colon	IC Rsx	Yes	24	ND	0	0
						Sig Rsx					
D.	285	27 F	23	12	Colon, anus	Anal	Yes	22	ND	0	ND
E.	307	35 M	31	12	Colon, SB	Anal	Yes	34	ND	34	ND
F.	253	27 F	17	6	Colon, SB	Anal	No	ND	ND	0	ND
					Anal	SB Rsx					
						IC Rsx					
G.	282	25 M	22	13	SB and Colon	SB Rsx (2)	No	93	ND	65	74
						Sig Rsx					
H.	250	15 M	23	8	Anus, SB	SB Rsx (2)	No	191	ND	94	97
I.	265	31 F	23	10	SB and Colon	Sig Rsx	No	208	78	255	72
						SB Rsx					
J.	298	37 M	22	6	Colon, anus	None	No	47	30	0	0
K.	256	16 M	23	1.5	Small bowel	None	No	83	172	75	175
L.	298	27 M	29	14	Colon, anus	Cecal Rsx	No	0	24	48	30
M.	207	25 F	20	12	SB and colon	Ilectomy	No	36	30	30	35
						Proctocolectomy					
N.	210	18 F	29	12	Ileum, colon	None	Yes	36	175	31	135
O.	264	28 M	22	10	jej, ileum	Stricture	No	45	32	52	20
						Ile Rsx (2)					
P.	199	27 F	18	8	Colon	Part colect	No	16	47	0	21
Q.	233	16 M	24	8	Colon, anus	None	No	ND	ND	37	64
R.	191	24 F	17	6	Duod, colon	None	No	19	19	6	8
S.	101	21 M	23	6	Colon.	None	No	21	53	13	12
T.	221	29 M	21	9	ileum, colo-anal	Div colost	No	131	45		
U.	91	42 F	17	8	Colon, SB	Colectomy	No	25	0		
						SB rsx (3)					

SB-small bowel; Rsx-resection; Sig-sigmoid; IC-ileocecal; jej-jejunum; ile-ileal; part colect-partial colectomy; Div colost-diverting colostomy; ND-not done.
From Oyama et al.[39] and Craig RM and Burt.[44]

Rigorous scoring was not performed as part of this analysis, as the colonoscopies were often performed off site, by their gastroenterologists, frequently in other states. Comparisons of Fig. 118.1 to 118.4 with the endoscopic findings sometimes showed disparities; some patients were in remission in terms of inflammatory indices, CDAI, and CSI, yet had persistent colonoscopic abnormalities.

As is evident from inspecting the Figs. 118.1 to 118.4, the patients usually had marked improvement over the first year following HSCT. Most patients also had marked improvement in

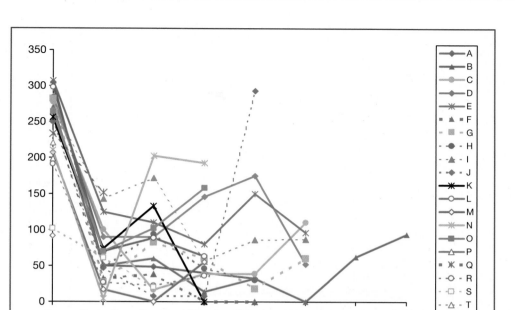

FIGURE 118.1 • CDAI, Crohn's disease activity index versus time. Upper bounds for *P* values for the time intervals compared to baseline: 6 months < 0.001; 1 year < 0.001; 2 years < 0.001; 3 years < 0.001; 4 years < 0.001.

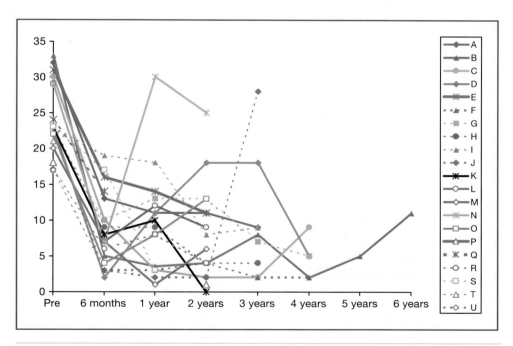

FIGURE 118.2 • Severity index versus time. Upper bounds for *P* values for the time intervals compared to baseline: 6 months < 0.001; 1 year < 0.001; 2 years < 0.001; 3 years 0.006; 4 years < 0.001.

symptoms, as reflected in CDAI and CSI. Occasionally patients had a short-lived response (D, N, Q).

It is difficult to define remission precisely as some might have no symptoms of the disease yet have some laboratory or colonoscopic findings. In addition, two patients required surgery for stricturing disease but had little or no evidence of inflammatory illness (patients K, O), and one patient (S) required a surgical resection for colovesicle fistula, yet improved in all other respects. If remission is defined as a patient with minimal or no symptoms of CD, off corticosteroids, with a CDAI < 150 and a

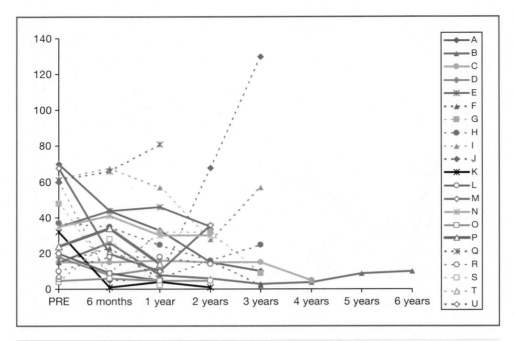

FIGURE 118.3 • Sedimentation rate versus time. Upper bounds for *P* values for the time intervals compared to baseline: 6 months 0.1; 1 year < 0.02; 2 years < 0.01; 3 years < 0.5; 4 years 0.004.

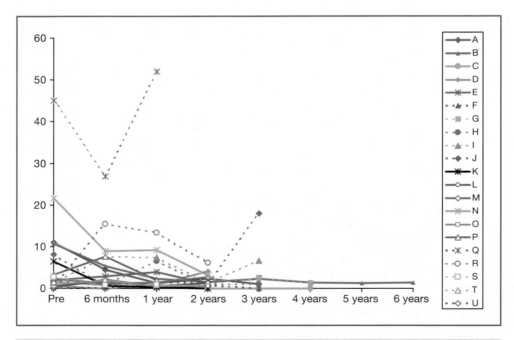

FIGURE 118.4 • C-reactive protein versus time. Upper bounds for *P* values for the time intervals compared to baseline: 6 months < 0.8; 1 year < 0.7; 2 years < 0.1; 3 years < 0.8; 4 years < 0.2.

CSI < 12, it is reasonable to consider the patient to be in remission even if he or she required surgery. Those who have had a relapse and have required surgery are described in Table 118.3. By this definition, some are currently in remission even though they had a relapse or required some surgery. The more exact placement of the clinical expression of disease is best seen in the Figures 118.1 to 118.4. Defining clinical remission this way,

the intervals post-HSCT are 6 years for 1 patient, 5 years for 6 patients, 4 years for 2 patients, 3 years for 4 patients, 2 years for 2 patients, and 1 year for 2 patients. Four are still in relapse, 3 at 5 years and 1 at 4 years post-HSCT. A modified Kaplan-Meyer plot of percentage in remission is presented in Fig. 118.5. Note that the plot begins at 6 months, as none of the patients were in remission at time 0; the denominators (total number of patients

TABLE 118.3 Relapses and Surgical Requirement Post-HSCT[a]

Subject	Relapse	Yrs p HSCT	Surgery	Yrs p HSCT	Cigarettes
C	Small Bowel	3 ½	Ileal resect	1	Yes
			Ileal resect	3 ½	
D	Colon	2	Colectomy	3	Yes
E	Colon	3 ½	None		Yes
F	Small bowel	1	None		No
J	Colon	2	Colectomy	3	No
K	None		Ileal resect	2	No
L	Colon	2	None		No
M	Small bowel	1	None		No
N	Colon	1	Colectomy	2	Yes
O	None		Stricture resect	2	No
Q	Colon, anus	1	Colectomy	1	No
S	None		Div colostomy	1	No

From Oyama et al.[39] and Craig RM and Burt.[44]

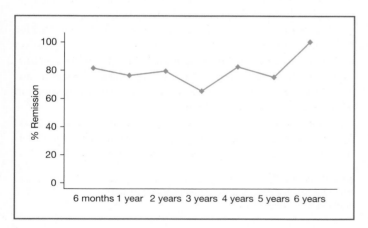

FIGURE 118.5 • Modified Kaplan-Meyer plot of patients in remission (percentage) versus time. The denominators (total patients at each time interval) are 21 at 6 months, 21 at 1 year, 19 at 2 years, 17 at 3 years, 11 at 4 years, 8 at 5 years, and 1 at 6 years.

at each interval) vary, as the accession times were not identical; and the remissions did not consistently fall, as some who relapsed went into remission.

Eight relapses occurred, 3 patients at 1 year, 3 patients at 2 years, and 2 patients at 3.5 years post-HSCT. Each clinically worsened following marked clinical improvement, reflected in a rise in CDAI and CSI. Resumption of cigarette smoking occurred in four patients. Each required reinstitution of therapy for CD and some required surgery. Therapy seemed to be more effective than that pretransplant. For example, patient F had a mild relapse that required infliximab, which has brought her into remission for the past 3 years, whereas she failed infliximab pretransplant. In addition, those requiring surgery following their relapse have overall done well (patients D, J, N, Q). Finally, the 4 patients who remain in relapse (patients C, E, L, and M) are faring much better than pre HSCT, evident from their most recent CDAI of 214, 96, 110, and 66, respectively. These are the only four currently requiring systemic corticosteroids.

Eight patients required some surgical procedure following the HSCT, for late or progressive small-bowel stricture (patient C a consequence of relapse; patients K and O, stricturing without relapse), total proctocolectomy for severe recurrent or resistant disease (patients D, J, N, and Q), or diverting colostomy for colovesicle fistula (patient S, who continued to have bowel improvement, yet had recurrent urosepsis).

Fistulae and strictures tended to resolve more slowly than other manifestations of CD. One patient had a pretransplant colovesicle fistula that persisted after HSCT and required a diverting colostomy due to recurrent urinary tract infections. A second required a colectomy 1 year following HSCT for severe rectosigmoid fistulizing disease, anorectal pain, and rectosigmoid stricturing. Three others had severe anorectocutaneous fistulae with gradual, but incomplete, improvement. One had severe anovulvar fistulae that gradually, completely resolved over 3 years.

Regarding stricture, one patient had a severe colonic stricture that completely resolved, and he is in clinical remission 6 years post-HSCT. One has had recurrent stricturing disease accompanying inflammatory recurrence (C). Two had progressive ileal strictures that required surgical resection (K, O), but no pathologic evidence of inflammation, and each has been in clinical remission post surgery. One had severe anorectal stricturing that completely resolved, permitting a take-down of her ileostomy with restoration of bowel continuity.

The above experience has recently been duplicated by an Italian group in five patients with refractory CD, who underwent HSCT following immune ablation, though unselected cells were administered (not CD34-enriched stem cells).[45] The authors argue that the CD34 selection process may not be necessary. Finally, there is another case report of a patient who received immune ablation and HSCT for refractory CD who also entered clinical remission.[46]

● CONCLUSION

We and others have found an increased incidence of antibodies to *Saccharomyces cerevesiae* (ASCA) in patients with Crohn's disease.[39,44] However, the presence of the antibody does not seem to confer an increased severity of illness, and the antibody may precede clinical illness for years. Although most of our patients had ASCA prior to their HSCT, the ASCA levels generally did not change following transplant, nor did they predict severity of illness (Table 118.2).

Other processes are probably involved in CD pathogenesis, including inappropriate counterregulatory functions, insufficient apoptosis of engaged lymphocytes, and impaired secretion of counterinflammatory cytokines from Treg cells and other lymphocytes. This promotes continued inflammatory activity that does not turn off. Our patients did have a robust rise in their T-reg cells from pre- to post-HSCT, lending support for a role for these cells in the salutary effect that we have observed. However, we did not find a correlation between the pre- or post-HSCT T-reg cells and relapse, possibly due to the small patient cohort (13 patients) analyzed.

Review of Figures 118.1 to 118.4 shows the striking improvement evident initially and the time of relapse and recovery in some. It is not clear why the improvement in the CRP and sedimentation rate is less apparent than that of the CDAI and CSI. We found the newer severity index (Table 118.1, Ref. 39) a more useful index in following our patients, as it reflects a more global assessment. However, there is a general correspondence between the two indices, validating the newer index (Figs. 118.1 and 118.2). The CSI is a more reliable index, as it allows for improved assessment of disease activity for small-bowel disease, which is not associated with as much diarrhea as colonic disease, allows for better scoring of patients with ileostomy, is more inclusive in terms of more measurements of disease activity, and is less subjective in terms of diarrhea, well-being, abdominal pain, and presence or absence of an abdominal mass. Patient U, for example, had the lowest CDAI upon entry, 91, yet met the CDI criterion of 17. The severity of her illness is evidenced by her having required four prior surgical procedures, including a proctocolectomy. In addition, she was ravaged with severe abdominal pain and had extensive inflammatory involvement of her small bowel on radiographs.

Most of patients receiving autologous HSCT have shown immediate or gradual improvement, though there have been relapses and some have required stricture removal or colectomy from relapse or worsening stricture. None has died from the procedure. It is not surprising that relapses have occurred in some. On the other hand, treatment-free remissions for as long as 6 years have been achieved, raising the possibility that autologous HSCT may have reset the patient's own immune system to its predisease status.

If clinical remission is defined as having minimal symptoms, not requiring corticosteroids, and having a CDAI < 150 and CSI < 12, only 4 of the treated patients are currently in relapse, though 9 have had clinical relapse. A modified Kaplan-Meyer clinical remission curve to describe the patients' clinical courses (Fig. 118.5) shows a rather striking improvement during the first 1 to 2 years, prior to the onset of relapses with remission rates of 75% to 100% at each study interval. It should be understood that these patients had been subjected to continuous disease for years prior to HSCT. Even those who remain in relapse are pleased with the temporary relief they obtained, and their postrelapse CDAI and CSI are improved over their pretransplant levels. Furthermore, the relapsed patients were more responsive to usual therapy following relapse, often entering remission again, as evident from the CDAI and CSI curves. Finally, some have had long-term, treatment-free responses, in contradistinction to their pre-HSCT courses.

Both cyclophosphamide and GCSF have been shown to have a salutary effect on CD, without stem-cell support.[47] The ultimate treatment effect of immune ablation and autologous HSCT predominantly comes from the immunosuppressive and cytoreductive effects of this conditioning regimen. The infusion of autologous HSC shortens the post-HSCT neutropenic interval, thereby making the procedure safer.

Currently, we believe this procedure should be reserved for those refractory patients who fulfill the inclusion and exclusion criteria outlined by our investigation, preferably within a clinical study, allowing for reporting results to the medical community. Although longer follow-up is needed, further investigation of autologous HSCT for CD appears warranted.

There is currently a multicenter, randomized trial in progress to test the efficacy of this procedure, comparing the mobilization procedure to the full conditioning plus HSCT.[48]

Editor's note (TMB): There is an excellent follow-up report of stem-cell transplantation for patients with refractory Crohn's disease by Burt, RK, Craig, RM, et al. in Blood 2010;110:6123–6132.

References

1. Bamias G, Nyce MR, De La Rue SA, Cominelli F. New concepts in the pathophysiology of inflammatory bowel disease. *Ann Intern Med.* 2005;143(12):895–904.

2. Fiocchi C. Inflammatory bowel disease: etiology and pathogenesis. *Gastroenterology.* 1998;115(1):182–205.

3. Mardini HE, Gregory KJ, Nasser M, et al. Gastroduodenal Crohn's disease is associated with NOD2/CARD15 gene polymorphisms, particularly L1007P homozygosity. *Dig Dis Sci.* 2005;50(12):2316–2322.

4. Hawn TR, Verbon A, Lettinga KD, et al. A common dominant TLR5 stop codon polymorphism abolishes flagellin signaling and is associated with susceptibility to legionnaires' disease. *J Exp Med.* 2003;198(10):1563–1572.

5. Ogura Y, Bonen DK, Inohara N, et al. A frameshift mutation in NOD2 associated with susceptibility to Crohn's disease. *Nature.* 2001;411(6837):603–606.

6. Cuthbert AP, Fisher SA, Mirza MM, et al. The contribution of NOD2 gene mutations to the risk and site of disease in inflammatory bowel disease. *Gastroenterology.* 2002;122(4):867–874.

7. Lala S, Ogura Y, Osborne C, et al. Crohn's disease and the NOD2 gene: a role for paneth cells. *Gastroenterology.* 2003;125(1):47–57.

8. Watanabe T, Kitani A, Strober W. NOD2 regulation of Toll-like receptor responses and the pathogenesis of Crohn's disease. *Gut.* 2005;54(11):1515–1518.

9. Chamaillard M, Iacob R, Desreumaux P, Colombel JF. Advances and perspectives in the genetics of inflammatory bowel diseases. *Clin Gastroenterol Hepatol.* 2006;4(2):143–151.

10. Rao SS, Cann PA, Holdsworth CD. Clinical experience of the tolerance of mesalazine and olsalazine in patients intolerant of sulphasalazine. *Scand J Gastroenterol.* 1987;22(3):332–336.

11. Bernstein LH, Frank MS, Brandt LJ, Boley SJ. Healing of perineal Crohn's disease with metronidazole. *Gastroenterology.* 1980;79(2):357–365.

12. Present DH, Korelitz BI, Wisch N, Glass JL, Sachar DB, Pasternack BS. Treatment of Crohn's disease with 6-mercaptopurine. A long-term, randomized, double-blind study. *N Engl J Med.* 1980;302(18):981–987.

13. Markowitz J, Grancher K, Kohn N, Lesser M, Daum F. A multicenter trial of 6-mercaptopurine and prednisone in children with newly diagnosed Crohn's disease. *Gastroenterology.* 2000;119(4):895–902.

14. Willoughby JM, Beckett J, Kumar PJ, Dawson AM. Controlled trial of azathioprine in Crohn's disease. *Lancet.* 1971;2(7731):944–947.

15. Kozarek RA, Patterson DJ, Gelfand MD, Botoman VA, Ball TJ, Wilske KR. Methotrexate induces clinical and histologic remission in patients with refractory inflammatory bowel disease. *Ann Intern Med.* 1989;110(5):353–356.

16. Brynskov J, Freund L, Rasmussen SN, et al. A placebo-controlled, double-blind, randomized trial of cyclosporine therapy in active chronic Crohn's disease. *N Engl J Med.* 1989;321(13):845–850.

17. Sandborn WJ, Present DH, Isaacs KL, et al. Tacrolimus for the treatment of fistulas in patients with Crohn's disease: a randomized, placebo-controlled trial. *Gastroenterology.* 2003;125(2):380–388.

18. Stallmach A, Wittig BM, Moser C, Fischinger J, Duchmann R, Zeitz M. Safety and efficacy of intravenous pulse cyclophosphamide in acute steroid refractory inflammatory bowel disease. *Gut.* 2003;52(3):377–382.

19. Present DH, Rutgeerts P, Targan S, et al. Infliximab for the treatment of fistulas in patients with Crohn's disease. *N Engl J Med.* 1999;340(18):1398–1405.

20. Farmer RG, Whelan G, Fazio VW. Long-term follow-up of patients with Crohn's disease. Relationship between the clinical pattern and prognosis. *Gastroenterology.* 1985;88(6):1818–1825.

21. Lapidus A, Bernell O, Hellers G, Löfberg R. Clinical course of colorectal Crohn's disease: a 35-year follow-up study of 507 patients. *Gastroenterology.* 1998;114(6):1151–1160.

22. Loftus EV Jr, Silverstein MD, Sandborn WJ, Tremaine WJ, Harmsen WS, Zinsmeister AR. Crohn's disease in Olmsted County, Minnesota, 1940–1993: incidence, prevalence, and survival. *Gastroenterology.* 1998;114(6):1161–1168.

23. Persson PG, Bernell O, Leijonmarck CE, Farahmand BY, Hellers G, Ahlbom A. Survival and cause-specific mortality in inflammatory bowel disease: a population-based cohort study. *Gastroenterology.* 1996;110(5):1339–1345.

24. Jess T, Winther KV, Munkholm P, Langholz E, Binder V. Mortality and causes of death in Crohn's disease: follow-up of a population-based cohort in Copenhagen County, Denmark. *Gastroenterology.*

2002;122(7):1808–1814.

25. Jess T, Loftus EV Jr, Harmsen WS, et al. Survival and cause specific mortality in patients with inflammatory bowel disease: a long term outcome study in Olmsted County, Minnesota, 1940–2004. *Gut.* 2006;55(9):1248–1254.

26. Lichtenstein GR, Feagan BG, Cohen RD, et al. Serious infections and mortality in association with therapies for Crohn's disease: TREAT registry. *Clin Gastroenterol Hepatol.* 2006;4(5):621–630.

27. Wolters FL, Russel MG, Sijbrandij J, et al. Crohn's disease: increased mortality 10 years after diagnosis in a Europe-wide population based cohort. *Gut.* 2006;55(4):510–518.

28. Lopez-Cubero SO, Sullivan KM, McDonald GB. Course of Crohn's disease after allogeneic marrow transplantation. *Gastroenterology.* 1998;114(3):433–440.

29. Drakos PE, Nagler A, Or R. Case of Crohn's disease in bone marrow transplantation. *Am J Hematol.* 1993;43(2):157–158.

30. Ditschkowski M, Einsele H, Schwerdtfeger R, et al. Improvement of inflammatory bowel disease after allogeneic stem-cell transplantation. *Transplantation.* 2003;75(10):1745–1747.

31. Talbot DC, Montes A, Teh WL, Nandi A, Powles RL. Remission of Crohn's disease following allogeneic bone marrow transplant for acute leukaemia. *Hosp Med.* 1998;59(7):580–581.

32. Castro J, Bentch HL, Smith L, et al. Prolonged clinical remission in patients with inflammatory bowel disease after high dose chemotherapy and autologous blood stem cell transplantation. *Blood.* 1996;88 (suppl 1):133a.

33. Burt RK, Marmont A, Oyama Y, et al. Randomized controlled trials of autologous hematopoietic stem cell transplantation for autoimmune diseases: the evolution from myeloablative to lymphoablative transplant regimens. *Arthritis Rheum.* 2006;54(12):3750–3760.

34. Oyama Y, Traynor A, Craig R, Barr W, Rosa R, Burt R. Treatment related mortality (TRM) and overall mortality (OM) in patients undergoing autologous hematopoietic stem cell transplantation (HSCT) for autoimmune diseases, a single center experience. *Blood.* 2003;102(suppl 1):986a.

35. Friedenstein AJ, Chailakhjan RK, Lalykina KS. The development of fibroblast colonies in monolayer cultures of guinea-pig bone marrow and spleen cells. *Cell Tissue Kinet.* 1970;3(4):393–403.

36. Uccelli A, Pistoia V, Moretta L. Mesenchymal stem cells: a new strategy for immunosuppression? *Trends Immunol.* 2007;28(5):219–226.

37. Ringdén O, Uzunel M, Rasmusson I, et al. Mesenchymal stem cells for treatment of therapy-resistant graft-versus-host disease. *Transplantation.* 2006;81(10):1390–1397.

38. Khalil PN, Weiler V, Nelson PJ, et al. Nonmyeloablative stem cell therapy enhances microcirculation and tissue regeneration in murine inflammatory bowel disease. *Gastroenterology.* 2007;132(3):944–954.

39. Oyama Y, Craig RM, Traynor AE, et al. Autologous hematopoietic stem cell transplantation in patients with refractory Crohn's disease. *Gastroenterology.* 2005;128(3):552–563.

40. Castro J, Bentch H, Smith L, et al. Autologous bone marrow transplantation for non-Hodgkin's lymphoma resulting in long-term remission of coincidental Crohn's disease. *Br J Haematol.* 1998;103:651–652.

41. Söderholm JD, Malm C, Juliusson G, Sjödahl R. Long-term endoscopic remission of crohn disease after autologous stem cell transplantation for acute myeloid leukaemia. *Scand J Gastroenterol.* 2002;37(5):613–616.

42. Scimè R, Cavallaro AM, Tringali S, et al. Complete clinical remission after high-dose immune suppression and autologous

hematopoietic stem cell transplantation in severe Crohn's disease refractory to immunosuppressive and immunomodulator therapy. *Inflamm Bowel Dis.* 2004;10(6):892–894.

43. Musso M, Porretto F, Crescimanno A, Bondì F, Polizzi V, Scalone R. Crohn's disease complicated by relapsed extranodal Hodgkin's lymphoma: prolonged complete remission after unmanipulated PBPC autotransplant. *Bone Marrow Transplant.* 2000;26(8):921–923.

44. Craig RM, Burt R. Autologous hematopoietic stem cell transplantation and immune ablation in refractory Crohn's disease. A six year follow-up. *Gastroenterology.* 2008;134:A14P.

45. Cassinotti A, Annaloro C, Ardizzone S, et al. Autologous haematopoietic stem cell transplantation without CD34+ cell selection in refractory Crohn's disease. *Gut.* 2008;57(2):211–217.

46. Kreisel W, Potthoff K, Bertz H, et al. Complete remission of Crohn's disease after high-dose cyclophosphamide and autologous stem cell transplantation. *Bone Marrow Transplant.* 2003;32(3):337–340.

47. Korzenik JR, Dieckgraefe BK, Valentine JF, Hausman DF, Gilbert MJ; Sargramostim in Crohn's Disease Study Group. Sargramostim for active Crohn's disease. *N Engl J Med.* 2005;352(21):2193–2201.

48. Hawkey CJ. Stem cell transplantation for Crohn's disease. *Best Pract Res Clin Haematol.* 2004;17(2):317–325.

Bowel Rest, Enteral and Parenteral Nutrition in IBD Patients

119

Jason Hemming and Rosemarie L. Fisher

The basis of the use of bowel rest in patients with Crohn's disease (CD) has its origin in several theories. Along the path for the search for the etiology of CD, there have been multiple instances where the possibility of an intraluminal antigen, be it bacterial, viral, food, or other, has been seriously considered. With this consideration, it only made sense that the idea of "putting the bowel to rest" might add to our therapeutic armamentarium. By taking away the antigenic stimulus, one might stop the progression or exacerbation of the disease process. However, as the antigen is unknown, one would have to stop giving anything by mouth, thus putting the bowel to rest.

It must also be considered that any nutrients delivered to the intestinal tract do, as part of normal physiology, stimulate various gastrointestinal hormones, increase luminal secretions, stimulate gastrointestinal motility, and augment mucosal permeability. Therefore, by removing these stimulating effects of intraluminal nutrients, one would be able to have a positive effect on the course of disease. Lastly, as evidence continues to grow about the normal and pathogenic physiologic role of intestinal bacteria in inflammatory bowel disease (IBD), the role bowel rest plays in altering the microbiota in patients with IBD must be considered.

What is an obvious problem to this approach, however, is that unless the patient receives some form of parenteral nutrition while putting the bowel to rest, malnutrition is either going to occur or worsen. In addition, as we have progressed in our understanding of the role of nutrition in the maintenance of the gastrointestinal mucosa and the role of various nutrients in cellular function. It has become less clear that putting the bowel to rest will result in any benefit to the patient or alter the course of disease, especially in the current era of increased immunologic and biologic therapy.

Is there evidence, however, that bowel rest is helpful in any patient with CD, and is there any evidence that, in fact, it may be harmful to this patient group? What follows, will attempt to delineate the evidence for and against the use of bowel rest and our approach to the use of bowel rest in patients with CD. However, one must ask, what is the definition of "bowel rest?" Is it actually "nothing by mouth" or may it include the use of elemental diets, which in the view of some clinicians, is equivalent to bowel rest? In addition, one must consider the use of bowel rest in both the short-term (acute disease) and long-term, or home, total parenteral nutrition (TPN) in these patients.

PHYSIOLOGIC EFFECTS OF BOWEL REST

Although the above theories about the benefits of bowel rest all seem quite reasonable, we have data from in vitro and in vivo studies, including postoperative studies, demonstrating that excluding nutrients from the lumen of intestine will result in mucosal atrophy and may result in further malabsorption and perhaps even bacterial translocation, or movement of bacteria across the luminal mucosal border. This might result in sepsis. One must be very careful to distinguish what role malnutrition itself plays in mucosal atrophy, as opposed to the absence of luminal nutrients, and the accompanying hormonal stimuli. Early studies compared the effects of bowel rest with what was effectively starvation. We know from studies in developing countries, that severe malnutrition will result in intestinal mucosal changes. Comparing intravenous and oral feeding to rats, there is a decrease in mucosal weight, mucosal protein, and enzyme content in those feed intravenously.[1] In vivo, patients with short bowel syndrome who are fed orally postoperatively, as opposed to being maintained on TPN, in a well-nourished state, have a more rapid, and higher rate of adaptive changes in the remaining small bowel.

More recently, several studies have challenged the importance of intraluminal nutrients in the maintenance of mucosal function. Resection of the distal bowel in rats has been shown to result in hyperplasia of a more proximal bowel. Enteral amino acids given alone were not incorporated into the proliferative zone of the intestinal crypt unless intravenous amino acids were administered as well. A more recent study, randomizing 67 patients undergoing major gastrointestinal surgery to either TPN or total enteral nutrition for 7 days postoperatively showed no clinical benefit in either systemic parameters or intestinal permeability parameters that were measured.[2]

The physician must continue to contemplate the effects of bowel rest on the normal or postoperative gut versus the increased permeability of CD. Despite great advancements, it is still unknown if a primary mucosal permeability disorder allows penetration of antigenic stimuli or if the presence of such luminal stimulants lead to increased permeability. In one case, bowel rest may increase mucosal permeability causing further systemic problems, whereas in the other, the removal of the stimulus should lead to an improvement in pathology and systemic complications.

It is well established that there is an increased mucosal permeability in patients with CD. Hollander and colleagues[3,4] found increased permeability in patients with inactive disease and in healthy relatives, thereby suggesting that the defect may be primary in nature. Teahon et al.[5] on the other hand, found no real difference between first-degree relatives with CD and healthy controls. Lastly, it has also been shown that first-degree relatives have an exaggerated increase in permeability after treatment with agents (e.g., nonsteroidal anti-inflammatory drugs) that alter mucosal permeability.

If we assume that the increased permeability is primary (because of CD and not malnutrition), and if it is also correct that the lack of luminal nutrients leads to further abnormalities in mucosal function, then putting the bowel to rest may only result in further injury. However, as the primary defect in CD remains unknown and the physiologic effects of bowel rest still unclear, perhaps the only way to evaluate its role of bowel rest in the treatment of CD is to review the clinical data to date.

● CLINICAL EXPERIENCE

TPN and "Nothing by Mouth" as Primary Therapy

The available data on the use of TPN and bowel rest for the primary treatment of CD are difficult to summarize to reach some conclusions. Many of the studies are retrospective and uncontrolled. The numbers of patients are commonly small and the criteria for remission are inconsistent. The idea of bowel rest as a treatment for active CD has been debated since the early 1980s, yet there still remains no clear-cut answers to questions regarding the efficacy of this approach. Overall, it is seen that approximately 64% (40–90%) of patients with CD will enter some form of remission after 3 to 6 weeks of TPN and taking "nothing by mouth." The subsequent relapse rate has been noted to be between 28% and 85% at 1 year and 40% and 60% at 2 years after primary therapy.[6] Furthermore, lower remission rates have been consistently reported in patients

having the penetrating disease, colonic involvement, or ulcerative colitis.

An earlier prospective but uncontrolled trial studied the effects of TPN, bowel rest, and no other medications in patients judged to be refractory to medical therapy. Thirty patients were kept "nothing by mouth" and on TPN for 3 months. On completion, 25 patients avoided surgery but there was a cumulative recurrence rate of 60% over 2 years and 85% after 4 years; rates four times higher than after surgery at that same institution. Thus prompting the authors to state that TPN is not as beneficial as surgery in this group of medically unresponsive patients.[7]

The best data to date examining the use of TPN and bowel rest comes from a multicenter, prospective, controlled trial published by Greenberg et al.[8] Fifty-one patients with active CD unresponsive to medical therapy were randomized to either TPN and "nothing by mouth," a defined polymeric tube feeding, or a standard oral diet supplemented by partial parental nutrition for 21 days. At 3 weeks and at 1-year follow-ups, there was no difference in either the remission rate, the avoidance of surgery or symptomatic improvement among the three groups. By concluding that there was no advantage in the use of bowel rest as opposed to good nutritional support, it raised the question as to whether the response to TPN and "nothing by mouth" was not as much secondary to the use of bowel rest but to the supply of adequate nutrition.

The 2001 American Gastroenterological Association technical review on Parenteral Nutrition concluded that bowel rest is not needed to achieve remission in active CD and that TPN is equivalent to enteral nutrition (EN) in the treatment of active small bowel CD.[9] Although this is a relatively old guideline, there has not been a new evidence to contradict this and so, the recommendations appropriately remain.

TPN and "Nothing by Mouth" as Adjunctive Therapy

The use of TPN as adjunctive therapy to standard drug therapy cannot be questioned if the patient is unable to take in adequate nutrients to maintain their energy and protein stores. This may be seen in cases where there is either bowel obstruction secondary to chronic scarring or acute inflammation. It may also be appropriate in the patient who enters the hospital with an acute exacerbation and no obstruction but severe malnutrition and an inability to tolerate oral nutrients or tube feedings.

Editor's note (TMB): It may also provide time for immunomodulator therapy to become effective including Crohn's colitis (Sitzmann, Converse, Bayless. *Gastroenterology.* 1990;99: 1647–1652).

Elemental Diets as a Substitute for Bowel Rest

Elemental diets were first used in CD to provide preoperative nutritional support. A prospective uncontrolled study by Voitk et al.[10] first suggested a primary therapeutic effect of elemental diet in the clinical improvement of patients awaiting surgery. Its use was first proposed for the same reason as to the use of bowel rest: less antigenic stimulation to the intestine. Beyond lower antigenicity, elemental diets may effect favorable changes in the intestine mucosa, encourage an anti-inflammatory cytokine profile and allow those with near total obstruction to tolerate oral feeding.

Elemental nutrition's support of an anti-inflammatory condition has been suggested by observed changes in endoscopic activity and cytokine profiles. In a short-term study of 28 patients after 4 weeks of elemental diet, endoscopic and histologic healing was observed in 44% and 19% and 39% and 20% in the terminal ileum and the colon, respectively. Elevated levels of interleukin (IL)-1β, IL-1 receptor antagonist (IL-1ra), IL-6, IL-8, and tumor necrosis factor-α observed prior to treatment returned to control levels after treatment.[11] The same group continued to follow patients and found that at 1 year, those that continued to receive long-term enteral support had significantly improved clinical remission rates, endoscopic activity, and inflammatory cytokine profiles as compared to a nonrandomized control group.[12] Of importance, the enteral group was allowed to eat as they pleased in addition to receiving EN.

Since the publication of Greenberg's study, researchers continue to investigate the role of EN support in CD. A substantial number of trials have compared elemental diets to conventional steroids; wherein most show a greater rate of induction of remission with steroids. Several well-done meta-analyses confirm these findings by demonstrating a superiority of corticosteroid therapy. A recent 2007 Cochrane review stated that, corticosteroid therapy is more effective than EN for inducing remission of active CD, with a pooled odds ratio of 0.33. Relapse rates at 12 months were similar at approximately 65%.[13]

Although EN seems inferior to corticosteroids, the low adverse effect profile makes it an attractive candidate for treating CD. Primary nutrition treatment would be beneficial in patients' refractory to corticosteroids or those that have other underlying conditions that make corticosteroids a less favorable option. This is particularly true in the pediatric population and thus we will leave more detailed discussion to the clinical use of elemental diets to subsequent chapters.

Pediatric CD Therapy

The authors find that despite clinical efficacy and minimal adverse effects, the use of EN is largely limited in adults with CD because of low palatability, poor acceptance of either oral or tube feeding, and inconvenience that lead to low compliance and high dropout rates from therapy.

Polymeric and Other Enteral Formulations

On the issue of formulation, all systemic reviews including the most recent Cochrane analysis have demonstrated no statistically significant differences based on nitrogen source whether elemental, semielemental or polymeric protein formulation. Further studies have investigated the importance of fat composition based on the hypothesis that the proportion or type of fat could affect the production of proinflammatory mediators. In this same Cochrane review a nonsignificant trend favoring very low fat content was described, but not recommended. The possibility that fat composition may have an immunomodulator or anti-inflammatory effect in active CD warrants further exploration.

Bowel Rest as Therapy for Fistulous Disease

There is data that shows that bowel rest and TPN will result in the long-term closure of non-Crohn's related enterocutaneous fistulas in some patients. However, this does not appear to be the case for patients with fistulizing CD. An initial review cited an overall closure rate of 38% but a much lower maintenance of closure after reintroduction of oral nutrition. A study from Japan, treated 22 fistulae with either bowel rest and TPN or enteral alimentation. None of the internal fistulae closed and only 42% of the external fistulae closed. The reopening rate after nutritional therapy was 88.9%, as compared to 53.8% in those requiring surgery.[14] The introduction of infliximab and other biologic therapies has dramatically changed the management and natural history of fistulous disease, greatly minimizing the number of patients using bowel rest and TPN to manage their disease. The only recent study addressing nutritional therapy and infliximab use, retrospectively showed that for 97 patients the efficacy of infliximab after 2 weeks was no different for those on enteral alimentation, TPN or an ad libitum diet.[15]

Home TPN in CD

In CD, the most common indication for home TPN is chronic intestinal failure secondary to short bowel syndrome usually in the setting of multiple small bowel resections. Home TPN is also effective in a smaller group of patients with multiple strictures, fistulae, or complications of standard medical therapy, who are not yet surgical candidates. Several databases from around the world have provided the opportunity to follow-up on these patients.

In the United States, the OLEY Registry collected data on more than 4000 patients between 1985 and 1995. In examining survival and complication rates, Howard and Hassan[16] reviewed the data on 562 patients with CD. The mean age of patients was 36 with a 1-year survival of 96%. Sixty percent had established complete rehabilitation, defined as the ability to sustain normal age-related activities, with another 38% reaching partial rehabilitation status at 1 year. The complication rate per year (those that required hospitalization) was 0.9 related to the TPN and 1.1 for non-TPN causes. A similar review from the Mayo Clinic showed that in their 225 patients on home TPN, 22.2% had IBD and short bowel syndrome. This population had a much younger mean age at institution of treatment, longer median duration of treatment, and overall better survival, at 5 years.[17] Further studies, despite not establishing an association of TPN and increased body weight or decreased frequency of further surgery, have shown significantly increased quality of life, serum albumin, and transferrin levels, and a reduction in requirements for oral steroids.

Editor's note (TMB): Improved nutrition status and less disease activity is a preoperative benefit in the markedly malnourished patient. There is a separate chapter on preoperation nutritional supplementation.

Complications

Although the use of bowel rest and TPN in this group is without question, it is associated with significant morbidity and potentially life-threatening complications. Complications can be categorized as catheter-related, gastrointestinal, renal, or metabolic. In a retrospective series of 41 Crohn's disease patients on home TPN (total of 121 patient-years), 58.5% of them had one or more TPN-related complication requiring hospitalization. The reasons for hospitalizations included catheter-related sepsis (79.2%), mechanical problems (62.5%) and dehydration, or electrolyte imbalance (20.8%). There were eight deaths in total, only 7% of which directly related to catheter-related sepsis.[18] A 2007 Canadian review of 150 patients receiving home TPN (47 with CD) showed similar rates of hospitalizations and catheter-related sepsis.[19]

● SUMMARY

The above information appears to result in an individual decision about the use of nutritional support and bowel rest in adult patients with IBD. The easiest decision is when patients have short bowel syndrome either due to disease or surgery, are unable to take life-sustaining nutrients orally, or have uncontrollable diarrhea or obstruction. The decision then is a matter of nutrition support and not a therapeutic decision with regards to the IBD. Use of nutrition support, either enteral or parenteral, in these authors opinions, then becomes a matter of adjunctive therapy, and not primary. Further trials utilizing various nutritional immunomodulators such as arginine or glutamine would be beneficial in helping to determine the use of nutrition support as primary therapy. However, the variablilty of disease location, spontaneous remission rates, and patient acceptance, may make this an extremely difficult process.

References

1. Hughes CA, Dowling RH. Speed of onset of adaptive mucosal hypoplasia and hypofunction in the intestine of parenterally fed rats. *Clin Sci.* 1980;59(5):317–327.

2. Reynolds JV, Kanwar S, Welsh FK, et al. 1997 Harry M. Vars Research Award. Does the route of feeding modify gut barrier function and clinical outcome in patients after major upper gastrointestinal surgery? *JPEN J Parenter Enteral Nutr.* 1997;21(4):196–201.

3. Hollander D, Vadheim CM, Brettholz E, Petersen GM, Delahunty T, Rotter JI. Increased intestinal permeability in patients with Crohn's disease and their relatives. A possible etiologic factor. *Ann Intern Med.* 1986;105(6):883–885.

4. Hollander D. Crohn's disease–a permeability disorder of the tight junction? *Gut.* 1988;29(12):1621–1624.

5. Teahon K, Smethurst P, Levi AJ, Menzies IS, Bjarnason I. Intestinal permeability in patients with Crohn's disease and their first degree relatives. *Gut.* 1992;33(3):320–323.

6. Dieleman LA, Heizer WD. Nutritional issues in inflammatory bowel disease. *Gastroenterol Clin North Am.* 1998;27(2):435–451.

7. Elson CO, Layden TJ, Nemchausky BA, Rosenberg JL, Rosenberg IH. An evaluation of total parenteral nutrition in the management of inflammatory bowel disease. *Dig Dis Sci.* 1980;25(1):42–48.

8. Greenberg GR, Fleming CR, Jeejeebhoy KN, Rosenberg IH, Sales D, Tremaine WJ. Controlled trial of bowel rest and nutritional support in the management of Crohn's disease. *Gut.* 1988;29(10):1309–1315.

9. Koretz RL, Lipman TO, Klein S; American Gastroenterological Association. AGA technical review on parenteral nutrition. *Gastroenterology.* 2001;121(4):970–1001.

10. Voitk AJ, Echave V, Feller JH, Brown RA, Gurd FN. Experience with elemental diet in the treatment of inflammatory bowel disease. Is this primary therapy? *Arch Surg.* 1973;107(2):329–333.

11. Yamamoto T, Nakahigashi M, Umegae S, Kitagawa T, Matsumoto K. Impact of elemental diet on mucosal inflammation in patients with active Crohn's disease: cytokine production and endoscopic and histological findings. *Inflamm Bowel Dis.* 2005;11(6):580–588.

12. Yamamoto T, Nakahigashi M, Saniabadi AR, et al. Impacts of long-term enteral nutrition on clinical and endoscopic disease activities and mucosal cytokines during remission in patients with Crohn's disease: a prospective study. *Inflamm Bowel Dis.* 2007;13(12):1493–1501.

13. Zachos M, Tondeur M, Griffiths AM. Enteral nutritional therapy for induction of remission in Crohn's disease. *Cochrane Database Syst Rev.* 2007;(1):CD000542.

14. Yamazaki Y, Fukushima T, Sugita A, Takemura H, Tsuchiya S. The medical, nutritional and surgical treatment of fistulae in Crohn's disease. *Jpn J Surg.* 1990;20(4):376–383.

15. Matsumoto T, Iida M, Kohgo Y, et al. Therapeutic efficacy of infliximab on active Crohn's disease under nutritional therapy. *Scand J Gastroenterol.* 2005;40(12):1423–1430.

16. Howard L, Hassan N. Home parenteral nutrition. 25 years later. *Gastroenterol Clin North Am.* 1998;27(2):481–512.

17. Scolapio JS, Fleming CR, Kelly DG, Wick DM, Zinsmeister AR. Survival of home parenteral nutrition-treated patients: 20 years of experience at the Mayo Clinic. *Mayo Clin Proc.* 1999;74(3):217–222.

18. Galandiuk S, O'Neill M, McDonald P, Fazio VW, Steiger E. A century of home parenteral nutrition for Crohn's disease. *Am J Surg.* 1990;159(6):540–544; discussion 544.

19. Raman M, Gramlich L, Whittaker S, Allard JP. Canadian home total parenteral nutrition registry: preliminary data on the patient population. *Can J Gastroenterol.* 2007;21(10):643–648.

Enteral Nutrition: Impact on Disease Activity and Growth in Pediatric IBD

120

Mary E. Sherlock and Anne M. Griffiths

Enteral feeding of formulated food can be used to correct or prevent malnutrition in inflammatory bowel disease (IBD). Its additional benefit as primary therapy in Crohn's disease was fortuitously discovered when patients given exclusive enteral nutrition preoperatively experienced improvement not only in their nutritional status as intended but also in clinical and laboratory parameters of intestinal inflammation. Thereafter enteral nutrition became an alternative to corticosteroids in the treatment of active Crohn's disease.

Patterns of use of enteral nutrition as therapy for Crohn's disease differ substantially around the world. Enteral nutrition has had a special place in the management of pediatric Crohn's disease, as a means of avoiding the growth-inhibiting (and other adverse) effects of corticosteroids. Nevertheless, in a survey of practice patterns, 62% of Western European pediatric gastroenterologists reported frequent use of enteral nutrition, in contrast to only 4% of their North American colleagues.[1] Such disparity is striking.

Treatment algorithms for Crohn's disease have changed. Increased and earlier use of biologic agents has reduced dependence on corticosteroids and has made mucosal healing a realistic goal. Nevertheless, for patients willing to accept dietary restrictions and comply with the demands of its therapeutic regimens, exclusive enteral nutrition remains a safe alternative option. This chapter will review the practical aspects of this therapy and discuss its place in the current treatment of pediatric IBD.

EFFICACY AS PRIMARY THERAPY OF ACTIVE CROHN'S DISEASE

Multiple adult and pediatric studies have compared enteral nutrition with corticosteroids in the treatment of active Crohn's disease, and data from such randomized controlled trials have been combined in meta-analyses.[2] Although corticosteroids are associated with a greater likelihood of induction of clinical remission, roughly 50% to 60% of patients treated with enteral nutrition in the clinical trial setting "respond," as judged by improvements in multi-item measures of disease activity and laboratory markers of inflammation.[2] As with all therapies, response rates vary depending on characteristics of the patient population.[2]

MUCOSAL IMPROVEMENT

It is well established that mucosal healing does not parallel clinical response to corticosteroids. In contrast, endoscopic healing may be achieved with anti-tumor necrosis factor (TNF)-α antibodies. Several pediatric groups have performed follow-up endoscopic assessments following exclusive enteral nutrition.[3,4] A retrospective comparative analysis reported greater endoscopic and histologic improvement in newly diagnosed pediatric patients treated with enteral nutrition, even though clinical response rate with corticosteroid therapy was comparable.[3] In comparison with prednisolone-induced clinical remission, this observational study also suggested a longer duration of clinical remission following attainment of mucosal healing with enteral nutrition.[3] In a prospective uncontrolled study of 65 children, Afzal et al.[4] reported post-treatment improvements in endoscopic and histologic mucosal assessments of patients with ileal or ileocolonic disease. Modern treatment paradigms call for interventions that achieve more than symptom control. The mucosal effects of enteral nutrition should continue to be examined, ideally in a prospective, randomized study, wherein those assessing the mucosal response are blinded to the treatment group.

PATIENT SELECTION

Anatomic Localization of Crohn's Disease

The site of intestinal inflammation in Crohn's disease may influence the likelihood of efficacy of enteral nutrition. We present it as a treatment option most confidently to patients with macroscopic inflammation located predominantly in the small intestine. Patients with Crohn's disease confined to the colon have generally been considered to respond less reliably,[2] although a recent report of experience in the pediatric IBD program in Glasgow, Scotland, refutes that observation.[5] Similarly, in a comparative trial employing elemental and polymeric formulae, Rigaud and colleagues[6] reported remission rates of 67% and 73%, respectively, in adult patients, despite the fact that two-thirds had isolated colonic disease. These observations support the use of enteral nutrition in active Crohn's disease involving predominantly, or even exclusively, the colon. Enteral nutrition has not, however, been used to treat active ulcerative colitis.

Duration of Crohn's Disease

Recent onset disease may be more responsive than disease of longer duration, as was evident in a pediatric multicenter study that stratified children according to disease duration prior to randomization.[7] Similarly, Day et al.[8] found remission rates of 80% in children with newly diagnosed Crohn's disease treated with enteral nutrition as a single therapy in comparison with remission rates of 58% of children with previously diagnosed Crohn's disease. It may be that the inflammation of recent onset is more amenable to anti-inflammatory treatments than disease that has established a chronic course. This may explain why, at least in smaller studies, children appear to have a greater response rate than their adult counterparts, given that their disease is more likely to be of shorter duration. A similar relationship between disease duration and response rates has also been observed in several multicenter trials of anti-TNF therapies.

● THERAPEUTIC REGIMENS

Exclusive Versus Supplementary Enteral Nutrition

To be successful, enteral nutrition should be administered as sole source nutrition. Allowance of regular food during treatment of active disease appears to compromise efficacy,[9] and may also render the child satiated, and less able to tolerate the desired amounts of formulated food. Oral intake of water and/or clear (see-through) fluids is allowed.

Mode of Administration

Liquid diets may be sipped orally (see discussion of palatability in later section), or administered via silastic nasogastric feeding tube (size 6 or 8 French). When a nasogastric feeding tube is used, most children learn to insert the tube by themselves at night and to administer the required volume of formula overnight. Ideally, the tube is removed each morning to facilitate normal daytime activities. When supplementary enteral nutrition over a period of months is contemplated, an indwelling gastrostomy tube may be inserted.

Target Volume and Calories

In the treatment of active Crohn's disease, enteral nutrition should be prescribed in the amount necessary to provide 100% of the patient's estimated caloric and protein requirements. Patients with Crohn's disease fail to downregulate their resting energy expenditure in the presence of malnutrition, likely due to effects of proinflammatory cytokines. Energy requirements may be calculated using normal predictive equations with the patient's ideal

Initial hourly infusion rate
20–40 mL/hour OR
1–2 mL/kg/hour
(using actual body weight)

Increasing enteral feeds
Increase by 10 cc every 6 to 8 hours
(as tolerated)
until 24-hour infusion goal rate is reached
(should take 36–48 hours to reach goal)

Cycling enteral feeds
Reduce the number of hours of enteral feeding
by 2–3 hours each night as tolerated. Divide
the total 24-hour goal volume by the desired
number of hours for the enteral feed to
determine the NG feed rate.

Final goal of overnight feeds
Feeds should run for 10–14 hours overnight
(dependent on lifestyle and tolerance).
Maximum feed rate is approximately
6–8 mL/kg/hour.

FIGURE 120.1 • Sample protocol for initiating exclusive enteral nutrition using formulated food.

body weight for height, or using the current weight with allowance for catch-up weight gain (approximately 20% extra calories).

Infusion rates should be increased in a stepwise manner considering individual tolerance. A sample protocol for the gradual increase to full feeds is given in Fig. 120.1. Most young patients aim ultimately to complete the necessary infusion over a 10-to-14-hour period each night.

Choice of Formula

Polymeric, peptide-based and amino-acid–based formulae have all been used to treat active Crohn's disease.[2] There is general agreement that the protein content of liquid diets does not influence efficacy.[2] Dietary lipids, however, can modulate inflammation by a variety of mechanisms that influence cellular production of cytokines and eicosanoids.[10] Excess n-6 polyunsaturated fatty acids (PUFAs) would be expected to attenuate the effect of enteral nutrition in treating Crohn's disease, whereas a relative increase in n-3 PUFAs might be beneficial.

Given the influence of fat content on efficacy, we recommend a conventional elemental liquid diet (because of the low-fat content) to optimize likelihood of response, if nasogastric tube feeding is to be employed. The treatment benefit of a low-fat—even n-3 PUFA-enriched—elemental diet, compared to a conventional polymeric diet, is admittedly small (<30% difference in response rates). Therefore, if a patient desires to drink (rather than enterally administer) formula, a polymeric liquid diet should be selected because of its greater palatability.

TABLE 120.1 Sample Order of Reintroduction to Solid Foods

Day of Introduction	Description of Foods	Examples of Foods
1–4	Low-fiber grains	– White flour breads/bagels/buns/plain pasta/roti/flatbread/rice – Plain crackers, pretzels, plain cookies (e.g., arrowroot, digestive) – Hot cereals: cream of wheat – Cold cereals (dry): low fiber, low fat (e.g., no granola) – Plain muffins without nuts or dried fruit
5–9	Low-fat/fiber meat and alternative sources	– Plain and tender cuts of chicken/turkey/lamb/veal/beef/pork – Low-fat fish – Smooth low-fat peanut butter (limited amounts) – Tofu – Eggs (prepared with little to no fat) – Note: avoid fried, cured, and processed meats; regular fat peanut butter, dried or canned peas, beans, lentils
10–14	Low-fiber vegetables and fruit	– Raw fruits without membrane and skin – All canned/stewed fruits without skin and seeds – Tender, cooked vegetables, no skins/seeds – Note: vegetables and fruit should be prepared using low-fat cooking methods – Soups with allowed meat, veg, rice, noodles (avoid highly seasoned soups, cream soups)
15–17	Low-fat dairy products	– Low-fat milks, yogurts, cheeses
18	Regular diet as tolerated	– Increase fat and fiber gradually to assess tolerance

Duration of Exclusive Enteral Nutrition

The required duration of exclusive enteral nutrition necessary to treat active inflammation has not been well defined. Improvements in clinical and laboratory parameters occur quickly, often by 2 weeks. Most gastroenterologists including ourselves, however, suggest continuing the therapy for a minimum of 4 to 6 weeks— longer if the child has not yet reached his/her ideal weight.

Reintroduction of Solid Food

Although some clinicians have investigated the merits of a specific exclusion diet following induction of clinical remission by exclusive enteral nutrition, we simply reintroduce foods gradually. It is prudent, particularly if the patient is known to have a relatively stenosed segment of intestine, to offer a low-fiber diet initially following completion of the enteral nutrition regimen. A sample order of food reintroduction is given in the Table 120.1.

● MAINTENANCE OF CLINICAL REMISSION FOLLOWING EXCLUSIVE ENTERAL NUTRITION

One of the limitations of liquid diet therapy, as with all medical treatments for Crohn's disease, has been the observed tendency for symptoms to recur promptly following its cessation. In most studies 60% to 70% of patients experience a relapse within 12 months of stopping enteral nutrition.[6]

Early introduction of an immunomodulatory drug such as azathioprine or methotrexate is one option for controlling Crohn's disease after an initial period of exclusive enteral nutrition. Two nutritional strategies can also be considered to maintain remission: firstly, "cyclical exclusive enteral nutrition," meaning nocturnal infusion of a liquid diet and avoidance of regular food 1 month out of 4[11]; or secondly, "supplementary enteral nutrition," that is, continuation of nocturnal nasogastric feeding four to five times weekly as supplement to an unrestricted ad lib daytime diet.[12] In a nonrandomized trial by Wilschanski and colleagues,[12] supplemental nocturnal enteral nutrition, with a "usual" diet during daytime was associated with improved growth and prolonged clinical remission in pediatric patients. We find this strategy to be well accepted by motivated patients, who enjoy the weight optimization and enhanced energy that accompany sustained provision of good nutrition. In a prospective study assessing supplementary liquid diet therapy, Takagi and colleagues randomized patients to receive either an unrestricted diet or a diet whereby 50% of daily calories were from an elemental diet and the remaining 50% from regular diet. Those receiving half their daily calories from an elemental diet had a lower relapse rate of 35% versus 64% of those on regular diet.[13]

● MECHANISM OF ACTION OF ENTERAL NUTRITION AS PRIMARY THERAPY

A therapy is more likely to be accepted, if the mechanism by which it ameliorates intestinal inflammation is understood. The mode of action of enteral nutrition remains conjectural. Hypotheses have included overall nutritional repletion, provision of important specific micronutrients to the diseased intestine, elimination of dietary antigen uptake, diminution of intestinal synthesis of inflammatory mediators via reduction in dietary fat, and alteration of intestinal microbial flora. Most recent research has focused on the role of lipids in modulating intestinal inflammation, with some studies attempting to explore the importance of changes in the enteric flora observed with enteral nutrition.

Clinical trials employing formulae with disparate fat contents, however, have yielded conflicting results. Response rates among patients treated by Bamba and colleagues[14] decreased as the amount of soybean oil (predominantly linoleic acid, an n-6 PUFA) in the elemental formula was increased. A well-designed multicenter European study, however, was stopped early because of a low remission rate in one of the enterally fed groups.[10] Sixty-seven percent of compliant patients treated with a diet high in linoleate (n-6 PUFA) and low in oleate (monounsaturated fatty acids) achieved remission compared with only 27% of those compliant with a formula low in linoleate and high in oleate.[10] These two clinical trials, and earlier ones, suggest that the magnitude of response to enteral nutrition is influenced by lipid composition, but the relative importance of specific fatty acids seems variable. More importantly, although amount and type of fat may modulate inflammatory pathways, the therapeutic success achieved with a variety of both polymeric (usually high fat) and elemental (usually low fat) formulae suggests that efficacy does not depend solely on fat content.

Effects of enteral nutrition on the gut microbial flora deserve further exploration, in light of the now well-established role of microbes in the pathogenesis of Crohn's disease. Molecular approaches to the identification of bacterial species are now available. A small study among children with Crohn's disease demonstrated that the enteric microflora is modified during and after a course of exclusive enteral nutrition.[15] Alterations in bacterial populations may modify interactions with the intestinal epithelium, thereby leading to modulation of inflammation. It is as yet unclear, however, whether the observed changes in the intestinal flora occur as a direct response to the administration of exclusive enteral nutrition, or merely as a consequence of decreased inflammation.

● FACILITATION OF LINEAR GROWTH WITH ENTERAL NUTRITION

Pathophysiology of Linear Growth Impairment

Impairment of linear growth commonly complicates pediatric Crohn's disease both prior to diagnosis and during follow-up. The major contributing (and interrelated) factors are the direct growth-inhibiting effects of proinflammatory cytokines produced by the inflamed intestine and chronic undernutrition.[16] Inappropriate use of chronic corticosteroid therapy will also impede linear growth.

Chronic Caloric Insufficiency

Growth requires energy. Multiple factors contribute to undernutrition in IBD. However, reduced intake, rather than excessive losses or increased needs, is generally the major cause.

Deliberate food restriction avoids symptoms. More importantly, cytokine-mediated disease-related anorexia can be profound. Whereas clinical studies have demonstrated that significant intestinal fat malabsorption is uncommon in most forms of Crohn's disease, leakage of protein is frequent.

Direct Cytokine Effects

Multiple cytokines contribute to the inflammation in IBD including TNFα, interferon (IFN)-γ, and many interleukins (IL; including IL-6, IL-12, IL-17, and IL-23). As has been recently reviewed, these inflammatory cytokines inhibit linear growth through pathways that involve the growth hormone/insulin growth factor (IGF)-1 axis as well as through other pathways.[16] Further, cytokines appear to alter gonadotropin releasing hormone secretion patterns and impair end-organ responsiveness to circulating testosterone, thereby compounding the effects of undernutrition in delaying progression through puberty.

Corticosteroid Suppression of Linear Growth

The growth-suppressive effects of glucocorticoids are multifactorial, and include central suppression of growth hormone release, decreased hepatic transcription of growth hormone receptor, such that production of IGF-1 is decreased, and decreased IGF-1 binding in cartilage. Hence exogenous corticosteroids create a state of functional growth hormone deficiency. Growth, particularly in prepubertal children, can be impaired by relatively modest daily doses of prednisone (3–5 mg/m^2). Chronic use is clearly deleterious. There is not good evidence, however, that restricted short-term use of steroids for treatment of active Crohn's disease at first presentation is detrimental to long-term growth.

● TREATING CROHN'S DISEASE TO FACILITATE GROWTH

Treatments that spare chronic steroid use and that induce and sustain mucosal healing will be associated with reduced cytokine production, which in turn leads to improved appetite and weight gain and enhanced linear growth. Hence significant improvements in weight and linear growth are observed during infliximab maintenance therapy, even in children with otherwise chronically active disease unresponsive to other therapies.[17] Observed improvement in linear growth with enteral nutrition reflects both provision of adequate calories and reduced intestinal inflammation. Several studies have documented gains in height velocity as well as in weight, as long as nutritional therapy is continued beyond the short induction phase.[12] Resumption of normal linear growth during enteral nutrition maintenance regimens is a marker of therapeutic success, that is, an indication that healing of inflammation as well as provision of nutrients has been achieved. Conversely, if a child merely gains weight but does not grow in height, it can be assumed that the inflamed intestine is not healing, and that other methods of treating the inflammation must be adopted.

The Place of Enteral Nutrition in Current Treatment Paradigms

In the former era of Crohn's disease treatment, when corticosteroids were the drugs most capable of rapidly inducing clinical remission, it could certainly be argued that enteral nutrition was a desirable alternative in treating active disease. The growth-inhibiting and other side effects of chronic corticosteroid therapy in children, together with the lack of mucosal healing achieved, made exclusive enteral nutrition attractive as primary therapy despite the demanding regimens of diet restriction.

Corticosteroids, however, are no longer the mainstay of treatment of active inflammation, offering little more than short-term symptom relief in responsive patients. Anti-TNFα antibodies have the potential to rapidly treat symptoms and to heal diseased bowel, thus moving the goals of therapy beyond symptom control. Normal health and growth are restored even among children with extensive Crohn's disease, chronically active despite other medical treatments.[17] Our practice has changed with the advent of biologic therapies.

Treatment Algorithms

For children newly diagnosed with Crohn's disease, the specific treatment algorithms we recommend depend on the disease phenotype. Despite some conflicting experience, as described earlier, our observation has been that enteral nutrition is particularly useful among young patients with predominantly small bowel disease. Patients with extensive small bowel disease commonly present with impaired linear growth. For this subgroup of children, and for those with less extensive ileal disease but significant weight loss, we encourage enteral nutrition as primary therapy rather than corticosteroids. If the response to induction therapy is good as anticipated, we encourage a maintenance regimen of supplementary enteral nutrition, particularly for patients with extensive small bowel disease. When colonic disease is extensive and severe, our clinical practice is to initiate corticosteroid therapy, but to add anti-TNFα therapy early if the response is incomplete. Other pediatric gastroenterologists report satisfying responses to enteral nutrition in the setting of predominant colitis, but our preference is to aim for the mucosal healing that we believe to be more reliably achieved with anti-TNFα therapy. The presence of significant perianal fistulizing disease is an indication for first-line anti-TNFα therapy in combination with antibiotics.

The benefits of biologic therapies are clear. In our practice anti-TNFα therapy, rather than enteral nutrition, has become the most commonly employed treatment for children with steroid-refractory or steroid-dependent inflammatory Crohn's disease. As pediatric gastroenterologists, however, we pay close attention to—and inform families of—associated risks as well as benefits. Data concerning adverse events convince us that hepatosplenic T-cell lymphoma, specifically, and other lymphomas and neoplasms, are being observed more frequently in children and adolescents treated with thiopurines alone, or with both thiopurines and anti-TNFα agents, than would be expected to occur in healthy individuals of the same age. Although the absolute risks are small, there is no doubt the increased risk is attributable to the drug(s) employed. The benefits and risks of therapy as well as the risks of ineffectively treated disease must always be weighed.

Editor's note (TMB): This very thoughtful chapter focuses on mucosal healing as a goal of therapy. Are we doing patients a disservice when we settle for less? Balancing benefits and risks should be a theme in our decision making as well.

References

1. Levine A, Milo T, Buller H, Markowitz J. Consensus and controversy in the management of pediatric Crohn disease: an international survey. *J Pediatr Gastroenterol Nutr.* 2003;36(4):464–469.

2. Griffiths AM, Ohlsson A, Sherman PM, Sutherland LR. Meta-analysis of enteral nutrition as a primary treatment of active Crohn's disease. *Gastroenterology.* 1995;108(4):1056–1067.

3. Berni Canani R, Terrin G, Borrelli O, et al. Short- and long-term therapeutic efficacy of nutritional therapy and corticosteroids in paediatric Crohn's disease. *Dig Liver Dis.* 2006;38(6):381–387.

4. Afzal NA, Davies S, Paintin M, et al. Colonic Crohn's disease in children does not respond well to treatment with enteral nutrition if the ileum is not involved. *Dig Dis Sci.* 2005;50(8):1471–1475.

5. Buchanan E, Gaunt WW, Cardigan T, Garrick V, McGrogan P, Russell RK. The use of exclusive enteral nutrition for induction of remission in children with Crohn's disease demonstrates that disease phenotype does not influence clinical remission. *Aliment Pharmacol Ther.* 2009;30(5):501–507.

6. Rigaud D, Cosnes J, Le Quintrec Y, René E, Gendre JP, Mignon M. Controlled trial comparing two types of enteral nutrition in treatment of active Crohn's disease: elemental versus polymeric diet. *Gut.* 1991;32(12):1492–1497.

7. Griffiths AM. Enteral nutrition in the management of Crohn's disease. *JPEN J Parenter Enteral Nutr.* 2005;29(4 suppl):S108–S112; discussion S112.

8. Day AS, Whitten KE, Lemberg DA, et al. Exclusive enteral feeding as primary therapy for Crohn's disease in Australian children and adolescents: a feasible and effective approach. *J Gastroenterol Hepatol.* 2006;21(10):1609–1614.

9. Johnson T, Macdonald S, Hill SM, Thomas A, Murphy MS. Treatment of active Crohn's disease in children using partial enteral nutrition with liquid formula: a randomised controlled trial. *Gut.* 2006;55(3):356–361.

10. Gassull MA, Fernández-Bañares F, Cabré E, et al.; European Group on Enteral Nutrition in Crohn's Disease. Fat composition may be a clue to explain the primary therapeutic effect of enteral nutrition in Crohn's disease: results of a double blind randomised multicentre European trial. *Gut.* 2002;51(2):164–168.

11. Belli DC, Seidman E, Bouthillier L, et al. Chronic intermittent elemental diet improves growth failure in children with Crohn's disease. *Gastroenterology.* 1988;94(3):603–610.

12. Wilschanski M, Sherman P, Pencharz P, Davis L, Corey M, Griffiths A. Supplementary enteral nutrition maintains remission in paediatric Crohn's disease. *Gut.* 1996;38(4):543–548.

13. Takagi S, Utsunomiya K, Kuriyama S, et al. Effectiveness of an 'half elemental diet' as maintenance therapy for Crohn's disease: A randomized-controlled trial. *Aliment Pharmacol Ther.* 2006;24(9):1333–1340.

14. Bamba T, Shimoyama T, Sasaki M, et al. Dietary fat attenuates the benefits of an elemental diet in active Crohn's disease: a randomized, controlled trial. *Eur J Gastroenterol Hepatol.* 2003;15(2):151–157.

15. Leach ST, Mitchell HM, Eng WR, Zhang L, Day AS. Sustained modulation of intestinal bacteria by exclusive enteral nutrition used to treat children with Crohn's disease. *Aliment Pharmacol Ther.* 2008;28(6):724–733.

16. Walters TD, Griffiths AM. Mechanisms of growth impairment in pediatric Crohn's disease. *Nat Rev Gastroenterol Hepatol.* 2009;6(9):513–523.

17. Walters TD, Gilman AR, Griffiths AM. Linear growth improves during infliximab therapy in children with chronically active severe Crohn's disease. *Inflamm Bowel Dis.* 2007;13(4):424–430.

Gastroduodenal Crohn's Disease | 121

Robert S. Burakoff

Twenty to fifty percent of patients with Crohn's disease will show evidence of gastroduodenal involvement on imaging, endoscopy, or histology.[1–3] However, clinically significant involvement of the stomach or duodenum occurs in fewer than 4% of patients with Crohn's disease.[2–4] Most of the patients who have gastroduodenal Crohn's disease have simultaneous ileocolonic disease, and most who appear to have isolated gastroduodenal disease at diagnosis will develop distal disease over time. It is possible that gastroduodenal Crohn's disease is under-recognized given frequent resolution of symptoms with treatment of ileocolonic disease or diagnosis of symptoms as other etiologies such as peptic ulcer disease or gastroesophageal reflux disease.[4]

● SYMPTOMS

Common symptoms in patients with clinically significant gastroduodenal Crohn's disease include postprandial epigastric pain and nausea. Additional symptoms include weight loss, early satiety, and anorexia. More continuous pain associated with nausea and vomiting can indicate the presence of gastric outlet obstruction secondary to gastroduodenal stricture formation. Less commonly, gastroduodenal Crohn's can cause gastrointestinal bleeding, usually in the form of chronic anemia, but also possibly hematemesis or melena. Gastrocolic fistulae can develop, often due to active colonic disease, resulting in feculent vomiting. Pancreatitis can also be a complication of duodenal Crohn's disease. Symptoms of gastroduodenal Crohn's disease can be similar to those from peptic ulcer disease, gastritis, gastroesophageal reflux disease, or side effects from Crohn's disease–related medications (such as 5-aminosalicylic acid [5-ASA], prednisone, 6-mercaptopurine, azathioprine, and metronidazole). In addition, symptoms can be treated by the medications used for ileocolonic disease and therefore may not be recognized.

● DIAGNOSIS

Diagnosis of gastroduodenal Crohn's disease is based on symptoms, radiology, endoscopy, and histologic findings. The antrum and the duodenum are most frequently involved. Criteria for the diagnosis of gastroduodenal Crohn's disease adapted from Nugent and Roy include either (a) histologic presence of non-caseating granulomatous inflammation of the stomach or duodenum with or without concomitant Crohn's disease in the remaining gastrointestinal tract, and without evidence of other systemic granulomatous disorders or (b) documented Crohn's disease elsewhere in the gastrointestinal tract and radiographic and/or endoscopic findings of diffuse inflammatory changes of the stomach or duodenum consistent with Crohn's disease.[5] There is a broad differential diagnosis for the often nonspecific findings of gastroduodenal Crohn's disease that include *Helicobacter pylori*, peptic disease, eosinophilic gastroenteritis, Wegener's granulomatosis, and other causes of granulomas, Zollinger-Ellison syndrome, lymphoma, and adenocarcinoma.

Radiologic Findings

Most of the findings are best seen with double-contrast radiography, although computerized tomography will identify some abnormalities as well. Common radiologic findings in gastroduodenal Crohn's disease are ulcerations, mucosal nodularity ("cobblestoning"), thickened folds, and strictures and narrowing of the antrum and duodenum. A "pseudo-Billroth-I" appearance can occur when the stomach and duodenum are involved.[1,2] The "Ram's horn" sign is a funnel-shaped deformity of the antrum and duodenal bulb.[1,2] Intramural fissures can also be observed in the duodenum, similar to those in the ileum. Poor gastric emptying can be assessed with a gastric emptying study. Gastrocolic fistulae are best diagnosed by a barium enema.

Endoscopic Findings

There are many nonspecific endoscopic findings in gastroduodenal Crohn's disease, which include erythema, friability, granularity, erosions, ulcers, thickened folds, mucosal nodularity ("cobblestoning"), fistulae, strictures, luminal narrowing, and lack of distensibility. Similar to more distal Crohn's disease, "notching of Kerckring's folds" can be seen in the duodenum, and this is a relatively specific sign of Crohn's disease.[1] Ulcerations in gastroduodenal Crohn's disease are often aphthous and linear, unlike the often round ulcers in peptic ulcer disease.[2] Several Japanese studies have suggested that bamboo-joint-like appearance of lesions in the gastric body and cardia may be unique to gastroduodenal Crohn's disease.[6] Multiple biopsies should be obtained in any area of endoscopic abnormality because the majority of the endoscopic findings are nonspecific and can be patchy.

Histologic Findings

Noncaseating granulomas are not always seen in gastroduodenal biopsies in Crohn's disease. In multiple case series, they were found in 5% to 83% of biopsies.[2] The most common findings are nonspecific and focally distributed acute and chronic inflammation.[1] Other pathologic features include mucosal edema, crypt abscesses, erosions, ulcers, and fibrosis. Importantly, *H. pylori* should be evaluated for in a patient with Crohn's disease and upper gastrointestinal symptoms.

⬤ MANAGEMENT OF GASTRODUODENAL CROHN'S DISEASE

Medical Therapy

If *H. pylori* is diagnosed, it should be treated to see if the symptoms and lesions respond. An attempt should also be made to determine whether the patient's symptoms are due to nonsteroidal anti-inflammatory drugs or medical therapy for Crohn's disease. One should attempt to decrease or even temporarily withdraw the primary drug therapy for Crohn's disease to determine if one of these medications is the offending agent.

Most patients with Crohn's disease do not need specific medical management of their gastroduodenal Crohn's disease as treatment of their ileocolonic Crohn's often determines their treatment and improves their upper gastrointestinal symptoms. Treatment of gastroduodenal Crohn's disease should be based on the severity of the patient's associated symptoms. Unfortunately, no controlled prospective data exist on the use of any drug on the primary treatment of gastroduodenal Crohn's disease, and, therefore, most of the recommendations are based on small case series and clinical experience.

A combined approach of acid suppression with a proton-pump inhibitor and anti-inflammatory therapy is often the initial treatment for nonobstructing gastroduodenal Crohn's disease.[2–4] Proton-pump inhibitors alone may improve symptoms, especially if there is a component of irritation by gastric acid, but does not control the underlying inflammatory process. The 5-ASA compounds, although frequently used in ileocolonic disease, are generally not good agents for the treatment of gastroduodenal Crohn's disease as most of the release systems deliver the active compound to more distal bowel. Pentasa (Ferring-Shire Pharmaceuticals, Wayne, Pennsylvania) is partially released in the stomach and proximal small bowel and, hence, could potentially have some benefit, but there have been no trials to support this. Gastroduodenal Crohn's disease has been shown to respond well to corticosteroids.[5,7] There is minimal data for budesonide, the topically active corticosteroid with

minimal systemic absorption, for this indication. There are case reports supporting the use of azathioprine and 6-mercaptopurine for maintenance of remission in gastroduodenal Crohn's disease.[7,8] Infliximab may also have a role in the treatment of refractory gastroduodenal Crohn's disease, similar to that of ileocolonic Crohn's disease.[9,10]

Endoscopic Therapy

For patients with gastroduodenal strictures causing obstruction, endoscopic balloon dilatation can help prevent or delay the need for surgery. Short strictures are the best candidates for balloon dilatation, and progressive dilatation is most successful in achieving symptomatic relief. Symptoms are often recurrent and frequent dilatations are often needed to provide long-term symptomatic relief.[11]

Surgical Therapy

Surgery for gastroduodenal Crohn's disease is usually reserved for patients with clinically significant obstruction. Approximately one-third of patients with gastroduodenal Crohn's disease eventually require surgery. Surgery is less commonly required for persistent pain, bleeding, perforation, or fistulas. There is a chapter by Dr. Jeffrey Milson on this subject, which provides more detailed information.

References

1. van Hogezand RA, Witte AM, Veenendaal RA, Wagtmans MJ, Lamers CB. Proximal Crohn's disease: review of the clinicopathologic features and therapy. *Inflamm Bowel Dis.* 2001;7(4):328–337.

2. Kefalas CH. Gastroduodenal Crohn's disease. *Proc (Bayl Univ Med Cent).* 2003;16(2):147–151.

3. Mottet C, Juillerat P, Pittet V, et al. Upper gastrointestinal Crohn's disease. *Digestion.* 2007;76(2):136–140.

4. Tremaine WJ. Gastroduodenal Crohn's disease: medical management. *Inflamm Bowel Dis.* 2003;9(2):127–128; discussion 131.

5. Nugent FW, Roy MA. Duodenal Crohn's disease: an analysis of 89 cases. *Am J Gastroenterol.* 1989;84(3):249–254.

6. Kuriyama M, Kato J, Morimoto N, Fujimoto T, Okada H, Yamamoto K. Specific gastroduodenoscopic findings in Crohn's disease: Comparison with findings in patients with ulcerative colitis and gastroesophageal reflux disease. *Dig Liver Dis.* 2008;40(6):468–475.

7. Miehsler W, Püspök A, Oberhuber T, Vogelsang H. Impact of different therapeutic regimens on the outcome of patients with Crohn's disease of the upper gastrointestinal tract. *Inflamm Bowel Dis.* 2001;7(2):99–105.

8. Korelitz BI, Adler DJ, Mendelsohn RA, Sacknoff AL. Long-term experience with 6-mercaptopurine in the treatment of Crohn's disease. *Am J Gastroenterol.* 1993;88(8):1198–1205.

9. Knapp AB, Mirsky FJ, Dillon EH, Korelitz BI. Successful infliximab therapy for a duodenal stricture caused by Crohn's disease. *Inflamm Bowel Dis.* 2005;11(12):1123–1125.

10. Odashima M, Otaka M, Jin M, et al. Successful treatment of refractory duodenal Crohn's disease with infliximab. *Dig Dis Sci.* 2007;52(1):31–32.

11. Van Assche G, Vermeire S, Rutgeerts P. Endoscopic therapy of strictures in Crohn's disease. *Inflamm Bowel Dis.* 2007;13(3):356–358; discussion 362.

Crohn's Jejunoileitis | 122

Kim L. Isaacs

Crohn's disease involvement of the jejunum is often underrecognized in patients with Crohn's disease. In childhood, involvement of the jejunum is associated with an aggressive disease course.[1] With recent advances in imaging techniques such as magnetic resonance (MR) and computed tomography (CT) enterography, jejunal disease is diagnosed in up to 20% of pediatric patients and 4% of adult patients with Crohn's disease.[2,3] It is important to distinguish jejunoileitis related to Crohn's disease from other forms of jejunoileitis (e.g., such as jejunoileitis seen with celiac disease). Diagnosis and early treatment of jejunoileitis may decrease the morbidity and need for surgical intervention, as well as identify patients who are likely to have a more aggressive and complicated disease course.

Editor's note (TMB): It is important to note that although jejunoileitis is lumped with upper gastrointestinal involvement as L4 in the Montreal classification, it is best considered separately from esophageal, gastric, and duodenal Crohn's disease.

● DIFFERENTIAL DIAGNOSIS

Jejunal ulcerations may be caused by Crohn's disease, bacterial infections, ischemia, radiation, vasculitis, drugs, neoplasm, and can be seen as a complication of celiac disease. The inflammatory process may be limited to the mucosa or be transmural, leading to jejunal stricture formation.[4] Small intestinal injury from nonsteroidal anti-inflammatory drugs (NSAIDs) is likely the most common of these entities and should be considered in the appropriate clinical setting. More than 50% of patients taking NSAIDs have mucosal damage to the small intestine. This is characterized by ulceration, erosions, erythema, and diaphragm like strictures.[5] Infections such as tuberculosis can affect the small bowel with a granulomatous process that mimics Crohn's disease. Patients with malignancy of the small bowel may present with obstructive symptoms, fever, and abdominal pain similar to patients with Crohn's disease. In patients with celiac disease, complications include loss of response to a gluten-free diet and ulcerative jejunitis that may then progress to an enteropathy-associated T-cell lymphoma.[6] Part of this spectrum may include

the rare entity of nongranulomatous ulcerative jejunoileitis, in which, patients present with fever, pain, steatorrhea and protein-losing enteropathy. Patients tend to be older than those presenting with proximal gastrointestinal Crohn's disease. These patients tend to do poorly with a rapid downhill course.[7]

Editor's note (TMB): There is a separate chapter on Ulcerative Jujunoileitis as well as information on lymphocytic enterocolitis in the chapter on microscopic colitis.

● DIAGNOSIS

Patients with Crohn's disease involving the small intestine typically present with abdominal pain, diarrhea, weight loss and anemia. Nausea and vomiting may be seen as obstructive symptoms in patients with severe stricturing disease. Children with significant small bowel disease exhibit disrupted linear growth and delayed puberty. Proximal small bowel disease is more commonly seen in children. Upper gastrointestinal involvement is more frequent in patients with jejunoileitis, seen in over 50% of patients at presentation.[2] Patients with jejunoileitis tend to have a more aggressive disease course, requiring early intervention with immune-active therapy. Early onset, aggressive, and stricturing disease appears to be associated with specific disease-susceptibility loci such as NOD2/CARD15 variants.[8] Evaluation of NOD2 allelic variation remains a research tool and is not routinely assessed as part of the initial clinical evaluation of patients with Crohn's disease.

In patients presenting with symptoms of Crohn's disease, initial assessment includes physical examination with close attention to growth and development parameters in children, laboratory evaluation (Table 122.1),[9] and assessment of the condition of the small bowel and colon.

Anemia is a common finding in Crohn's disease, and elevated platelets pose as a clue to an ongoing inflammatory process. Nonspecific parameters such as C-reactive protein level or an erythrocyte sedimentation rate, may provide information about the ongoing inflammation. A low albumin helps identify patients with a protein-loosing enteropathy and may help

---

TABLE 122.1 Laboratory Evaluation

- Complete blood count
- Electrolytes
- Albumin
- C-reactive protein or sedimentation rate
- Stool studies—bacterial culture, *C. difficile* toxin, giardia and cryptosporidiosis, if travel history—comprehensive ova and parasite exam
- Other: Fecal calprotectin—noninvasive measure to assess degree of bowel inflammation.[9]

TABLE 122.2 Small Bowel Studies Sensitivity and Specificity

Examination	Sensitivity (%)	Specificity (%)
Capsule endoscopy[11a]	83	53
CT enterography[11a]	67	100
MR enterography[12b]	67	98
Small bowel follow-through[11a]	67	100
Ileocolonoscopy (small bowel visualization ileum only)[11a]	50	100

[a] Adapted from Solem et al.[11] Four-way comparison trial looking at each of these modalities in evaluation of Crohn's disease.
[b] Sensitivity and specificity reported for mucosal ulcerations.

---

identify the sicker patient. Serological tests to identify antibodies that may be present in patients with inflammatory bowel disease (ANCA, ASCA, anti CBIR-, anti-OmpC, anti-I2) are not tremendously useful diagnostically but may help to identify patients who are likely to have a more severe disease course. The degree of immune response to microbial antigens has been shown to be associated with more aggressive disease phenotypes, in children with Crohn's disease.[10] In patients presenting with malabsorption, assessment of fat-soluble vitamin levels and micronutrients will help identify patients who would benefit with supplements.

Initial endoscopic evaluation includes colonoscopy with intubation of the terminal ileum and upper endoscopy or push enteroscopy. Biopsies should be performed. Endoscopic findings in patients with Crohn's disease may include, scattered aphthous ulcerations or deeper more confluent ulcerations. Biopsies may show granulomatous inflammation in up to 50% of patients with Crohn's disease.

There are several modalities that can be used for evaluation of the small bowel (Table 122.2).[11,12] These include the traditional upper gastrointestinal/small bowel follow through (UGI/SBFT) barium radiograph, CT and MR enterography, push enteroscopy, and capsule endoscopy.[11] The UGI/SBFT demonstrates mucosal detail, length of small bowel involvement, fistulous disease, and luminal diameter. UGI/SBFT is best for an advanced luminal disease and cannot show disease activity or extraluminal disease. CT enterography has high sensitivity towards detecting small bowel Crohn's disease, with an advantage of looking at extraluminal disease. Increased exposure to ionizing radiation limits this technique, comparison studies are performed especially when repeated. MR enterography technique have been shown to be comparable to CT, with excellent demonstration of wall thickening, mural enhancement, and vascular engorgement representing inflammation.[13] A recent prospective, blinded, four-way trial demonstrated that the sensitivity of SBFT, CT enterography, MR enterography, and capsule endoscopy are similar towards the diagnosis of small bowel Crohn's disease.[11] In terms of the radiologic evaluation of the small bowel, method of choice is guided by local expertise and the type of information required from the examination. MR enterography should be considered as the procedure of choice, if repeated evaluations are necessary.

Editor's note (TMB): There is a separate chapter in Volume I on imaging techniques and another on endoscopic capsule use.

Endoscopic assessment of the small bowel allows for direct visualization of the mucosa to assist in making the diagnosis. Therapeutic intervention can be considered in tissue samples obtained using push enteroscopy and single and double balloon enteroscopy.[14] Obtaining tissue is important, when trying to exclude a number of disease processes in the differential diagnosis including lymphoma, tuberculosis, ulcerative jejunitis associated with celiac disease, and vasculitis. Capsule endoscopy allows identification of mucosal ulceration in patients with early Crohn's disease, where the degree of damage is inadequate to be evident in radiologic studies. The sensitivity of capsule endoscopy in the patient (high-risk) population, with other clinical and laboratory features suggestive of Crohn's disease was high. In one single center study, a group of patients with suspected Crohn's disease with abnormal capsule endoscopy (greater than three ulcers) were followed for 12 months looking for other supporting criteria to make a new diagnosis of Crohn's disease.[15] In this study, the sensitivity of capsule endoscopy for the diagnosis of Crohn's disease was 77% and the specificity was 89%. There was a high-negative predictive value for the negative examinations. In the setting of suspected Crohn's disease, the capsule retention rate was reported to be 1.5%.[16] This may be more of a concern in the evaluation of patients with jejunoileitis, due to the increased incidence of stricturing disease in this population. In patients with obstructive symptoms, the use of the patency capsule prior to the standard capsule may detect the patients who are likely to develop capsule retention. Single and double balloon enteroscopy allows for deep intubation of the small bowel by inflating and deflating the balloon/s that allows the small bowel to be "sleeved" over the endoscope.[14] These techniques may allow direct visualization of the involved tissue with targeted biopsy of the abnormalities. In the case of patients with short-segment strictures of the jejunum, balloon dilation with or without steroid injection into the stricture may lead to improved symptoms. There may be an increased risk of perforation of the small bowel with deep endoscopic techniques in patients with Crohn's disease, due to tension on the diseased bowel during the procedure.

Editor's note (TMB): There is a chapter on double balloon enteroscopy and dilatation.

If diagnosis is still unclear, surgical sampling or resection of the diseased segment may be required to exclude infection or lymphoma.

TREATMENT

Most studies looking at children presenting with jejunoileal involvement suggest a more aggressive disease course. Children with jejunoileitis have lower weight and height scores than patients without jejunal involvement.[1] There is a greater degree of fistulization, stricture formation, and need for surgery than the nonjejunoileal presentation of Crohn's disease.[1] These

findings suggest that early and an aggressive therapy should be strongly considered in this population (Table 122.3).[17]

Standard therapy over many years has involved an escalation of milder therapies including 5-amino salicylates to more aggressive therapies such as the antimetabolites; 6-mercaptopurine and azathioprine or antitumor necrosis factor (anti-TNF) therapy (infliximab, adalimumab, and certolizumab), that modulate the immune system. The difficulty has been in identifying the patient population that has aggressive disease behavior, where the benefits of therapy outweigh the risk of early immune modulation. An aggressive therapy is warranted in a patient population with jejunoileitis. Markowitz and colleagues[18] demonstrated that early addition of 6-mercaptopurine to an induction regimen of corticosteroids, significantly decreased the need for long-term steroids and thus improving the rates of remission maintenance. In an observational study of children with moderate to severe Crohn's disease, those treated with immunomodulators, within the first 3 months of diagnosis had decreased steroid usage and a decreased number of hospitalizations.[19] There is clinical trial evidence (SONIC) that in patient's who are immunomodulator naïve, early combination therapy with azathioprine and infliximab are more likely to achieve a steroid-free remission than with infliximab or azathioprine monotherapy with 26-week remission rates of 56.8%, 44.4%, and 30/6%, respectively.[20] The patient presenting with jejunoileitis may be a candidate for this approach. The short- and long-term risks of infection and malignancy need to be factored in to the therapeutic decisions. In young males, the reports of an increased incidence of hepatosplenic T-cell lymphoma in patients on combination therapy with azathioprine/6-MP and anti-TNF therapy[21] may favor monotherapy with immune-active medications rather than the combination therapy described in the SONIC trial.

Nutritional therapy is of clear benefit in patients with severe malabsorption associated with significant small bowel disease or short bowel syndrome. Nutritional therapy in these patients can improve weight and correct the significant nutrient deficiencies

TABLE 122.3 Medical Therapy of Crohn's Jejunoileitis[a]

5-Aminosalicylates: These have no role in the treatment of Crohn's jejunoileitis—most of the available agents are released in the distal ileum and colon bypassing the proximal small bowel. Pentasa (Shire Pharmaceuticals) is available for release in the small bowel but has no clinical trial data to show efficacy in proximal small bowel Crohn's disease. Based on meta-analyses, looking at the use of these agents in Crohn's disease, the effect would be mild at best and is not appropriate for aggressive proximal disease.

Steroids/immunomodulators: Systemic corticosteroids are useful in the induction of remission of extensive jejunoileal Crohn's disease. This includes prednisone and parenteral steroids. Ileal release budesonide (Entocort) is not likely to be of benefit due to its release characteristics in the distal small bowel. Once steroids are initiated—an immunomodulator such as 6-mercaptopurine or azathioprine should be initiated at the same time. If the enzyme that metabolizes this class of drugs, thiopurine methyltransferase is normal full weight based dosing of 6-mercaptopurine (1–1.5 mg/kg) or azathioprine (2–2.5 mg/kg) can be initiated early in the course of treatment.

Antitumor necrosis factor (anti-TNF) agents: This class of drugs can be considered in the induction of remission in patients with jejunoileal Crohn's disease. The aggressiveness of this disease phenotype supports the use of aggressive immune-active therapy. Induction of remission with dual therapy (anti-TNF plus immunomodulator) may lead to the highest remission rates but overall risk of therapy should be evaluated in context of the overall clinical presentation. Other treatment strategies include, induction of remission with dual therapy followed by withdrawal of the one the agents (anti-TNF or immunomodulator) after a period of time to allow for maintenance therapy with a single agent or induction of remission and maintenance with the anti-TNF agent alone. How to effectively use this class of drugs for induction of remission and long-term therapy is currently in evolution.

[a]From Lichtenstein et al.[17]

TABLE 122.4 Nutritional Supplements to Consider[a]

Supplement	Dose
Calcium carbonate	1000–1500 mg/day
Vitamin D (cholecalciferol)	800 IU/day
Magnesium	300 mg/day
Folic acid	800 µg/day
Vitamin B12 (based on levels)	1 mg/day Sublingually Monthly parenteral B12 if needed
Docosahexaenoic acid and eicosapentaenoic acid	1 g/day Total

[a]From Moorthy et al.[22]
Look for fat-soluble vitamin deficiency—A, D, K, and E and replace as needed.
Look for zinc deficiency and replace as needed.

that are sometimes seen (Table 122.4). There are studies that suggest that nutritional therapy has a role in the primary treatment of small bowel disease in up to 50% of patients involved in the trial.[2] Both the enteral and the polymeric formulations have benefited patients but unfortunately, they do not sustain remission once the nutritional therapy is discontinued. A 60% to 70% relapse rate was evident after discontinuation of enteral feedings.[2] Enteral nutritional therapy has been used more extensively in children than in adults, likely in part due to patient acceptance. This form of therapy requires the nightly placement of a nasogastric feeding tube for administration of the feeds. Total parenteral nutrition has not been shown to be superior to enteral therapy, in terms of, treating small bowel Crohn's disease; however, it may be superior in correcting nutritional deficits in patients with severe short bowel syndrome. Patient nutritional counseling may be beneficial in identifying foods that patients can tolerate, that will also provide enough nutrients to sustain weight. Vitamin levels should be checked in patients with malabsorption and replaced appropriately.[22]

Editor's note (TMB): There is a separate chapter on enteral nutrition in pediatric patients.

In patients who require surgical intervention, stricturoplasty instead of resection should be considered in the appropriate patients. Strictures are common in patients with jejunoileal disease and if the amount of small bowel removed can be limited by treating strictures with stricturoplasty, the development of short bowel syndrome may be delayed or avoided in these patients. Stricturoplasty can be done successfully and safely in patients with jejunoileitis.[23] Referral should be made to a surgeon who is experienced in this technique.

● SUMMARY

Jejunoileal Crohn's disease most commonly presents in children, and has an aggressive disease course. Early diagnosis and treatment are important. In a patient presenting with Crohn's disease elsewhere, or signs and symptoms of upper small bowel

Crohn's disease evaluation of the proximal small bowel should be performed. CT and MR enterography, capsule endoscopy, and deep enteroscopy may increase diagnostic yield. Other causes of jejunal disease should be considered including NSAID damage and small bowel lymphoma. Once the diagnosis of Crohn's jejunoileal disease is made immune-active, therapy should be initiated early in the disease course.

References

1. Attard TM, Horton KM, DeVito K, et al. Pediatric jejunoileitis: a severe Crohn's disease phenotype that requires intensive nutritional management. *Inflamm Bowel Dis.* 2004;10(4):357–360.

2. Cuffari C, Dubinsky M, Darbari A, Sena L, Baldassano R. Crohn's jejunoileitis: the pediatrician's perspective on diagnosis and management. *Inflamm Bowel Dis.* 2005;11(7):696–704.

3. Darbari A, Sena L, Argani P, Oliva-Hemker JM, Thompson R, Cuffari C. Gadolinium-enhanced magnetic resonance imaging: a useful radiological tool in diagnosing pediatric IBD. *Inflamm Bowel Dis.* 2004;10(2):67–72.

4. LePane CA, Barkin JS, Parra J, Simon T. Ulcerative jejunoileitis: a complication of celiac sprue simulating Crohn's disease diagnosed with capsule endoscopy (PillCam). *Dig Dis Sci.* 2007;52(3):698–701.

5. Higuchi K, Umegaki E, Watanabe T, et al. Present status and strategy of NSAIDs-induced small bowel injury. *J Gastroenterol.* 2009;44(9):879–888.

6. Biagi F, Lorenzini P, Corazza GR. Literature review on the clinical relationship between ulcerative jejunoileitis, coeliac disease, and enteropathy-associated T-cell. *Scand J Gastroenterol.* 2000;35(8):785–790.

7. Freeman M, Cho SR. Non-granulomatous ulcerative jejunoileitis. *Am J Gastroenterol.* 1984;79(6):446–449.

8. Ahmad T, Armuzzi A, Bunce M, et al. The molecular classification of the clinical manifestations of Crohn's disease. *Gastroenterology.* 2002;122(4):854–866.

9. Canani R, Terrin G, Rapacciuolo L, et al., Faecal calprotectin as reliable non-invasive marker to assess the severity of mucosal inflammation in children with inflammatory bowel disease. *Dig Liver Dis.* 2008;40:547–553.

10. Dubinsky M, Lin Y, Dutridge D, et al. Serum immune responses predict rapid disease progression among children with Crohn's disease: immune responses predict disease progression. *Am J Gastroenterol.* 2006;101:360–367.

11. Solem C, Loftus E, Fletcher J, et al. Small-bowel imaging in Crohn's disease: a prospective, blinded, 4-way comparison trial. *Gastrointest Endosc.* 2008;68: 255–266.

12. Masselli G, Casciani E, Polettini E, Gualdi G. Comparison of MR enteroclysis with MR enterography and conventional enteroclysis in patients with Crohn's disease. *Eur Radiol.* 2008;18(3):438–447.

13. Ippolito D, Invernizzi F, Galimberti S, Panelli M, Sironi S. MR enterography with polyethylene glycol as oral contrast medium in the follow-up of patients with Crohn disease: comparison with CT enterography. *Abdom Imaging.* 2010;35(5):563–570.

14. Bourreille A, Ignjatovic A, Aabakken L, et al. Role of small-bowel endoscopy in the management of patients with inflammatory bowel disease: an international OMED-ECCO consensus. *Endoscopy.* 2009;41(7):618–637.

15. Tukey M, Pleskow D, Legnani P, et al. The utility of capsule endoscopy in patients with suspected Crohn's disease. *Am J Gastroenterol.* 2009;104:2734–2739.

16. Lewis BS. Expanding role of capsule endoscopy in inflammatory bowel disease. *World J Gastroenterol.* 2008;14(26):4137–4141.

17. Lichtenstein G, Hanauer S, Sandborn W. Management of Crohn's disease in adults. *Am J Gastroenterol.* 2009;104:465–483.

18. Markowitz J, Grancher K, Kohn N, Lesser M, Daum F. A multicenter trial of 6-mercaptopurine and prednisone in children with newly diagnosed Crohn's disease. *Gastroenterology.* 2000;119(4):895–902.

19. Punati J, Markowitz J, Lerer T, et al.; Pediatric IBD Collaborative Research Group. Effect of early immunomodulator use in moderate to severe pediatric Crohn disease. *Inflamm Bowel Dis.* 2008;14(7):949–954.

20. Sandborn W, Rutgeerts P, Reinisch W, et al. SONIC: a randomized, double-blind, controlled trial comparing infliximab and infliximab plus azathioprine to zathioprine in patients with Crohns's disease naive to immunomodulators and biologic therapy. *Inflamm Bowel Dis.* 2008;14(3):S1.

21. Mackey A, Green L, Leptak C, Avigan M. Hepatosplenic T-cell lymphoma associated with infliximab use in young patients treated for inflammatory bowel disease: update. *J Pediatr Gastroenterol Nutr.* 2009;48:386–388.

22. Moorthy D, Cappellano KL, Rosenberg IH. Nutrition and Crohn's disease: an update of print and Web-based guidance. *Nutr Rev.* 2008;66(7):387–397.

23. Fazio VW, Galandiuk S. Strictureplasty in diffuse Crohn's jejunoileitis. *Dis Colon Rectum.* 1985;28(7):512–518.

Management of Internal and External Fistulas in Crohn's Disease | 123

Richard P. MacDermott, Miguel Regueiro, and
William J. Tremaine

INTRODUCTION

Thirty-five percent to forty percent of patients with Crohn's disease will develop fistulas.[1,2] These fistulas are due to the tracking of transmural inflammation from one loop of bowel to another epithelial-lined organ or skin. Fistulas originate from an area of active Crohn's disease involving the stomach, duodenum, small bowel, colon, rectum, or anus.[3-7]

Fistulas in Crohn's disease are classified as internal or external.[3-7] Internal fistulas extend from one loop of diseased bowel and terminate in an adjacent loop of bowel or organ. The most common types of internal fistulas include enteroenteric, enterovesical, and rectovaginal fistulas.[3-7] External fistulas extend from diseased small intestine, colon, rectum, or anus and terminate on the skin. The most common types of external fistulas include enterocutaneous, perianal, or parastomal fistulas.[3-7]

In this chapter, we will discuss current management strategies for internal and external fistulas in Crohn's disease. We will not discuss perianal fistulas in this chapter, because the management of perianal fistulas is covered in separate chapters in this book. We will also attempt to avoid reiterating what has been previously published in comprehensive and well-written review articles.[3-7] Case studies will be used to illustrate common presentations and management approaches to internal and external fistulas.

OVERALL APPROACH TO FISTULIZING CROHN'S DISEASE

The diagnoses and management of fistulas in Crohn's disease requires close cooperation among gastroenterology, radiology, and surgery. The treatment of fistulas is directed at the active Crohn's disease, the fistula tracks, and complications such as abscesses and strictures. First, it is important to determine the extent and severity of active Crohn's disease involving the small bowel, colon, rectum, and the anus, using endoscopic and radiologic imaging techniques. Second, the fistula tracks need to be characterized with regard to the directions that the fistulas head and the terminal points of exit of the fistulas, using standard endoscopic and radiologic imaging techniques plus fistulography. Third, it is critical to make certain that possible abscesses have been identified using computed tomography (CT) and magnetic resonance imaging (MRI). Fourth, abscesses need to be drained prior to medical therapy. Fifth, fistulas proximal to intestinal strictures that cause partial obstruction require surgery. Sixth, fistulas that cause few or low-grade symptoms and that are not associated with abscesses or strictures can be treated with medical therapy.

The choice of the most appropriate treatment for Crohn's disease fistulas depends on the type of fistula, the extent and severity of concomitant inflammation, and the presence of complications such as an abscess or stricture.[3-7] The standard medical therapy of fistulas in Crohn's disease includes antibiotics, such as ciprofloxacin and metronidazole; immunomodulators, such as 6-mercaptopurine (6-MP) and azathioprine; and biologics, such as infliximab or adalimumab.[3-13] Surgery is required for fistulas that are refractory to medical therapy, and for fistulas associated with a complication, such as an abscess and/or a stricture.[14-20]

ENTEROENTERIC FISULAS

Case No. 1

This case presents a 26-year-old female, with a 10-year history of severe small bowel Crohn's disease, referred for treatment with biologic therapy due to severe chronic abdominal pain, intermittent nausea and vomiting, weight loss, and very severe diarrhea. On CT enterography, the patient had multiple loops of small bowel involved with Crohn's disease plus multiple strictures. Due to the complex, obstructing Crohn's disease in the small bowel, surgery was elected as the initial approach. At the time of surgery, the severely involved, multiple loops of small bowel were resected. In addition, a previously unrecognized fistula from the ileum to the sigmoid colon was also resected. The patient was then treated with adalimumab for active Crohn's disease that remained in the jejunum and which had not been resected.

Comment on Case No. 1

This case illustrates a common problem encountered with enteroenteric fistulas: their presence is often not apparent until the time of surgery. In this case, the patient's severe symptoms had been attributed to the extensive small bowel Crohn's disease. In actuality, her severe diarrhea was due to bypassing most of the small bowel and colon by the ileum to sigmoid fistula. This is a common scenario in which the fistula emanates from a portion of intestine just proximal to a stricture. As such, rather than presenting with obstructive symptoms due to the stricture, these patients often present with high output diarrhea from the fistula. Therefore, a high index of suspicion must be maintained for Crohn's disease patients with symptoms that may be due to enteroenteric fistulas.

Discussion of Case No. 1

Enteroenteric fistulas are common in Crohn's disease and include any connection or track between two loops of intestine.[3–7] Enteroenteric fistulas typically form due to active Crohn's disease involving one loop of bowel that penetrates into adjacent healthy intestine or colon.[3–7] The most common Crohn's disease enteroenteric fistulas are ileoileal and ileocecal fistulas, which are often asymptomatic and usually are unexpectedly detected on imaging studies of the intestine.[3–7] Ileoileal or ileocecal fistulas that do not bypass long segments of intestine usually do not cause major symptoms, unless complicated by an abscess, and usually do not require surgery.[3–7]

In contrast, duodenocolic and ileosigmoid fistulas are less common, but are often very dramatic due to the severe presenting symptoms.[3–7] Duodenocolic and ileosigmoid fistulas can cause excessive diarrhea and severe malabsorption for two reasons: large portions of the small bowel and/or colon are bypassed[3–7] and the abnormal connection with the colon fosters small intestinal bacterial overgrowth.

The presence of enteroenteric fistulas raises two major concerns: firstly, the possibility that an abscess is present that is part of the process and secondly, the possibility that a Crohn's disease stricture is present that may have triggered the development of the fistulas. Thus, careful abdominal imaging and endoscopic studies are needed to look for the presence of abscesses and strictures.

Periodic broad-spectrum antibiotics may relieve symptoms that are due to small intestinal bacterial overgrowth. Surgery is indicated for fistulas with associated abscesses or strictures.[14] However, every attempt should be made to resolve abscesses prior to surgery. To reduce the chance that the patient might require a diverting ostomy, abscesses larger or equal to 2 cm in diameter may be drained with a percutaneous catheter by an interventional radiologist. Smaller abscesses can be treated with broad-spectrum antibiotics. Serial imaging at 2-week intervals can be performed to confirm that the abscess is resolved. At the time of surgery, the diseased loop of intestine from which the fistula emanates is resected, the fistula is resected (taken down), and the loop of bowel into which the fistula terminates is repaired or resected.[14] In addition, the strictured segment of intestine can be resected and any residual abscess can be drained.[14]

Medical therapy for enteroenteric fistulas needs to be directed at both the active Crohn's disease and the fistulas. Medical therapies include immunomodulators such as 6-MP or azathioprine and/or biologics such as infliximab or adalimumab.[3–13] Due to associated complications of strictures or abscesses, it has been observed that internal fistulas respond less well to biologics than perianal fistulas and often require resective surgery.[12]

● ENTEROVESICAL FISTULAS

Case No. 2

This case presents a 21-year-old male with Crohn's disease of the terminal ileum and sigmoid colon for 2 years, who had been previously treated (by his insistence), with growth hormone, testosterone, and intermittent steroids. The patient was referred due to a history of two recent urinary tract infections and passing air during urination. CT scan demonstrated air in the bladder plus adjacent sigmoid colonic wall thickening. The patient was treated with antibiotics for the urinary tract infections and he "felt better." He did not want to see a surgeon, because his father had undergone multiple surgeries for Crohn's disease and the patient did not want to have surgery for his Crohn's disease. The patient refused treatment with immunomodulators or biologics due to fear of immunosuppression.

Comments on Case No. 2

This case demonstrates the common experience that enterovesical fistulas can present without severe symptoms: merely recurrent urinary tract infections and the feeling of passing air in the urine. It is important to obtain a pelvic CT or MRI scan to demonstrate evidence of a colovesical or enterovesical fistula. Sometimes imaging will not define an enterovesical fistula and a high level of suspicion should remain if patients have persistent pneumaturia or urinary tract infections. In these cases repeat imaging may detect a fistula that was previously not identified. Although surgical evaluation may be recommended, patients often wish to defer definitive treatment unless absolutely necessary, because of a wish to protect their bladder.

Discussion of Case No. 2

The reported incidence of enterovesical fistulas in Crohn's disease ranges from 2% to 8%.[3–7] Enterovesical fistulas are the result of transmural inflammation that tracks to the bladder, usually originating from a diseased loop of ileum or sigmoid colon. The presence of enterovesical fistulas also raises the concern of the potential presence of a pelvic abscess.[3–7] Patients who develop enterovesical fistulas often have symptoms of urinary frequency, dysuria, pneumaturia, and urinary tract infections.

Fecaluria and/or hematuria provide evidence of complicated fistulas due to Crohn's disease.[3–7] In one series of patients with enterovesical fistulas, cystoscopy was more sensitive than CT scan at identifying the fistulas (74% vs. 52%).[19]

Medical therapy for enterovesical fistulas includes antibiotics to treat urinary tract infections, immunomodulators, and biologics. Surgery is recommended if the Crohn's disease is refractory to medications or a complication such as recurrent urosepsis or an abscess develops.[15] However, the timing of surgery for enterovesical fistulas is a complex decision involving the preferences of the patient as well as the gastroenterologist and surgeon.[15] The surgical management of an enterovesical fistula involves dissection of the bladder away from the diseased bowel, resection of the inflamed bowel, and decompression of the bladder with a Foley catheter to let the defect from the fistula close or, in some cases, oversewing of the bladder defect caused by the fistula.[15]

RECTOVAGINAL FISTULAS

Case No. 3

This case presents a 23-year-old female with severe Crohn's disease of the colon and small bowel for 6 years. The patient presented with severe, chronic abdominal pain and severe diarrhea. She also had intermittent feces per vagina and severe dyspareunia. The patient had an excellent response to induction and maintenance therapy with infliximab with resolution of all of her symptoms. One year later, she developed severe nausea and vomiting that was initially thought to be due to an exacerbation of her Crohn's disease, secondary to loss of response to infliximab. Blood work revealed that the patient was unexpectedly pregnant and 7 months later she delivered by C-section.

Comments on Case No. 3

This case highlights the very troublesome symptoms that commonly occur with rectovaginal fistulas, including passage of feces through the vagina and dyspareunia. This patient fortunately responded very well to infliximab and therefore surgery was not needed.

Discussion of Case No. 3

Rectovaginal fistulas have been estimated to occur in approximately 10% of women with anal and/or rectal Crohn's disease.[3–7] Rectovaginal fistulas usually emanate from a deep ulcer due to Crohn's disease in the anterior anus or in the rectum. Common symptoms include passing air alone or passing air in combination with mucopurulent or fecal drainage from the vagina. Additional common symptoms include dyspareunia, perineal pain, and recurrent yeast infections.[3–7] Endoscopic evaluation of both the anus and rectum followed by pelvic MRI or pelvic CT scan plus examination under anesthesia by a surgeon is needed to determine the anatomic tracks of the fistulas. Even with these techniques, small fistulas may not be identifiable.

In general, patients with mild to moderate symptoms can be treated with medical therapy.[3–13] Improvement has been observed in some patients with rectovaginal fistulas, following treatment with 6-MP, azathioprine, infliximab,

and adalimumab.[3–13] Complete closure of rectovaginal fistula with anti-tumor necrosis factor agents can occur, but, more commonly, patients notice a decrease in symptoms rather than complete resolution. Most patients will consider occasional passage of vaginal air a significant and acceptable outcome of medical therapy. However, patients with severe symptoms may require surgery, either with an attempt at closure of the fistula or proctectomy and ostomy placement.[16,17] Unfortunately, surgical repair of fistulas with mucosal advancement flaps are successful in no more than 50% of patients.[20] No matter what treatment approaches are used, recurrence rates are very high. Following surgical repair, the active Crohn's disease from which the rectovaginal fistulas originate usually requires medical therapy with immunomodulator and/or biologic therapy to help prevent recurrence of the rectovaginal fistulas.

ENTEROCUTANEOUS FISTULAS

Case No. 4

The case presents a 48-year-old male with a history of four resections for severe recurrent gastroduodenal and small bowel Crohn's disease. He presented with severe dehydration, malnutrition, and weight loss due to five active enterocutaneous fistulas, which originated from recurrent gastroduodenal and jejunal Crohn's disease. Infliximab induction and maintenance therapy for 1 year resulted in one of the fistulas closing, three fistulas exhibiting significantly decreased drainage, and one fistula with no response. Most importantly, the patient no longer had dehydration and was able to maintain a normal nutritional status. The patient was particularly pleased because prior to infliximab therapy, after drinking coffee, his abdominal wall barrier dressings would be soaked within 15 minutes, whereas after infliximab therapy the dressings did not need to be changed for 2 to 3 hours.

Comments on Case No. 4

One aspect of enterocutaneous fistulas that this case demonstrates is that not all fistulas present in the same patient will have the same response to medical therapy. Many patients with enterocutaneous fistulas may also have fistulas elsewhere, such as perianal fistulas. Successful treatment of enterocutaneous fistulas does not necessarily mean the complete closure of all fistulas. The medically important goal of successful therapy is improvement of severe clinical problems such as malnutrition, dehydration, and recurrent skin infections. The goal that is important to the patient is restoration of an acceptable quality of life, which may be achieved without complete closure of all the enterocutaneous fistulas, as was the case with this patient.

Discussion of Case No. 4

Enterocutaneous fistulas rarely develop spontaneously and are most commonly due to active Crohn's disease.[3–7] Early postoperative enterocutaneous fistulas (within 7–14 days of surgery) are usually due to an anastomotic leak or breakdown, and require surgical repair.[18] In contrast, late enterocutaneous fistulas (3 or more months following surgery) usually emanate from recurrent Crohn's disease at the anastomotic site with tracking to the previous incision site.[18] Enterocutaneous fistulas may be complicated by an abscess or the high output of small intestinal contents, which can lead to dehydration, breakdown of skin, and electrolyte imbalance. Enterocutaneous fistulas that have a low output and which are not complicated by abscess formation are appropriate for treatment with immunomodulator and/or biologic therapy.[3–13] However, as is the case with all internal fistulas, enterocutaneous fistulas may respond less well to immunomodulators and/or biologics than perianal fistulas.[12]

● PARASTOMAL FISTULAS

Case No. 5

The case presents a 37-year-old female with a history of a colectomy for ulcerative colitis, a failed J-pouch due to Crohn's disease, and the placement of a Koch pouch. The patient presented due to intermittent severe peristomal pain and a fistula near the Koch pouch nipple valve, which intermittently (1–2 weeks per month) demonstrated drainage of large amounts of purulent material. When drainage from the fistula site occurred, the severe pain near the pouch nipple valve decreased, and then the pain gradually increased over the following 2 to 3 weeks. Abdominal CT scan and fistulogram demonstrated an intraabdominal abscess, between the skin and the ileum, immediately proximal to the Koch pouch. The patient underwent surgery with resection of recurrent Crohn's disease and a stricture in the neoterminal ileum immediately proximal to the Koch pouch, reconstruction of the Koch pouch, and placement of the new Koch pouch on the opposite side of the abdomen. The patient was then begun on maintenance therapy with adalimumab.

Comments on Case No. 5

This case demonstrates that, very often, an abscess may be the source of fistulas and/or may develop secondary to a fistula. Therefore, evaluation of fistulas requires careful imaging with both CT scans and fistulography. Immunomodulators and biologics should not be given in the presence of an abscess. Abscesses may be drained percutaneously by an interventional radiologist. A well-demarcated and walled-off abscess can be managed surgically, as in this case. If there is no abscess present and there is active Crohn's disease in the neoterminal ileum or stoma, parastomal fistulas may respond to immunomodulator and/or biologic therapy.

Discussion of Case No. 5

Patients with Crohn's disease who undergo a proctocolectomy with an ileostomy may develop parastomal fistulas years after the initial surgery.[3–7] Early postoperative parastomal fistulas, that is, "surgical" fistulas that present within 3 to 7 days of surgery are usually due to technical problems, with resultant injury to the neoterminal ileum, and therefore require immediate reoperation.[3–7] Most parastomal fistulas occur late (3 or more months following surgery) and usually are the consequence of recurrent Crohn's disease at the stoma or neoterminal ileum.[3–7] Although there are no prospective studies evaluating medical therapy for parastomal fistulas, fistulas that arise in combination with active intestinal Crohn's disease should be treated

with immunomodulators and/or biologic therapy. Parastomal fistulas that are complicated by an abscess or stricture and/or that are refractory to immunomodulator and biologic therapy require surgery. Surgery for noninfected parastomal fistulas usually involves a simple revision of the stoma, whereas surgery for multiple fistulas with or without an abscess usually requires resection of the neoterminal ileum and relocation of the stoma.

● CONCLUSION

Internal and external Crohn's disease fistulas present a challenge to the clinician and also to the patient. A multidisciplinary approach that includes the radiologist, surgeon, and gastroenterologist is important. Fortunately, many internal and external fistulas are either asymptomatic or cause only low-grade symptoms and therefore do not require aggressive medical or surgical therapy, but rather may be managed with antibiotics and antidiarrheal medications.[3–7] The use of immunomodulators and biologics has improved our treatment of internal and external fistulas for many patients with Crohn's disease. However, unlike the excellent response of perianal fistulas to medical therapy, internal fistulas are less responsive to immunomodulators and/or biologics and often require surgery, especially if such complications as an abscess or stricture are also present.[14–20]

References

1. Schwartz DA, Loftus EV Jr, Tremaine WJ, et al. The natural history of fistulizing Crohn's disease in Olmsted County, Minnesota. *Gastroenterology.* 2002;122(4):875–880.

2. Cosnes J, Cattan S, Blain A, et al. Long-term evolution of disease behavior of Crohn's disease. *Inflamm Bowel Dis.* 2002;8(4):244–250.

3. Lichtenstein GR. Treatment of fistulizing Crohn's disease. *Gastroenterology.* 2000;119(4):1132–1147.

4. Levy C, Tremaine WJ. Management of internal fistulas in Crohn's disease. *Inflamm Bowel Dis.* 2002;8(2):106–111.

5. Present DH. Crohn's fistula: current concepts in management. *Gastroenterology.* 2003;124(6):1629–1635.

6. Judge TA, Lichtenstein GR. Treatment of fistulizing Crohn's disease. *Gastroenterol Clin North Am.* 2004;33(2):421–454, xi.

7. Osterman MT, Lichtenstein GR. Infliximab in fistulizing Crohn's disease. *Gastroenterol Clin North Am.* 2006;35(4):795–820.

8. Present DH, Rutgeerts P, Targan S, et al. Infliximab for the treatment of fistulas in patients with Crohn's disease. *N Engl J Med.* 1999;340(18):1398–1405.

9. Sands BE, Anderson FH, Bernstein CN, et al. Infliximab maintenance therapy for fistulizing Crohn's disease. *N Engl J Med.* 2004;350(9):876–885.

10. Lichtenstein GR, Yan S, Bala M, Blank M, Sands BE. Infliximab maintenance treatment reduces hospitalizations, surgeries, and procedures in fistulizing Crohn's disease. *Gastroenterology.* 2005;128(4):862–869.

11. Colombel JF, Schwartz DA, Sandborn WJ, et al. Adalimumab for the treatment of fistulas in patients with Crohn's disease. *Gut.* 2009;58(7):940–948.

12. Ricart E, Panaccione R, Loftus EV, Tremaine WJ, Sandborn WJ. Infliximab for Crohn's disease in clinical practice at the Mayo Clinic: the first 100 patients. *Am J Gastroenterol.* 2001;96(3):722–729.

13. Sands BE, Blank MA, Patel K, van Deventer SJ; ACCENT II Study. Long-term treatment of rectovaginal fistulas in Crohn's disease: response to infliximab in the ACCENT II Study. *Clin Gastroenterol Hepatol.* 2004;2(10):912–920.

14. Melton GB, Stocchi L, Wick EC, Appau KA, Fazio VW. Contemporary surgical management for ileosigmoid fistulas in Crohn's disease. *J Gastrointest Surg.* 2009;13(5):839–845.

15. Sonnenberg A, Gavin MW. Timing of surgery for enterovesical fistula in Crohn's disease: decision analysis using a time-dependent compartment model. *Inflamm Bowel Dis.* 2000;6(4):280–285.

16. Andreani SM, Dang HH, Grondona P, Khan AZ, Edwards DP. Rectovaginal fistula in Crohn's disease. *Dis Colon Rectum.* 2007;50(12):2215–2222.

17. Löffler T, Welsch T, Mühl S, Hinz U, Schmidt J, Kienle P. Long-term success rate after surgical treatment of anorectal and rectovaginal fistulas in Crohn's disease. *Int J Colorectal Dis.* 2009;24(5):521–526.

18. Poritz LS, Gagliano GA, McLeod RS, MacRae H, Cohen Z. Surgical management of entero and colocutaneous fistulae in Crohn's disease: 17 year's experience. *Int J Colorectal Dis.* 2004;19(5):481–485; discussion 486.

19. Solem CA, Loftus EV Jr, Tremaine WJ, Pemberton JH, Wolff BG, Sandborn WJ. Fistulas to the urinary system in Crohn's disease: clinical features and outcomes. *Am J Gastroenterol.* 2002;97(9):2300–2305.

20. Hull TL, Fazio VW. Surgical approaches to low anovaginal fistula in Crohn's disease. *Am J Surg.* 1997;173(2):95–98.

Colonoscopic Screening and Surveillance in Chronic Crohn's Colitis

124

Peter H. Rubin

It has long been standard practice that patients with ulcerative colitis (UC) of more than 8 years' duration should undergo colonoscopy every year or so, with circumferential mucosal biopsies taken every 10 cm as well as from strictures and any other suspicious areas. More recently, the same protocol has been recommended for patients with chronic Crohn's disease (CD) of the colon.

That patients with chronic Crohn's colitis had a heightened risk of dysplasia and cancer had been suggested by a number of case reports and limited retrospective studies. Sachar had prophesized as early as 1983 that "when cases of ulcerative and Crohn's colitis of similar anatomical extent are followed for similar durations of time, the two diseases may ultimately prove to have similar increases in risk for colorectal cancer."

Several studies from Europe, Scandinavia, and Australia, mostly population based, did not find an increase in cancer in CD patients. These studies were limited, however, in not focusing on the subpopulation at greatest risk, namely, those with chronic, anatomically extensive colitis.

Weedon and colleagues reported that colorectal cancer was more likely in Crohn's colitis than in the general population, with standardized incidence ratio of 26.6. Similarly Gillen et al. comparing UC and CD found that the cumulative incidence of colorectal cancer was elevated similarly in extensive, chronic UC and CD.

It was the work of Friedman and colleagues that established in prospective longitudinal studies on large cohorts of Crohn's patients that the risk of finding dysplasia or cancer in chronic CD colitis is comparable to that in chronic UC. Friedman et al.'s (1991) study of an 18-year screening and surveillance colonoscopy experience comprised 663 colonoscopies in 259 patients with chronic Crohn's colitis involving at least one third of the colon. Overall some degree of dysplasia or cancer was found in 16% of this cohort. By life-table analysis it was determined that the probability of detecting dysplasia or cancer after a negative screening colonoscopy was 22% by the fourth surveillance examination, comparable to that in chronic UC. Risk factors for

dysplasia or cancer included age greater than 45 and change in symptomatology as the indication for colonoscopy.

Friedman et al. have reexamined these data 7 years later, with these patients now having had 1424 colonoscopic examinations. The cumulative risk of detecting a first finding of dysplasia or cancer after a negative screening colonoscopy is 25% by the tenth surveillance examination, thus corroborating her earlier findings.

Interestingly, Friedman et al.'s data did not identify duration of disease per se as a risk factor. But chronicity in CD may be more difficult to determine than is possible with UC. The first symptoms of CD are often subtle and may not even be primarily gastrointestinal. This is true especially when onset is in childhood and in the elderly. In these patients the delay between symptom onset and diagnosis may be considerable, leading to an underestimation of duration of disease. Furthermore it may be that parameters other than duration and anatomic extent may influence incidence of dysplasia. These include the possible protective effect of chronic suppressive medication with mesalamines or immunomodulators and the degree of mucosal healing achieved as determined both macroscopically and microscopically.

● SCREENING/SURVEILLANCE PROTOCOL

On the basis of these findings, it would seem prudent that the profile of patients with CD of the colon who should be enrolled in a screening/surveillance colonoscopy protocol should be as follows:

- Crohn's colitis of greater than 8 years' duration (perhaps calculated from onset of symptoms rather than date of diagnosis)
- childhood onset,
- diagnosis made after age 45,
- active symptoms, and
- coexisting sclerosing cholangitis.

The studies by Friedman et al. were restricted to those patients with Crohn's colitis involving at least one third of the colon. It has not been established what screening and surveillance algorithm to recommend for those CD patients with lesser colonic mucosal extent, such as that limited to the ileocecal area or with scattered aphthous lesions or with involvement only of the rectosigmoid. Extrapolating from our experience in UC it would seem reasonable to survey these patients less frequently, perhaps every 5 years.

● PERSISTANT AND RECTAL CD

There are a number of disturbing reports of cancers, sometimes multifocal, arising in patients with persistent anorectal CD. Of particular concern are those patients with chronic, severe, perineal, fistulous, and perianal disease. The relative risk of anal and rectal cancer in CD is elevated at least 10-fold over the general population. Rectal adenocarcinomas or anal squamous carcinomas may be difficult to diagnose endoscopically because the anal verge is not optimally accessed with conventional end-viewing instruments. Deep, submucosal biopsies obtained during examination under anesthesia may be required. The role of endoscopic ultrasonography in these patients has not been established.

Another challenging, now seldom found, subgroup of chronic CD patients are those who had undergone bypass surgery with ileotransverse colon anastomosis without resection of right colon and terminal ileum. This was a common surgical approach about 40 years ago. These and other patients who have had partial colon resection remain at risk and should be followed with surveillance colonoscopy, with every attempt made to enter the bypassed portion of the colon.

● COLONIC STRICTURE

There is some controversy about what to recommend for patients with chronic Crohn's colitis when the colon has become strictured and complete colonoscopy cannot be accomplished. In UC any stricture that precludes complete colonoscopy is considered an ominous finding for neoplasia, mandating colectomy. In the protocol followed by Friedman et al. whenever stricturing was encountered that prevented passage of the conventional colonoscope, a thin-caliber (pediatric) instrument was used. This increased complete screening and surveillance examinations by 16% and 33%, respectively, leading to about 90% complete examinations and detected dysplasia or cancer in 5 additional patients. For the remaining 10% of patients with incomplete colonoscopies the protocol followed by Friedman et al. did not mandate colon resection but rather used single-contrast barium enemas to visualize the impassable strictures and proximal colon.

As stricturing is a common feature of benign CD the protocol followed by Friedman, perhaps supplemented by CT enterography, still seems reasonable, presuming that no dysplasia has been detected elsewhere in the endoscopically accessible colon.

● RESPONSE TO FINDING DYSPLASIA

The response to finding dysplasia in CD has tended to be the same as that recommended in UC. When dysplasia is encountered on endoscopy in either UC or CD a key macroscopic determinant is whether the dysplastic biopsies have been obtained from flat or polypoid mucosa. If the dysplasia is polypoid and amenable to colonoscopic polypectomy, colectomy can be avoided, provided that separate biopsies throughout the colon and circumferential to the polypectomy site are negative for dysplasia and the patient is called back for a colonoscopy within several months to document by biopsies a "clean colon." The follow-up examinations should then be done annually.

The development of chromoendoscopy has altered this screening and surveillance paradigm somewhat, providing the possibility of increased detection of polypoid morphology in what may have appeared to be flat mucosa when viewed with conventional white-light endoscopy. Some advocates of chromoendoscopy have proposed taking only "targeted" biopsies: sampling only areas that appear elevated after application of dye sprays and not obtaining random biopsies throughout the colon. But this has not yet been accepted as standard of care in the United States. In Crohn's colitis chromoendoscopy interpretation may be difficult in the setting of the "cobble stone" and pseudopolypoid lesions of CD. At present I do not use chromoendoscopy routinely in Crohn's colitis patients, unless prior evaluation has detected polypoid dysplasia.

As the progression from "indefinite" to "low-grade" to "high-grade" dysplasia to cancer is not a reliable sequence, most gastroenterologists recommend surgical resection for all but indefinite dysplasia when the dysplasia has been detected in nonpolypoid mucosa.

But recommending colon resection in CD is a more complicated and momentous decision than in UC. In UC the standard surgery is total colectomy, with either ileopelvic anal anastomosis (IPAA) or end ileostomy or Brooke ileostomy. The UC patient after total colectomy is, by definition, cured of UC and the threat of colon cancer averted. In CD, however, the option of an (IPAA) is at best controversial, and not feasible, if there is a documented presence of ileal or perineal disease. Total proctocolectomy with end ileostomy may lead to poor healing of the perineum around the proctectomy. Furthermore, because CD is notorious for recurring after surgery, colectomy cannot assure cure, as is possible when used in UC. Whether to perform segmental resection or subtotal colectomy with rectal Hartman closure depends on the anatomic distribution of the CD and surgeon-patient preference. If rectum is retained it remains at risk for dysplasia or cancer and must be surveyed every year or so with proctoscopy and biopsies.

● SUMMARY

In summary, patients' with chronic Crohn's colitis involving at least one third of the colon should be enrolled in colonoscopic screening and surveillance programs identical to those recommended for patients with chronic UC. The approach to dysplasia in polypoid and "flat" mucosa is the same as in UC, though the surgical options with CD may differ from those offered to patients with UC. Unlike UC, encountering strictures that are not passable with thin-caliber endoscope may not necessitate colon resection. Colonoscopic surveillance in Crohn's patients with lesser anatomic colonic involvement probably can be less rigorous, though there is concern about those with chronic anorectal disease.

Small Bowel Stenosis in Crohn's Disease | 125

Dahlia Awais and Peter D.R. Higgins

EPIDEMIOLOGY

Crohn's disease is classified into three phenotypes of disease behavior: inflammatory (B1, nonpenetrating, nonstricturing), stricturing (B2, stenotic), and penetrating (B3, fistulas, and abscesses).[1] Although this is the standard classification, it is important to note that the stricturing and penetrating categories have significant overlap; most fistulae/penetrating complications arise from a stenosis.[2,3] Epidemiologic data on stricture occurrence in Crohn's disease is rather limited. However, data suggest that stricturing disease is less common than penetrating disease and the incidence of stricturing disease increases with the disease duration therefore suggesting that after a decade of disease, about one-third of patients with Crohn's disease will have a stricture.[4]

A 5-year prospective follow-up of a cohort of 646 patients found that penetrating disease was far more common than stricturing disease and identified a 12% risk for stricture 5 years after diagnosis and an 18% risk 20 years after diagnosis.[5] In a retrospective analysis of 297, patients with Crohn's disease, the incidence of stricturing disease increased over time, with a 10% rate of stricturing disease at diagnosis, but this increased to 30% after 10 years of disease.[4] Over 10 years of follow-up, 27% of the patients initially characterized as having inflammatory phenotype had developed stricturing disease.[4] Despite advances in our understanding of Crohn's disease and increased use of immunosuppressants and biologics, the frequency of strictures and the need for surgery in Crohn's disease has not significantly decreased.[6–9]

RISK FACTORS FOR STRICTURING DISEASE

Small bowel strictures are important complications of Crohn's disease that can lead to surgery. There is great interest in identifying patients at high risk for future stricturing disease. Identifying predictors of disease behavior could possibly lead to early-targeted interventions to change the natural history of the disease. With the goal of identifying important risk factors for complicated diseases, genetic, environmental, immunologic, and other disease features have been evaluated.

Several studies have identified disease severity, small bowel disease, and disease duration as important risk factors for the development of strictures. A prospective cohort study found disease location to be the most important predictor of disease behavior, and stricturing disease was associated with small bowel involvement (ileal or jejunal), absence of colonic involvement, and absence of anal disease.[5] An analysis of the TREAT Registry identified duration of disease, disease severity, ileal disease, and new corticosteroid use as significant predictors of intestinal stricture, stenosis, or obstruction.[10] It is believed that the combination of disease severity and duration (moderate chronic or severe acute inflammation) is a risk factor for stricture development, and that inflammation appears necessary for initiating fibrotic stenosis.[11]

The role of genes, including NOD2/CARD15, and serologic markers such as ASCA (antisaccharomyces cerevisiae antibodies) in prognosticating stricture risk remain unclear.[12–14] Although there is consensus that NOD2/CARD15 status is associated with small bowel disease and young age at disease onset, whether or not it is also an independent risk factor for fibrostenosing disease is arguable due to inconsistent data.[12,14,15] A recent meta-analysis of genetic studies found that the predictive ability of NOD2 status for complicated disease was poor, with a sensitivity of 36% and a specificity of 73%.[16] ASCA serologies are frequently associated with Crohn's disease and higher antibody levels have been associated with both fibrostenosing and penetrating Crohn's disease[17]; however, in a multivariate analysis, ASCA status was not identified as an independent predictor of disease behavior.[14] Other serologic markers including antibodies to the outer membrane porin C of *Escherichia coli* (OmpC), *Pseudomonas fluorescens*-associated sequence I2 (anti-I2), and flagellin CBir1 (anti-CBir1) have been studied and appear to be associated with complicated disease[18,19]; however, their ability to predict future disease behavior remains unclear. Furthermore, no prospective studies have proven that any interventions can change the natural history of patients who have a high risk of fibrostenotic Crohn's disease.

There is evidence that disease location, duration, and degree of inflammation are risk factors for stricture formation. The role of potential genetic or serologic markers remains unclear. Currently available data does not allow us to predict which patients with Crohn's disease will develop fibrotic strictures, or to act on this information even if it were available.

Editor's note (TMB): Having a relative with stenosing Crohn's disease increases the risk of stenosis in the next affected first degree relative. Bayless, et al. *Gastroenterology.* 1996;111:573–579.

PATHOGENESIS

The pathogenesis of fibrotic stricture development in Crohn's disease is poorly understood.[20,21] Chronic inflammation and recurrent intestinal wound healing are believed to play a central role in stricture formation; however, the exact physiological pathways involved are unclear, and it remains puzzling why some patients have frequent strictures, and others remain affected. Fibrosis is believed to be the result of "excessive wound healing" triggered by severe or chronic inflammation,[11] and inflammatory cells, cytokines, and mesenchymal cells. All likely play a role in the ultimate development of fibrosis.[22] Mesenchymal cells including fibroblasts, myofibroblasts, and smooth muscle cells are believed to participate in the fibrogenesis process as they produce components of the extracellular matrix.[11] An imbalance between extracellular matrix synthesis and degradation may contribute to the accumulation of fibrosis.[23] The role of specific cytokines continues to be studied. Particular cytokines involved in wound healing, including transforming growth factor-β1 and interleukin-13, appear to be pro-fibrotic.[23] Animal models of intestinal fibrosis have been developed and continue to be studied to improve our understanding of the pathogenesis of stricture formation.[24–26]

Editor's note (TMB): A recent paper from Targon, et al at Cedar Sinai looks at the role of innate immunity as well as acquired immunity in ileal stenosis.

DIAGNOSTIC EVALUATION— DISTINGUISHING INFLAMMATORY FROM FIBROTIC

Patients with Crohn's disease who present with obstructive symptoms including postprandial abdominal pain, distension, and nausea and vomiting require further evaluation to assess for obstruction or partial obstruction. If obstruction or partial obstruction is suspected, it is also important to evaluate the underlying cause, which in Crohn's disease can be secondary to inflammatory narrowing, fibrotic stricture, combined inflammation and fibrosis, cancer, or adhesive disease from previous surgeries. This characterization is essential in selecting the appropriate treatment. The initial clinical impression does not always correlate with radiographic findings, and imaging can add important information to a physician's assessment.[27] Radiographic imaging including computed tomography (CT) enterography and magnetic resonance (MR) enterography, which allow for detailed visualization of the small bowel, can be very helpful in this diagnostic evaluation. Clinical indices and laboratory markers are often less informative.[28]

On imaging, pre-stenotic dilation (luminal widening proximal to the narrowing) is generally not seen in purely inflammatory stenosis and is suggestive of a fixed fibrotic stricture.[29] Mucosal enhancement and increased vascularity (comb sign) on CT enterography or MR enterography are highly correlated with active inflammation and can be helpful in distinguishing between an inflammatory narrowing and fibrotic stricture.[30,31] These imaging modalities are also helpful in identifying the location as well as the length of involved bowel, which are important considerations for management. Historically, small bowel follow through was the imaging modality of choice for the evaluation of active Crohn's disease; however, CT enterography, and MR enterography are better at detecting inflammation, provide more comprehensive imaging, and are today's preferred imaging modalities.[32] When choosing between CT and MRI for the evaluation of small bowel stenosis in Crohn's disease, consideration should be given to local expertise, patient age, and patient radiation exposure.[33]

Ultrasound, which is more commonly used in Europe in the evaluation of Crohn's disease, may also be able to distinguish inflammation from fibrosis.[28] Contrast enhanced ultrasound and ultrasound elasticity imaging have promise in Crohn's disease and may provide useful information in the differentiation of inflammatory versus fibrotic narrowing; however, more studies are needed.[34]

THERAPEUTIC OPTIONS

The appropriate treatment of a stricture depends on many factors. As indicated above, appropriate characterization of the stricture as primarily inflammatory or primarily fibrotic can be very helpful. Although more aggressive medical management can be successful in the setting of an inflammatory stricture and may avoid or delay surgery, it is unlikely to be of benefit if the stricture is largely fibrotic, in which case options include surgical resection, strictureplasty, and balloon dilation. Surgical resection has been the traditional treatment for strictures, but a course of repeated extensive bowel resections can lead to short bowel syndrome. Therefore, effort should be taken to avoid or limit bowel resection when possible. Bowel can often be conserved with through-the-scope (TTS) balloon dilation or strictureplasty, and these alternatives to resection should be considered in the appropriate candidate.

Editor's note (TMB): There are separate chapters on enterography, or balloon dilatation, and on strictureplasty.

If evidence suggests the narrowing is primarily inflammatory, medical therapy should be pursued. This may include initiation of steroids, a biologic, or an immunomodulator. Despite early concerns that rapid healing induced by infliximab could cause stricture formation, the data do not support this, and there is no evidence that infliximab is a major risk factor for stricture formation.[10,35,36] Although patients who receive infliximab may be more likely to develop strictures, this does not appear to be due to infliximab itself, but rather to other patient factors including disease severity, which made them appropriate candidates for infliximab.[10] Infliximab is not contraindicated in the presence of strictures, but is most effective when inflammation is the major cause of stenosis. Although not harmful, *per se,* it is ineffective in the setting of significant fibrosis, and may be especially effective after the surgical removal of strictures.[37]

If evidence suggests the narrowing is primarily fibrotic, options including balloon dilation and surgery should be considered. Although data are limited and there have been no randomized controlled trials, TTS balloon dilation is considered a safe and effective treatment for both simple, short postsurgical anastomotic strictures including primary, nonanastomotic, short fibrotic strictures in Crohn's disease. A systematic review of endoscopic dilation in Crohn's disease identified 13 retrospective studies in which a total of 353 strictures were dilated in 347 patients. A majority of the strictures were postsurgical, anastomotic strictures. The procedure was technically successfully in 86% of patients and 68% of those patients had avoided surgery by study end (mean follow-up 33 months). There was an overall 58% long-term success rate. Surgery was ultimately required in 42% of patients who underwent an attempt at dilation. More than one-third of patients remained surgery-free after only one dilation session. The overall mean complication rate was 2%, in which the majority were bowel perforations; however, reported complication rates including bleeding and perforation that ranged from 0% to 18%.[38] Data regarding TTS dilation for primary nonanastomotic strictures are particularly limited. Although there is more literature on the dilation of anastomotic strictures, data suggest it is equally safe and effective for the treatment of primary, nonanastomotic strictures.[39] Appropriate stricture selection is important, and endoscopic balloon dilation for short strictures that are less than or equal to 4 cm in length have been associated with the best outcomes.[38] Steroid injection into the stricture after dilation appears to be safe and it may be an useful adjunct to dilation; however, to date, there are only three retrospective studies, the largest of which had 17 patients,[40–42] and only a single small randomized controlled trial has been published, which found no benefit to steroid injection.[43]

Although data suggest that endoscopic balloon dilation is safe and effective in appropriately selected strictures, there have been no randomized trials comparing different dilation approaches, there are no specific guidelines regarding optimal dilation technique or timing or re-treatment in Crohn's disease, and there is wide variation in published practice. Variations exist in the maximum balloon diameter used, like whether serial dilations or a single dilation is performed in a session, duration of balloon insufflation during a dilation session, and frequency of dilation.[38]

For symptomatic fibrotic strictures that are not amenable, or not responding to endoscopic therapy, surgical options include resection or strictureplasty. Strictureplasty preserves intestinal length while increasing the diameter of the lumen. This is particularly advantageous for patients with a prior history of repeated resection and those at risk for short bowel syndrome. Strictureplasty is generally contraindicated in the presence of active perforating disease. Although there are no randomized controlled trials comparing strictureplasty to resection, strictureplasty is considered safe and effective and time to recurrence is believed to be comparable to that of resection.[44]

● FUTURE DIRECTIONS

Although the medical therapy of Crohn's disease includes a number of anti-inflammatory agents, our medical armamentarium does not yet include therapies which can treat or prevent the occurrence of fibrostenosis. As our understanding of the pathogenesis of fibrostenotic strictures deepens, we hope to see the development of effective local or systemic antifibrotic medications for the treatment of fibrostenosing Crohn's disease.

References

1. Gasche C, Scholmerich J, Brynskov J, et al. A simple classification of Crohn's disease: report of the Working Party for the World Congresses of Gastroenterology, Vienna 1998. *Inflamm Bowel Dis.* 2000;6(1):8–15.

2. Kelly JK, Preshaw RM. Origin of fistulas in Crohn's disease. *J Clin Gastroenterol.* 1989;11(2):193–196.

3. Oberhuber G, Stangl PC, Vogelsang H, Schober E, Herbst F, Gasche C. Significant association of strictures and internal fistula formation in Crohn's disease. *Virchows Arch.* 2000;437(3):293–297.

4. Louis E, Collard A, Oger AF, Degroote E, Aboul Nasr El Yafi FA, Belaiche J. Behaviour of Crohn's disease according to the Vienna classification: changing pattern over the course of the disease. *Gut.* 2001;49(6):777–782.

5. Cosnes J, Cattan S, Blain A, et al. Long-term evolution of disease behavior of Crohn's disease. *Inflamm Bowel Dis.* 2002;8(4):244–250.

6. Jones DW, Finlayson SR. Trends in surgery for Crohn's disease in the era of infliximab. *Ann Surg.* 2010;252(2):307–312.

7. Cosnes J, Nion-Larmurier I, Beaugerie L, Afchain P, Tiret E, Gendre JP. Impact of the increasing use of immunosuppressants in Crohn's disease on the need for intestinal surgery. *Gut.* 2005;54(2):237–241.

8. Poritz LS, Rowe WA, Koltun WA. Remicade does not abolish the need for surgery in fistulizing Crohn's disease. *Dis Colon Rectum.* 2002;45(6):771–775.

9. Cannom RR, Kaiser AM, Ault GT, Beart RW Jr, Etzioni DA. Inflammatory bowel disease in the United States from 1998 to 2005: has infliximab affected surgical rates? *Am Surg.* 2009;75(10):976–980.

10. Lichtenstein GR, Olson A, Travers S, et al. Factors associated with the development of intestinal strictures or obstructions in patients with Crohn's disease. *Am J Gastroenterol.* 2006;101(5):1030–1038.

11. Rieder F, Brenmoehl J, Leeb S, Schölmerich J, Rogler G. Wound healing and fibrosis in intestinal disease. *Gut.* 2007;56(1):130–139.

12. Abreu MT, Taylor KD, Lin YC, et al. Mutations in NOD2 are associated with fibrostenosing disease in patients with Crohn's disease. *Gastroenterology.* 2002;123(3):679–688.

13. Lesage S, Zouali H, Cézard JP, et al.; EPWG-IBD Group; EPIMAD Group; GETAID Group. CARD15/NOD2 mutational analysis and genotype-phenotype correlation in 612 patients with inflammatory bowel disease. *Am J Hum Genet.* 2002;70(4):845–857.

14. Louis E, Michel V, Hugot JP, et al. Early development of stricturing or penetrating pattern in Crohn's disease is influenced by disease location, number of flares, and smoking but not by NOD2/CARD15 genotype. *Gut.* 2003;52(4):552–557.

15. Vermeire S. NOD2/CARD15: relevance in clinical practice. *Best Pract Res Clin Gastroenterol.* 2004;18(3):569–575.

16. Adler J, Rangwalla S, Higgins PDR. *The Prognostic Power of NOD2 Genotype for Complicated Crohn's Disease: A Meta-Analysis,* in *Digestive Disease Week.* Chicago, IL: American Gastroenterological Association; 2009. p. 251.

17. Vasiliauskas EA, Kam LY, Karp LC, Gaiennie J, Yang H, Targan SR. Marker antibody expression stratifies Crohn's disease into immunologically homogeneous subgroups with distinct clinical characteristics. *Gut.* 2000;47(4):487–496.

18. Mow WS, Vasiliauskas EA, Lin YC, et al. Association of antibody responses to microbial antigens and complications of small bowel Crohn's disease. *Gastroenterology.* 2004;126(2):414–424.

19. Targan SR, Landers CJ, Yang H, et al. Antibodies to CBir1 flagellin define a unique response that is associated independently with complicated Crohn's disease. *Gastroenterology.* 2005;128(7):2020–2028.

20. Powell DW, Mifflin RC, Valentich JD, Crowe SE, Saada JI, West AB. Myofibroblasts. II. Intestinal subepithelial myofibroblasts. *Am J Physiol.* 1999;277(2 Pt 1):C183–C201.

21. Powell DW, Mifflin RC, Valentich JD, Crowe SE, Saada JI, West AB. Myofibroblasts. I. Paracrine cells important in health and disease. *Am J Physiol.* 1999;277(1 Pt 1):C1–C9.

22. Burke JP, Mulsow JJ, O'Keane C, Docherty NG, Watson RW, O'Connell PR. Fibrogenesis in Crohn's disease. *Am J Gastroenterol.* 2007;102(2):439–448.

23. Rieder F, Fiocchi C. Intestinal fibrosis in inflammatory bowel disease: progress in basic and clinical science. *Curr Opin Gastroenterol.* 2008;24(4):462–468.

24. Grassl GA, Valdez Y, Bergstrom KS, Vallance BA, Finlay BB. Chronic enteric salmonella infection in mice leads to severe and persistent intestinal fibrosis. *Gastroenterology.* 2008;134(3):768–780.

25. Lawrance IC, Wu F, Leite AZ, et al. A murine model of chronic inflammation-induced intestinal fibrosis down-regulated by antisense NF-kappa B. *Gastroenterology.* 2003;125(6):1750–1761.

26. Rigby RJ, Hunt MR, Scull BP, et al. A new animal model of postsurgical bowel inflammation and fibrosis: the effect of commensal microflora. *Gut.* 2009;58(8):1104–1112.

27. Higgins PD, Caoili E, Zimmermann M, et al. Computed tomographic enterography adds information to clinical management in small bowel Crohn's disease. *Inflamm Bowel Dis.* 2007;13(3):262–268.

28. Maconi G, Carsana L, Fociani P, et al. Small bowel stenosis in Crohn's disease: clinical, biochemical and ultrasonographic evaluation of histological features. *Aliment Pharmacol Ther.* 2003;18(7):749–756.

29. Sorrentino D. Role of biologics and other therapies in stricturing Crohn's disease: what have we learnt so far? *Digestion.* 2008;77(1):38–47.

30. Bodily KD, Fletcher JG, Solem CA, et al. Crohn Disease: mural attenuation and thickness at contrast-enhanced CT enterography–correlation with endoscopic and histologic findings of inflammation. *Radiology.* 2006;238(2):505–516.

31. Koh DM, Miao Y, Chinn RJ, et al. MR imaging evaluation of the activity of Crohn's disease. *AJR Am J Roentgenol.* 2001;177(6):1325–1332.

32. Lee SS, Kim AY, Yang SK, et al. Crohn disease of the small bowel: comparison of CT enterography, MR enterography, and small-bowel follow-through as diagnostic techniques. *Radiology.* 2009;251(3):751–761.

33. Brenner DJ, Hall EJ. Computed tomography–an increasing source of radiation exposure. *N Engl J Med.* 2007;357(22):2277–2284.

34. Migaleddu V, Quaia E, Scano D, Virgilio G. Inflammatory activity in Crohn disease: ultrasound findings. *Abdom Imaging.* 2008;33(5):589–597.

35. Pallotta N, Barberani F, Hassan NA, Guagnozzi D, Vincoli G, Corazziari E. Effect of infliximab on small bowel stenoses in patients with Crohn's disease. *World J Gastroenterol.* 2008;14(12):1885–1890.

36. Sorrentino D, Terrosu G, Vadalà S, Avellini C. Fibrotic strictures and anti-TNF-alpha therapy in Crohn's disease. *Digestion.* 2007;75(1):22–24.

37. Regueiro M, Schraut W, Baidoo L, et al. Infliximab prevents Crohn's disease recurrence after ileal resection. *Gastroenterology.* 2009;136(2):441–50.e1; quiz 716.

38. Hassan C, Zullo A, De Francesco V, et al. Systematic review: Endoscopic dilatation in Crohn's disease. *Aliment Pharmacol Ther.* 2007;26(11–12):1457–1464.

39. Atreja A, Dwivedi S, Lashner B, Vargo JJ, Shen B. Short and long-term outcomes of endoscopic stricture dilation for primary and anastomotic strictures in patients with crohn's disease. *Gastroenterology.* 2010;138(5):S528–S529.

40. Brooker JC, Beckett CG, Saunders BP, Benson MJ. Long-acting steroid injection after endoscopic dilation of anastomotic Crohn's strictures may improve the outcome: a retrospective case series. *Endoscopy.* 2003;35(4):333–337.

41. Ramboer C, Verhamme M, Dhondt E, Huys S, Van Eygen K, Vermeire L. Endoscopic treatment of stenosis in recurrent Crohn's disease with balloon dilation combined with local corticosteroid injection. *Gastrointest Endosc.* 1995;42(3):252–255.

42. Singh VV, Draganov P, Valentine J. Efficacy and safety of endoscopic balloon dilation of symptomatic upper and lower gastrointestinal Crohn's disease strictures. *J Clin Gastroenterol.* 2005;39(4):284–290.

43. East JE, Brooker JC, Rutter MD, Saunders BP. A pilot study of intrastricture steroid versus placebo injection after balloon dilatation of Crohn's strictures. *Clin Gastroenterol Hepatol.* 2007;5(9):1065–1069.

44. Yamamoto T, Fazio VW, Tekkis PP. Safety and efficacy of strictureplasty for Crohn's disease: a systematic review and meta-analysis. *Dis Colon Rectum.* 2007;50(11):1968–1986.

Colonic Strictures in Crohn's Disease Patients

126

Keely Parisian and Bret A. Lashner

In theory, Crohn's disease (CD) begins as an inflammatory-type disease. The natural history of disease and following some medical therapies, inflammation gradually subsides and fibrous strictures are left behind.[1] Clinically important strictures can develop in up to 40% of patients with small bowel disease and up to 15% in patients with large bowel disease. Anastomotic strictures can be seen in up to half of the patients following ileocolectomy. Although most strictures in CD patients are in the small bowel, colonic strictures are often symptomatic and offer some unique opportunities for medical and surgical treatment.

PATHOGENESIS

Most colonic strictures are fibrous in nature and are caused by the exuberant deposition of collagen from fibroblasts. The exact mechanism of cytokine signaling to these cells is not known, but transforming growth factor (TGF)-β has been identified as a key factor in cicatrix formation.[2,3] Also, mutations in the NOD2/CARD15 gene and other genes, such as a gene near the IL12B gene, are associated with the stricturing disease.[4] However, not all studies have linked NOD2/CARD15 with stricturing disease.[5]

More recently, serologic markers have been touted as being prognostically important. A 796-patient pediatric cohort examined the relationship between CD behavior, NOD2/CARD15 mutations, and serologic markers related to inflammatory bowel disease (IBD).[6] Anti-*Saccharomyces cerevisiae* antibodies (ASCA), anti-OmpC, and anti-CBir1 antibodies, but not NOD2/CARD15, were associated with stricturing disease, internal penetrating disease, and the need for surgery. Perinuclear antineutrophil cytoplasmic antibodies was protective for strictures. Furthermore, the greater the number of separate antibodies that were positive, the higher was the risk for both stricturing and internal penetrating disease. Patients with multiple positive antibodies (i.e., ASCA and anti-CBir1) should be considered for anti-inflammatory therapy, even biologic therapy, before strictures and fistulas develop.

Editor's note (TMB): At this time, we do not have evidence that immunomodulators or biologic therapy will prevent small bowel strictures.

Cigarette smoking is felt to be associated with a more aggressive form of CD that leads to early surgery, stricturing, and penetrating disease. In a large epidemiologic study from Scotland, current smokers with CD had less colonic disease than nonsmokers.[7] Also, smokers were no more likely than nonsmokers to develop stricturing or penetrating disease. Patients with isolated colonic disease developed strictures less often and at a slower rate than patients with ileal disease. From this study, nonsmoking was associated with the development of colonic disease, but did not influence the rate of stricture development.

Perianal lesions in CD entail a variety of manifestations and include anal and rectal strictures. In a study of 202 patients with CD, 54% had evidence of perianal disease but only 9% had evidence of an anorectal stricture.[8] Interestingly, colonic strictures, especially rectal strictures, are associated with penetrating disease. In contrast to the evolution of colonic strictures, anal and rectal strictures are postulated to arise as a result of inflammation and fibrosis secondary to fistula and abscess formation.[9] As such, affected patients may require a different diagnostic approach and treatment strategy.

DIFFERENTIAL DIAGNOSIS

Colorectal cancer is a complication of extensive Crohn's colitis, and can be mistaken for a benign colonic stricture.[10] Prior to the institution of any therapy for colonic strictures, strictures must be extensively biopsied to be certain that they are benign. Unlike in ulcerative colitis patients, the vast majority of strictures, over 93%, in CD patients have no neoplasia, but still must be biopsied.[11,12] In rare cases, metastatic cancer to the colon can mimic stricturing CD.[13] The detection of neoplasia, cancer or dysplasia, should prompt a recommendation for either a segmental colectomy or a total proctocolectomy.

The differential diagnosis of colonic strictures in CD patients includes colonic tuberculosis,[14] diverticulosis,[15] nonsteroidal anti-inflammatory drug-induced stricture,[16] and endometriosis.[17] Ruling out these diagnoses can be done with appropriate testing. CT enterography has an accuracy for detecting surgically-proven stricture formation of 83%.[18] Positron emission tomography/computed tomography (PET/CT) has a high sensitivity for detecting segments of bowel with deep ulceration; it is not as sensitive for detecting fibrous strictures.[19] Virtual colonoscopy has been shown to be highly sensitive and specific for detecting anastomotic recurrence, including strictures, of CD.[20]

In summary, strictures of the colon in CD patients can be detected with colonoscopy, CT enterography, or virtual colonoscopy. Several items on the differential diagnosis must be considered, but all strictures should be extensively biopsied to be certain that there is no neoplastic tissue.

MEDICAL THERAPY

Medical therapy for colonic strictures is very limited. Balloon dilation is often effective and discussed in a separate Chapter. Intestinal strictures have been proposed as a complication of infliximab use, but a study from a large database could not confirm this adverse effect. Although there were twice as many events of stenosis, stricture, or obstruction in patients treated with infliximab compared to those not treated with infliximab (1.95 events/100 patient-years vs. 0.99 events/100 patient-years, $P < 0.001$), the effect may have been confounded.[21] On multivariable analysis, CD severity, disease duration, ileal disease, and corticosteroid use were significant risk factors for strictures, not infliximab use.

Some patients with colonic strictures can have both an inflammatory and fibrous component to it. Anti-inflammatory medications, like infliximab, may provide clinically beneficial effects, such as relieving obstructing symptoms and allowing for a small segmental surgical resection.[22] Intralesional injection of low-dose infliximab into the distal and medial portions of a colonic stricture, including an anastomotic stricture, was found to be successful in about half of patients whose strictures were refractory to systemic anti-inflammatory therapy.[23,24] In a 13-patient randomized clinical trial, CD patients with ileocolic anastomotic strictures were randomized to receive submucosal triamcinalone 40 mg injection versus placebo after balloon dilation, and followed for 1 year.[25] Re-dilation was needed in 5/7 triamcinalone-treated patients and only 1/6 placebo-treated patients. Even though the study was small and the results were not significant, there is a strong suggestion that steroid injection at the time of balloon dilation is not likely to be helpful, and for unknown reasons may be harmful. The unique situation of an ileal pouch outlet stricture is believed to be caused by reactivation of IBD, either CD or ulcerative colitis, in the rectal cuff. Both balloon dilation and mesalamine suppositories may be therapeutic.[26,27]

In summary, medical therapy for colonic strictures is very limited. Patients with colonic strictures should be given a trial of anti-inflammatory therapy, like infliximab, to see if some benefit can be obtained prior to balloon dilation. Intralesional infliximab could be of benefit, but steroid injection does not appear to help.

SURGICAL THERAPY

Surgery is necessary in patients with colonic strictures who have symptomatic, benign obstructive disease and who do not

TABLE 126.1 Site of Colonic Stricture and Treatment

Colonic Stricture	Rectal Stricture
Anti-inflammatory therapy (i.e., infliximab)	Anti-inflammatory therapy (i.e., infliximab)
Intralesional infliximab	Antibiotics and drainage if underlying sepsis
Endoscopic balloon dilation	Finger or balloon dilation
Strictureplasty, segmental resection, total colectomy	Total proctocolectomy

respond to balloon dilation or medical therapy.[28] The decision for a strictureplasty, segmental resection, total colectomy, or total proctocolectomy depends on specific disease features. In general, preservation of colonic length and the ileocecal valve should be considered since there may be less postoperative diarrhea and better quality of life. Anastomoses or strictureplasties in the transverse colon near the second portion of the duodenum should be avoided—recurrence may lead to a difficult to treat fistula to the upper gastrointestinal tract.

Perianal strictures may dictate the extent of surgery in addition to alternate medical and endoscopic therapy (Table 126.1). In a study of CD patients having colonic surgery, total proctectomy was found to be significantly more necessary (26% vs. 3.7%) in patients with perianal disease than in patients without perianal disease.[29] Furthermore, the rate of healing following surgery was significantly lower ($P = 0.01$) in patients with perineal involvement compared to patients without perineal involvement. The study suggests that perianal lesions in CD may precipitate a more extensive surgical intervention and a worse outcome.

Strictureplasties of the colon are rarely done since resections are a more simple procedure.[30] In one series, only 7% of strictureplasties in CD patients were performed in the colon.[31] However, repeat surgery was needed in 20% of those who had strictureplasty compared to 44% in patients who had resection. In another series comparing colonic strictureplasty to colonic resection, the recurrence rate (36% for strictureplasty vs. 24% for resection), postoperative morbidity (16% vs. 22%), and Inflammatory Bowel Disease Questionnaire (IBDQ) quality-of-life scores (177 vs. 182) were not significantly different between groups.[32] Ultimately, the specific surgical procedure is made by the surgeon, often at the time of surgery, when there is a clear view of the affected bowel.[33]

CONCLUSION

The complex interplay of cell signaling pathways and the natural history of CD are paramount to the formation of colonic strictures. All colonic strictures should be extensively biopsied to be certain that neoplasia is not present. Also, anti-inflammatory therapy is advised to be certain that there is not an inflammatory component to the fibrous stricture. Patients with continuing obstructive symptoms despite anti-inflammatory therapy should be considered for surgery with either a strictureplasty or a resection. Research into the pathogenesis of fibrosis in CD is essential to find novel anti-fibrotic therapies that can prevent these serious complications.

References

1. Cosnes J, Cattan S, Blain A, et al. Long-term evolution of disease behavior of Crohn's disease. *Inflamm Bowel Dis.* 2002;8(4): 244–250.

2. Di Sabatino A, Jackson CL, Pickard KM, et al. Transforming growth factor beta signalling and matrix metalloproteinases in the mucosa overlying Crohn's disease strictures. *Gut.* 2009;58(6):777–789.

3. Lang M, Schlechtweg M, Kellermeier S, et al. Gene expression profiles of mucosal fibroblasts from strictured and nonstrictured areas of patients with Crohn's disease. *Inflamm Bowel Dis.* 2009;15(2):212–223.

4. Henckaerts L, Van Steen K, Verstreken I, et al. Genetic risk profiling and prediction of disease course in Crohn's disease patients. *Clin Gastroenterol Hepatol.* 2009;7(9):972–980.e2.

5. Shaoul R, Karban A, Reif S, et al. Disease behavior in children with Crohn's disease: the effect of disease duration, ethnicity, genotype, and phenotype. *Dig Dis Sci.* 2009;54(1):142–150.

6. Dubinsky MC, Kugathasan S, Mei L, et al. Increased immune reactivity predicts aggressive complicating Crohn's disease in children. *Clin Gastroenterol Hepatol.* 2008;6(10):1105–1111.

7. Aldhous MC, Drummond HE, Anderson N, Smith LA, Arnott ID, Satsangi J. Does cigarette smoking influence the phenotype of Crohn's disease? Analysis using the Montreal classification. *Am J Gastroenterol.* 2007;102(3):577–588.

8. Keighley MR, Allan RN. Current status and influence of operation on perianal Crohn's disease. *Int J Colorectal Dis.* 1986;1(2):104–107.

9. Fields S, Rosainz L, Korelitz BI, Panagopoulos G, Schneider J. Rectal strictures in Crohn's disease and coexisting perirectal complications. *Inflamm Bowel Dis.* 2008;14(1):29–31.

10. Sigel JE, Petras RE, Lashner BA, Fazio VW, Goldblum JR. Intestinal adenocarcinoma in Crohn's disease: a report of 30 cases with a focus on coexisting dysplasia. *Am J Surg Pathol.* 1999;23(6):651–655.

11. Lashner BA, Turner BC, Bostwick DG, Frank PH, Hanauer SB. Dysplasia and cancer complicating strictures in ulcerative colitis. *Dig Dis Sci.* 1990;35(3):349–352.

12. Yamakazi Y, Ribeiro MB, Sachar DB, Aufses AH, Jr, Greenstein AJ. Malignant strictures in Crohn's disease. *Am J Gastroenterol.* 1991;86:882–885.

13. Zenda T, Taniguchi K, Hashimoto T, et al. Metastatic colon cancer mimicking Crohn's disease. *Ann Diagn Pathol.* 2007;11(6):427–432.

14. Madani TA. Colonic tuberculosis clinically misdiagnosed as anorexia nervosa, and radiologically and histopathologically as Crohn's disease. *Can J Infect Dis.* 2002;13(2):136–140.

15. Sultan K, Fields S, Panagopoulos G, Korelitz BI. The nature of inflammatory bowel disease in patients with coexistent colonic diverticulosis. *J Clin Gastroenterol.* 2006;40(4):317–321.

16. Thiéfin G, Beaugerie L. Toxic effects of nonsteroidal anti-inflammatory drugs on the small bowel, colon, and rectum. *Joint Bone Spine.* 2005;72(4):286–294.

17. Yantiss RK, Clement PB, Young RH. Endometriosis of the intestinal tract: a study of 44 cases of a disease that may cause diverse challenges in clinical and pathologic evaluation. *Am J Surg Pathol.* 2001;25(4):445–454.

18. Vogel J, da Luz Moreira A, Baker M, et al. CT enterography for Crohn's disease: accurate preoperative diagnostic imaging. *Dis Colon Rectum.* 2007;50(11):1761–1769.

19. Louis E, Ancion G, Colard A, Spote V, Belaiche J, Hustinx R. Noninvasive assessment of Crohn's disease intestinal lesions with (18)F-FDG PET/CT. *J Nucl Med.* 2007;48(7):1053–1059.

20. Biancone L, Fiori R, Tosti C, et al. Virtual colonoscopy compared with conventional colonoscopy for stricturing postoperative recurrence in Crohn's disease. *Inflamm Bowel Dis.* 2003;9(6):343–350.

21. Lichtenstein GR, Olson A, Travers S, et al. Factors associated with the development of intestinal strictures or obstructions in patients with Crohn's disease. *Am J Gastroenterol.* 2006;101(5):1030–1038.

22. Sorrentino D, Avellini C, Beltrami CA, Pasqual E, Zearo E. Selective effect of infliximab on the inflammatory component of a colonic stricture in Crohn's disease. *Int J Colorectal Dis.* 2006;21(3):276–281.

23. Swaminath A, Lichtiger S. Dilation of colonic strictures by intralesional injection of infliximab in patients with Crohn's colitis. *Inflamm Bowel Dis.* 2008;14(2):213–216.

24. Biancone L, Cretella M, Tosti C, et al. Local injection of infliximab in the postoperative recurrence of Crohn's disease. *Gastrointest Endosc.* 2006;63(3):486–492.

25. East JE, Brooker JC, Rutter MD, Saunders BP. A pilot study of intrastricture steroid versus placebo injection after balloon dilatation of Crohn's strictures. *Clin Gastroenterol Hepatol.* 2007;5(9):1065–1069.

26. Shen B, Fazio VW, Remzi FH, et al. Endoscopic balloon dilation of ileal pouch strictures. *Am J Gastroenterol.* 2004;99(12):2340–2347.

27. Shen B, Lashner BA, Bennett AE, et al. Treatment of rectal cuff inflammation (cuffitis) in patients with ulcerative colitis following restorative proctocolectomy and ileal pouch-anal anastomosis. *Am J Gastroenterol.* 2004;99(8):1527–1531.

28. Figg RE, Church JM. Perineal Crohn's disease: an indicator of poor prognosis and potential proctectomy. *Dis Colon Rectum.* 2009;52(4):646–650.

29. Figg RE, Church JM. Perineal Crohn's disease: an indicator of poor prognosis and potential proctectomy. *Dis Colon Rectum.* 2009;52(4):646–650.

30. Yamamoto T, Fazio VW, Tekkis PP. Safety and efficacy of strictureplasty for Crohn's disease: a systematic review and meta-analysis. *Dis Colon Rectum.* 2007;50(11):1968–1986.

31. Futami K, Arima S. Role of strictureplasty in surgical treatment of Crohn's disease. *J Gastroenterol.* 2005;40(suppl 16):35–39.

32. Broering DC, Eisenberger CF, Koch A, et al. Strictureplasty for large bowel stenosis in Crohn's disease: quality of life after surgical therapy. *Int J Colorectal Dis.* 2001;16(2):81–87.

33. Ozuner G, Fazio VW, Lavery IC, Milsom JW, Strong SA. Reoperative rates for Crohn's disease following strictureplasty. Long-term analysis. *Dis Colon Rectum.* 1996;39(11):1199–1203.

Enteroscopy in the Evaluation and Treatment of Crohn's-Related Small Bowel Strictures

127

Patrick I. Okolo III and Lissette Musaib-Ali

Following the development of double-balloon enteroscopy (DBE) in 2001,[1] augmented methods of small bowel enteroscopy have enabled a significant expansion of both diagnostic evaluation and endoluminal therapy in the midgut (ampulla of Vater to the ileocecal valve). Prior to this development, push enteroscopy was the only practical alternative to intraoperative enteroscopy, which was reserved for exceptional circumstances only. Push enteroscopy could reliably examine 50 to 150 cm beyond the ligament of Treitz using an oral approach.[2–5] In contrast, augmented enteroscopy using balloon-assisted enteroscopy or spiral enteroscopy allows for deeper examination of the mid gut using an oral (anterograde) or (retrograde) approach alone or in combination. Total enteroscopy (endoscopic examination of the entire small bowel) can be achieved via the oral route in 25% to 40% of patients.[6] When both routes are combined, total enteroscopy can be achieved in up to 75% of patients.[7,8]

In principle, augmented enteroscopy relies on the use of balloon or overtube to pleat and stabilize the small bowel to allow for deep evaluation of the mid gut using a flexible endoscope. There are three clinically available methods of performing augmented enteroscopy.

a) Double-balloon enteroscopy
b) Single-balloon enteroscopy
c) Spiral enteroscopy

Double-Balloon Enteroscopy

This was first described by Yamamoto and colleagues[1] in 2001. DBE refers to endoluminal examination of the small bowel using a double-balloon endoscope. DBE achieves deep and sometimes complete intubation of the small bowel by pleating the bowel onto a 2-m long, flexible endoscope accompanied by an overtube. Both the endoscope and the accompanying overtube have balloons at their distal ends. Using sequential inflation and deflation of these two balloons, combined with instrument insertion (push) and retraction (pull), deep access of the small intestine can be achieved via the oral and anal routes, alone or in combination.

Single-Balloon Enteroscopy

Single-balloon enteroscopy (SBE) refers to endoluminal examination of the small bowel using a single-balloon endoscope.[6] This flexible 2-m long scope does not utilize a balloon at its distal end but rather relies on fixation using tip angulation. An accompanying silicone overtube allows for sequential inflation and deflation with scope insertion and retraction maneuvers to achieve deep intubation of the small intestine.

Spiral Enteroscopy

Spiral enteroscopy is a relatively more recently developed technique of augmented enteroscopy.[9,10] A dedicated enteroscope is passed through and coupled with a single-use overtube equipped with helical spirals at its distal end. The overtube can be rotated independently of the enteroscope to achieve linear motion by pleating the small bowel. The enteroscope can be uncoupled from the overtube and inserted/retracted to further augment the extent of insertion. A recently introduced modification of the overtube now allows for retrograde enteroscopy using this technique.

There is a paucity of data comparing the different methods of augmented enteroscopy in most clinical situations including Crohn's disease (CD). The clinical scenario and the availability of local expertise should drive the choice of technique.

ROLE OF ENTEROSCOPY IN TREATMENT OF CROHN'S STRICTURES

Crohn's-related small bowel strictures are often problematic from both the standpoint of diagnosis and treatment. One of the pivotal decisions to be made after a stricture is delineated is to determine its potential etiology and, most importantly, to exclude malignancy. Augmented enteroscopy allows endoluminal access to small bowel strictures so they can be visualized and biopsied. Crohn's strictures may be multiple in nature,[11] difficult to define, or come to light precipitously by retention of a capsule.[12,13]

Augmented enteroscopy provides a first line nonoperative option for the treatment of Crohn's patients with intestinal strictures. Using a balloon to dilate the appropriate stricture, symptomatic relief can be achieved. In addition, tattooing the site can also be helpful should subsequent surgical management be necessary. In the right clinical setting, endoscopic stents can be placed in the mid–small intestine, for example, in palliative situations with malignant strictures. The ability to gain greater depth of insertion allows for integration of standard endoscopic maneuvers in previously hard-to-reach areas and has extended the gastroenterologist ability to offer endoluminal options for the treatment of Crohn's-related strictures.

PREREQUISITES FOR DILATATION OF CROHN'S STRICTURE USING DEEP ENTEROSCOPY

Small bowel imaging to demonstrate the position and characteristic of the stricture is often necessary. Although most small bowel series will suffice for most situations, some patients will undergo enterography using computed tomography or magnetic resonance imaging. A stricture may be identified by a retained endoscopic capsule performed for evaluation of Crohn's or obscure gastrointestinal bleeding.

Following the decision to proceed with dilatation, the operator must have a mastery of deep enteroscopy. This assures the highest likelihood of technical success. The endoscopist must be able to navigate to the site of luminal compromise by an anterograde or retrograde approach and then assess the length and appearance of the stricture. Table 127.1 demonstrates the accessories and technical component necessary to perform stricture dilatation in the setting of deep enteroscopy.

TABLE 127.1 Equipment Checklist for Deep Enteroscopy Dilatation of Crohn's Strictures

- Small bowel imaging—small bowel series. The role of CT/MR enterography is evolving
- Device (deep)-assisted enteroscopy system
- Hydrostatic balloon—preferably wire guided
- Hydrophilic or hybrid guidewire
- Fluoroscopy may be necessary to assess the length of strictures

MR, magnetic resonance; CT, computed tomography.

TECHNIQUE OF STRICTURE DILATATION IN DEEP ENTEROSCOPY

The patient is positioned in a comfortable position—it may be necessary to change from left lateral decubitus to supine or prone when fluoroscopy is critical or following orotracheal intubation. General anesthesia is not necessary but relatively deeper sedation using propofol or augmented conscious sedation is often necessary. The approach is decided a priori depending on the clinical situation. The patient should receive nothing by mouth for at least 10 hours and will have a full colon preparation in the case of a retrograde approach. A high-quality bowel preparation facilitates the procedure, and a split dosing may be associated with improved results.[14–16]

Solo navigation to the stricture is necessary to treat most strictures. A method using a balloon tipped decompression tube to assist navigation to the stricture has also been described[17] and may be useful in difficult circumstances. Antispasmodics such as glucagon and/or a gentle lavage with dilute simethicone may be necessary to enhance visualization. The stricture is inspected to exclude any features that would dampen enthusiasm for endoscopic therapy. These findings include severe mucosal changes that suggest profound inflammation, tortuousity or a contiguous fistula, or other breach in mural integrity. The stricture is identified endoscopically. Strictures in the small bowel have a luminal diameter of 8 mm or less. The enteroscopes used for most deep enteroscopy are larger than 9 mm and may not traverse many of these strictures. Whenever possible, the stricture should be positioned *en face* manner to allow for further delineation. When it isn't possible to position the stricture en face, a special 2800 mm ERCP catheter (Wilson Cook, Winston Salem, North Carolina) facilitates the position and subsequent passage of a hybrid guidewire across the stricture. In an en face position, it is possible to delineate the entire length of the stricture by injecting contrast directly through the catheter with the endoscope balloon inflated (in the case of DBE) or using an inflated wire-guided hydrostatic balloon (when performing spiral or SBE). These balloons prevent retrograde spillage of contrast and allows delineation of the stricture length. If the stricture is traversed using an ERCP accessory in the manner described earlier, contrast is injected in the normal distal bowel as the catheter is withdrawn thus allowing delineation of the stricture. Strictures longer than 5 cm are considered unsuitable for endoscopic dilatation.[8,18]

A hydrostatic balloon is passed across the stricture and is situated ideally with its (hydrostatic balloon) midportion in the stricture. A slow progressive inflation allows the balloon to remain situated in the stricture and prevent forward displacement of the balloon during inflation. The balloon is inflated with water up to the balloon diameter and the appropriate pounds per square inch setting. The balloon is inflated in the stricture for 60 seconds and then deflated under direct visualization. A second dilatation is unnecessary during the same session and perhaps should be avoided. The median balloon diameter used for dilation in most studies ranges from 15 to 17 mm, though more aggressive dilatation has been described (range 12–20 mm), whereas others have described more aggressive approach with a balloon up to 25 mm diameter. Perforation rates of 10% have been reported with these aggressive techniques.[19]

Adenocarcinoma of the small bowel is rare but appears to be more frequent in CD.[20–22] Rarely, a Crohn's stricture may be malignant and, when appropriate, enteral stent placement using deep enteroscopy[23] may obviate the need for surgery in patients who are unsuitable candidates for surgery.

OUTCOMES OF STRICTURE DILATATION USING DEEP ENTEROSCOPY

Endoscopic dilatation of Crohn's-related strictures in the small bowel may be followed by (a) technical and clinical success, (b) technical but no clinical success, and (c) no technical or clinical success. Complication rates while performing endotherapy for Crohn's-related strictures may be increased in contrast to standard small bowel and are an important consideration during decision making.

Although there is a paucity of high-grade evidence for endoscopic therapy in Crohn's-related small bowel strictures, there is a growing body of experience with the use of these techniques.[7,8,17,18,24–27] In the study conducted by Pohl et al., the role of DBE in 19 Crohn's disease patients was evaluated. All the patients in this study were clinically symptomatic. There were 28 strictures found on deep enteroscopy in patients with symptomatic small bowel strictures secondary to CD. DBE detected 28 strictures, of which 75% (21/28) were primary, and 25% (7/28) were anastomotic. Prior to dilation, the strictures in this study were 1 to 4 cm long and the diameter ranged from 5 to 8 mm. On inspection, 9 of 19 patients were considered immediately unsuitable for balloon dilatation (severe inflammatory changes or angulation). Ten patients underwent 15 procedures to address 13 identified strictures. The response rate to endoscopic dilation in terms of technical success is variable but ranges from 8 of 19 to 8 of 11 in reported series. It is important to remember that these results assume a per-patient-intention-to-treat approach. Some of the patients had more than one stricture, and some strictures were not amenable to endoscopic therapy because solo navigation was impeded due to anatomic factors such as severe angulation or adhesive disease.

The outcomes from these interventions appear to be durable. Long-term success as defined by the absence of symptoms appears to be between 60% and 80%.[8,19] Over a 3-year horizon, approximately 66% of patients will avoid surgical resection or stricturoplasty following balloon dilatation of Crohn's-related strictures. Ten to twenty percent of patients may develop recurrent symptoms and may require a repeat procedure or referral for surgical stricturopalsty.[19] This almost parallels the stricturoplasty experience where up to 25% of patients may require a repeat surgical procedure following the index surgical stricturoplasty over a 3-month follow-up period.

Perforation

Perforation remains a significant risk in performing dilatation of Crohn's strictures during deep enteroscopy. Deep enteroscopy with balloon dilation of strictures has a reported perforation risk of 0% to 3%.[28] There are reports of 10% perforations, especially of anastomotic strictures.

In a reported multicenter US Experience with 2254 patients, the risk appeared to be higher in these patients undergoing retrograde examinations in the face of surgically altered anatomy.[29] Endoscopists performing such procedures are well aware of this risk; and although there is heightened risk in patients with CD and strictures, they are not by themselves prohibitive. As with all advanced therapeutic procedures, a deliberative approach includes proper weighing of risk and benefit. This heuristic balance helps to yield optimal results.

CONCLUSION

Deep enteroscopy heralded by the advent of DBE has extended the endoscopist role in the management of many diseases of the small intestine. The ability to reach lesions and perform therapeutic maneuvers has improved treatment potential for patients with Crohn's-related strictures. This approach should be preferentially explored as a treatment option in CD patients who have stricturing disease of the small intestine. This chapter reviews the limits of length and risk of perforation.

Editor's note (TMB): Double balloon enteroscopy has proven helpful in removing retained video endoscopic capsules in patients with Crohn's Disease. (Okolo et al., ASGE video session, DDW 2011.)

References

1. Yamamoto H, Sekine Y, Sato Y, et al. Total enteroscopy with a nonsurgical steerable double-balloon method. *Gastrointest Endosc.* 2001;53(2):216–220.
2. Ogoshi K, Hara Y, Ashizawa S. New technic for small intestinal fiberoscopy. *Gastrointest Endosc.* 1973;20(2):64–65.
3. Foutch PG, Sawyer R, Sanowski RA. Push-enteroscopy for diagnosis of patients with gastrointestinal bleeding of obscure origin. *Gastrointest Endosc.* 1990;36(4):337–341.
4. Pennazio M, Arrigoni A, Risio M, Spandre M, Rossini FP. Clinical evaluation of push-type enteroscopy. *Endoscopy.* 1995;27(2):164–170.
5. Perez-Cuadrado E, Macenlle R, Iglesias J, Fabra R, Lamas D. Usefulness of oral video push enteroscopy in Crohn's disease. *Endoscopy.* 1997;29(8):745–747.
6. Tsujikawa T, Saitoh Y, Andoh A, et al. Novel single-balloon enteroscopy for diagnosis and treatment of the small intestine: preliminary experiences. *Endoscopy.* 2008;40(1):11–15.
7. Yamamoto H, Kita H, Sunada K, et al. Clinical outcomes of double-balloon endoscopy for the diagnosis and treatment of small-intestinal diseases. *Clin Gastroenterol Hepatol.* 2004;2(11):1010–1016.
8. Pohl J, May A, Nachbar L, Ell C. Diagnostic and therapeutic yield of push-and-pull enteroscopy for symptomatic small bowel Crohn's disease strictures. *Eur J Gastroenterol Hepatol.* 2007;19(7):529–534.
9. Akerman PA, Agrawal D, Cantero D, Pangtay J. Spiral enteroscopy with the new DSB overtube: a novel technique for deep peroral small-bowel intubation. *Endoscopy.* 2008;40(12):974–978.
10. Buscaglia JM, Dunbar KB, Okolo PI 3rd, et al. The spiral enteroscopy training initiative: results of a prospective study evaluating the Discovery SB overtube device during small bowel enteroscopy (with video). *Endoscopy.* 2009;41(3):194–199.
11. Sunada K, Yamamoto H, Kita H, et al. Clinical outcomes of enteroscopy using the double-balloon method for strictures of the small intestine. *World J Gastroenterol.* 2005;11(7):1087–1089.

12. Cheifetz AS, Lewis BS. Capsule endoscopy retention: is it a complication? *J Clin Gastroenterol.* 2006;40(8):688–691.

13. Fry LC, Carey EJ, Shiff AD, et al. The yield of capsule endoscopy in patients with abdominal pain or diarrhea. *Endoscopy.* 2006;38(5):498–502.

14. Aoun E, Abdul-Baki H, Azar C, et al. A randomized single-blind trial of split-dose PEG-electrolyte solution without dietary restriction compared with whole dose PEG-electrolyte solution with dietary restriction for colonoscopy preparation. *Gastrointest Endosc.* 2005;62(2):213–218.

15. Picchio M, Gallinaro L, Ceci F, et al. Comparison of standard polyethylene glycol and two doses of oral sodium phosphate solution in precolonoscopy bowel preparation: a randomized controlled trial. *Acta Gastroenterol Belg.* 2008;71(1):15–20.

16. Abdul-Baki H, Hashash JG, Elhajj II, et al. A randomized, controlled, double-blind trial of the adjunct use of tegaserod in whole-dose or split-dose polyethylene glycol electrolyte solution for colonoscopy preparation. *Gastrointest Endosc.* 2008;68(2):294–300; quiz 334, 336.

17. Yano T, Yamamoto H, Kita H, et al. Technical modification of the double-balloon endoscopy to access to the proximal side of the stenosis in the distal colon. *Gastrointest Endosc.* 2005;62(2):302–304.

18. Despott EJ, Gupta A, Burling D, et al. Effective dilation of small-bowel strictures by double-balloon enteroscopy in patients with symptomatic Crohn's disease (with video). *Gastrointest Endosc.* 2009;70(5):1030–1036.

19. Couckuyt H, Gevers AM, Coremans G, Hiele M, Rutgeerts P. Efficacy and safety of hydrostatic balloon dilatation of ileocolonic Crohn's strictures: a prospective longterm analysis. *Gut.* 1995;36(4):577–580.

20. Munkholm P. Review article: the incidence and prevalence of colorectal cancer in inflammatory bowel disease. *Aliment Pharmacol Ther.* 2003;18(suppl 2):1–5.

21. Palascak-Juif V, Bouvier AM, Cosnes J, et al. Small bowel adenocarcinoma in patients with Crohn's disease compared with small bowel adenocarcinoma de novo. *Inflamm Bowel Dis.* 2005;11(9):828–832.

22. Dossett LA, White LM, Welch DC, et al. Small bowel adenocarcinoma complicating Crohn's disease: case series and review of the literature. *Am Surg.* 2007;73(11):1181–1187.

23. Lennon AM, Chandrasekhara V, Shin EJ, Okolo PI 3rd. Spiral-enteroscopy-assisted enteral stent placement for palliation of malignant small-bowel obstruction (with video). *Gastrointest Endosc.* 2010;71(2):422–425.

24. Pérez-Cuadrado E, Molina Pérez E. Multiple strictures in jejunal Crohn's disease: push enteroscopy dilation. *Endoscopy.* 2001;33(2):194.

25. Keuchel M. Double balloon (push-and-pull) enteroscopy: breakthrough in the management of small intestinal strictures in Crohn's disease? *Eur J Gastroenterol Hepatol.* 2007;19(7):523–525.

26. Kobayashi K, Haruki S, Sada M, Katsumata T, Saigenji K. Single-balloon enteroscopy. *Nippon Rinsho.* 2008;66(7):1371–1378.

27. Manes G, Imbesi V, Ardizzone S, Cassinotti A, Pallotta S, Porro GB. Use of double-balloon enteroscopy in the management of patients with Crohn's disease: feasibility and diagnostic yield in a high-volume centre for inflammatory bowel disease. *Surg Endosc.* 2009.

28. Mensink PB, Haringsma J, Kucharzik T, et al. Complications of double balloon enteroscopy: a multicenter survey. *Endoscopy.* 2007;39(7):613–615.

29. Gerson LB, Tokar J, Chiorean M, et al. Complications associated with double balloon enteroscopy at nine US centers. *Clin Gastroenterol Hepatol.* 2009;7(11):1177–1182, 1182.e1.

Endoscopic Treatment of Crohn's Primary and Anastomotic Stenoses

128

Richard A. Kozarek

Historically, treatment of gastrointestinal stenoses with dilation had been limited to accessible anatomic areas, primarily the esophagus or anorectum. With the advent of endoscopically or radiographically placed polyethylene balloons, a variety of gastric, colonic, biliary, and anastomotic strictures have become amenable to such therapy. The basic goals of stricture dilation include luminal enlargement in a safe and efficacious fashion and prevention of restenosis.[1] In the setting of Crohn's disease, the latter may include corticosteroids or mesalamine as well as immunosuppressive or biologic therapy following dilation of a colonic or anastomotic stricture.

It remains uncertain what the mechanisms of luminal enlargement are with many of the available dilating systems. Two basic theories have been espoused for stricture dilation: circumferential "stretch" versus stricture "split."[1] The former presupposes considerable elasticity to circumferential fibrous tissue; the latter presupposes an inherent stenosis rigidity in which dilation is effected by one or several longitudinal tears. Although it appears naïve to believe that a 3-mm diameter anastomotic or inflammatory stricture can be dilated to 10 or 15 mm without a significant laceration of scirrhous tissue and potentially of muscle, there are no good gross anatomic or histologic studies available postdilation.

● TECHNIQUE

Whether passed through a colonoscope, endoscope, or a single- or double-balloon enteroscope, the use of a through-the-scope dilator requires endoscopic approximation of the stricture size and selection of a balloon that is several mm larger. Both balloon and dilator shaft should be coated with silicone, and negative pressure may be required by means of a 10- to 20-mL syringe, particularly when reusing a balloon. These measures, as well as avoiding excessive angulation of the endoscopic tip, allow dilator passage until all or part of the balloon is visualized. The balloon is centered in the stenotic anastomosis or stenosis using endoscopic and, at times, concomitant fluoroscopic control. The latter also helps prevent damage of more proximal bowel wall related to excessive pressure of the balloon tip or extreme balloon angulation.

Although air can be used for inflation, a 10% or 25% contrast solution allows better visualization fluoroscopically and a more uniform balloon dilation. Technical efficacy in dilation requires obliteration of the balloon waist and ranges between 30 and 45 lb/in^2 (2–3 atm) for 10- and 15-mm balloons, respectively[1] (Fig. 128.1). More recently, continuous radial expansion dilators, with balloon diameter defined by the pressure delivered, have been marketed. Ranging in size from 6 to 8, 8 to 10, 10 to 12, 12 to 15, 15 to 18, and 18 to 20 mm in diameter, these balloons are 5.5 cm in length and can be passed over an 0.035-in guidewire. There are no data that demonstrate 2 minutes of continued inflation are advantageous over 15 seconds once a balloon waist has been effaced. I generally use 30 to 60 seconds of dilation and subsequently redilate a second or third time after repositioning of the balloon. Once dilation has been effected, complete evacuation of the balloon and straightening of the scope tip are required to allow retrieval. Additional larger dilating balloons can subsequently be used, but the degree of luminal enlargement in a single session remains a matter of common sense and is contingent on size of the initial stenosis, presence and degree of ulceration, and patient discomfort with initial dilation. As such, the ultimate goal is to dilate with a 15-mm balloon followed by complete endoscopic inspection of more proximal or distal bowel contingent upon whether the dilation is to be done colonoscopically or per os. This goal sometimes requires two or three dilating sessions separated by a several-day interval if the obstruction is acute or several-week interval if it is chronic.

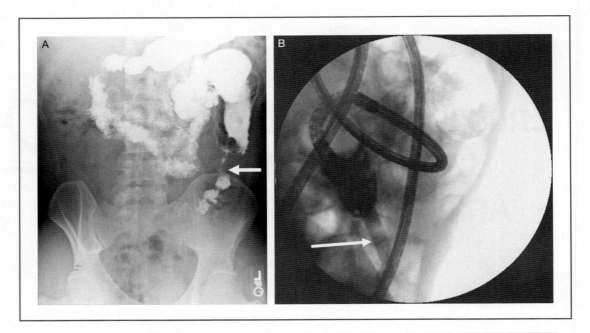

FIGURE 128.1 • Arrow demonstrates single high-grade jejunal stricture (A) with proximal small-bowel dilation treated 10- to 12-mm continuous radial expansion balloon dilation (B).

In addition to balloon dilation, three additional endoscopic methods of treating Crohn's stenoses have been described but applied sparingly. The first includes multiple radial cuts in short strictures using either a contact-tip laser or electrocautery, techniques previously applied to "defiant" lower esophageal rings.[2]

The second includes circumferential (4-quadrant) corticosteroid injections using a sclerotherapy needle.[3] The latter, applied to refractory keloids or esophageal reflux stenoses, usually entails injection of 40 to 100 mg of triamcinolone either concomitantly or in lieu of dilation.

Finally, fully covered self-expanding metal stents (SEMS) have been successfully placed to effect a sustained dilation. Such stents can be retrieved after several weeks if they do not pass spontaneously.[4]

● DISCUSSION

Table 128.1 synopses multiple series using balloon dilation for Crohn's disease strictures, both primary and anastomotic. Although the vast majority of stenoses can now be dilated, particularly with the advent of double-balloon enteroscopy, dilation therapy is far from a perfect technology. As such, stricture recurrence has ranged from 10% at 19 months to as high as 62% at 5 years. Moreover, surgery for failed symptomatic improvement or recurrent stricture approximates 25% and has been as high as 59% as reported in the paper by Thomas-Gibson et al.[10] Add to this a small but definite procedure-related perforation and bleeding rates, one recognizes the delicate balance required to use dilation as a therapeutic tool: proper patient selection (it is inappropriate to dilate fistulizing strictures or patients with a 20-cm long, primary or anastomotic stenosis), appropriate selection of a balloon diameter (inflating an 18-mm balloon with a 2-mm diameter, deeply ulcerated stricture cannot end well), and proper treatment of the underlying Crohn's disease (many of these patients with recurrent obstructive disease respond better to TNF inhibitors, natalizumab, or other immunosuppressive agents, than to 5-ASA preparations or steroids).

Corticosteroid injection has been added to balloon dilation by some practitioners (Table 128.1), usually injecting a long-acting preparation into the splits or tears following balloon dilation on the basis of success achieved using this technique for refractory radiation, caustic, and aced-peptic strictures. I personally inject stenoses every cm or so using 5-mg aliquots of triamcinolone up to a maximum of 50 mg in a single session if a previous dilation session led to no, or only short-lived, improvement. Results of steroid injection have been variable. Brooker et al. noted a sustained remission after a single procedure in 50% of their patients treated with dilation and steroids,[12] whereas Singh et al. noted a 76.5% overall success rate at a mean follow-up of 18.8 months in 17 patients.[14] There was a 10% stenosis recurrence in patients undergoing concomitant steroid injection compared to 31% in patients undergoing balloon dilation alone. In the only controlled trial reported to date, East et al. performed a pilot study randomizing seven patients to balloon dilation plus 40 mg of triamcinolone injection to balloon dilation and placebo injection of anastomotic ileocolonic strictures.[17] Not only did steroid injection fail to decrease the need for or interval of redilation, there was also a trend toward a worse outcome with steroid injection. The authors cautioned that the use of this technique should be carefully considered until more data are available.

TABLE 128.1 Comparison of the Performance Characteristics of Published Series of at Least 10 Patients Undergoing Endoscopic Balloon Dilation of Intestinal Strictures Due to Crohn's Disease

Reference	Number		Stricture Location	Success (%) per patient (per stricture)	Complications (%)		Median Follow-Up (months)	Stricture Recurrence (%)	Surgery for Stricture (%)
	Patients	Strictures Dilated			Bleeding	Perforation			
Bloomberg et al. (1991)[5]	27	137	—	66 (NR)	0	7	15	33	NR
Breysem et al. (1992)[6]	18	18	IC, C	78 (78)	0	0	25	33	27
Junge and Zuchner (1994)[7]	10	11	I, I-I, C	80 (82)	9	0	17	13	NR
Couckuyt et al. (1995)[8]	55	78	I, I-I, IC, I-Ca, C	62 (73)	0	11	33	62 at 5 years	38 at 5 years
Dear and Hunter (2001)[9]	22	71	—	73 (NR)	0	0	44	33	27
Thomas-Gibson et al. (2003)[10]	59	124	I-I, C, I-Ca, pouch-ileal	77 (82)	2	5	30	59	59
Sabate et al. (2003)[11]	38	53	J, I, C, IC	84 (89)	3	3	23	36 at 1 year / 60 at 5 years	26 at 1 year / 43 at 5 years
Morini et al. (2003)[12]	43	45	I, I-I, I-C, I-Ca	79 (76)	5.8	0	64	37	26
Brooker et al. (2003)[13]	14	26+		50 (80)	0	0	16	29	21
Singh et al. (2005)[14]	17	29**	D, I, I-C, C	77 (97)	0	10	19	10 vs. 31**	24
Ferlitsch et al. (2006)[15]	46	73	I, C, I-C	85 (82)	5	3	21	62	28
Ajlouni et al. (2007)[16]	37	83	I, C, I-C, I-Ca, I-I	84 (90)	3	0	21	26	13

†Included 20 strictures into which corticosteroids were injected.
**Included a comparison of 11 strictures having corticosteroid injection with 18 having no corticosteroids.
C, primary colonic stricture; I, primary ileal stricture; I-C, ileocolonic; I-Ca, ileocecal; I-I, stricture at ileo-ileal anastomosis; J, primary jejunal stricture; NR, not reported.
Reprinted with permission from Ajlouni Y, Iser JH, Gibson PR. Endoscopic balloon dilatation of intestinal strictures in Crohn's disease: safe alternative to surgery. *J Gastroenterol Hepatol.* 2007;22(4):489.

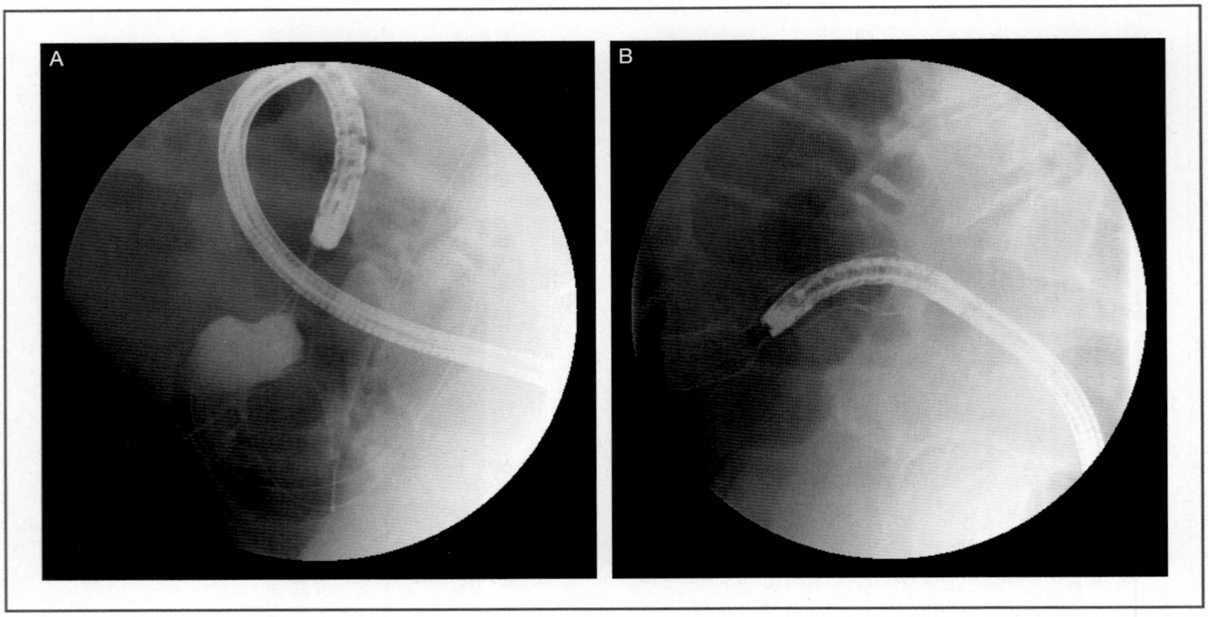

FIGURE 128.2 • High-grade colonic obstruction in high-risk patient with refractory sigmoid stenosis (A) treated with self-expandable metal stent (SEMS) (B). Prosthesis removed at 6 weeks.

TABLE 128.2 Factors Associated with Improved Procedural/Clinical Success in Balloon Dilation of Crohn's Strictures

Short stenoses (<5 cm)
Balloon diameter
Fibrotic vs. inflammatory stenosis
Adequate control of inflammatory process (? immunosuppressives/biologics)

TABLE 128.3 Factors Unproven to Affect the Efficacy of Balloon Dilation for Crohn's Disease

Small bowel vs. colonic site*
Anastomotic vs. primary stenosis
Steroid injection
Oral steroids/mesalamine
Radial electrocautery
Self-expandable metal stent

*Assumes endoscopic access.

Two other techniques have been sparingly applied in the treatment of refractory Crohn's disease strictures: radial cuts with a needle-knife sphincterotome and the placement of SEMS. From the former standpoint, Rolny et al. dilated 27 patients with anastomotic Crohn's disease strictures, 2 of whom developed acute perforation from radial incisions with electrocautery.[2] I neither utilize nor recommend this technique. From the latter standpoint, SEMS have been occasionally inserted into benign stenoses, including Crohn's disease, as a bridge to elective surgery in acute left-colon obstruction (Fig. 128.2). In the largest series to date, Small et al. placed SEMS in 23 patients with benign colorectal obstruction, only one of whom, however, had Crohn's disease.[4] Major complications occurred in 38%, including 4 patients who had reobstruction; 2, migration; and 2, perforation. It is obvious that these results are suboptimal, and routine SEMS placement cannot be routinely recommended for Crohn's disease strictures at this time.

Tables 128.2 and 128.3 depict factors within my own practice as well as those gleaned from a critical review of the literature that have the potential to affect efficacy of balloon dilation for Crohn's stenoses.

CONCLUSIONS

The ability to dilate a Crohn's stenosis does not imply that dilation is the procedure of choice in every case. For instance, patients with concomitant fistulous disease, patients in whom neoplasia cannot be ruled out, and patients with multiple strictures or a long stenosis are better handled with surgical resection or stricturoplasty (Fig. 128.3). Moreover, to maintain efficacy, subsequent medical control of the gut inflammation is essential. Whether this is immunosuppressive, or some combination of mesalamine, steroids, or antibiotics, must be individualized to the patient in question.

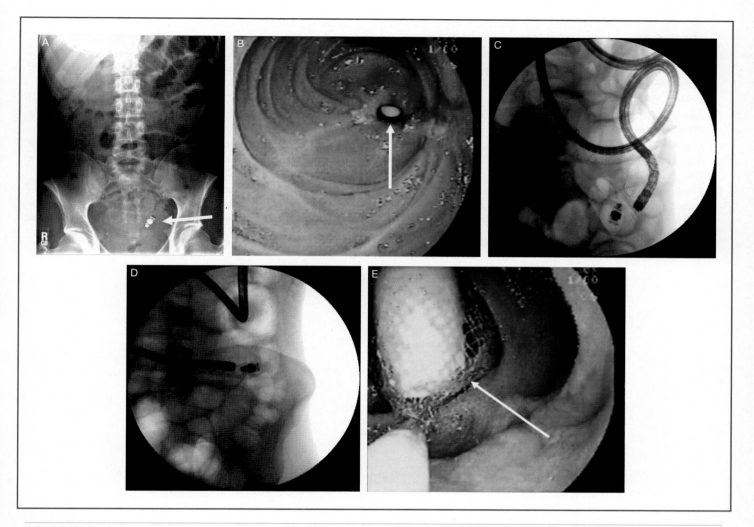

FIGURE 128.3 • Arrow demonstrates small-bowel PillCam™ in series of stenoses in patient with jejunal CD (A) (B). Capsule removed with Roth net using double-balloon enteroscope (C, D, E). Given the number and length of stenoses, patient underwent segmental small-bowel resection rather than attempt at balloon dilation.

Editor's note (TMB): Stricture Dilatation: In a May 2011 DDW abstract (No. 853, A 208), A. Gustavsson et al. described a large series of 776 dilatations in 178 patients with structuring CD. Eighty percent were anastamotic. Surgical resection was postponed, for an average of 3.4 years, in half of the patients and was avoided in the other half. The complication rate was 5.3%.

References

1. Lord JD, Kozarek RA. Gastrointestinal dilation and stent placement. In: Yamada T, Alpers DH, Owyang C, Powell DH, Kalloo A, eds. *Textbook of Gastroenterology,* 5th ed. Oxford: Blackwell; 2008:2958–2973.

2. Rolny P. Anastomotic strictures in Crohn's disease: a new field for therapeutic endoscopy. *Gastrointest Endosc.* 1993;39(6):862–864.

3. Lavy A. Steroid injection improves outcome in Crohn's disease strictures. *Endoscopy.* 1994;26(4):366.

4. Small AJ, Young-Fadok TM, Baron TH. Expandable metal stent placement for benign colorectal obstruction: outcomes for 23 cases. *Surg Endosc.* 2008;22(2):454–462.

5. Blomberg B, Rolny P, Järnerot G. Endoscopic treatment of anastomotic strictures in Crohn's disease. *Endoscopy.* 1991;23(4):195–198.

6. Breysem Y, Janssens JF, Coremans G, Vantrappen G, Hendrickx G, Rutgeerts P. Endoscopic balloon dilation of colonic and ileocolonic Crohn's strictures: long-term results. *Gastrointest Endosc.* 1992;38(2):142–147.

7. Junge U, Züchner H. [Endoscopic balloon dilatation of symptomatic strictures in Crohn's disease]. *Dtsch Med Wochenschr.* 1994;119(41):1377–1382.

8. Couckuyt H, Gevers AM, Coremans G, Hiele M, Rutgeerts P. Efficacy and safety of hydrostatic balloon dilatation of ileocolonic Crohn's strictures: a prospective long-term analysis. *Gut.* 1995;36(4):577–580.

9. Dear KL, Hunter JO. Colonoscopic hydrostatic balloon dilatation of Crohn's strictures. *J Clin Gastroenterol.* 2001;33(4):315–318.

10. Thomas-Gibson S, Brooker JC, Hayward CM, Shah SG, Williams CB, Saunders BP. Colonoscopic balloon dilation of Crohn's strictures: a review of long-term outcomes. *Eur J Gastroenterol Hepatol.* 2003;15(5):485–488.

11. Sabaté JM, Villarejo J, Bouhnik Y, et al. Hydrostatic balloon dilatation of Crohn's strictures. *Aliment Pharmacol Ther.* 2003;18(4):409–413.

12. Morini S, Hassan C, Lorenzetti R, et al. Long-term outcome of endoscopic pneumatic dilatation in Crohn's disease. *Dig Liver Dis.* 2003;35(12):893–897.

13. Brooker JC, Beckett CG, Saunders BP, Benson MJ. Long-acting steroid injection after endoscopic dilation of anastomotic Crohn's strictures may improve the outcome: a retrospective case series.

Endoscopy. 2003;35(4):333–337.

14. Singh VV, Draganov P, Valentine J. Efficacy and safety of endoscopic balloon dilation of symptomatic upper and lower gastrointestinal Crohn's disease strictures. *J Clin Gastroenterol.* 2005;39(4):284–290.

15. Ferlitsch A, Reinisch W, Püspök A, et al. Safety and efficacy of endoscopic balloon dilation for treatment of Crohn's disease strictures. *Endoscopy.* 2006;38(5):483–487.

16. Ajlouni Y, Iser JH, Gibson PR. Endoscopic balloon dilatation of intestinal strictures in Crohn's disease: safe alternative to surgery. *J Gastroenterol Hepatol.* 2007;22(4):486–490.

17. East JE, Brooker JC, Rutter MD, Saunders BP. A pilot study of intrastricture steroid versus placebo injection after balloon dilatation of Crohn's strictures. *Clin Gastroenterol Hepatol.*

Surgery for Crohn's Colitis

PART

X

Surgery for Crohn's Colitis

Indications and Procedures for Surgery of Small-Bowel Crohn's Disease

129

Sharon L. Stein and Fabrizio Michelassi

The etiology of Crohn's disease is unknown, and no curative treatment has yet been discovered. Despite substantial advances in medical treatments, relapses, complications, and recurrences are frequent, and the overwhelming majority of patients ultimately require a surgical resection. More concerning is that 50% of patients will require additional surgeries during their lifetime. Multiple resections increase the risk of inadequate intestinal length leading to nutritional and fluid deficiencies. The goals of surgery are, therefore, to treat symptoms and complications of the disease while minimizing the magnitude of the surgical intervention. This chapter will cover the indications for surgical treatment of Crohn's disease, operative treatment for small-bowel disease, and surgical strategies for intestinal preservation.

● INDICATIONS FOR SURGICAL INTERVENTION

Medical Failure

The most common indication for surgical intervention in Crohn's disease had been medically refractory disease. Progression of disease may render patients symptomatic despite best medical therapy. Chronic weight loss, diarrhea, or abdominal pain may be indications to consider surgical therapy. Steroids, which may be used during an acute Crohn's disease flare, have not been shown to be successful in maintenance therapy. Failure to wean from steroids occurs in up to 30% of patients and may require surgical intervention. Patients may experience side effects or intolerance to steroids or other medications despite efficacy in treatment. Immunologics such as 6-mercaptopurine and azathioprine may result in pancreatitis, hepatitis, and bone marrow suppression. Patients may develop intolerance or reactions to biologics. As new medications are discovered to treat Crohn's disease, side-effect profiles escalate and may be unacceptable to some patients. Inability to maintain treatment secondary to side effects, intolerance, or patient desire is an indication to consider surgical options.

Editor's note (TMB): The advent of anti-TNF agents has decreased the need for surgery for active luminal disease.

Intestinal Obstruction

Patients with Crohn's disease often develop symptoms of chronic obstruction, including nausea, anorexia, diarrhea, and obstipation. Acute treatment of obstruction includes bowel rest, antibiotics, and nasogastric tube insertion. Approximately 50% of patients with inflammatory disease will respond acutely to treatment with immunosuppressants and bowel rest. Stricturing disease is less likely than inflammatory disease to improve with conservative management, and patients with continued symptoms despite medical therapy warrant surgical intervention (Fig. 129.1). Acute obstruction is a less common presentation of Crohn's disease and standard surgical evaluation of etiology, including adhesions from prior surgery, should be used.

Editor's note (TMB): There are separate chapters on small bowel and on colonic stenosis.

Sepsis

Abscess and Inflammatory Mass

Patients with Crohn's disease may present with an abscess from a contained perforation. Patients with generalized peritoneal signs should undergo immediate laparotomy, but most patients present with less definitive findings. On physical exam, a phlegmon or mass may be palpated. Leukocytosis and electrolyte disturbances are common. Radiographic evaluation consists of an upright chest radiograph to rule out a pneumoperitoneum and computed tomography scan to identify an inflammatory mass or abscess. In stable patients, initial management includes fluid resuscitation, administration of antibiotics, bowel rest, and percutaneous drainage if an abscess is present. Most patients will

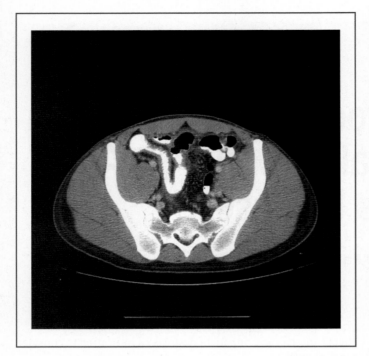

FIGURE 129.1 • Computed tomography demonstrating long segment of ileitis in patients with Crohn's disease. Patient failed medical management and require laparoscopic ileocectomy for treatment. Printed with Permission of New York Presbyterian Hospital, Weill Cornell Medical School.

ultimately undergo a resection, but initial nonoperative management allows for resolution of inflammation and minimizes resection of affected but otherwise healthy bowel.

Editor's note (TMB): There is a separate chapter on the management of intraabdominal abscesses.

Fistula

Enteroenteric Fistula

Fistulization occur in up to 30% of patients. Enteroenteric fistulization is often asymptomatic and discovered incidentally during surgery. Signs of complicated Crohn's disease, including abscess or local fistulization apparent on CT scan, may be indicators of more extensive abdominal involvement, and patients should be aware that additional findings may be encountered intraoperatively. Bowel-to-bowel fistulas typically become symptomatic only when associated with significant fecal diversion. When long segments of small intestine are bypassed, loss of absorptive intestinal surface area may occur, resulting in diarrhea, enteropathy, and protein wasting. Disease from the terminal ileum frequently fistulizes to the sigmoid, whereas the duodenum is more likely to be involved in recurrent disease from the neoterminal ileum. Intraoperative treatment of a fistula consists of resection of the primarily diseased bowel and assessment recipient segment. Typically, the recipient side of the fistula is not diseased. In this case, the recipient side is refreshed and closed primarily, or a wedge resection and repair are performed. Only if the recipient appears diseased should this be resected as well.

Enterocutaneous, Enterovaginal, and Enterovesical Fistulas

Enterocutaneous fistulas may occur in as much as 15% of patients (Fig. 129.2). Resection of the diseased bowel and appropriate drainage of the fistula track should be sufficient for treatment in primary disease. Many patients with enterocutaneous fistulas have complicated surgical histories, with multiple prior resections and loss of abdominal domain. Treatment in these cases may require nutritional, medical, and surgical optimization, including total parental nutrition, pharmacologic treatment, and diversion of fecal stream. Biologic therapy, such as infliximab, has been shown to have significant short-term success, but recurrence is common in this population and surgical intervention may ultimately be necessary.

Enterovaginal fistulas occur in women who have had prior hysterectomies. Malodorous drainage may be noted, and irritation of perineal skin from incontinence of vaginal discharge may be noted. When symptomatic fistulas arise from the small bowel, options include treatment with biologic therapy or primary resection. Crohn's disease may also fistulize to the bladder. Typical symptoms include fecaluria and pneumaturia. Recurrent urinary infections may result in pyelonephritis, in which case surgery is warranted to prevent renal dysfunction from repeat infections. The bladder can be closed with simple repair, and a Foley catheter is left in place postoperatively to avoid bladder over distention.

Hemorrhage

Acute hemorrhage is a rare complication of Crohn's disease. Identifying the source of bleeding may be difficult. Colonoscopy can demonstrate bleeding from the colon or terminal ileum, but it fails to assess small-bowel hemorrhage. Tagged red-blood-cell studies and angiography may identify the source in the mobile small intestines but may lead to difficulties in localization during surgical exploration. If the site of bleeding is noted during angiography, a catheter may be left in situ to help identify the source intraoperatively. Capsule endoscopy may be used for chronic bleeding but is not appropriate for acute hemorrhage. In a patient with unidentified bleeding source, an on-table enteroscopy can be performed, with the endoscopist examining the bowel lumen while the surgeon manipulates the intestines over the scope to increase visualization.

Cancer or Suspicion of Cancer

Patients with Crohn's disease are at increased risk of gastrointestinal cancers. Colon cancer is the most common gastrointestinal malignancy in Crohn's disease, though cancers of the small intestine have also been reported. Site of neoplasia includes areas of inflammation and stenosis; any questionable loop of bowel should be resected or biopsied to determine possible neoplastic involvement. Appropriate treatment includes segmental resection with en bloc lymph-node resection.

Growth Retardation

Children with Crohn's disease may suffer from growth retardation secondary to malnutrition associated with chronic active disease. Up to 25% of children may be affected. Steroids have

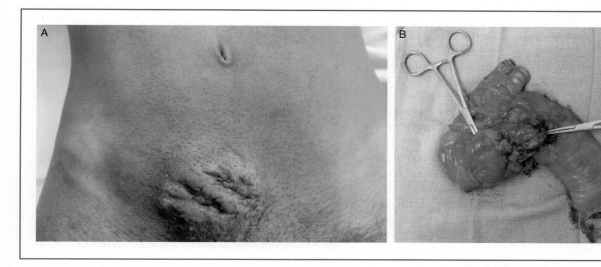

FIGURE 129.2 • (A) Enterocutaneous fistula in Crohn's disease. Patient with recurrent, untreated ileocecal disease, presented with fistula to anterior abdominal wall and drainage. Ileocecal resection was performed with open packing of the anterior abdominal wall. (B) Gross resection specimen demonstrating internal fistulas between ileum and colon. Printed with Permission of New York Presbyterian Hospital, Weill Cornell Medical School.

also been shown to alter growth in children and are a consideration. Studies have demonstrated that surgical resection may minimize long-term growth retardation and should be considered in surgically appropriate patients.

SURGICAL TREATMENT OF CROHN'S DISEASE

Preoperative Preparation

Prior to elective surgical intervention, evaluation of the entire gastrointestinal tract is performed to assess extent of disease, create an appropriate operative plan, and counsel the patient regarding surgical options. The small-bowel assessment includes endoscopic and radiographic studies. Upper endoscopy evaluates the esophagus, stomach, and proximal duodenum but fails to provide information about the more distal small bowel. This may be supplemented with a small-bowel follow-through to elucidate the presence of mucosal and stricturing disease in the jejunum and ileum. Alternatively, computed tomography and computed tomographic enterography can be used to assess both intralumenal and extralumenal disease, including the presence of extralumenal abscess and phelgmons. Oral and IV contrast are routinely used. Patients who have had prior ileocecal resections may benefit from a contrast enema study that evaluates the neoileum and ileocolonic anastomosis or colonoscopy with ileal intubation that assesses the terminal ileum and provides biopsies for pathologic assessment.

Patients who require surgery emergently or urgently may be unable to undergo additional diagnostic studies. Often a CT with oral and IV contrast may be the only preoperative assessment. In these cases, both the patient and surgeon must be prepared for intraoperative evaluation and therapeutic treatment as appropriate.

The surgeon should have a thorough knowledge of medications commonly used in Crohn's disease, to appropriately treat the patient preoperatively. Steroid-dependent patients will require perioperative stress doses of steroids to prevent adrenal insufficiency. Data regarding preoperative use of methotrexate and infliximab are mixed, with some studies reporting increased rate of perioperative complications. Consideration of discontinuing these medications prior to surgery is appropriate and should be discussed with the patient and gastroenterologist. Biologics such as infliximab may take as long as 8 to 12 weeks for serum levels to return to normal. Other medications such as 5-ASA derivatives, 6-MP, and azathioprine have not been associated with increased perioperative complications.

Editor's note (TMB): Questions about increased sepsis after colonic surgery in patients on anti-TNF agents are discussed in other chapters.

Fluid and electrolyte abnormalities should be addressed prior to surgery. Patients with chronic disease may have significant metabolic derangements on presentation. Fluid resuscitation and correction of electrolyte imbalance should be performed preoperatively. Profound anemia and coagulopathies should be treated. In rare cases of severe malnutrition, patients may benefit from preoperative nutritional supplementation prior to undergoing surgery.

Patients undergoing elective surgery may be considered for preoperative bowel preparation. Although recent data have demonstrated the safety of anastomosis in unprepped bowel, the authors continue to use mechanical bowel preparation in selected cases. In complicated disease, a more extensive resection than predicted by preoperative imaging may be necessary. Bowel preparation allows for intraoperative examination of lumenal surfaces, while using techniques such as colonoscopy. In addition, should a diversion be necessary, a bowel preparation will reduce the fecal load between the stoma and anastomosis and will help to mediate the possible complications should an anastomotic leak occur.

Operative Strategy

The initial phase in a surgical procedure for Crohn's disease is a total abdominal exploration with assessment of intestinal involvement. Despite preoperative imaging, it is not uncommon to discover additional involved intestine intraoperatively. The entire length of small intestine from ligament of Treitz to ileocecal valve should be examined. Signs of disease such as creeping fat, corkscrewing, hyperemia, thickened mesentery, and intestinal dilation are recorded in the operative record. If stricture or narrowing is noted in the proximal or mid small bowel, the distal bowel is assessed for synchronous lesions. Surgical treatment of an upstream occlusion can render downstream narrowing symptomatic in the early postoperative period, leading to symptoms of early recurrence. Adhesions from prior operations, fistulas, or abscess formation may complicate operative exploration and hinder assessment, but a thorough evaluation must be performed as concomitant disease is common.[1,2]

Intestinal Resection

Intestinal resection of severely diseased segments continues to be the most common surgical procedure performed in patients with Crohn's disease. Ileocecal involvement is the most common location and traditionally treated with an ileocectomy. Several studies have demonstrated that resection should be limited to severe disease. Resection of microscopic or minimal disease does not decrease recurrence rates or prevent recurrence. In addition, resection of addition length of small bowel may increase the possibility of short-gut syndrome. The most seriously diseased segment, including areas with fistula or abscess formation, is resected. Resection is performed to soft, pliable tissue that will allow for the performance of a stapled or handsewn anastomosis. Although staplers have been demonstrated to be safe and perhaps decrease recurrence rates in Crohn's disease, performance of a handsewn anastomosis may be necessary in a setting of intestinal luminal-size discrepancy, or diseased bowel, to ensure a secure anastomosis. Construction of an ample anastomosis is important: The most common site of recurrence is proximal to a prior anastomosis.

Preservation of innocent bystander loops is enhanced by preoperative treatment of inflammatory disease with antibiotics and bowel rest. Normal bowel may abut diseased segments, and operating during the acute period may result in resection of secondarily involved intestine. A rest period, at times with TPN, prior to surgery may help reduce length of resection. Closed-suction drains are left in abscess cavities and removed when drainage decreases typically 2 to 3 days after surgery.

Editor's note (TMB): There is a chapter on perioperative nutrition.

Strictureplasty

Strictureplasty techniques were first described in the treatment of small-bowel Crohn's disease in the 1980s by Lee and Papaioannou. Techniques were borrowed from tubercular surgeries in which a narrowing in the small bowel was retailored to create a larger lumenal opening (Fig. 129.3). Strictureplasties are commonly used to prevent extended resection of long lengths of disease bowel, especially if resection would leave 100 cm or less of nondiseased bowel. These patients may be left with short-gut syndrome requiring parental nutritional supplementation

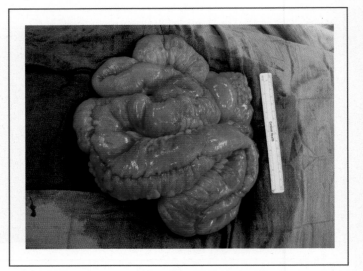

FIGURE 129.3 • Strictureplasty: intraoperative photo demonstrate a long side-to-side isoperistaltic strictureplasty. The severely diseased segments of intestine have been apposed to relatively normal segments, allowing for restoration of fecal stream without resection of intestinal length. Printed with Permission of New York Presbyterian Hospital, Weill Cornell Medical School.

and significant protein and fluid enteropathy. In addition, strictureplasty is appropriate in the setting of recurrent disease, which often occurs at the site of a prior intestinal anastomosis. Strictureplasty has been shown to be safe in duodenal, small-bowel, ileocolic disease and active disease. They are contraindicated in the presence of generalized sepsis, long unyielding segments of disease, and in the presence of cancer or dysplasia.

The main advantage of strictureplasty is the preservation of normal segments of bowel that abut intermittent strictures. Often strictures are small skip lesions, and it may be difficult or impossible to preserve intervening normal intestines. In addition, there is increased evidence that the acuity of the disease decreases at the site of the strictureplasty and the disease becomes quiescent postoperatively. Endoscopic and radiographic studies demonstrate a normal lumenal appearance on follow-up studies. Whether this correlates with a simultaneous restoration of absorptive function has not yet been established. The incidence of postoperative recurrence is lower at a strictureplasty site than at the site of an intestinal resection.[3–5] Techniques for resection will be covered in a separate chapter within the text.

Intestinal Bypass

Although bypass procedures were once performed routinely to simplify operations on patients with Crohn's disease, they are no longer performed regularly. Initially, it was believed that bypassed segments were at increased risk of malignant transformation, but this is not supported in the literature. As surgeons have gained experience and confidence in operating on Crohn's disease patients, resection and strictureplasty have become the mainstays of treatment. Bypass procedures are still performed for duodenal obstruction, which may otherwise require pancreaticoduodenectomy or biliary bypass.

● APPROACH

Several studies have demonstrated the efficacy and safety of laparoscopic surgery in patients with Crohn's disease.[6,7] Laparoscopy results in shorter hospital stays, decreased pain requirement, and decreased rates of complications. In addition, cosmetic benefits may be considerable, especially in a young, body-conscious population of Crohn's disease patients. However, laparoscopy in Crohn's disease can be a challenging task and should be performed by experienced laparoscopic surgeons. Significant adhesions from previous surgical interventions or disease, thickened mesentery, abscess, and fistulas complicate Crohn's disease and may require a traditional open approach. Attempts to perform minimally invasive surgery should never compromise the completeness of abdominal exploration, assessment of disease, and appropriate options for treatment.

Postoperative Care

Postoperatively, patients with Crohn's disease may require special treatment. In the case of an abscess or perforation, the patient will be kept on antibiotics postoperatively until signs of infection have dissipated. In patients with poor nutrition, parental supplementation may be indicated. Patients on steroids chronically require stress doses to prevent adrenal suppression. Although data are not yet definitive, there appears to be a correlation with patients taking biologics preoperatively and an increased rate of infectious complications postoperatively. These patients should be monitored closely in the early postoperative period. Appropriate consultation with gastroenterology should be obtained to evaluate the patient for risk of postoperative recurrence and consideration of early immunoprophylaxis therapy.

Editor's note (TMB): The chapter on efforts to prevent postoperative recurrences includes the use of anti-TNF agents to provide postoperative care for selected patients.

References

1. Fichera A, Lovadina S, Rubin M, et al. Patterns and operative treatment of recurrent Crohn's disease: a prospective longitudinal study. *Surgery.* 2006;140(4):649–654

2. Fichera A, Michelassi F. Surgical treatment of Crohn's disease. *J Gastrointest Surg.* 2007;11(6):791–803.

3. Hurst RD, Michelassi F. Strictureplasty for Crohn's disease: techniques and long-term results. *World J Surg.* 1998;22:359–363.

4. Lesperance K, Martin MJ, Lehmann R, et al. National trends and outcomes for the surgical therapy of ileocolonic Crohn's disease: a population based analysis of laparoscopic versus open approaches. *J Gastrointest Surg.* 2009;13:1251–1259.

5. Michelassi F. Side-to-side isoperistaltic strictureplasty for multiple Crohn's strictures. *Dis Colon Rectum.* 1996;39(3):345–349.

6. Michelassi F, Tashieri A, Tonelli F, et al. An international, multicenter, prospective, observational study of the side-to-side isoperistaltic strictureplasty in Crohn's disease. *Dis Colon Retum.* 2007;50(3):277–284.

7. Stocchi L, Milsom JW, Fazio VW. Long-term outcomes of laparoscopic versus open ileocolic resection for Crohn's disease: follow-up of a prospective randomized trial. *Surgery.* 2008;144(4):622–627.

Pediatric IBD Surgery | 130

Cathy E. Shin

Inflammatory bowel disease (IBD) occurs relatively frequently in the pediatric population and presents unique challenges in this age group. The definitions of ulcerative colitis (UC) and Crohn's disease (CD) in the general population have been reviewed in other chapters and are equally applicable to the pediatric population. Approximately 25% to 30% of patients with CD and 20% of patients with UC present before the age of 20. The challenge of treating children and adolescents with IBD relates to the fact that they are constantly changing both physically and psychologically.

Therefore, therapy for pediatric IBD is multimodal and encompasses medicines, nutritional support, psychological treatment, and ultimately, surgery. From the pediatric surgical point of view, the correct diagnosis and surgical treatment is crucial for a successful outcome, which we define as treating the child's symptoms, improving quality of life and preventing cancer.

DIAGNOSIS

The diagnosis of pediatric IBD should be suspected in almost any patient with chronic gastrointestinal (GI) symptoms. The diagnosis is supported initially by the presence of a family history of IBD and weight loss or failure to thrive in combination with novel laboratory evidence to support an IBD diagnosis. However, a definitive diagnosis requires endoscopic and radiographic evaluation.

The work up for pediatric IBD includes

- history and physical
- family history
- growth chart, pubertal staging, and bone age
- hematologic and biochemical studies
- stools for bacterial pathogens, ova and parasites, *C. difficile* toxin
- imaging studies
- endoscopy (including capsule) with biopsies.

Unfortunately, there is no gold standard for the diagnosis of pediatric IBD. The diagnosis is often difficult, as the presenting symptoms can be quite vague. Some children present with abdominal pain and depression and are, therefore, referred to a psychologist rather than to a pediatric gastroenterologist. Such delay in diagnosis accounts for the high incidence of growth failure in pediatric IBD. In fact, growth failure may be the presenting symptom in the absence of any specific GI symptoms.[1] Following the growth curve is, therefore, essential in the monitoring of pediatric IBD.

Radiologic evaluation is often helpful to image the small and large bowel as well as bone age to record the degree of developmental delay. A GI contrast series is helpful in CD patients with strictures and fistula formation (Fig. 130.1 and 130.2). Recent advances in imaging include computed tomography

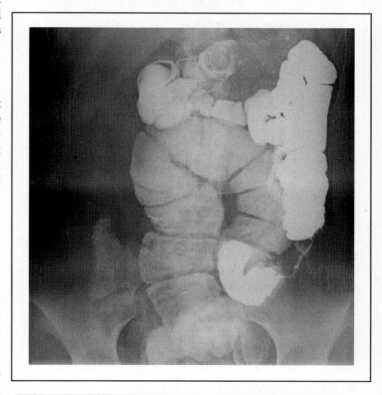

FIGURE 130.1 • 14y with Crohn's Disease jejunal- sigmoid fistula.

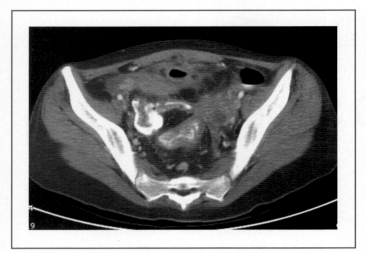

FIGURE 130.2 • 16y with Crohn's Disease inflammatory mass with abscess formation.

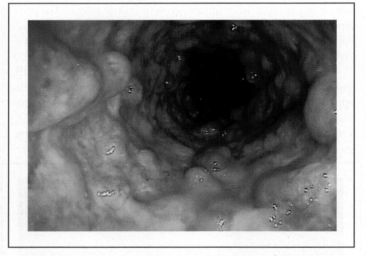

FIGURE 130.3 • 13y Crohn's Disease psuedopolyps seen in colonoscopy.

scans, which are excellent for distinguishing fibrostenotic from inflammatory strictures, and magnetic resonance imaging (MRI), which has become increasingly helpful in the diagnosis and management of perianal CD.

Despite advances in serologic testing and imaging, however, endoscopic biopsy is essential to confirm the clinical diagnosis. Colonoscopy is the usual endoscopic examination of choice in suspected cases of IBD (Fig. 130.3). When CD is suspected, the colonoscopy should include visualization of the terminal ileum. The classic findings of UC and CD on endoscopy and histology have been reviewed in detail elsewhere and are similar in children and adults.[2]

INDETERMINATE COLITIS

Although less common, indeterminate colitis (IC) should be considered in the differential of pediatric IBD. IC is generally characterized by early onset in the first years of life and rapid progression to pancolitis. The definition has changed throughout the years, but this remains a legitimate diagnosis and should be considered before irreversible surgical treatment is performed.[3] Because a high incidence of pouch failure after total proctocolectomy with ileoanal anastomosis (IAA) has been described in patients with IC, perhaps a subtotal colectomy and ileostomy with preservation of the rectum should be considered to allow for analysis of the entire specimen for a definite diagnosis.[4,5] It has recently been suggested that patients with IC who are anti-*Saccharomyces cerevisiae* antibody positive are more likely to have CD, which obviously has the potential to alter the surgical approach.

In spite of advances in diagnostic tools in radiology, endoscopy, and pathology, a small population of children initially diagnosed with UC may later exhibit the characteristics of CD. There is a chance that, after surgical correction of UC or IC, signs and symptoms of CD may emerge. In one study, low body weight and body mass index at the time of surgery was observed more often in children with UC who subsequently manifested CD in the postoperative period.[6]

SURGICAL MANAGEMENT

Therapy for pediatric IBD is multimodal, and surgery is just part of a successful outcome. In our institution, both children and parents are educated about the surgical options well in advance and encouraged to talk to other children and families that have already gone through such procedures.

More specifically, most pediatric surgeons would agree that the severely diseased IBD patients should undergo surgical treatment while the epiphyses are still open to allow for optimal growth and development. In view of the cumulative side effects of mediations to treat IBD, the option for surgery in children should be considered when symptoms require prolonged intense therapy. The concept of surgery involving bowel resections, pouch creations, and ileostomies at a critical time of physical and emotional development often deters both children and parents.

The ostomy is a source of embarrassment for the child and important to address as a young child and teenager. Consultation with the enterostomal therapist and ability to talk to other IBD children with ostomies help to alleviate some of the mystery and fear of the surgery: This is invaluable. The options of the appliance on the left or right, above or below the belt, and skin care are all reviewed well in advance. The purpose of preoperative stoma-site marking is to select an appropriate location in an area of the abdomen for surgical placement of a stoma and is best marked while the child is in a sitting position. A poorly located stoma may result in pouching problems, increase potential for leakage, and place undue hardship and emotional trauma on the pediatric patient. The ideal stoma site is located below the umbilicus, within the rectus muscle, away from scars, creases, bony prominences, umbilicus, and belt line, on the summit of the infraumbilical fat mound, and visible to the patient. Optimal stoma-site placement will promote self-care and rehabilitation of the patient. Patients undergoing stoma formation have to make major physical and psychologic adjustments following surgery, but the concept of a temporary stoma is stressed again and again.

In the specific case of ileal pouch-anal anastomosis (IPAA) in teenage boys, there is a risk of sexual dysfunction, which is imperative to discuss preoperatively. Teenage boys are often embarrassed, and often a conversation to review the anatomy and risk of sexual function helps with their anxiety. The risks of erection dysfunction, retrograde ejaculation, and bladder function are rare, but important to discuss.[7]

Moreover, it is understood that female children undergoing an open IPAA will experience reduced fertility; however, there maybe some benefit from laparoscopic technique. Historically, pelvic adhesions and possible injury to the parasympathetic or sympathetic plexus would, potentially impair sexual function and fertility. More recently, improvements in laparoscopic surgery may potentially improve both sexual function and reproductive ability by reducing pelvic adhesions. However, there are no strong data to support this yet. However, it is generally understood that young women after IBD pelvic surgery have a higher incidence of impaired fertility than do patients who are nonoperatively managed. Also, some studies suggest that there is a higher incidence of dyspareunia after surgery, but this does not affect overall sexual function. Lastly, if pregnancy does occur, Caesarean section should be considered in patients with scarred, rigid perineum.[8] Majority of the pelvic surgeries performed for pediatric IBD are performed during their "reproductive years." Advising young female IBD patients and their patients about their reproductive ability is an important part of preoperative consultation.

I personally prefer a minimally invasive approach to surgery in children afflicted with IBD. As in adults, the benefits of using a laparoscopic approach are well described, including smaller incisions, less pain, faster recovery, and earlier return of bowel function. Although there are some disadvantages, ultimately the satisfaction of the child and family and successful functional outcome are the principal goals. At the same time, it is of the utmost importance that the surgeon has the clinical judgment to know when to convert to open technique.

PEDIATRIC LAPAROSCOPY

The following details some of the general principles of pediatric laparoscopy in children with IBD. Preoperatively, nutritional optimization is crucial; obtaining a serum prealbumin level may be useful in gauging optimal timing of surgery. Corticosteroids are continued but weaned as much as possible. Bowel preparation is usually entails a clear liquid diet 2 days prior to surgery and GoLYTELY the night prior to surgery (in the absence of obstruction). The child is positioned on a beanbag and the legs are placed in stirrups, with the perineum at the break of the table. An orogastric tube and a Foley catheter are inserted. Both arms are tucked. Sequential compression devices and warming blankets are used if appropriate. Intravenous antibiotics are essential preoperatively and at intervals intraoperatively.

Usually a rigid sigmoidoscopy is performed to assess whether the distal rectum is involved by the inflammatory process. The abdomen is prepared and draped. The use of a minimally invasive surgical room is helpful to allow multiple camera angles and monitor positions. Also, steep-Trendelenburg and reverse-Trendelenburg positions can improve the exposure. The number of trocars and position depends on the planned procedure. Most of the ports are 5 mm in size. If there is an ostomy being performed, this site is used as one of the port placements. Intraabdominal pneumoperitoneum pressure is limited to 15 mm Hg. The abdominal cavity is inspected for concomitant disease gently with the use of atraumatic 5-mm bowel graspers. Dissection is performed with hook-cautery or energy-based devices. The dissection and mobilization should always be initiated in a normal area—advancing toward the diseased segment. Again, conservative resection of grossly abnormal-appearing intestine is all that is usually necessary in CD. The principle of traction and countertraction is applied. Bowel resection is usually performed with a laparoscopic linear stapler. The anastomosis is performed either laparoscopically, sewn intracorporeally, or with a circular stapler (the completeness of the "doughnuts" is always checked.) If the anastomosis is in the rectum, it is tested by insufflating air into the rectum with the pelvic cavity filled with water. During the creation of the stoma site, the fascia underneath is incised laparoscopically. A stoma stricture can occur if the trocar incision is not extended. These general principles of minimally invasive surgery apply to both adults and children.[9,10]

SURGICAL MANAGEMENT OF UC

Historically, in 1933, Nissen described a 10-year-old child with familial adenomatous polyposis on whom he performed a total proctocolectomy with ileoanal anastomosis IAA. Several years later, Ravitch and Sabiston demonstrated that it was possible to remove rectal mucosa, leaving the muscle, pulling ileum through the muscular cuff, and restoring continuity by suturing to the dentate line. The outcomes were poor, and not until 1977 was IAA readdressed. Dr. Lester Martin, a pediatric surgeon, published the results of IPAA in a series of 17 children operated on for UC. The functional outcomes were good, and the procedure was successful in 15 children. This publication renewed interest in the possibility of restoring continence following proctocolectomy.

What followed was a decade of experimentation with various pouch configurations before the J-pouch configuration was accepted as the standard operative technique because of ease of construction and efficiency of evacuation. The surgical cure for UC was called restorative proctocolectomy or IPAA.[11]

In contrast to adults, the clinical presentation of UC is more often severe in children. Approximately 30% of patients with UC undergo surgery within the first 10 years of their illness, of which a substantial number have surgery for refractory disease during the initial presentation. Fortunately, with early diagnosis and improved medical management, children with UC rarely present as requiring emergent procedures for megacolon, bleeding, or perforation. Medical therapy for UC often relieves symptoms temporarily, but UC can rarely be cured without surgical resection of the diseased intestine. Unlike CD, UC is potentially curable with surgery. Therefore, surgery is often indicated in children with recurrent severe disease. Even if the disease is responsive to medical therapy, growth retardation from recurrent bouts of disease and the requisite use of corticosteroids may justify surgery. Intractable chronic disease, usually steroid dependent or resistant, is the most common indication for elective surgery. There is also a general consensus that the presence of dysplasia, even low grade, in flat mucosa is also an indication for colectomy. On rare occasions, severe pyoderma gangrenosum has prompted colectomy, but extracolonic manifestations of UC are generally managed without surgery. Some other indications for surgery would include limitations to child's lifestyle and activities and, most important, a desire for improved quality of life. This includes stress over limited physical and social activities and missing school days.

Among pediatric surgeons, the type of pouch or a pouch at all is controversial. Straight and J-pouch ileoanal anastomoses are associated with considerable morbidity; the straight one results in higher stool frequency, and the J pouch is associated with increased risk of pouchitis. Generally, it is found that over time, problems improved from both operations, and function was equally good. J-pouch patients had consistently lower stool frequency and better continence rates. Continence was excellent regardless of the technique.[11–13]

Editor's note (TMB): There is a chapter on ileal-pouch surgery in children and adolescents in the first edition of this book.

Stapled Anastomosis

Stapled anastomosis without mucosectomy confers functional benefit when compared with handsewn anastomosis and mucosectomy. There is evidence to suggest that disease control is superior when mucosectomy is performed, but this is not as strong as the evidence for better function when mucosectomy is avoided. As such, in my opinion, the procedure of choice is the stapled approach. However, situations exist where mucosectomy is indicated: those at high risk of cuff dysplasia and at high risk of inflammation of the cuff (patients in whom severe preexisting distal rectal inflammation is present). The use of the J pouch and avoiding the mucosectomy in such patients would require life-long surveillance of the rectal mucosa for dysplasia.[14]

Staged Procedures

Although some surgeons are tempted to perform a one-stage IPAA, I prefer to separate the procedure into two stages, with a diverting ileostomy for approximately 2 to 3 months to minimize the risk of pouch leak and infection. The patient is counseled that the recovery time is often protracted without a diverting ileostomy. This procedure, if done correctly, is the best chance for a improving the child's quality of life; therefore, I would be more conservative in my approach.[15,16]

Summary

To briefly summarize our laparoscopic technique, this approach involved a completely laparoscopic, intracorporeal proctocolectomy followed by an open-stapled ileal J-pouch construction and stapled anastomosis. Typically, this procedure involved a four-port technique in a diamond configuration. First, a lateral-to-medial approach is used to mobilize the entire colon. In most cases, the omentum is preserved during transverse colon mobilization and the mesocolon is divided using bipolar cautery (Ligasure, ValleyLab, Boulder, CO) with careful identification, isolation, and division of the ileocolic vessels. Once the intracorporeal proctocolectomy (as low as possible and thus leaving a few centimeters of rectal mucosa in situ) is completed, a low transverse suprapubic incision is made for colon extraction (Fig. 130.4), a 12-cm J pouch is formed, and an end-to-

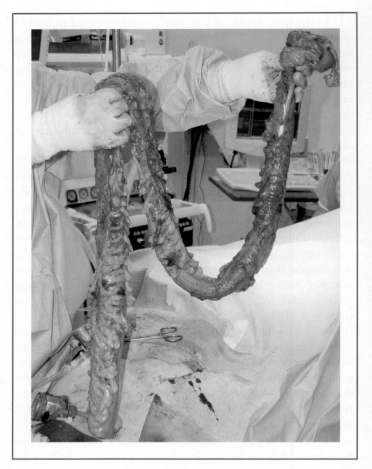

FIGURE 130.4 • 12y with UC undergoing laparoscopic proctocolectomy and J pouch ileoanal anastomosis with removal of colon via small low transverse incision.

end stapled intracorporeal anastomosis is made between the anal canal and the pouch using an circular intestinal stapler. A diverting ileostomy is performed at the preoperatively marked ostomy site/trocar site.

Pelvic Complications

In certain cases, the proctocolectomy with IPAA can be performed as a single procedure, though most pediatric surgeons use the multiple-stage approach. The temporary ileostomy minimizes the risk of leak and pelvic sepsis. The pelvic complications are usually associated with worsened functional outcomes, and in my opinion, a conservative, staged approach is superior. Other complications may include anastomotic stenosis, fistula, intestinal obstruction, wound complications, and pouchitis.[16]

Postoperative Period

Intravenous corticosteroids are tapered quickly, and a low oral dose is maintained. Most children are discharged after 4 to 5 days as long as they are comfortable with the ostomy. They return to full activity within 2 weeks. During these several weeks, the children are advised to understand and record what types of food may loosen stools more than others. After approximately 2 to 3 months, depending on their clinical course, the children are taken back to the operating room for examination under anesthesia, sigmoidoscopy, and ostomy reversal. The anastomosis is gently dilated and if pouch appears healthy, then the ostomy takedown is performed.

Pouchitis

Of course, as in adults, pouchitis is the most frequent complication after the IPAA, with reported incidence as high as 20% to 50%. However, pouchitis is more severe in children. Presenting symptoms of pouchitis include increased stool frequency and urgency, liquid consistency of stool, anal bleeding, malaise, anorexia, abdominal cramps, and a low-grade fever. Symptoms alone are not diagnostic of pouchitis; they must occur in association with specific endoscopic and histopathologic findings. The mechanism of pouchitis seems to be related to bacterial colonization of the pouch. As in adults, treatment with antibiotics is usually successful; alternative treatment modalities include pouch washouts with tap water and cortisone retention enemas. In extreme cases, diverting ileostomy maybe necessary for children with chronic pouchitis that may cause delayed growth and development.[4]

Other Issues

Patients with endoscopic inflammation of the rectal cuff in the absence of pouchitis are classified as having *cuffitis*, which is essentially persistence of the preexisting colitis in the residual rectal tissue. Patients with similar symptoms but with no pouchitis or rectal-cuff inflammation are classified as having a functional disorder termed *irritable pouch syndrome*. The diagnosis of CD should be entertained in patients with refractory pouchitis, especially those with ulceration and/or stenosis of the pouch inlet and inflammatory involvement of the afferent ileum. Finally, anastomotic stricture should be treated immediately with aggressive Hegar rectal dilations. Routine sigmoidoscopy and exam under anesthesia is important to monitor for all these postoperative complications.

Editor's note (TMB): There are several chapters on pouch outcomes in the first edition of this book.

Pouch Removal

In children with IPAA, approximately 15% will require removal of the J pouch and permanent ileostomy. Disappointingly, in a quarter of the children who require J-pouch removal, the diagnosis is later found to be CD instead of UC. Some pediatric surgeons will recommend that the J pouch be taken down, if the diagnosis of CD involving the pouch is established. However, the majority of these children can medically be managed like a CD patient and keep the IPAA. Only in extreme cases should the J pouch be removed.

Surveillance

All these children require life-long surveillance of the remaining rectal mucosa, and the risk of carcinoma increases with time. As in adults, the development of carcinoma is at least 10 years from the onset of UC. Therefore, surveillance of the ileal-pouch mucosa should begin at 10 years from the onset of disease (not the IPAA) in patients at risk. In children, if the child is diagnosed at age 7, the first evaluation should occur at age 17. A surveillance schedule should include annual biopsies from the anal transitional zone and the ileal pouch itself, with the recognition that accurate identification of the zone can be difficult after surgery. Because of this, it is ideal for the operating surgeon to perform this evaluation on a yearly basis.[14]

● SURGICAL MANAGEMENT OF CD

CD is an absolute contraindication to IPAA owing to increased postoperative complications and long-term failure. Pouch loss may be expected in 10% to 12% of all patients, but the risk increases to 33% in those patients with recrudescent CD. That being said, 70% of these IPAA patients is not infrequently performed in patients initially diagnosed with UC and subsequently determined to have CD do not develop serious postoperative complications and up to 90% retain their pouch in the absence of ileal or perianal disease. Also, anti-tumor necrosis factor (anti-TNF) therapy has been a promising factor in treatment of pouch retention. The presence of perianal CD and skip lesions within the small bowel are specific contraindications to IPAA, though the incidence and extent of small-bowel loss with pouch excision differs little from that occasioned by recurrent ileitis in patients with an ileostomy. IPAA is usually successful in patients with IC, but approximately 30% of cases will manifest overt CD within 10 years of operation.

The incidence of CD has risen during the past decade, especially in the very young (aged <2 years). Within the pediatric IBD population, usually it is easier to rule out UC in a patient with CD than CD in a child with UC. In most children, the onset of CD is after the age of 10 years but may present at any age. Specific to pediatric CD, there is commonly a significant diagnostic delay, usually longer than a year between the presentation of symptoms and the definitive diagnosis. These children usually present with growth failure (10%–40%) and abdominal pain due to stricture disease. Family history of IBD is often present. Presence of serologic markers may help identify Crohn's patients. Work-up should include endoscopy for both upper and lower GI tract with ileal intubation . Also contrast series (upper GI and small-bowel follow-through) or CT or MRI enterography should detail the entire length of the small bowel for strictures and fistulas. As mentioned previously, the capsule "endoscope" can be placed during upper endoscopy in children as young as 2 years of age, though the risk of capsule retention should always be considered, especially in patients with strictures. Studies have shown that histology of the upper tract may confirm a diagnosis of CD that would otherwise have been missed in up to 30% of the cases. Some children with CD may present with extraintestinal manifestations (arthritis, erythema nodosum, pyoderma gangrenosum, iritis, and uveitis) before any overt bowel involvement.

Surgical Intervention

As many as 80% of patients with CD will require at least one operation in the course of their disease. Unfortunately, unlike in UC, there is no definitive surgical cure for CD, because CD has the potential to involve the entire GI tract. Pediatric surgeons are only able to provide palliative care and treatment focused on specific complications of the disease. In the past several decades, novel drug therapies have significantly reduced the need for surgical therapy in CD. True surgical emergencies are rare in CD; toxic megacolon or massive GI bleeding is rare. As in adults, pediatric CD surgery is limited to children who are refractory to medical therapy. Sometimes, when medical therapy is poorly tolerated, surgery is the only option.

The more common indications for surgery in CD are relative and can usually be done electively. These include intractability to medical therapy with steroid dependency or resistance, complex fistulae, abdominal abscesses, refractory disease, and growth retardation in children. The main principle again is to treat the affected intestine only. In the past, patients with CD on average underwent at least 4 to 5 bowel resections during their lifetime, and if diagnosed in childhood, even more often. As in adults, radical resections are not necessary and often times will leave the child with short-gut syndrome. Intestinal resections or stictureoplasties are limited to a diseased segment of bowel. Asymptomatic, isolated skip lesions are left alone.

Having said this, there are rare cases when a major bowel resection is required. When CD has affected a large portion of the intestine and surgery is the only option, the affected intestine must be resected and care must be taken to spare the rectum if possible. The typical surgical solution in these pediatric cases is colectomy and ileorectal anasotmosis in one or two stages.

As in pediatric UC patients, initial diagnostic laparoscopic evaluation of the peritoneal cavity with care to inspect the entire length of intestine to identify other potential diseased areas is an important first step. After a thorough exploration with the camera, the procedure is either performed laparoscopically or converted to an open procedure.

The laparoscopic technique involves mobilization of the diseased segment with a stapled intracorporeal anastomosis. Intracorporeal stay sutures are used to align the two segments of bowel, and two small enterotomies are made to allow the two arms of the endoscopic stapling device. Once the stapling device is engaged, the result is a 3- to 4-cm functional end-to-end anastomosis. The remaining enterotomy and mesenteric defect is closed with suture, and the specimen is brought out via the umbilical incision.

In many patients with CD, there is a large inflammatory mass that is imaged preoperatively, and, if needed, use of ureteral stents will facilitate intraoperative dissection. The margins for the resection, again, are gross only. There is no correlation between presence of microscopic CD and recurrence. The fistulas can be simply transected and the resulting defect closed with two layers.

Stricturoplasty

Small-bowel obstruction from CD is usually a result of stricture formation. Again, the treatment of choice is antiinflammatory medications and immunotherapy. However, refractoriness to medical therapy or growth failure will lead some children to operation. The most conservative surgical approach allowing sparing of bowel is strictureplasty.[17] Short strictures should be treated by Heineke-Mikiulicz strictureplasty. As in adults, this procedure can be performed laparoscopically as well. This procedure involves a longitudinal incision across the stricture and

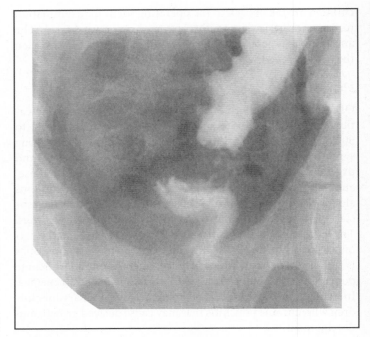

FIGURE 130.5 • 9 y with CD and significant sigmoid colonic stricture

1 to 2 cm of normal bowel on either side of the stricture, followed by closure of the incision transversely with a single layer of polydioxanone (PDS) suture. For longer strictures, a Finney side-to-side anastomosis can be performed. This too can be performed laparoscopically. The stricture is treated with a longitudinal enterotomy that is folded onto itself. Opposing layers of intestine are sutured to each other in a side-to-side anastomosis fashion with PDS suture. The complications from strictureplasty include leak and bleeding, as in adults. The recurrence rate from strictureplasty is the same for bowel resection. There is statistically no difference in recurrence between the two types of strictureplasties. These surgical techniques help in resolving the recurrent episodes of bowel obstruction while conserving the maximum possible bowel length.

In addition, there are a small number of CD strictures in the colon (Fig. 130.5) that may warrant surgical intervention. As mentioned earlier, strictureplasty is useful in the small bowel; however, the experience and outcomes are limited in the large bowel. Because there is little danger of short gut with a limited colon resection for a colonic stricture, these strictures are usually treated with resection rather than a strictureplasty.

In pediatric surgery, massive bowel resections for other pediatric intestinal disease have been performed and have resulted in short-gut syndrome. However, in CD this is avoided as much as possible. Just as in adult patients, saving bowel length in children is equally possible when strictureplasty is used. Because children are diagnosed early with CD, every effort is made to preserve bowel length. These children are at risk for needing multiple surgeries in their lifetimes.

Perianal Disease

Children with CD perianal disease suffer from skin tags, fissures, fistulas, and abscesses.[18] These lesions may present before, during, or after intestinal manifestations of CD. There is no correlation between the clinical progression of perianal symptoms and the intestinal course. Often, these perianal complications are asymptomatic. As in other manifestations of CD, perianal disease is treatable with medications, and surgery is reserved for complications. However, the management of these lesions remains controversial and sometimes very difficult.

Again, the approach is a conservative surgical approach. MRI, proctosigmoidosocopy, and exam under anesthesia by a pediatric surgeon can best delineate perianal disease. Approximately 10% of children newly diagnosed with CD have fistulas and/or abscesses at diagnosis. The majority of these lesions resolve within a year, without any surgical intervention.[19]

The most common perianal complication in pediatric CD is a perianal abscess requiring incision and drainage and debridement. The abscess is opened in a cruciate figure and then packed loosely with gauze, with the gauze removed slowly in the next 24 to 48 h. I have not used fibrin glue, but there are a number of reports of successful closures with this modality. Infrasphincteric fistulas in ano are difficult to treat in children, as is the case with adults, and require fistulotomy or fistulectomy. Diverting colostomy may be useful in speeding recovery time in the case of difficult wounds. Again pediatric CD surgery is very conservative; therefore, aggressive fissurectomy is not recommended. The fissures are generally treated medically. With high recurrence rate and poor wound healing in pediatric CD, fissures should be treated with dietary restriction, total parenteral nutrition (TPN), or diverting colostomy.

Complications

Complications after surgical treatment of children with CD are similar to those in adults. There are the usual anastomotic leaks, sepsis, and fistula formations. Unfortunately, the main and typical complication of CD is recurrence of the disease itself. However, the recurrence risk is not related to the indication for surgery, the clinical presentation, or the age of presentation, sex, or time from onset of the CD. There is a consensus that recurrence rate is highest in CD children with perianal disease and lowest in CD children with a diverting stoma. Unfortunately, a small percentage of pediatric CD patients end up with a permanent stoma.

As in pediatric UC, duration of *colonic* disease is the most important factor in assessing a child for risk of cancer. Also like in UC, it is estimated that the risk of cancer increases 1% per year after the first 10 years of diagnosis. Children with CD have a higher risk than children with UC.

● CONCLUSIONS

Unfortunately, the incidence of pediatric IBD is increasing. Diagnosis and differentiation between the various forms of IBD remains difficult, but great strides have been made with the advent of new imaging studies and serologic markers. Treatment has benefitted from more extensive research in adult IBD patients, but the goals of reversing growth retardation and achieving normal physical development distinguish the management of pediatric IBD. Ultimately, after years of treatment as a child, the adolescent's care must be transferred from the

pediatric to the adult services. It is important that the pediatric IBD team anticipate the transfer of medical and surgical care to an adult institution and adult gastroenterologist and surgeon. Good communication is key to a smooth transition and good clinical outcome.[20] Our goal as pediatric gastroenterologists and pediatric surgeons is to prepare the child with IBD for adulthood. IBD is a difficult diagnosis for the child and parents, and we have many tools at our disposal to ease their symptoms and improve their quality of life.

References

1. Alexander F, Sarigol S, DiFiore J, et al. Fate of the pouch in 151 pediatric patients after ileal pouch anal anastomosis. *J Pediatr Surg.* 2003;38(1):78–82.

2. Ceriati E, Deganello F, De Peppo F, et al. Surgery for ulcerative colitis in pediatric patients: functional results of 10-year follow-up with straight endorectal pull-through. *Pediatr Surg Int.* 2004;20(8):573–578.

3. Cornish JA, Tan E, Teare J, et al. The effect of restorative proctocolectomy on sexual function, urinary function, fertility, pregnancy and delivery: a systematic review. *Dis Colon Rectum.* 2007;50(8):1128–1138.

4. Delaney CP, Remzi FH, Gramlich T, Dadvand B, Fazio VW. Equivalent function, quality of life and pouch survival rates after ileal pouch-anal anastomosis for indeterminate and ulcerative colitis. *Ann Surg.* 2002;236(1):43–48.

5. Dubinsky M. Special issues in pediatric inflammatory bowel disease. *World J Gastroenterol.* 2008;14(3):413–420.

6. Dutta S, Rothenberg SS, Chang J, Bealer J. Total intracorporeal laparoscopic resection of Crohn's disease. *J Pediatr Surg.* 2003;38(5):717–719.

7. Evers EA, Pfefferkorn MD, Steiner SJ. Factors predictive of Crohn disease following colectomy in medically refractory pediatric colitis. *J Pediatr Gastroenterol Nutr.* 2009;48(3):283–286.

8. Fonkalsrud, EW. Ulcerative colitis. In O'Neil, Rowe, Grosfeld, Fonkalsrud, Coran, eds. *Pediatric Surgery.* 5th ed. 1998.

9. Escher JC. Transition from pediatric to adult health care in inflammatory bowel disease. *Dig Dis.* 2009;27(3):382–386.

10. Habal FM, Ravindran NC. Management of inflammatory bowel disease in the pregnant patient. *World J Gastroenterol.* 2008;14(9):1326–1332.

11. Kayton ML. Cancer and pediatric inflammatory bowel disease. *Semin Pediatr Surg.* 2007;16(3):205–213.

12. Keljo DJ, Markowitz J, Langton C, et al. Course and treatment of perianal disease in children newly diagnosed with Crohn's disease. *Inflamm Bowel Dis.* 2009;15(3):383–387.

13. Markel TA, Lou DC, Pfefferkorn M, et al. Steroids and poor nutrition are associated with infectious wound complications in children undergoing first stage procedures for ulcerative colitis. *Surgery.* 2008;144(4):540–545; discussion 545.

14. Meier AH, Roth L, Cilley RE, Dillon PW. Completely minimally invasive approach to restorative total proctocolectomy with j-pouch construction in children. *Surg Laparosc Endosc Percutan Tech.* 2007;17(5):418–421.

15. Palder SB, Shandling B, Bilik R, Griffiths AM, Sherman P. Perianal complications of pediatric Crohn's disease. *J Pediatr Surg.* 1991;26(5):513–515.

16. Rice HE, Chuang E. Current management of pediatric inflammatory bowel disease. *Semin Pediatr Surg.* 1999;8(4):221–228.

17. Romano C, Famiani A, Gallizzi R, Comito D, Ferrau' V, Rossi P. Indeterminate colitis: a distinctive clinical pattern of inflammatory bowel disease in children. *Pediatrics.* 2008; 122(6):e1278–e1281.

18. Seetharamaiah R, West BT, Ignash SJ, et al. Outcomes in pediatric patients undergoing straight vs J pouch ileoanal anastomosis: a multicenter analysis. *J Pediatr Surg.* 2009;44(7):1410–1417.

19. Yamamoto T, Fazio VW, Tekkis PP. Safety and efficacy of stricture-plasty for Crohn's disease: a systematic review and meta-analysis. *Dis Colon Rectum.* 2007;50(11):1968–1986.

Perioperative Nutrition Support | 131

Vishal Bhagat and Michael D. Sitrin

Nutritional therapy has become an integral part of the treatment of patients with inflammatory bowel disease (IBD). It must be appreciated, however, that nutritional treatments are used for various purposes in these patients, such as reversal of nutritional deficits due to IBD, primary treatment of the inflammatory disorder, prevention of complications associated with IBD surgery, or management of gut failure. The goals of nutritional therapy should clearly be established at the outset, as these will determine the most appropriate type and duration of treatment. In this chapter, issues related primarily to nutrition and surgical management of IBD will be discussed.

● TOTAL PARENTERAL NUTRITION PRIOR TO IBD SURGERY

One of the most common questions regarding nutritional management of IBD concerns perioperative nutritional support for the patient undergoing elective surgery. Poor wound healing, infections of various types, anastomotic leaks, prolonged ileus, decubitus pressure sores, and increased mortality are frequent postoperative complications in malnourished patients. In the past, many IBD patients would receive a course of preoperative total parenteral nutrition (TPN) prior to elective surgery on the assumption that this would decrease postoperative complications and permit excellent bowel preparation for the procedure. Relatively scant data from controlled clinical trials are available on the impact of preoperative TPN specifically on IBD surgery. Collins et al. reported that TPN decreased postoperative complications in patients undergoing protocolectomy or proctectomy.[1]

Studies of perioperative nutrition support in general, however, have raised some important issues regarding the utility of preoperative TPN. A landmark, large, cooperative, multicenter trial conducted in Veterans Administration (VA) hospitals explored the role of perioperative nutrition support in patients undergoing major elective abdominal or thoracic operations. Overall, patients who received a 7- to 15-day period of preoperative TPN support did not have fewer postoperative complications than those who did not receive nutrition therapy and, in fact, had significantly more postoperative infections.[2] A recent review of published studies concluded that routine use of perioperative TPN is not beneficial.[3]

Nutritional Assessment

More detailed examination of the benefits and risks of preoperative nutrition support has called attention to the importance of nutritional assessment in the appropriate selection of patients for preoperative nutrition support. Further analysis of the VA cooperative study data was performed by stratifying the patients according to their nutritional status. A Subjective Global Assessment that uses data from the history and bedside physical examination and a Nutrition Risk Index that considers body weight and serum albumin were used for nutritional assessment. Both techniques have been extensively validated as predictors of postoperative morbidity and mortality. Patients with severe malnutrition who received preoperative TPN had significantly fewer noninfectious complications and no increase in postoperative infections, compared to those who did not receive nutrition support. In contrast, patients with borderline or mild malnutrition who received preoperative TPN had more postoperative infections than did those who did not receive intravenous feedings and were not protected from noninfectious complications such as anastomosis leaks, respiratory failure, cardiac complications, wound dehiscences, and so on. The higher postoperative infection rate in those receiving TPN was not explained as solely caused by catheter-related infections but mainly by more episodes of pneumonia and empyema. This VA cooperative study has been criticized by some who note that many of the patients treated with TPN received excessive intravenous energy intakes, putting them at higher risk for hyperglycemia, which can interfere with neutrophil function and predispose them to infection. Others have claimed that use of intravenous lipid emulsions to provide a substantial portion of the energy intake promoted infections. A meta-analysis of prospective randomized controlled trials showed an increase in septic and metabolic complications related to overnutrition in patients undergoing gastrointestinal surgery.[4] Nevertheless, other analyses of perioperative TPN also have quite consistently demonstrated an increase in postoperative infections in mild to moderately malnourished patients who received TPN.[3]

These observations emphasize the importance of performing a nutritional assessment of patients with IBD prior to surgery. Various assessment techniques and tools can be used, each with their own advantages and disadvantages. In a prospective evaluation of 200 patients undergoing gastrointestinal surgery, the Nutrition Risk Score that includes body mass index, weight loss, appetite, dysphagia, and severity of disease was the best predictor of postoperative complications.[5] A large prospective, preoperative risk assessment study demonstrated that serum albumin is a single best indicator of postoperative complications.[6] Although the causes of increased infection risk in TPN are at present controversial and uncertain, current data support the use of preoperative TPN only in patients with substantial protein-calorie malnutrition.

OPTIMAL DURATION AND TIMING OF TPN

The optimal duration of TPN prior to elective surgery is also often debated. Faced with a severely cachectic patient with complex IBD, the surgeon often is tempted to request prolonged parenteral nutrition, ranging from weeks to months, prior to operating on these high-risk individuals. Christie and Hill[7] have studied the physiologic effects of nutritional repletion of patients with IBD awaiting surgical treatment. They observed rapid improvements in the function of respiratory and other muscles and increased levels of serum proteins within 1 week after initiation of TPN. These occurred at a time before significant changes in body composition could be demonstrated, and subsequent further improvements in physiologic function and repletion of body cell mass progressed very slowly. It is likely that the rapid gain of physiologic function following parenteral nutrition reflected enhanced cellular metabolism. Studies have shown that 5 to 7 days of preoperative TPN in malnourished patients undergoing gastrointestinal surgery (including IBD surgery) reduced postoperative complications and mortality compared to those who did not receive preoperative TPN. A longer duration of preoperative TPN may not be beneficial and would significantly increase medical costs.[3,8,9] TPN begun preoperatively should be continued in the immediate postoperative period.

In contrast to the beneficial effects of early postoperative enteral nutrition (see the following), TPN given only postoperatively has generally been shown to increase infectious complications. Hence, it should be delayed for 5 to 7 days in patients in whom optimal, postoperative, oral, or enteral feeding cannot be achieved after surgery because of ileus or other complications.[3] It may be reasonable to start TPN in the immediate postoperative period in patients with severe malnutrition if adequate enteral nutrition is unlikely to be achieved.

Using a case-control methodology, Lashner et al. reported that CD patients who received short-term preoperative TPN had somewhat smaller resections than did matched patients who were not nutritionally treated prior to surgery.[10] In a prospective controlled trial of consecutive patients, Yamamoto et al. showed that nocturnal enteral nutrition reduced endoscopic recurrence of CD after ileal or ileocolic resection.[11] These observations need

to be confirmed before making any recommendations. It must be emphasized that urgently needed surgery when complications of IBD such as abscess, perforation, or high-grade obstruction are suspected should not be delayed in the hope of improving the patient's nutritional status and surgical outcome.

ENTERAL NUTRITION SUPPORT

Few controlled clinical trials have been performed specifically comparing preoperative TPN with enteral nutrition support of patients with IBD. Patients with UC and CD often tolerate tube feedings very well, and enteral nutrition support can provide both effective nutritional repletion and excellent bowel preparation in these patients. Furthermore, enteral nutrition support may avoid the postoperative infectious complications associated with current TPN regimens in those with mild-to-moderate malnutrition. González-Huix et al.[12] compared enteral versus parenteral nutrition as adjunctive therapy with acute UC patients treated with corticosteroids. Remission rate and need for colectomy were similar in both the groups. In those who required colectomy, postoperative infections and complications of nutrition support were more common with parenteral nutrition.

In contrast to deleterious effects of TPN (as mentioned previously), enteral nutrition is beneficial in the immediate postoperative period in reducing infectious complications and duration of hospital stay in patients undergoing gastrointestinal surgery and should be started within 24 to 48 h. It is not necessary to wait for return of bowel sounds.[3] Enteral nutrition should be the first choice for perioperative nutritional rehabilitation, and TPN should be reserved for those with very short-bowel, high-grade obstruction, certain types of fistulas, and those who do not tolerate tube feedings.

IMMUNOMODULATORY ENTERAL NUTRITION AND HUMAN GROWTH HORMONE THERAPY

Malnutrition-induced suppression of the immune system is believed to be one of the major factors responsible for postoperative complications and mortality. Arginine, glutamine, omega-3-fatty acids, vitamin C, vitamin E, and nucleotides are believed to have immunomodulatory effects. A recent review of published studies concluded that perioperative immunomodulatory nutrition reduces postoperative infectious complications and length of hospital stay in patients undergoing elective gastrointestinal surgery compared to standard tube feeding formulas.[3] Two subsequent prospective randomized controlled trials, however, have failed to show any benefit.[13] There is also a concern for worsening hemodynamic instability in patients with sepsis, with the use of an arginine-containing formula. Moreover, it is unclear which of the above-mentioned supplements are responsible for beneficial effects. In conclusion, further studies are required before recommending routine use of perioperative immunomodulatory nutrition.

Combining perioperative nutrition support with human growth hormone in UC patients undergoing total colectomy preserved limb lean-tissue mass, increased postoperative muscular strength, and reduced long-term postoperative fatigue in one randomized controlled study.[14] Further studies are needed to confirm the role of human growth hormone therapy in patients with IBD undergoing surgery.

FISTULAE

Gastrointestinal fistulae are among the most difficult complications in patients with CD. Patients with fistulae are often very malnourished, due to the severity of the IBD, loss of nutrients through the fistulae track secretions, and predisposition for small-bowel bacterial overgrowth and malabsorption. Several groups have examined the effect of TPN and bowel rest on fistula healing in CD. Some have reported high rates of healing, whereas others found that fistulae rarely closed and stayed healed after TPN. These disparate results largely can be explained by recognizing that there are different types of fistulae in patients with CD. Postoperative fistulae occur due to anastamotic leaks or leaks at the site of drainage tubes and generally are not associated with active IBD. These types of fistulae have high healing rates and generally close with 30 days or less of TPN and bowel rest. In contrast, enterocutaneous and enteroenteric fistulae due to CD per se generally originate from areas of active disease proximal to a site of obstruction, and perianal fistulae usually occur in the context of active rectal CD. These types of fistulae have poorer response to TPN and bowel rest. Although they frequently will close temporarily, they commonly reopen once oral food intake resumes. Overall, long-term closure of these fistulae occurs in less than 30% of patients, and surgical treatment usually is needed. Because of the high prevalence of severe malnutrition in patients with fistulae, nutritional therapy may play an important adjunctive role prior to corrective surgery. Some experts have suggested use of somatostatin/octreotide that has antisecretory and antimotility properties in conjunction with parenteral nutrition to promote faster healing of postoperative fistulae and to reduce the number of complications, but placebo-controlled trials have failed to show any benefit.[15] There are no controlled studies of use of these agents in fistulae related to CD.

Fistula-track secretions often contain large amounts of certain micronutrients, such as zinc and vitamin C, which are important for wound healing. This has prompted some to recommend additional supplementation of these nutrients, though the benefit of this approach on fistula healing has not been proven.

Enteral nutrition support also has been successfully used to manage fistulae in CD, though the reported series are small and controlled comparisons with TPN have not been performed. Elemental formulas are nearly completely absorbed in the proximal small bowel and generally are well tolerated in patients with fistulae from more distal intestine. In addition, fistulae from stomach, duodenum, or proximal jejunum often can be bypassed by placing a feeding tube distal to the origin of the fistula, and tube feedings generally will not increase fistula output. Enteral nutrition support has been reported to improve perianal fistulae, but healing often is not complete.

Editor's note (TMB): There is a separate chapter in this section on management of abdominal fistulae and an earlier chapter on bowel rest for Crohn's disease. There is also an excellent chapter on enteral nutrition in adolescents with Crohn's disease.

NUTRITIONAL MANAGEMENT OF THE SHORT-BOWEL SYNDROME

The short-bowel syndrome (SBS) occurs when there is <200 cm of bowel remaining after extensive small-bowel resection in patients with CD. Those patients at greatest nutritional risk generally have a jejunocolic or an ileocolic anastomosis with <60 cm of residual small intestine or an end jejunostomy with <115 cm of residual small intestine. It has been suggested that intestinal failure is better defined in terms of fecal energy loss rather than residual bowel length. Patients can be grouped into two distinct subgroups: those with colon in continuity, and those without colon in continuity. In patients with SBS, the colon becomes an important nutritional organ by absorbing energy in the form of short-chain fatty acids as well as sodium and water.

Most patients will require TPN immediately after extensive small-bowel resection, while postoperative complications are addressed and metabolic issues stabilized. Attempts should be made as soon as appropriate to wean patients who have sufficient absorptive capacity when they are taken off TPN. Maximal adaptation of the residual intestine may take as long as 1 to 2 years. Nutritional therapy should be introduced gradually with the goal of providing patients approximately 25 to 30 kcal/kg body weight per day and 1.0 to 1.5 g/kg per day of protein. There is no benefit of high-fat low-carbohydrate or low-fat high-carbohydrate diets in patients with severe short-gut syndrome or patients with small-bowel stomas. Simple carbohydrates should be avoided to prevent dumping of syndrome-like symptoms.

A low-fat diet can only be recommended in patients with moderate small-bowel resection with colon in continuity to prevent steatorrhea and calcium oxalate stone formation, but it should not impair their energy intake. Soluble fiber is fermented to short-chain fatty acids by colonic bacteria and serves as an additional energy source in patients with colon in continuity. Small amounts of medium-chain triglycerides are absorbed by the colon and may be included in the diet as an additional energy source. Dietary oxalate should be restricted and supplemental calcium used in patients with residual colon in continuity to prevent calcium-oxalate renal-stone formation.

Glucose-polymer-based oral rehydration solutions (ORS) should be used to prevent dehydration and electrolyte disturbances and to reduce TPN fluid requirements. High-dose H2 antagonists and proton-pump inhibitors reduce gastric fluid secretion and fluid losses during the first 6 months postenterectomy. Fluid losses usually require long-term control with antimotility agents, such as loperamide or diphenoxylate. If these are ineffective, especially in patients without colon in continuity, use of codeine sulfate or tincture of opium may be necessary. Rarely, subcutaneous octreotide is required. It should be used only if fluid intravenous requirements are more than 3 L/day because postresection intestinal adaptation may be impaired and the risk for cholelithiasis may be increased. Magnesium deficiency can occur in patients with ileal resection despite a normal serum concentration. However, magnesium supplementation is problematic and often requires parenteral administration. Iron is absorbed in duodenum and, in the absence of gastrointestinal bleeding, is not routinely required as a supplement. Deficiency of fat-soluble vitamins (A, D, E, and K) and trace elements (zinc, selenium) can occur and often require supplementation. Water-soluble vitamin deficiency is rare.[16]

Patients with CD and SBS and/or active disease are sometimes supported by home TPN. Home TPN can lead to excellent rehabilitation with low mortality. It can improve quality of life, reduce steroid requirements, and replenish nutritional needs. Despite these benefits, home TPN is associated with significant morbidity due to catheter-related sepsis, catheter occlusion, venous thrombosis, dehydration, and electrolyte derangements. Metabolic bone disease and liver dysfunction, which can progress to liver failure, are severe complications of home TPN. Home TPN also does not prevent relapses of the disease, and there is no reduction in surgical procedures.[17] Therefore, every effort should be made to wean the patients off TPN. Although results are not consistent in all randomized controlled trials, human recombinant growth hormone therapy may improve absorptive function and facilitate parenteral nutrition weaning in patients with SBS.[18] Optimal clinical benefits appear to be achieved when human growth hormone therapy is combined with specialized oral diet and perhaps glutamine. Glucagon-like peptide-II (GLP-II) is secreted from L cells of terminal ileum. It has been postulated that relative lack of jejunal hypertrophy following ileal resection may be at least partly related to the resection of GLP-II-producing L cells. In preliminary small studies, teduglutide (ALX-0600), a dipeptidyl peptidase IV–resistant GLP-2 analogue, has shown significant improvement in intestinal absorption in patients with SBS with or without colon.[19] Controlled clinical studies are ongoing to look for potential effects of this drug in reducing TPN dependence in patients with SBS. Intestinal transplantation is an option for patients who cannot be weaned off TPN and with severe complications of home TPN (such as liver failure) requiring discontinuation. At present, results are not satisfactory to justify intestinal transplantation in patients stable on home TPN.[20]

Editor's note (TMB): There is a separate chapter on short-bowel syndrome and intestinal transplantation.

References

1. Collins JP, Oxby CB, Hill GL. Intravenous aminoacids and intravenous hyperalimentation as protein-sparing therapy after major surgery. A controlled clinical trial. *Lancet.* 1978;1(8068):788–791.

2. The Veterans Affairs Total Parenteral Nutrition Cooperative Study Group. Perioperative total parenteral nutrition in surgical patients. *N Engl J Med.* 1991;325:525–532.

3. Martindale RG, McClave SA, Vanek VW, et al. Guidelines for the provision and assessment of nutrition support therapy in the adult critically ill patient: Society of Critical Care Medicine and American Society for Parenteral and Enteral Nutrition: Executive Summary. *Crit Care Med.* 2009;37(5):1757–1761.

4. Torosian MH. Perioperative nutrition support for patients undergoing gastrointestinal surgery: critical analysis and recommendations. *World J Surg.* 1999;23(6):565–569.

5. Schiesser M, Kirchhoff P, Müller MK, Schäfer M, Clavien PA. The correlation of nutrition risk index, nutrition risk score, and bioimpedance analysis with postoperative complications in patients undergoing gastrointestinal surgery. *Surgery.* 2009;145(5):519–526.

6. Daley J, Khuri SF, Henderson W, et al. Risk adjustment of the postoperative morbidity rate for the comparative assessment of the quality of surgical care: results of the National Veterans Affairs Surgical Risk Study. *J Am Coll Surg.* 1997;185(4):328–340.

7. Christie PM, Hill GL. Effect of intravenous nutrition on nutrition and function in acute attacks of inflammatory bowel disease. *Gastroenterology.* 1990;99(3):730–736.

8. Rombeau JL, Barot LR, Williamson CE, Mullen JL. Preoperative total parenteral nutrition and surgical outcome in patients with inflammatory bowel disease. *Am J Surg.* 1982;143(1):139–143.

9. Yao GX, Wang XR, Jiang ZM, Zhang SY, Ni AP. Role of perioperative parenteral nutrition in severely malnourished patients with Crohn's disease. *World J Gastroenterol.* 2005;11(36):5732–5734.

10. Lashner BA, Evans AA, Hanauer SB. Preoperative total parenteral nutrition for bowel resection in Crohn's disease. *Dig Dis Sci.* 1989;34(5):741–746.

11. Yamamoto T, Nakahigashi M, Umegae S, Kitagawa T, Matsumoto K. Impact of long-term enteral nutrition on clinical and endoscopic recurrence after resection for Crohn's disease: A prospective, non-randomized, parallel, controlled study. *Aliment Pharmacol Ther.* 2007;25(1):67–72.

12. González-Huix F, Fernández-Bañares F, Esteve-Comas M, et al. Enteral versus parenteral nutrition as adjunct therapy in acute ulcerative colitis. *Am J Gastroenterol.* 1993;88(2):227–232.

13. Klek S, Kulig J, Sierzega M, et al. Standard and immunomodulating enteral nutrition in patients after extended gastrointestinal surgery–a prospective, randomized, controlled clinical trial. *Clin Nutr.* 2008;27(4):504–512.

14. Kissmeyer-Nielsen P, Jensen MB, Laurberg S. Perioperative growth hormone treatment and functional outcome after major abdominal surgery: a randomized, double-blind, controlled study. *Ann Surg.* 1999;229(2):298–302.

15. Makhdoom ZA, Komar MJ, Still CD. Nutrition and enterocutaneous fistulas. *J Clin Gastroenterol.* 2000;31(3):195–204.

16. Buchman AL, Scolapio J, Fryer J. AGA technical review on short bowel syndrome and intestinal transplantation. *Gastroenterology.* 2003;124(4):1111–1134.

17. Galandiuk S, O'Neill M, McDonald P, Fazio VW, Steiger E. A century of home parenteral nutrition for Crohn's disease. *Am J Surg.* 1990;159(6):540–544; discussion 544.

18. Jeejeebhoy KN. Management of short bowel syndrome: avoidance of total parenteral nutrition. *Gastroenterology.* 2006;130(2 suppl 1):S60–S66.

19. Jeppesen PB, Sanguinetti EL, Buchman A, et al. Teduglutide (ALX-0600), a dipeptidyl peptidase IV resistant glucagon-like peptide 2 analogue, improves intestinal function in short bowel syndrome patients. *Gut.* 2005;54(9):1224–1231.

20. Pironi L, Forbes A, Joly F, et al. Survival of patients identified as candidates for intestinal transplantation: a 3-year prospective follow-up. *Gastroenterology.* 2008;135(1):61–71.

Laparoscopic Resection for Crohn's Disease | 132

Hien T. Nguyen and Anne Lidor

Crohn's disease is a transmural inflammatory disease of unknown origin that can affect any portion of the gastrointestinal tract, with a variable degree of inflammation that can also involve adjacent organs. Treatment for this disease begins with anti-inflammatory medications, although some experts feel that rapid progression to immunomodulators minimizes steroid dependency. When medication treatment fails to control the sequelae of inflammatory changes, surgical treatment oftentimes becomes necessary.

Indications for surgical intervention for Crohn's disease include bleeding, perforation, obstruction, and intractability to medical treatment. Of these, the most common indication for surgery is obstruction and the most common procedure is an ileocecectomy. The benefits of laparoscopic surgery are especially relevant in IBD patients with associated malnourishment and immunosuppression by minimizing wound size, as well as financial benefits in terms of resolution of ileus, narcotic use, and hospital stay. However, the pathology of Crohn's disease has typically been thought to make a laparoscopic approach more difficult, mostly due to the presence of inflammatory changes, thickened mesentery, fistulas, abscesses, and adhesions.

Over the last decade, laparoscopic surgical resection has gained popularity as definitive surgical treatment for Crohn's disease. As early as 1995, McFadden et al.[1] published successful laparoscopic ileocececotomies, sigmoid colectomies, and takedown of transverse colonic fistulas with feasible and safe results. More recently, a meta-analysis study by Tan and Tjandra[2] to determine the safety and feasibility of laparoscopic surgery in Crohn's disease patients found that laparoscopic surgery takes longer to perform when compared to open surgery, with a mean difference of approximately 25 minutes. However, laparoscopic surgery has significant short-term benefits compared to open surgery, including more rapid return of bowel function, earlier tolerance of oral intake, shorter hospitalization by 1.82 days, and overall lower morbidity.

Long-term outcomes of laparoscopic versus open ileocolic resection for Crohn's disease have also been studied recently by Fazio et al.[3] This prospective randomized trial followed 56 patients who had an ileocecectomy. Average follow-up was 10.5 years with

almost half of the patient population receiving a laparoscopic operation. Incisional hernia repair was needed in 4% of laparoscopic patients versus 14% in open cases. More patients required multiple operations after an open surgery than laparoscopic operation. The overall recurrence rate was 52%, with no significant differences between laparoscopic and open surgery with regard to medication to treat Crohn's disease, recurrence rates, and need for abdominal operation for recurrent Crohn's disease. The authors concluded that laparoscopic resection is at least comparable to open resection in the treatment of ileocolic Crohn's disease.

Emergent surgery for Crohn's disease may be indicated when patients present with frank peritonitis, intra-abdominal abscess not amenable to percutaneous drainage, toxic colitis, megacolon, or delayed presentation for long-standing obstruction that may lead to bowel ischemia and subsequent perforation. In situations where sepsis or instability is suspected, laparoscopic surgery should be substituted by a generous midline incision to allow quick and efficient surgical intervention.

TECHNIQUE

Preoperative Evaluation

The identification of a surgical disease in Crohn's patients is usually made when clinical findings are associated with a CT scan, small bowel series, or colonoscopy findings, suggesting acute or intractable disease. Malnutrition is commonly found in this patient population, and total parenteral nutrition should be considered during the perioperative process. A clean-contaminated or contaminated procedure is likely, due to the resection of intestine. As such, preoperative antibiotics with adequate coverage of Gram-negative aerobes and anaerobes are given. Patients on immunosuppressive steroid therapy should be continued during surgery.

Patient positioning for laparoscopic surgery must take into consideration the possibility of conversion to a midline laparotomy. All pressure points are padded and a Foley catheter is placed. If the disease process involves the sigmoid or rectum, patients are placed in a modified lithotomy position with legs placed in stirrups to allow the use of a transanal end-to-end anastomosis (EEA) stapler. Gross inflammation of the terminal ileum or sigmoid colon may warrant the preoperative placement of a ureteral stent to facilitate the identification and protection of the ureter during dissection.

Operative Specifics

After appropriate preparation, a periumbilical cutdown technique is used to place a Hasson trocar, and the abdomen is insufflated to 15 mm Hg. Additional trocars can be placed in the suprapubic and upper midline positions to allow a triangulated approach to the surgical target. The small bowel should be run to evaluate for strictures and the colon is assessed for pathology. Affected bowel to be resected is gently mobilized laterally to medially with care taken to identify important adjacent structures such as significant blood vessels and the ureter. An ileocecectomy requires the mobilization of the terminal ileum, cecum, and ascending colon. The lateral peritoneal attachment of the ascending colon is sharply divided with the aid of a hemostatic device such as Harmonic scalpel or Ligasure. Dissection continues to include the entire hepatic flexure to allow easy mobilization of the ileocecal specimen. Thickened, foreshortened mesentery is commonly encountered and the border of resection is chosen to allow excision of the entire inflamed ileocecal junction with accompanying edematous, thickened mesentery and creeping mesenteric fat. The mesentery of the specimen can be divided intra-abdominally with a laparoscopic stapling device or a LigaSure (Valleylab, Boulder, CO). Otherwise, the entire specimen can be eviscerated by enlarging the periumbilical midline trocar incision. Once this is accomplished, mesenteric division can occur extra-abdominally along with division of the proximal and distal ends of the specimen. Extra-abdominal resection allows palpation of the specimen to determine appropriate margins. Resection of bowel should extend to grossly normal tissue, and mesenteric vascular division should be performed close to bowel to avoid injury to adjacent structures, unless malignancy is a consideration. At this point, reanastomosis between the remaining ileum and ascending colon can be performed with a side-to-side stapled or handsewn anastomosis. Care must be taken to close the mesenteric defect.

Indication for Colectomy

Even though fulminant or toxic colitis is more common in ulcerative colitis, up to 20% of patients with Crohn's disease can present with this diagnosis. In this situation, a total colectomy with an end ileostomy and stapled rectal stump may be indicated. Prior to committing to this operation, a preoperative proctosigmoidoscopy should be performed to ensure normal-appearing rectal mucosa to allow adequate healing after transection and stapling of the rectum. Otherwise, a total proctocolectomy may be indicated. Unlike ulcerative colitis, an ileal pouch anal anastomosis should be avoided due to the possibility of anal involvement in Crohn's inflammation. Laparoscopic total colectomy is possible if the mesentery is not too foreshortened and the inflammatory changes still allow safe mobilization of the colon and protection of adjacent structures, such as the duodenum and ureters. Otherwise, conversion to open surgery is suggested.

Indication for Stricturoplasty

Surgical intervention for Crohn's disease is not intended to be curative because of the recurrent nature of the disease. As such, the philosophy is always to be conservative with bowel resection. In situations where isolated small bowel strictures are the cause for intervention, focal stricturoplasty with bowel preservation is performed. For lesions less than 10 cm, a longitudinal incision is made on the antimesenteric border of the affected small bowel, and then closed transversely with an absorbable running suture. Longer strictures can be addressed by creating a U-shaped anastomosis after the longitudinal incision. There is potential for malignant degeneration at these stricture sites, and biopsies should be sent for frozen section intraoperatively. Stricturoplasty can be safely performed laparoscopically, adhering to the same basic principles of laparoscopic bowel surgery.

Fistula Repair

The transmural nature of Crohn's disease oftentimes causes fistula formation with adjacent structures, such as the bladder or adjacent bowel. Dissection of a colovesicular fistula can be difficult, and in these situations dissection should remain close to the bowel and the bladder opening is closed with absorbable suture. Enteroenteric fistulas can sometimes be stapled across.

Mobilization of the inflamed tissue may lead to moderate bleeding, and blood clots should be evacuated and meticulous hemostasis should be obtained. Spillage of bowel contents should prompt copious irrigation of the operative field. The routine placement of a drain is usually not necessary. The midline fascial defect is closed with interrupted suture followed by irrigation of the abdominal wound, skin reapproximation, and injection of local anesthesia. Trocar site fascial defects greater than 1 cm should also be closed with a transfascial stitch.

Conversion to Open

The advancement and familiarity of minimally invasive surgery allows surgeons to provide this option to patients with comparable results to open surgery. Because of the complexity of the pathology, laparoscopic surgery for Crohn's disease is often performed by trained specialists in the field. However, it is the prudent surgeon that recognizes the need to convert to open surgery when indicated to safely perform the operation.

In a study to determine the reasons for conversion from laparoscopic to open surgery for Crohn's disease, Bayless et al.[4] prospectively analyzed 110 patients undergoing laparoscopic intervention for Crohn's-related diseases such as obstruction, failure of medical management, fistula, and perineal sepsis. Conversion to open was defined as an incision greater than 5 cm. Forty percent of these patients required conversion to open due to adhesions, extent of inflammation, size of inflammatory mass, inability to dissect a fistula, or inability to assess anatomy. Factors associated with conversion were internal fistula as an indication for surgery, smoking, steroid administration, extracecal colonic disease, and preoperative malnutrition.

Postoperative Care

Early ambulation is encouraged. The Foley catheter is removed on postoperative day 1 and diet is advanced as tolerated. Many surgeons prefer ketorolac for pain relief, although some controversy exists to the potential proinflammatory effects of this medication. Patients are restarted on their preoperative medication regimen. Unlike open surgery, steroid users generally do not require stress-dosing after laparoscopic surgery.

Common postoperative complications include obstruction, wound infection, bleeding, and anastomotic leak. Most obstructions are due to postoperative ileus or edema at the anastomosis site. Nasogastric decompression may be necessary and should resolve most obstructions. Worsening abdominal pain, fever, and tachycardia are ominous signs for an anastomotic leak. Imaging studies are not reliable in diagnosing leaks, and a strong clinical suspicion should lead to reexploration.

References

1. Liu CD, Rolandelli R, Ashley SW, Evans B, Shin M, McFadden DW. Laparoscopic surgery for inflammatory bowel disease. *Am Surg.* 1995;61(12):1054–1056.

2. Tan JJ, Tjandra JJ. Laparoscopic surgery for Crohn's disease: a meta-analysis. *Dis Colon Rectum.* 2007;50(5):576–585.

3. Stocchi L, Milsom JW, Fazio VW. Long-term outcomes of laparoscopic versus open ileocolic resection for Crohn's disease: follow-up of a prospective randomized trial. *Surgery.* 2008;144(4):622–627; discussion 627–628.

4. Schmidt CM, Talamini MA, Kaufman HS, Lilliemoe KD, Learn P, Bayless T. Laparoscopic surgery for Crohn's disease: reasons for conversion. *Ann Surg.* 2001;233(6):733–739.

Additional Suggested Reading

1. Casillas S, Delaney CP. Laparoscopic surgery for inflammatory bowel disease. *Dig Surg.* 2005;22:135–142.

2. Young-Fadok TM, HallLong K, McConnell EJ, Gomez Rey G, Cabanela RL. Advantages of laparoscopic resection for ileocolic Crohn's disease: improved outcomes and reduced costs. *Surg Endosc.* 2001;15:450–454.

3. Schmidt CM, Talamini MA, Kaufman HS, Lilliemoe KD, Learn P, Bayless T. Laparoscopic surgery for Crohn's disease: reasons for conversion. *Ann Surg.* 2001;233(6):733–739.

Crohn's Disease: Strictureplasty | 133

Scott A. Strong

Crohn's disease is a chronic inflammatory condition of the alimentary tract that is characterized by recurring episodes of disease exacerbation. Although surgery is reserved for individuals with disease-associated complications or debilitating symptoms despite medical therapy, most patients will undergo an operation during their lifetime. Moreover, recrudescent or recurrent disease commonly mandates reoperation, and repeated resections predispose patients to the development of short-bowel syndrome. Operative techniques that spare bowel length have been adopted over the past three decades because they conserve intestine without adversely impacting operative morbidity and recurrence. Specifically, strictureplasty is a surgical procedure that safely addresses a symptomatic stricture without sacrificing the affected bowel.

● BACKGROUND

The occurrence of skip lesions in the small intestine was recognized soon after the earliest reports of regional ileitis were published. During that early era, patients with several short diseased segments located in the proximal small bowel were managed by one or more resections to eliminate all of the affected areas. However, concerns subsequently arose regarding imminent short-bowel syndrome when the recurrent nature of Crohn's disease was understood. Thus, operations were avoided for patients with extensive jejunoileitis, and these individuals were instead treated with anti-inflammatory medications and hyperalimentation.

Patients afflicted by intestinal tuberculosis, similar to those with small bowel Crohn's disease, occasionally suffer from obstructive intestinal symptoms related to multiple strictures of the jejunum and ileum. In 1977, Katariya and colleagues reported using a novel operative technique described as "stricture-plasty" in patients with multiple tuberculosis strictures; the procedure effectively ameliorated obstructive symptoms while safely preserving the affected small bowel.[1] Emmanoel Lee, of the John Radcliffe Hospital in Oxford, United Kingdom, successfully employed this nonresectional technique two years later in a 21-year-old woman with multiple small bowel strictures

caused by Crohn's disease. Lee and Papaioannou subsequently reported their experience in nine patients in whom strictureplasty was performed for extensive Crohn's disease of the small bowel.[2]

The surgeon caring for patients with Crohn's disease must understand the efficacy of appropriate medical therapy, consider the patient's long-term prognosis, and conserve small bowel whenever possible because repeated or massive resections can lead to short-bowel syndrome. Therefore, operative treatment is reserved for patients who develop disease complications or fail their medical therapy. At the time of laparotomy, only those segments considered to be contributing to the patient's constellation of symptoms merit operative attention. However, if strictures are identified at operation, regardless of whether the surgeon believes them to be symptomatic, strictureplasty should supplement the primary procedure. This approach is justified because experience has proven that strictureplasty adds little to the morbidity of resection, and reoperation following strictureplasty is more likely to be necessary for new symptomatic strictures than for restricturing of an old strictureplasty site; detailed information related to the these justifications is provided in later sections.

● TECHNIQUES

The strictureplasty procedure has been performed for strictures in multiple anatomic locations, including those arising in the jejunum/ileum, ileocolic anastomosis, ileocecal valve, duodenum, and colon. The type of strictureplasty employed is generally dictated by the length of the stricture, but the location of the stricture and the pliability of the affected bowel sometimes impact the choice of techniques. Relatively short (<10 cm) strictures are usually managed by a Heineke-Mikulicz strictureplasty. Medium (10–20 cm) strictures should be typically approached using a Finney strictureplasty, and long (>20 cm) strictures are best treated with a Michelassi strictureplasty. Other less commonly used techniques have also been reported. The Judd and Moskel-Walske-Neumayer strictureplasties are modified from the Heineke-Mikulicz procedure and used for

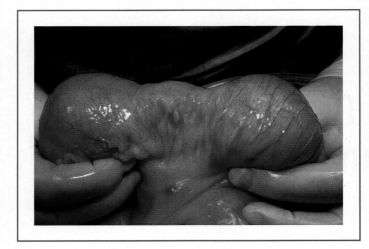

FIGURE 133.1 • Typical appearance of Crohn's disease of the small bowel.

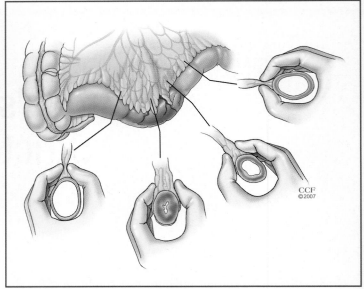

FIGURE 133.2 • Palpation of Crohn's disease of the terminal ileum.

complex short-length strictures.[3] A Judd strictureplasty may be employed when a fistula accompanies the stricture, whereas the Moskel-Walske-Neumayer strictureplasty might be warranted if the bowel proximal to the stricture is excessively dilated. If a medium-length stricture is encountered, a combination Heineke-Mikulicz and Finney strictureplasty can be used.[4] Alternatively, a double Heineke-Mikulicz-type strictureplasty[5] or Jaboulay strictureplasty[2] can be performed in this instance.

Regardless the type of planned strictureplasty, the operation is similarly begun through a laparoscopic or conventional approach. The stomach, duodenum, small intestine, and large bowel are carefully inspected. As the small bowel is distally traced from the duodenojejunal junction, suture tags are placed on segments affected by disease. In its classic form, Crohn's disease of the small bowel is easily recognizable (Fig. 133.1). The involved segment is characteristically indurated, thick-walled, and constricted with omentum or adjacent bowel loops occasionally adherent to the inflamed area. Skip lesions affecting short or long segments of small bowel occur in approximately 20% of cases.

In jejunoileal disease, thickening of the mesenteric margin of the bowel, a fierce serositis or "corkscrew" appearance of the serosal vessels, and fat encroachment or wrapping on the sides of the intestinal wall are commonly seen. The scalloped appearance of the normal bowel mesentery is lost, as the fat deposition between the terminal branches of the marginal vessels is excessive. The proximal bowel above the strictured segment is commonly dilated and this bowel may be thickened because of muscular hypertrophy that accompanies chronic obstruction.

In some cases, these classic findings are absent. In these instances, the best guide to disease location is palpation along the mesenteric margin, as the margin of a diseased segment is invariably thickened in response to an overlying mesenteric ulcer (Fig. 133.2). Even subtly strictured segments are easily recognized by this marginal thickening of the mesenteric angle. If doubt exists or the surgeon is inexperienced with strictureplasty, then calibration is a reasonable alternative for identifying strictured segments. Methods to quantify the caliber of a stricture through an open enterotomy include passage of a standard marble (16.5-mm diameter), 2-cm bougie, or Foley catheter with the balloon inflated to a 2-cm diameter. However, all of these techniques are time consuming and may contribute to intraoperative contamination.

At the completion of each strictureplasty, a radiopaque titanium clip is applied to the mesenteric fat adjacent to the closure site. A single clip is applied at the most proximal site and an increasing number of clips are placed at each subsequent strictureplasty site as the surgeon distally progresses along the bowel length. These markers allow for future identification of strictureplasty sites during contrast radiography of the small bowel.

Heineke-Mikulicz Strictureplasty

The Heineke-Mikulicz strictureplasty is commenced by making a linear antimesenteric incision that is proximally and distally extended 1 to 2 cm beyond the stricture (Fig. 133.3). The wound edges are carefully inspected and any bleeding is meticulously controlled with electrocautery. The accompanying mesenteric ulcer is scrutinized and then selectively biopsied to exclude an unrecognized malignancy. Stay sutures are placed on both sides of the enterotomy at the midpoint of the enterotomy site, and lateral traction is applied to convert the longitudinal enterotomy into a transverse defect. The wound is transversely closed using an interrupted single layer of sutures.

Finney Strictureplasty

The Finney strictureplasty is employed for reasonably supple bowel affected by a medium-length stricture. The bowel is again longitudinally opened as with a Heineke-Mikulicz procedure, and then folded on itself into a U-shape. A side-to-side two-layer anastomosis is then created with absorbable sutures (Fig. 133.4). The posterior portion of the strictureplasty is closed with a continuous suture, incorporating all layers of the bowel wall. Additional interrupted sutures are placed at 1- to 2-cm intervals. The anterior layer is closed in a similar fashion while

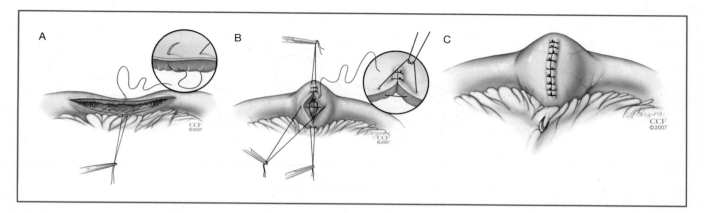

FIGURE 133.3 • A–C Heineke-Mikulicz strictureplasty used in short (<10 cm) length strictures.

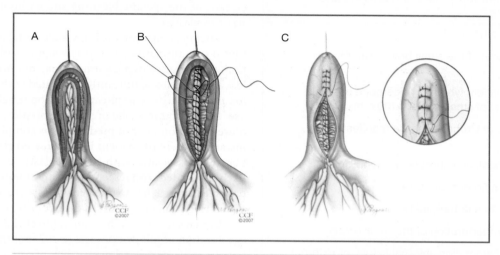

FIGURE 133.4 • A–C Finney strictureplasty used in medium (10–20 cm) length strictures.

carefully inverting the mucosal layer, particularly at the apices of the enterotomy. One of the concerns voiced regarding a Finney strictureplasty is that of bacterial overgrowth in the resultant large, diverticulum-like sac that extends from the intestine. In addition, recurrent stricturing tends to occur within the afferent limb of bowel just proximal to the Finney-type diverticulum.

Michelassi Strictureplasty

Long strictures provide technical challenges in completing a Finney strictureplasty. Similarly, unless the bowel is supple enough to bend into a U-shape and still allow for a tension-free anastomosis, leakage and sepsis are likely to occur. In these instances, a Michelassi strictureplasty[6] is performed using absorbable sutures to create a two-layer side-to-side isoperistaltic anastomosis encompassing the entire strictured segment; the outer closure incorporates the seromuscular layers and the inner closure is full-thickness in nature (Fig. 133.5). The bowel is opened as with the other procedures and then divided at its midpoint. The normal bowel proximal to the stricture is joined to the diseased bowel immediately distal to the division. The anastomosis is continued until the diseased bowel immediately proximal to the division is sutured to the normal bowel distal to the entire diseased segment. Care is taken to assure that stenotic areas of one segment align with

dilated areas of the other segment wherever possible. In some cases, a thickened or indurated mesentery precludes tension-free alignment of the two segments; a safe anastomosis can only be created by excising the middle segment of the diseased bowel prior to creating the isoperistaltic anastomosis.

● OUTCOMES

Many centers have conducted comprehensive studies on patients undergoing strictureplasty. The typical patient treated by strictureplasty presents with symptoms related to small bowel obstruction unresponsive to medical therapy. Nearly two-thirds of patients will undergo synchronous resection, most have three separate segments treated by strictureplasty, and more than 250 cm of small bowel remains after the procedure. Six months postoperatively, nearly all patients note relief of their obstructive symptoms and average 10 kg of weight gain. Furthermore, 80% patients have discontinued steroid therapy with the remainder averaging less than 10 mg of daily prednisone.[7]

The technique of the strictureplasty procedure is based upon incising and suturing diseased segments, and this raises natural concerns regarding suture-line healing and the occurrence of intra-abdominal sepsis. Aside from meticulous conduct

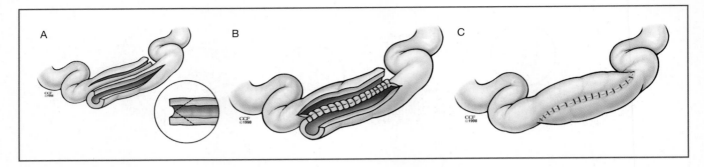

FIGURE 133.5 • A–C Michelassi strictureplasty used in long (>20 cm) length strictures.

TABLE 133.1 Strictureplasty: Indications and Contraindications

Indications for strictureplasty
diffuse involvement of the small bowel with multiple strictures
stricture(s) in a patient who has undergone previous major resection(s) of small bowel (>100 cm)
rapid recurrence of Crohn's disease manifested as obstruction
stricture in a patient with short bowel syndrome
nonphlegmonous fibrotic stricture
Contraindications to strictureplasty
free or contained perforation of the small bowel
phlegmonous inflammation, internal fistula, or external fistula involving the affected site
multiple strictures within a short segment
stricture in close proximity to a site chosen for resection
colonic strictures
hypoalbuminemia (<2.0 g/dL)

of the procedure, prevention of such complications lies with careful patient selection (Table 133.1).

A recent literature review by Yamamoto and colleagues[8] reported on 20 studies with 1057 patients undergoing jejunoileal strictureplasties; the majority of these procedures were Heineke-Mikulicz strictureplasties. An overall complication rate of 13% was noted, and these complications included: anastomotic leak, fistula, or abscess (4%); hemorrhage (3%); ileus (2%), and; bowel obstruction (1%). Approximately 78% of the septic events were related to a strictureplasty site and 44% of the affected patients required repeat laparotomy to successfully control the sepsis. Most instances of strictureplasty site bleeding will spontaneously cease without intervention. If hemorrhage persists, however, selective mesenteric angiography is performed and vasopressin is intra-arterially infused. In the rare event that bleeding is uncontrolled by the interventional radiologist or recurs, laparotomy is required to control the hemorrhage.

Unfortunately, if re-operation is necessary, it is difficult to be certain of the specific bleeding site without opening several strictureplasties.

Anemia, concomitant intra-abdominal abscess with peritoneal contamination, emergency surgery, older age at operation, preoperative hypoalbuminemia, and preoperative weight loss are variables significantly associated with an increased risk for perioperative complications.[8] Conversely, corticosteroid use, length, number, site of strictureplasties, and synchronous bowel resection are not predictors for complications. In those instances where the patient is at increased risk for septic complications associated with strictureplasty, an equivalent risk is likely associated with resection and anastomosis. Therefore, the preferred approach is to proceed with strictureplasty, but create a diverting stoma proximal to the operative site.

In that same review by Yamamoto et al.,[8] the range of average duration of follow-up was 2 to 107 months. Overall, symptomatic recurrence developed in 39% of patients and reoperative recurrence occurred in 30%. The pooled meta-analytical results of recurrence rate after strictureplasty demonstrated a combined recurrence rate of 23%. Their results after a meta-regression analysis of recurrence rate for variable study follow-up periods yielded a 5-year recurrence rate of 28%. Recurrence requiring reoperation at a previous strictureplasty site occurred in 10% of patients and the site-specific reoperation rate (number of strictureplasties requiring reoperation/total number of strictureplasties) was only 3%. These results are similar to the findings of Wibmer and associates[9] who reviewed 40 relevant articles dealing with strictureplasty at any anatomical site, and they found the median reoperative recurrence rate was 24% after a median follow-up of 46 months.

Short duration of disease, short interval since prior resection, and younger age are reported to be significant risk factors for recurrence; corticosteroid use, length, number, or site of strictureplasties, and nutritional status, do not impact recurrence.[8] However, a more recent report by Greenstein and associates[10] found that the number of strictures and the number of strictureplasties were both associated with reoperative recurrence. Specifically, the 5-year reoperation rates were 14% and 31% for patients with ≤8 strictures and patients with >8 strictures, respectively, and the 5-year reoperation rates were 14% and 33% for patients with ≤4 strictureplasties and patients with >4 strictureplasties, respectively. In multivariate regression, each additional stricture was associated with a 7% increase in recurrence and each additional strictureplasty was associated with a 23% increase in recurrence.

Compared to resection, patients undergoing strictureplasty alone tend to experience a lower incidence of postoperative complications.[11] However, reoperative recurrence after strictureplasty alone is more likely than after resection alone, and patients who have a resection experience a significantly longer recurrence-free survival than those individuals undergoing strictureplasty alone.[11] Interestingly, the 10-year site-specific cumulative reoperative recurrence rate for a strictureplasty and an anastomosis following resection are 7% and 18%, respectively.[12] Therefore, it appears that the risk for reoperative recurrence is more likely associated with disease behavior than the use of strictureplasty instead of resection and anastomosis.

Patients undergoing a Michelassi strictureplasty represent a select group, and the results associated with this procedure were reported in a study that accumulated the experience of six internationally recognized centers.[13] Overall, 184 patients underwent such a procedure and the average length of diseased bowel used for the strictureplasty was nearly 40 cm. One-fifth of the patients suffered an enteric fistula, but the incidence of hemorrhage and bowel obstruction were similar to that seen with Heineke-Mikulicz strictureplasty. The 5-year reoperative rate was 23%, and recurrence requiring reoperation at the previous Michelassi strictureplasty site occurred in only 7% of patients.

A few centers have reported on their experience with strictureplasty for stricturing of an ileocolic anastomosis, and the results have been acceptable compared to resection.[14–16] Specifically, the largest series contained 39 patients, and their rates of septic complications after strictureplasty versus resection were 3% and 13%, respectively.[16] Moreover, the 10-year cumulative reoperation rates at the ileocolic site were 66% and 54%, respectively.

Two reports describing significant numbers of strictureplasty for duodenal Crohn's disease have been published with mixed results. The first study from Birmingham, England reported no obvious advantages associated with duodenal strictureplasty over gastrojejunostomy. Furthermore, strictureplasty was associated with a higher incidence of early complications and recurrent stricturing.[17] In contrast, the Cleveland Clinic found duodenal strictureplasty to be safe and effective with potential physiologic advantages over gastrojejunostomy.[18] The difference between the two series may be explained by a longer follow-up period associated with the Birmingham report.

Strictureplasty has been described for colonic narrowing. Broering and associates[19] assessed the efficacy of strictureplasty versus resection in patients with obstructive Crohn's disease of the colon. The results were evaluated in terms of postoperative complications, surgical recurrence, and quality of life. Of 58 patients with colon disease, 29 underwent strictureplasty. Postoperative morbidity and quality of life were not significantly different between the two groups. The reoperative recurrence rate was 36% in those patients treated by strictureplasty and 24% in those managed by resection. However, 6% of colonic strictures are complicated by an underlying malignancy, and preservation of colon by strictureplasty does not seem to afford any distinct advantages. Therefore, symptomatic colonic strictures should likely be resected rather than treated by strictureplasty.

At least three case reports of malignancy arising in a strictureplasty site have been published.[20–22] Although the issue of routine biopsy remains controversial, most experts do not recommend routine biopsy, although biopsy should be performed if there is any suspicion of carcinoma.

● CONCLUSION

Strictureplasty remains relatively unchanged from its initial description almost three decades ago. Some variations have been suggested for relatively long strictures. Nearly all series attest to the short-term safety and efficacy of the technique, with long-term studies reporting competitive clinical and reoperative recurrence rates. The various techniques should be part of the armamentarium of any surgeon regularly managing patients with Crohn's disease.

References

1. Katariya RN, Sood S, Rao PG, Rao PL. Stricture-plasty for tubercular strictures of the gastro-intestinal tract. *Br J Surg.* 1977;64(7):496–498.
2. Lee EC, Papaioannou N. Minimal surgery for chronic obstruction in patients with extensive or universal Crohn's disease. *Ann R Coll Surg Engl.* 1982;64(4):229–233.
3. Gaetini A, De Simone M, Resegotti A. Our experience with strictureplasty in the surgical treatment of Crohn's disease. *Hepatogastroenterology.* 1989;36(6):511–515.
4. Fazio VW, Tjandra JJ. Strictureplasty for Crohn's disease with multiple long strictures. *Dis Colon Rectum.* 1993;36(1):71–72.
5. Sasaki I, Funayama Y, Naito H, Fukushima K, Shibata C, Matsuno S. Extended strictureplasty for multiple short skipped strictures of Crohn's disease. *Dis Colon Rectum.* 1996;39(3):342–344.
6. Michelassi F. Side-to-side isoperistaltic strictureplasty for multiple Crohn's strictures. *Dis Colon Rectum.* 1996;39(3):345–349.
7. Yamamoto T, Bain IM, Allan RN, Keighley MR. An audit of strictureplasty for small-bowel Crohn's disease. *Dis Colon Rectum.* 1999;42(6):797–803.
8. Yamamoto T, Fazio VW, Tekkis PP. Safety and efficacy of strictureplasty for Crohn's disease: a systematic review and meta-analysis. *Dis Colon Rectum.* 2007;50(11):1968–1986.
9. Wibmer AG, Kroesen AJ, Gröne J, Buhr HJ, Ritz JP. Comparison of strictureplasty and endoscopic balloon dilatation for stricturing Crohn's disease–review of the literature. *Int J Colorectal Dis.* 2010;25(10):1149–1157.
10. Greenstein AJ, Zhang LP, Miller AT, et al. Relationship of the number of Crohn's strictures and strictureplasties to postoperative recurrence. *J Am Coll Surg.* 2009;208(6):1065–1070.
11. Reese GE, Purkayastha S, Tilney HS, von Roon A, Yamamoto T, Tekkis PP. Strictureplasty vs resection in small bowel Crohn's disease: an evaluation of short-term outcomes and recurrence. *Colorectal Dis.* 2007;9(8):686–694.
12. Uchino M, Ikeuchi H, Matsuoka H, Matsumoto T, Takesue Y, Tomita N. Long-term efficacy of strictureplasty for Crohn's disease. *Surg Today.* 2010;40(10):949–953.
13. Michelassi F, Taschieri A, Tonelli F, et al. An international, multicenter, prospective, observational study of the side-to-side isoperistaltic strictureplasty in Crohn's disease. *Dis Colon Rectum.* 2007;50(3):277–284.

14. Tjandra JJ, Fazio VW. Strictureplasty for ileocolic anastomotic strictures in Crohn's disease. *Dis Colon Rectum.* 1993;36(12):1099–103; discussion 1103.

15. Taschieri AM, Cristaldi M, Elli M, et al. Description of new "bowel-sparing" techniques for long strictures of Crohn's disease. *Am J Surg.* 1997;173(6):509–512.

16. Yamamoto T, Allan RN, Keighley MR. Strategy for surgical management of ileocolonic anastomotic recurrence in Crohn's disease. *World J Surg.* 1999;23(10):1055–60; discussion 1060.

17. Yamamoto T, Bain IM, Connolly AB, Allan RN, Keighley MR. Outcome of strictureplasty for duodenal Crohn's disease. *Br J Surg.* 1999;86(2):259–262.

18. Worsey MJ, Hull T, Ryland L, Fazio V. Strictureplasty is an effective option in the operative management of duodenal Crohn's disease. *Dis Colon Rectum.* 1999;42(5):596–600.

19. Broering DC, Eisenberger CF, Koch A, et al. Strictureplasty for large bowel stenosis in Crohn's disease: quality of life after surgical therapy. *Int J Colorectal Dis.* 2001;16(2):81–87.

20. Marchetti F, Fazio VW, Ozuner G. Adenocarcinoma arising from a strictureplasty site in Crohn's disease. Report of a case. *Dis Colon Rectum.* 1996;39(11):1315–1321.

21. Jaskowiak NT, Michelassi F. Adenocarcinoma at a strictureplasty site in Crohn's disease: report of a case. *Dis Colon Rectum.* 2001;44(2):284–287.

22. Tonelli F, Bargellini T, Leo F, Nesi G. Duodenal adenocarcinoma arising at the strictureplasty site in a patient with Crohn's disease: report of a case. *Int J Colorectal Dis.* 2009;24(4):475–477.

Gastroduodenal Crohn's Disease: Surgical Management | 134

Edwin R. Itenberg and Jeffrey W. Milsom

INTRODUCTION

Involvement of the duodenum in Crohn's disease is rare, even more infrequent is primary disease of the stomach and duodenum. Using clinical and radiographic findings, it is estimated to occur in only about 0.5% to 4% of adults with Crohn's disease.[1] Most patients present with concurrent disease at other locations at the time of surgery or have a previous history of surgery for Crohn's disease. In one study involving 89 cases of duodenal Crohn's disease,[2] more than 80% of patients had preexisting or coincidental distal disease at presentation. At long-term follow-up, only 7/89 (8%) patients in this study had isolated duodenal disease.

PRESENTATION AND WORKUP

The most common symptom of gastroduodenal (GD) Crohn's disease is abdominal pain, usually epigastric in location. Symptoms are similar to peptic ulcer disease and are often managed similarly, with H2 blockers or proton pump inhibitors as first-line medical treatment. In addition, anti-inflammatory medications may be added as well. The correct diagnosis can be made from clinical, endoscopic, and radiographic features despite lack of histological evidence.[3]

Historically, barium upper gastrointestinal studies (UGIS) were used for diagnosis of GD Crohn's disease. These may show thickened folds, aphthous ulcers, deep longitudinal fissuring ulcerations, cobblestoning, and stricturing.[1] The "Ram's horn" sign can also be seen, as a tubular narrowing of the antrum, limited distensibility, and poor peristalsis giving a distinct conical narrowing.[4] UGIS also readily picks up fistulas involving the duodenum.[1] Endoscopy with biopsy remains the gold standard in the diagnosis of GD Crohn's disease. Endoscopic findings include patchy erythema, mucosal friability, thickened folds, linear and aphthous ulcers, and cobblestoning.[5]

SURGICAL OPTIONS—GENERAL PRINCIPLES

In one study, 37% of patients did not respond to medical therapy alone, and ultimately required surgery.[2] Indications for surgical intervention are usually due to obstructive symptoms, including postprandial pain (71–100%), weight loss (55–72%), and nausea and vomiting (32–72%). Less common indications for surgery are due to hemorrhage (usually chronic), as well as recurrent pancreatitis. A barium UGIS should be performed prior to surgery to evaluate extent of involvement and the degree of obstruction, and to look for any skip lesions.[6] In the study by Worsey et al.,[7] 12% of patients had greater than one stricture in the duodenum. A few options exist for surgical treatment; however, due to the rarity of this disease, no prospective trials show superiority of one treatment. In contrast to Crohn's disease at other sites, resectional surgery for GD Crohn's disease is associated with a substantially increased morbidity and therefore almost always avoided.[8]

SURGICAL OPTIONS—BYPASS

Traditionally, open bypass either by gastrojejunostomy or gastroduodenostomy combined with a truncal vagotomy was the preferred treatment option.[3,7] Addition of vagotomy is added to reduce the risk of marginal ulceration of the jejunal limb. A study from the Cleveland Clinic found that at long-term follow-up, 50% of patients who underwent bypass without vagotomy required reoperation for marginal ulcers.[3] Worsey et al.[7] recommends the addition of vagotomy to a bypass procedure based on their data, which shows only 2/21 patients who underwent bypass with vagotomy required reoperation for marginal ulcer. Other studies do not recommend performing vagotomy mainly because of the complications that are encountered postoperatively such as diarrhea, dumping syndrome, and delayed gastric emptying.[2,8–10] In the study by Shapiro et al.,[9] only 1/24 patients had vagotomy as part of gastrojejunostomy, and, at average of 58 months, no patients experienced clinically significant GD ulcers requiring operation. This is attributed to the more widespread use of proton pump inhibitors today. Modern therapy probably supports avoidance of at least truncal vagotomy.

SURGICAL OPTIONS— STRICTUREPLASTY

Strictureplasty has long been a widely accepted treatment option for Crohn's disease of the small bowel. The advantages of strictureplasty are that a vagotomy is not usually required, it obviates the need to mobilize and use jejunum that may otherwise be involved by Crohn's disease or adhesions from prior surgery, and a potential blind loop is not created.[2] However, for isolated disease of the duodenum, the results of strictureplasty have been mixed. In the study by Yamamoto et al.,[10] 13 patients underwent strictureplasty. After median follow-up of 143 months, they found that nine patients (69%) required reoperation. Three patients required early operation for anastomotic breakdown and fistula,[5] and prolonged obstruction.[4] Six patients ultimately required reoperation for restricture at the previous strictureplasty site. In comparison are the results from a study by Worsey et al.[7] in which 13 patients underwent strictureplasty. In all, 15 strictureplasties were performed in 13 patients—9 Heineke-Mickulicz and 6 Finney strictureplasties. At mean follow-up of 42 months, only 2 (15%) required repeat operation for complications or recurrence of GD Crohn's disease. This led the authors to conclude that strictureplasty is a safe and effective operation for GD Crohn's disease.

When performing strictureplasty, the duodenum should be fully mobilized using a Kocher maneuver. A Finney type strictureplasty is preferable, beginning proximal to the pylorus, and a hand-sewn anastomosis can be performed for optimal security of friable tissue. The entire duodenum, including the third and fourth portions, should be examined before performing the strictureplasty, to rule out additional strictures. This can be done either digitally or with an inflated foley catheter, and now we perform an upper endoscopy to assess the sutured duodenum before closing the abdomen. We also place an omental overlay if sufficient length is available to improve healing and prevent fistulization

ROLE OF LAPAROSCOPY

Laparoscopic surgery has only recently been offered as an option for patients with Crohn's disease of the duodenum.[9] In the study from the Mount Sinai Medical Center, 26 patients were operated on for intrinsic duodenal Crohn's disease. Of these patients, 11 had open bypass, 13 had laparoscopic bypass, and 2 had strictureplasty. Patients in the laparoscopic group resumed oral diet 3 days after surgery and were discharged at a mean of 6.9 days after surgery, as compared with 4.4 and 12.2 days after open bypass, respectively. At long-term follow-up (mean of 58 months) morbidity in the laparoscopic group was 8% compared to 45% in the open bypass group. Also, none of the patients developed marginal ulcers requiring reoperation.

Another option in laparoscopic treatment of Crohn's disease is strictureplasty. Although the anatomic location of the duodenum makes intracorporeal strictureplasty more difficult, much promise is being shown using robotic assistance in gastrointestinal (GI) surgery. In one study by Sonoda et al.,[11] completely intracorporeal strictureplasties were performed using the da Vinci surgical system in dogs. Their results showed improved dexterity compared to conventional laparoscopic surgery, and all strictureplasty sites healed without signs of sepsis.

FISTULAS

GD fistulas complicating Crohn's disease are rare, occurring in less than 1% of patients. A GD fistula is usually a result of primary disease elsewhere in the GI tract, most commonly in the transverse colon or as recurrence at the ileocolonic anastomosis after a resection. To prevent this, Wilk et al.[12] recommend placing the ileocolonic anastomosis as far away as possible from the duodenum and/or placing a piece of omentum between the duodenum and the anastomosis. In Yamamoto's study,[10] only 1 out of 11 fistulas closed with medical treatment, leading them to recommend surgical closure of GD fistulas because of their good long-term results. When the stomach or duodenum is not involved with Crohn's disease, treatment involves resection and primary closure of the diseased segment. If the defect is large, the preferred therapy is duodenojejunostomy, provided the jejunum is free of disease.

SUMMARY

In our experience, GD strictureplasty is the preferred option to bypass for GD Crohn's disease. Strictureplasties confer a physiologic advantage to bypass, as intestinal continuity is preserved, no vagotomy is necessary, and the possibility of a blind loop is eliminated. We prefer to avoid a bypass in these patients because it leaves behind residual disease and does not treat the underlying cause of symptoms. The role of laparoscopic and robotic surgery is quite promising in Crohn's disease, but at this time further investigations into their use are needed.

References

1. Reynolds HL Jr, Stellato TA. Crohn's disease of the foregut. *Surg Clin North Am.* 2001;81(1):117–135, viii.

2. Nugent FW, Roy MA. Duodenal Crohn's disease: an analysis of 89 cases. *Am J Gastroenterol.* 1989;84(3):249–254.

3. Ross TM, Fazio VW, Farmer RG. Long-term results of surgical treatment for Crohn's disease of the duodenum. *Ann Surg.* 1983;197(4):399–406.

4. Farman J, Faegenburg D, Dallemand S, Chen CK. Crohn's disease of the stomach: the "ram's horn" sign. *Am J Roentgenol Radium Ther Nucl Med.* 1975;123(2):242–251.

5. Kefalas CH. Gastroduodenal Crohn's disease. *Proc (Bayl Univ Med Cent).* 2003;16(2):147–151.

6. Salky B. Severe gastroduodenal Crohn's disease: surgical treatment. *Inflamm Bowel Dis.* 2003;9(2):129–30; discussion 131.

7. Worsey MJ, Hull T, Ryland L, Fazio V. Strictureplasty is an effective option in the operative management of duodenal Crohn's disease. *Dis Colon Rectum.* 1999;42(5):596–600.

8. Murray JJ, Schoetz DJ Jr, Nugent FW, Coller JA, Veidenheimer MC. Surgical management of Crohn's disease involving the duodenum. *Am J Surg.* 1984;147(1):58–65.

9. Shapiro M, Greenstein AJ, Byrn J, et al. Surgical management and outcomes of patients with duodenal Crohn's disease. *J Am Coll Surg.* 2008;207(1):36–42.

10. Yamamoto T, Bain IM, Connolly AB, Allan RN, Keighley MR. Outcome of strictureplasty for duodenal Crohn's disease. *Br J Surg.* 1999;86(2):259–262.

11. Sonoda T, Lee S, Whelan RL, et al. Robotically assisted small intestinal strictureplasty in dogs: a survival study involving 16 Heineke-Mikulicz strictureplasties. *Surg Endosc.* 2007;21(12):2220–2223.

12. Wilk PJ, Fazio V, Turnbull RB Jr. The dilemma of Crohn's disease: ileoduodenal fistula complicating Crohn's disease. *Dis Colon Rectum.* 1977;20(5):387–392.

Intraabdominal Abscesses in Crohn's Disease | 135

Akbar K. Waljee, Ryan W. Stidham, and Peter D. R. Higgins

EPIDEMIOLOGY AND PATHOGENESIS

Intraabdominal abscesses in patients with Crohn's disease (CD) generally result from a bowel perforation that is contained by adjacent structures, including nearby unaffected segments of bowel. These abscesses eventually occur in 10% to 30% of all patients with CD. Abscesses occur as a consequence of deep ulceration and transmural inflammation in combination with locally increased intraluminal pressure, which drives the initiation of a perforating fistula. When this perforation is contained by adjacent tissues, it becomes an intraabdominal abscess. Internal fistulae in CD are almost exclusively found adjacent to luminal strictures (though these strictures may not always be apparent on imaging studies) and most commonly occur adjacent to a loop of ileum. An epidemiologic estimate of the prevalence of nonperianal fistulae in CD patients in Olmsted County, Minnesota, found a prevalence rate of nonperianal fistulae of 12% at 10 years, and 24% by 20 years of disease.[1] The occurrence of intraabdominal abscess in CD appears to parallel the development of nonperianal fistulae, with an increasing prevalence with longer duration of disease.

CLINICAL PRESENTATION

The clinical presentation of abdominal abscesses is highly variable and can be modified by immunosuppressive therapy for CD. Patients can present with symptoms of abdominal pain with fevers and leukocytosis, or with a sign of a new, palpable abdominal mass. The presence of an area of localized redness, swelling, pain, and warmth can be found with abdominal-wall abscesses or incipient enterocutaneous fistulae (Fig. 135.1). More commonly, a deep intraabdominal or pelvic abscess presents as a vague, difficult-to-localize discomfort or mild pain, and systemic symptoms can predominate.

It is common for patients, particularly those on chronic steroids or immunomodulators, to present with more subtle malaise, low-grade fevers, decreased appetite, and fatigue. Increases in the white blood count, the erythrocyte sedimentation rate or CRP, and the platelet count in the absence of significant worsening of bowel symptoms can be helpful clues in patients on

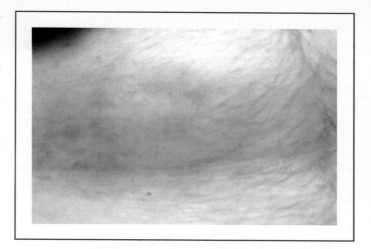

FIGURE 135.1 • Abdominal-wall abscess in Crohn's disease.

steroids without localizing symptoms. In contrast, anti-tumor necrosis factor (anti-TNFα) agents reduce the ability of the immune system to restrain abscesses, and patients on these agents often experience rapid growth of an abscess and local signs and symptoms with few systemic symptoms. Even in the presence of anti-TNFα agents, it is uncommon for abdominal abscesses in CD to present with overwhelming sepsis.

DIAGNOSIS AND PROGNOSIS

The physical exam is limited in the detection of an abdominal abscess deeper than the abdominal wall. Psoas abscesses present with the inability to stand up straight, pain on straight leg while raising it or with hip extension, with partial relief from hip flexion. In most cases, an elevated index of suspicion and an imaging study are required to detect abscesses. A study of patients in the emergency department that examined the symptoms and lab tests associated with intraabdominal abscesses found that anorexia, chills, and elevations in hematocrit, white blood cell count, and platelet count were most

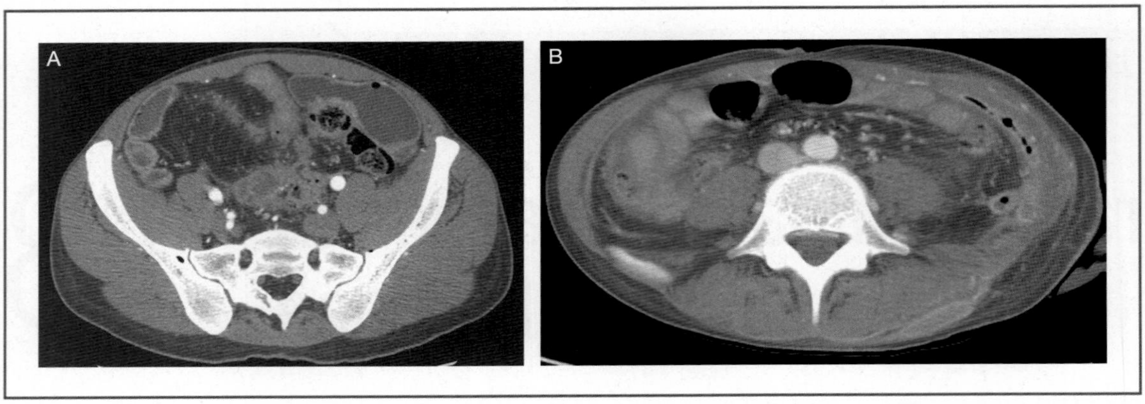

FIGURE 135.2 • (A) Single midline abscess in pelvis adjacent to major vessels. (B) Multiple small air–containing abscesses in the left abdominal wall.

predictive of intraabdominal abscess.[2] Given the frequency of abscesses and their often nebulous presentation when symptoms are masked by immune suppressants in CD, the need for accurate diagnosis and intervention is crucial. Maconi's prospective study has shown that standard oral contrast CT (computed tomography) and US (ultrasound) have comparable accuracy in detecting intraabdominal abscesses, though CT may have a higher specificity and positive predictive value. It is important to note that CT and US can miss up to 17% of intraabdominal abscesses that are small or deep within the abdominal cavity, and a single negative-imaging test (e.g., the-middle-of-the-night emergency-department CT scan) in a clinically suspicious setting should not necessarily close off this line of diagnostic thinking.[3]

In addition to CT and US, CT enterography (CTE) and MR enterography (MRE) have rapidly become popular in the diagnosis and monitoring of CD. Both of these cross-sectional imaging techniques use negative oral contrast, allowing better visualization of the bowel wall than is possible with standard CT. MRE has nearly the resolution of CTE, but, due to slower acquisition time, is more susceptible to motion (including peristaltic movement) artifacts. CTE and MRE are helpful for identifying abscesses and fistulae and provide accurate assessment of bowel inflammation and can identify nearby bowel strictures. The imaging study used should depend in part on local expertise, as CT, US, and MR appear to be comparable in accuracy, though CT may be the most specific of the three for abscess identification.[3]

The goals of whichever imaging study is used are (1) to assess for the presence of an abscess; (2) to determine whether the abscess location, size, and loculations allow a safe route for complete percutaneous drainage; (3) to determine whether there is an adjacent stricture or fistula contributing to the abscess; (4) to determine whether there is adjacent bowel inflammation contributing to the abscess; and (5) to establish a baseline for longitudinal assessment of the success of treatment and the readiness of the patient for immunosuppressive therapy. Communication with the diagnostic radiologist and the interventional radiology team that performs abscess drainage are important in obtaining all of the needed information from the baseline imaging study and formulating a plan for evacuation of the infectious material.

The characteristics of the abscess and the nearby bowel can help predict the likelihood of nonoperative success. Examples of a simple posterior midline abscess (2A) and a complex of left anterior abdominal wall abscesses (2B) are presented in Fig. 135.2. A complex, loculated abscess, or one that is in a location not amenable to percutaneous drainage, is more likely to require surgical intervention. An adjacent stricture or wide fistulae from the bowel to the abscess are both associated with an increased likelihood of requiring surgery. Finally, active inflammation in the adjacent bowel makes treatment difficult, as use of systemic antiinflammatory therapy, particularly with steroids or anti-TNFα agents (which act as "abscess fertilizers") will often contribute to the growth and persistence of an incompletely drained abscess.[4–6]

● PRINCIPLES OF THERAPY

Intraabdominal abscesses require removal of the infectious material; aspiration is usually sufficient for collections ≤ 3 cm, whereas catheter drainage is generally required for abscesses > 3 cm. Abscesses that connect to bowel via widely patent fistulae will often require drainage followed by elective surgery. Antibiotics are an important adjunct to removal of the infectious material, whereas antiinflammatory medications, particularly steroids and anti-TNFα agents, in the absence of successful abscess evacuation, often augment the growth of abscesses in CD.

There are numerous options in the treatment of intraabdominal abscesses associated with CD. Unfortunately, most of the available data are from retrospective case series, and no therapies have been evaluated with controlled trials in this patient population. We have to extrapolate largely from the results of case series, with conclusions tempered by the high probability of substantial selection bias in all of the published series. The options include surgical incision and drainage with antibiotics, percutaneous drainage with antibiotics, antibiotic therapy without drainage, combining one of these three options with antiinflammatory therapy, and/or combining one of these options with surgical resection of the diseased bowel.

ANTIBIOTIC THERAPY

Antibiotic therapy should be chosen to cover gram-negative rods and anaerobes, and initial parenteral delivery is generally used to maximize absorption in CD patients who often have active small-bowel inflammation. Ampicillin/sulbactam or piperacillin/tazobactam are often used initially, though penicillin allergy may require the use of metronidazole plus either ceftriaxone or levofloxacin. We aim to have antibiotics in the bloodstream before evacuation of infectious material is begun. Parenteral antibiotics are generally continued for 1 week or at least 2 days beyond defervescence and an improvement in the white blood cell count. Antibiotics can then be converted to once-daily or oral coverage to facilitate outpatient care. Oral antibiotics, which may include a quinolone plus metronidazole, amoxicillin clavulanate, or trimethoprim/sulfamethoxazole plus metronidazole, are generally continued until at least 3 days after the drainage catheter is removed and repeat imaging has confirmed that the cavity has been fully evacuated.

EVACUATION OF INFECTIOUS MATERIAL

A team approach to defining the optimal route for drainage of all infectious material is helpful. Location of abscesses near vessels can require alternate access routes for percutaneous drainage, and a transgluteal approach to pelvic fluid collections is often needed. Very small collections (diameter < 1 cm) may be difficult to access, whereas those with a diameter of 1 to 3 cm can often be effectively drained with an aspiration needle. Those greater than 3 cm in diameter will generally require placement of a 8 to 14 French catheter, with irrigation with 10 to 20 mL of sterile normal saline every 6 to 12 hours, depending on the size of the abscess and the thickness of the draining material. The output volume and character should be recorded between and with each irrigation and monitored for changes.[7,8]

Ideally, catheter output should become steadily less thick and purulent and decrease in volume over the first week. The patient should also defervesce over the first 3 days and have a fall in white blood cell count and erythrocyte sedimentation rate with successful drainage. A sudden cessation in output, or a failure to defervesce and have laboratory parameter improvement, is an indication for reimaging, as the catheter could be dislodged or kinked, or incompletely draining a portion of the abscess, and will require repositioning or placement of an additional drainage catheter. A sudden increase in fluid output may occur if a clogged catheter is reopened by irrigation, but this could also indicate a new or enlarging fistulous connection to bowel. A more watery, bilious, or feculent appearance with increased output is an indication for a sinogram, with contrast injected through the catheter to evaluate for a wide fistula from the abscess to the bowel.

An abscess drainage catheter can be removed after output becomes nonpurulent, decreases to <20 mL per day for 3 consecutive days, and repeat imaging confirms the resolution of the entire abscess. This required an average of 10.5 days (but increased up to 23 days) in Golfieri's series. Initial drainage was successful, without abscess recurrence in 74% of spontaneous Crohn's abscesses in this series, and an additional 10% could be successfully treated after recurrence, with a 16% overall failure rate.[9] It is important to emphasize that with large or complex abscesses, recurrence should be expected in 25% to 50% cases and can be successfully treated in approximately 40% of these recurrent cases with a second round of percutaneous drainage.

With high-resolution CT scanners, small abscesses < 1 cm in size are more likely to be found and reported than in the past. If these can be aspirated safely, they should be, but these are often detected as part of a cluster of small, undrainable abscesses adjacent to actively inflamed bowel proximal to a stricture. In this setting, therapy with antibiotics alone can be attempted and has been moderately successful in a retrospective series. Kim treated 20 CD patients with intraabdominal abscesses (average size 3.3 cm) with antibiotics alone when percutaneous drainage was not possible. Eighteen responded initially, and 13 of 20 achieved had no recurrence at 6 months without percutaneous drainage or surgery.[8]

MONITORING, CARE, AND FEEDING

Patients must be instructed on how to care for and irrigate drainage catheters before outpatient care is begun and need to be able to describe and record their abscess catheter output each day. Monitoring progress toward the resolution of an intraabdominal abscess requires regular imaging. This can be done with weekly CT scans as per Golfieri,[9] but this approach can result in substantial radiation exposure. It is often effective to use US or MRI, or less frequent CT for repeated evaluation, particularly with a complex collection that is likely to require a long treatment course. We typically perform follow-up imaging at 2-week intervals, unless there has been a change in catheter output to suggest that the catheter has been displaced or kinked or that a new enteric fistula has formed.

The restriction of diet to enteral formulas or total parenteral nutrition is controversial in the treatment of intraabdominal Crohn's abscesses, and minimal data are available to support dietary restriction. A few retrospective case series have suggested that TPN in patients kept NPO might be beneficial, but Greenberg's randomized controlled trial of TPN while NPO in CD found that this therapy did not significantly improve CD outcomes during hospitalization or at 1 year.[10] TPN is associated with an increased risk of line infections, which are of particular concern in immunosuppressed IBD patients. Central lines are also associated with an increased incidence of venous thromboembolism, which is further increased in IBD patients with active disease.[11] Given these risks and the substantial costs of TPN, a clear benefit to TPN and bowel rest needs to be demonstrated before this can be routinely recommended for CD patients with intraabdominal abscess.

Editor's note (TMB): There is a separate chapter on perioperative nutrition.

ANTIINFLAMMATORY THERAPY

Systemic steroid therapy and anti-TNFα therapy have both been strongly associated with increased skin and soft-tissue infections, wound infections, and increased incidence and growth of abscesses. The risk of infection in association with steroids is dose and duration related, with an odds ratio of 6.3 for infection with <20-mg prednisone per day and 18.9 for >40-mg prednisone per day.[12] The risk of infection also increases with a cumulative steroid dose of >700 mg. Several studies have shown an increased risk of surgical complications and infection in association with anti-TNFα therapy; the largest is from the British Society for Rheumatology Biologics Registry. With more than 10,000 patients, and more than 2000 surgeries, they were able to show that anti-TNFα therapy is associated with skin and soft-tissue infections and that the perioperative risk is strongest if anti-TNFα agents have been administered in the previous 2 weeks. The risk diminishes with a greater than 2-week window since dosing of the anti-TNFα and is reduced further if the anti-TNFα medication was administered more than 4 weeks prior to surgery.[4]

Systemic steroid and anti-TNFα therapies are usually avoided until complete drainage of the infectious material is confirmed with repeat imaging and catheter removal, or definitive surgery is performed. Some centers will initiate therapy with these agents within 24 to 48 hours after initial drainage is accomplished, if the radiologic team feels that the entire abscess cavity has been accessed and an effective drain is in place. This approach can be safe and effective, but it requires close monitoring to ensure that the drainage catheter remains in place and is not clogged or displaced before complete eradication of the access is achieved.

Thiopurines and *methotrexate* appear to pose substantially less risk of interfering with eradication of an abscess and can be initiated during abscess drainage, though their onset of action is delayed, and more rapidly acting nonsystemic agents may be needed in combination with one of these immunomodulators. Nonsystemic antiinflammatory therapies can be used immediately, including *budesonide* for the ileum and right colon and *mesalamine enemas* for the left colon. In our experience, budesonide can also be used for *upper tract inflammation*, if the patient opens the capsule and mixes the contents with applesauce, then chews the granules thoroughly before swallowing, which produces a more rapid release of budesonide, but may produce more systemic effects.

Surgical planning should also affect the choices and timing of antiinflammatory therapy. Many CD patients with intraabdominal abscesses will have strictures or large fistulae that will require elective surgery and at least 10% are likely to fail percutaneous drainage and antibiotic therapy. Ideally after removal of all infectious material, antiinflammatory therapy will be used to control bowel inflammation prior to surgery. This will minimize the friability of bowel used in creating an ostomy or an anastomosis, to reduce the risk of bowel leak and subsequent peritonitis or formation of new abscesses. Thiopurines and methotrexate do not appear to significantly increase the risk of infections or complications in the postoperative period, whereas current systemic steroids and recent (infusion or injection in prior 2–4 weeks) anti-TNFα agents have been associated with worse surgical outcomes.[4,13–15] If it is clear that surgery is likely in the near future and infectious material has been drained, effective control of bowel inflammation should be achieved with immunomodulators and/or biologics, and systemic steroids should be tapered to minimum doses. The scheduling of surgery should be targeted, when possible, for the trough period of anti-TNFα agent dosing.

SURGICAL THERAPY

Traditionally, intraabdominal abscesses caused by CD have been managed with surgical drainage and systemic antibiotic therapy coupled with resection of the involved inflamed or fibrotic segment of the bowel. Due to concerns about postoperative complications from contamination of the operative field by the abscess, this was often done as a two-stage surgical procedure, with initial surgical incision and drainage of the abscess, followed by a delayed bowel resection. This led to attempts to accomplish the first stage, drainage of infectious material, by a percutaneous route, enabling a single surgery and a primary reanastomosis. Even if percutaneous drainage is only partially effective, it may provide benefit in reducing the amount of infectious material in the operative field and in buying time to treat and control bowel-wall inflammation prior to surgery.

Numerous retrospective studies have reported success rates of percutaneous catheter drainage of Crohn's abscess ranging from 37% to 90%. Surgical therapy, though it offers more open access and can allow definitive therapy of the abscess and nearby strictured or fistulizing bowel, can have an abscess recurrence rate that is comparable to percutaneous drainage and is more likely than percutaneous drainage to lead to an enterocutaneous fistula. Immediate surgical approaches also often require substantial resection of adjacent bowel, putting patients at risk for future short-bowel syndrome. Although percutaneous drainage will fail to prevent recurrence of abscesses in some patients, and a number of patients will require surgery for strictures or fistulae irrespective of the abscess outcome, an initial medical approach has a number of attractive features. Initial antibiotics and attempts at percutaneous drainage are inexpensive and less invasive than surgery, evacuation of infectious material will reduce subsequent perioperative infectious risk, and drainage of infectious material allows subsequent antiinflammatory therapy, which can make elective CD surgery less complicated and often require less extensive resection of bowel.

The determination that medical therapy has failed can be difficult when there is partial improvement with antibiotic treatment and percutaneous drainage. In general, if at least 3 weeks of antibiotics and 2 attempts at percutaneous drainage have failed to demonstrate continuing progress on repeated imaging, surgical intervention is indicated. Occasionally, a complex, loculated collection will require multiple percutaneous interventions and drains over 30 to 60 days, but if the abscess has not improved in the interval since the previous imaging despite continuing effective drainage, maximum medical benefit has been achieved.[16,17]

MEDICAL THERAPY AFTER EFFECTIVE ABSCESS TREATMENT

A history of an intraabdominal abscess implies severe transmural inflammation and a contained perforation and is a powerful prognostic factor for a future of complicated CD. These patients should not rely on maintenance therapy with antibiotics, mesalamine, herbal therapies, or modified diets. Evidence from randomized controlled trials suggests that patients who

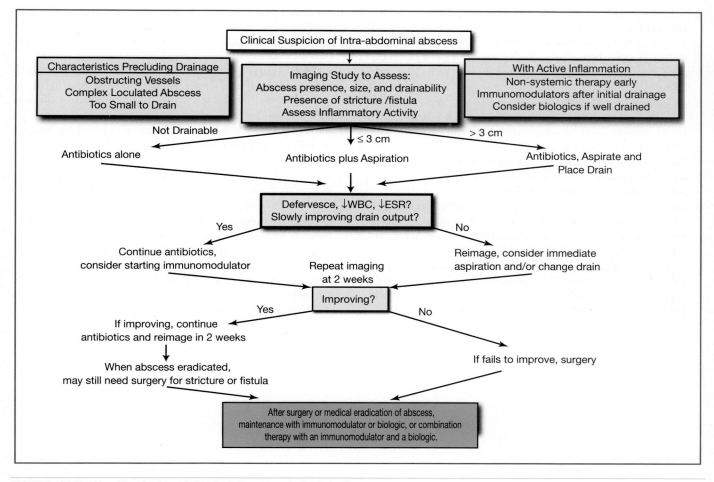

FIGURE 135.3 • Algorithm for intraabdominal abscesses in Crohn's disease.

have required surgical resection derive endoscopic and clinical benefit from 3 months of metronidazole and long-term aza-thioprine.[18] Regueiro's data suggest that initiation of infliximab is also very beneficial in preventing the recurrence of mucosal ulceration.[19] Furthermore, the SONIC trial data show that, in the subset of patients with active inflammation early in the disease course, combination therapy with azathioprine and inflix-imab is superior to biologic monotherapy.

At a minimum, these patients should receive 3 months of antibiotics and be started or continued on azathioprine 2.5 mg/kg. Methotrexate may have similar benefits, but there are limited data available in patients who have had intraabdom-inal abscesses. A full discussion with the patient should make it clear that these patients are at high risk for future complica-tions and should contrast the potential benefits of combination therapy with azathioprine and infliximab with the potential for long-term harm from recurrence of intraabdominal abscesses, perforation, peritonitis, and chronic bowel adhesions. An algo-rithm summarizing the diagnostic and therapeutic approach in this chapter is presented in Fig. 135.3.

References

1. Schwartz DA, Loftus EV Jr, Tremaine WJ, et al. The natural his-tory of fistulizing Crohn's disease in Olmsted County, Minnesota. *Gastroenterology*. 2002;122(4):875–880.

2. Freed KS, Lo JY, Baker JA, et al. Predictive model for the diagnosis of intraabdominal abscess. *Acad Radiol*. 1998;5(7):473–479.

3. Maconi G, Sampietro GM, Parente F, et al. Contrast radiol-ogy, computed tomography and ultrasonography in detect-ing internal fistulas and intra-abdominal abscesses in Crohn's disease: a prospective comparative study. *Am J Gastroenterol*. 2003;98(7):1545–1555.

4. Dixon WG, Watson K, Lunt M, Hyrich KL, Silman AJ, Symmons DP; British Society for Rheumatology Biologics Register. Rates of serious infection, including site-specific and bacterial intra-cellular infection, in rheumatoid arthritis patients receiving anti-tumor necrosis factor therapy: results from the British Society for Rheumatology Biologics Register. *Arthritis Rheum*. 2006;54(8):2368–2376.

5. Lichtenstein GR, Feagan BG, Cohen RD, et al. Serious infections and mortality in association with therapies for Crohn's disease: TREAT registry. *Clin Gastroenterol Hepatol*. 2006;4(5):621–630.

6. Dixon WG, Symmons DP, Lunt M, Watson KD, Hyrich KL, Silman AJ. Serious infection following anti-tumor necrosis factor alpha therapy in patients with rheumatoid arthritis: lessons from interpreting data from observational studies. *Arthritis Rheum*. 2007;56(9):2896–2904.

7. Ayuk P, Williams N, Scott NA, Nicholson DA, Irving MH. Management of intra-abdominal abscesses in Crohn's disease. *Ann R Coll Surg Engl*. 1996;78(1):5–10.

8. Kim DH, Cheon JH, Moon CM, et al. [Clinical efficacy of non-surgical treatment of Crohn's disease-related intraabdominal abscess]. *Korean J Gastroenterol.* 2009;53(1):29–35.

9. Golfieri R, Cappelli A, Giampalma E, et al. CT-guided percutaneous pelvic abscess drainage in Crohn's disease. *Tech Coloproctol.* 2006;10(2):99–105.

10. Greenberg GR, Fleming CR, Jeejeebhoy KN, Rosenberg IH, Sales D, Tremaine WJ. Controlled trial of bowel rest and nutritional support in the management of Crohn's disease. *Gut.* 1988;29(10):1309–1315.

11. Grainge MJ, West J, Card TR. Venous thromboembolism during active disease and remission in inflammatory bowel disease: a cohort study. *Lancet.* 2010;375(9715):657–663.

12. Aberra FN, Lewis JD, Hass D, Rombeau JL, Osborne B, Lichtenstein GR. Corticosteroids and immunomodulators: postoperative infectious complication risk in inflammatory bowel disease patients. *Gastroenterology.* 2003;125(2):320–327.

13. Mor IJ, Vogel JD, da Luz Moreira A, Shen B, Hammel J, Remzi FH. Infliximab in ulcerative colitis is associated with an increased risk of postoperative complications after restorative proctocolectomy. *Dis Colon Rectum.* 2008;51(8):1202–7; discussion 1207.

14. Selvasekar CR, Cima RR, Larson DW, et al. Effect of infliximab on short-term complications in patients undergoing operation for chronic ulcerative colitis. *J Am Coll Surg.* 2007;204(5):956–62; discussion 962.

15. Lopes JV, Freitas LA, Marques RD, Bocca AL, Sousa JB, Oliveira PG. Analysis of the tensile strength on the healing of the abdominal wall of rats treated with infliximab. *Acta Cir Bras.* 2008;23(5):441–446.

16. Strong SA, Koltun WA, Hyman NH, Buie WD. Practice parameters for the surgical management of Crohn's disease. *Dis Colon Rectum.* 2007;50(11):1735–1746.

17. Gutierrez A, Lee H, Sands BE. Outcome of surgical versus percutaneous drainage of abdominal and pelvic abscesses in Crohn's disease. *Am J Gastroenterol.* 2006;101(10):2283–2289.

18. D'Haens GR, Vermeire S, Van Assche G, et al. Therapy of metronidazole with azathioprine to prevent postoperative recurrence of Crohn's disease: a controlled randomized trial. *Gastroenterology.* 2008;135(4):1123–1129.

19. Regueiro M, Schraut W, Baidoo L, et al. Infliximab prevents Crohn's disease recurrence after ileal resection. *Gastroenterology.* 2009;136(2):441–50.e1; quiz 716.

Measures to Minimize Postoperative Recurrences of Crohn's Disease | 136

Paul J. Rutgeerts

BOWEL RESECTION

There is no doubt that resection of the diseased bowel in patients with Crohn's disease (CD) induces long-lasting remission and significantly improves the quality of life. Many patients even feel that surgery has been postponed too long in their case. Laparoscopy-assisted resections have rendered the surgical approach even less traumatic. Most clinicians however think that surgery should be advocated only in the presence of complications of the disease, including stenosis, abscess, and fistula. Intractable disease is generally not considered a surgical indication. Still there exist significant differences in policy concerning surgery between inflammatory bowel disease centers, with some referring almost every patient for resection early in the disease course and others delaying surgery as long as possible.

RECURRENCE AFTER RESECTION

The most important complication of bowel resection for CD is recurrence of the disease. It has become clear that nearly all patients will suffer recurrence of Crohn's lesions leading to new symptoms after a variable length of time. While new lesions can be detected early, long-term outcome is only improved if the condition is treated immediately after early detection or if recurrence is prevented.

PREVENTION OF RECURRENCE AFTER RESECTION

This chapter focuses on prevention of recurrence after "curative" resection, that is, after resection of all macroscopically diseased tissue. Local resections and bypass operations leaving macroscopic disease behind offer no chance of cure. It is also clear that radical surgery (large disease-free margins and removal of lymph nodes draining the region) does not protect against recurrence and is not necessary.[1,2]

We believe that prevention of recurrent CD after resection of the diseased bowel is a completely different situation from maintaining clinical remission with the diseased bowel in place. Therefore, combining studies on surgically induced and medically induced remission is not justified.[3]

The ultimate goal in the management of CD should be to heal the bowel lesions as early after diagnosis as possible with medical therapy, even if cure is not possible, to avoid surgery. It seems that early introduction of combined immunosuppression and anti-tumor necrosis factor (anti-TNF) therapy will make this goal achievable in some patients.

NATURAL HISTORY OF RECURRENT CD: PRESYMPTOMATIC PHASE

Systematic endoscopic study data are available only for the neoterminal ileum and ileocolonic anastomosis after ileal or ileocolonic resections. Recurrent lesions can be visualized as early as a few weeks to months after resection in the neoterminal ileum proximal to the anastomosis with a postanastomotic colon mostly free of macroscopic disease. It is not at all clear what makes the ileal mucosa so vulnerable to recurrent lesions. CD has been shown to be a disease affecting the entire intestine. In "normal" ileum, mucosal architectural changes, epithelial bridge formation, and goblet cell hyperplasia are present. Inflammatory lesions in the section margins are not predictive of recurrence, but perineural inflammatory changes at the section margins are.[4]

The combined presence of bacteria, luminal contents, and bile acids; the break in the mucosa of the suture; and reflux of colonic contents and the organization of the mucosal immune cells may be contributing factors.[5–7] Recently, an interesting animal model of Crohn's recurrence was described.[8]

TIME OF RECURRENCE

All systematic endoscopic and histologic studies are concordant and report early recurrent lesions in 70% to 80% of the patients in the first year after surgery.[9] Recurrence of tissue lesions generally precedes the appearance of recurrent clinical signs by several years, but eventually the majority of patients with lesions will develop relapse of CD symptoms. This evolution over time was not appreciated in early studies largely because X-rays of the small bowel were not sensitive enough for early detection.

PREDICTABILITY OF FOUR CLINICAL RECURRENCES

The severity and extent of tissue recurrence predicts the time to clinical relapse. Patients without lesions or presenting with only a few aphthous ulcers at ileocolonoscopy at 1 year are not at risk for early symptomatic relapse, but more than half of the patients presenting with diffuse aphthous or ulcerative ileitis will have symptomatic relapse within 1 to 3 years after operation.[9] Patients with ulcers confined to the immediate perianastomotic region are probably prone to develop a fibrotic stricture of the anastomosis.

There is convincing evidence that, in patients with postoperative recurrence, the evolution of CD mimics the natural evolution of CD at its onset. The evolution goes from preulcerative inflammation over aphthoid ulcers to more extensive ulceration and nodularity to result in complications, including stenosis and fissures, which can be complicated by abscesses and fistulae.[6] At a certain time, gastrointestinal symptoms recur, and it is conceivable that this symptom-free interval after surgery mirrors the presymptomatic phase at the onset of the disease.[10,11]

SYMPTOMATIC PHASE OF RECURRENT CD

For assessment of recurrence rates, an actuarial analysis has to be used. This implies the calculation of the number of patients with recurrent disease over the number of patients at risk in each year of follow-up allowing recurrence in previous years.

Symptoms recur after curative resection in about 10% of the patients per follow-up year if one looks at figures of older follow-up series. In the placebo groups of postoperative prevention drug studies, the symptomatic recurrence rates are higher and amount to 23% to 26% at 1 year and about 40% at 2 years.

The symptoms of recurrent disease are not always easily distinguishable from symptoms caused by postoperative state and choleraic diarrhea. The baseline is the state at 3 months after resection. Most patients have recovered completely by that time. The CD activity index as a measure of clinical disease activity has not been well validated in the postoperative setting.

DISEASE PATTERN PHENOTYPE

The pattern of CD remains unchanged after surgery in comparison with the preoperative situation. Patients presenting with perforating disease (abscesses and fistulae) before surgery tend to develop the same complications after resection and will have early recurrent symptoms. When the disease is characterized by fibrostenosis before operation, the chances are that the disease will again be structuring and will be more indolent after resection.[12]

A proportion of patients will have a more inflammatory type of disease that might or might not respond to anti-inflammatory therapy. It is also striking that the length of ileal involvement measured on small bowel X-ray examinations before and at the time of symptomatic recurrence is similar, whereas the extent of ileal lesions stays remarkably constant as long as the patient does not undergo a new resection. The need for repeated surgery due to complications of severe recurrence varies between 16% and 65% at 10 years overall.

RISK FACTORS FOR SYMPTOMATIC RECURRENCE AFTER RESECTION FOR CD

The only independent factors generally reproduced in multivariate analysis are location of the disease before surgery, the pattern of the disease, and smoking status.

Location of Diseased Segment

The anatomic site of bowel resection is without doubt an important determinant of recurrence. The highest rates are found after resection for ileocolitis or ileitis with ileocolonic anastomosis. Lower rates are found after colonic resection with colocolic anastomosis. Surprisingly, CD recurs also in the ileum after right colonic resection with ileocolonic anastomosis when the ileum was not diseased before surgery. The rate of symptomatic recurrence proximal to an ileostomy is lowest. It is not certain whether the rate is really lower or whether the evolution of recurrent lesions is slower. In all situations, a narrowed bowel seems to be associated with more inflammation.

Reoperation rates after resection with ileocolonic anastomosis range from 25% to 60% at 5 years and 42% to 91% at 15 years. The type of anastomosis, handsewn end to end versus stapled side to side, does not seem to influence the recurrence rates.[5,13–15]

After colocolic anastomosis, the recurrence rates range between 8.5% and 42% at 5 years and 22% and 40% at 15 years. Reoperation for end ileostomies still amounts to 25% at 5 years and 45% at 10 years.

The rate of recurrence of CD in the neoterminal ileum after ileorectal anastomosis seems comparable to that after more proximal ileocolonic anastomosis, but the disease more often spreads distally with anorectal complications as main manifestation.

Behavior of Disease Preoperatively

The behavior of CD is a good predictor of recurrence as described in studies by De Dombal and coauthors in Leeds and Greenstein et al. in New York.[12] De Dombal et al., in 1971, described a biphasic symptomatic recurrence graph but offered no clear explanation. The Mount Sinai investigators distinguished perforating indications for resection and nonperforating indications. Perforating indications included acute free perforation, subacute perforation with abscess formation, and chronic perforation with intestinal fistula formation. Nonperforating indications comprised intestinal obstruction, medical intractability, hemorrhage, and toxic dilation without perforation.

Operations for perforating indications in their retrospective analysis were followed by repeated resection twice as fast as operations for nonperforating indications. Time to first reoperation was 4.7 years in the perforating group and 8.8 years in the nonperforating group. Time to second reoperation averaged 2.3 years for perforating versus 5.2 years for nonperforating indications. Second operations in the perforating indication group were undertaken for perforating indications again in 64% of the patients with ileitis and 77% of the patients with ileocolitis. A third resection in patients with perforating indications for second resection was performed for perforating complications in 81% overall.[12]

Not all investigators have confirmed this dichotomy of CD behavior.[1]

Editor's note (TMB): The loss of clarity of clinical types begins when patients with radiologic and pathologic evidence of fistulas secondary to obstruction are reclassified as fistulizing or perforating lumina classification. This has badly confused the stratification of patients for postrecurrence studies.

Smoking Status

Generally, smoking has a deleterious effect on CD. The risk factor for clinical recurrence and reoperation generally reproduced is smoking. In an Italian series by M. Cottone in 1994, the 6-year recurrence-free rate after surgery was 60% (95% confidence interval (CI), 43–72%) for nonsmokers, 41% (95% CI, 11–70%) for ex-smokers, and 27% (95% CI, 17–37%) for smokers.

The need for repeated surgery 5 years after surgery averages 20% in nonsmokers versus 36% in smokers as shown by Sutherland et al.[16] in 1990. At 10 years, these rates amount to 41% and 70%, respectively. The risk is particularly high in female smokers with small bowel disease (odds ratio, 9.2).

The risk for excisional surgery associated with smoking is increased only in patients not given immunosuppressive drugs as shown by the French Getaid Group. It seems that the effect of smoking can be antagonized by long-term immunosuppression, but patients should of course be convinced to quit smoking.[17]

● PREVENTION OF EARLY TISSUE LESIONS

It is obvious that if one can prevent the recurrence of new lesions in the remaining bowel, symptomatic relapse will also be prevented. Eventually, this would lead to cure of the disease. Only one strategy has resulted in long-term disease-free perianastomotic region thus far. Diversion of intestinal contents through a proximal ileostomy protects the neoterminal ileum and ileocolonic anastomosis from recurrence, suggesting that luminal contents, probably the bacterial flora, trigger flares of CD. This is also strongly suggested by the finding that, in the same model, infusion of ileal contents through a normal diverted ileocolonic anastomosis induces inflammation characterized by mixed inflammatory infiltrate and cytokine upregulation already after 1 week.[7]

Prophylactic therapy after resection for CD should therefore aim primarily at keeping the remaining bowel completely free of CD. A second endpoint could be the prevention of symptomatic recurrence only. We are at present far from reaching the primary goal. Standard anti-inflammatory approaches with standard or topically acting glucocorticosteroids or 5-ASA formulations are not able to prevent tissue recurrence. Standard glucocorticosteroids or budesonide therefore should be tapered and discontinued within 4 weeks after resection. Studies with 5-ASA formulations suggest that in the short term the most severe endoscopic lesions can be prevented, but studies are not unequivocal.[18]

Nitroimidazole and Antibiotics

Nitroimidazole antibiotics, including metronidazole (20 mg/kg/day) or ornidazole (1 g per day), are effective in preventing endoscopic recurrence. They decrease overall endoscopic recurrence rates and prevent severe lesions from developing as long as they are taken by the patients. Troublesome side effects prohibit long-term use of these antibiotics. Data are scarce but seem to suggest that clinical relapse can also be prevented with these antibiotics.

Azathioprine and 6-Mercaptopurine

6-Mercaptopurine (6-MP) 50 mg/day is more effective than placebo to prevent endoscopic and radiologic recurrence after 1 and 2 years, and this treatment is also associated with clinical benefit.[19]

Infliximab

There is limited but strong evidence that infliximab is highly effective in preventing endoscopic recurrence of CD after ileocolonic resection for CD. In a study by Regueiro et al., the rate of endoscopic recurrence at 1 year was significantly lower in patients treated with infliximab (1 of 11 patients; 9.1%) compared with patients treated with placebo (11 of 13 patients; 84.6%) ($P = 0.0006$).[20]

● DRUG PREVENTION STRATEGIES FOR SYMPTOMATIC POSTOPERATIVE RECURRENCE

Meta-analyses have shown that corticosteroids, 5-ASA, and probiotics are not effective for the prevention of symptomatic postsurgical recurrence of CD.

A meta-analysis shows that azathioprine is effective in preventing symptomatic recurrence of CD postsurgery. Four controlled trials enrolled 433 patients and compared azathioprine ($n = 3$) or 6-MP ($n = 1$) with control arms (placebo with or without antibiotic induction therapy or mesalamine). In the overall analysis, purine analogs were more effective than control arms in preventing clinical recurrence at 1 year (mean difference, 95% CI: 8, 1–15%, $P = 0.021$, number needed to treat (NNT) = 13) and 2 years (mean difference, 95% CI: 13%, 2–24%, $P = 0.018$, NNT = 8). The rate of adverse events leading to drug withdrawal was higher in thiopurine-treated patients than in control arms (17.2% vs. 9.8%, respectively, $P = 0.021$).[19]

Infliximab decreases the symptomatic recurrence rate after surgery, but the difference with placebo did not reach significance because of the small number of patients. In the study by Regueiro et al., there was a nonsignificant higher proportion of patients in clinical remission in the infliximab group (8 of

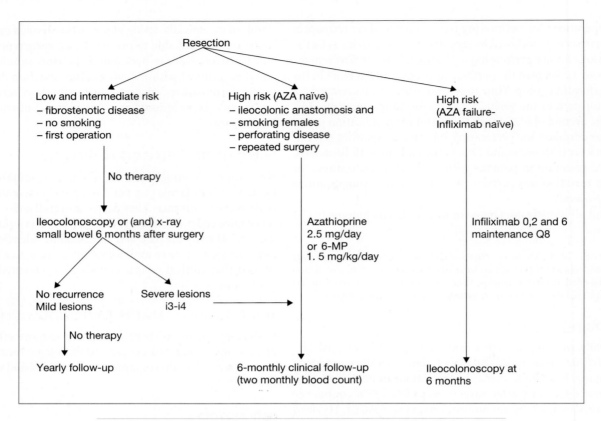

FIGURE 136.1 • Algorithm for the prophylaxis of Crohn's recurrence after resection.

10; 80.0%) at 1 year compared with the placebo group (7 of 13; 53.8%) (*P* = 0.38).[20]

PROPOSED ALGORITHM

At present, it is not justified to give all patients prophylactic medical therapy after curative bowel resection for CD. We propose an algorithm taking into account risk factors for early recurrent disease and response to treatments for CD administered before the operation (Fig. 136.1).

MANAGEMENT OF CLINICAL RECURRENCE OF CD AFTER RESECTION

It is imperative to treat patients with relapse due to disease recurrence in an aggressive manner. These patients may not have received prophylactic therapy or may have failed such therapy. It is always necessary to confirm recurrent lesions in the bowel using ileocolonoscopy or other imaging techniques. Progression of the disease must be prevented with all means because reoperation will lead to more functional loss and diarrhea, which becomes more difficult to treat. Many symptoms that then develop are not related to CD itself. If the patient has not previously received azathioprine, this drug is started at 2.5 mg/kg/day OM, and if necessary, for control of symptoms, steroids (we use the topically acting agent, budesonide) can be added for 3 to 6 months. If treatment with azathioprine is not effective or if the patient already received proper treatment with azathioprine before surgery, which was not

successful, infliximab is indicated certainly if the patient did not receive this previously. We propose to use combination therapy with infliximab and azathioprine for 6 months and to continue them with infliximab monotherapy. In case the patient already received infliximab previously, the decision to start this treatment again should depend on the response to the treatment earlier. Adalimumab may also be a good choice, but there are no data available on this drug in the postoperative situation.

CONCLUSION

Two strategies have been identified that allow efficacious prophylaxis of postoperative recurrence of CD after curative resection of the diseased bowel, including immunosuppression with azathioprine on the one hand and anti-TNF therapy with infliximab on the other hand. The way these treatments have to be used in that setting needs to be further explored. Currently, there is also an important place for assessment of mucosal lesions with endoscopy or X-rays in the planning of postoperative therapy.

Editor's note (TMB): As predicted, Professor Rutgeerts has distilled his wisdom and documented expressive and useful information for clinicians and patients. Thank you, Paul.

References

1. Cammà C, Giunta M, Rosselli M, Cottone M. Mesalamine in the maintenance treatment of Crohn's disease: a meta-analysis

adjusted for confounding variables. *Gastroenterology.* 1997;113(5):1465–1473.

2. D'Haens GR, Geboes K, Peeters M, Baert F, Penninckx F, Rutgeerts P. Early lesions of recurrent Crohn's disease caused by infusion of intestinal contents in excluded ileum. *Gastroenterology.* 1998;114(2):262–267.

3. Ferrante M, de Hertogh G, Hlavaty T, et al. The value of myenteric plexitis to predict early postoperative Crohn's disease recurrence. *Gastroenterology.* 2006;130(6):1595–1606.

4. Greenstein AJ, Lachman P, Sachar DB, et al. Perforating and non-perforating indications for repeated operations in Crohn's disease: evidence for two clinical forms. *Gut.* 1988;29(5):588–592.

5. Griffiths AM, Wesson DE, Shandling B, Corey M, Sherman PM. Factors influencing postoperative recurrence of Crohn's disease in childhood. *Gut.* 1991;32(5):491–495.

6. Lee EC, Papaioannou N. Recurrences following surgery for Crohn's disease. *Clin Gastroenterol.* 1980;9(2):419–438.

7. McLeod RS, Wolff BG, Steinhart AH, et al. Prophylactic mesalamine treatment decreases postoperative recurrence of Crohn's disease. *Gastroenterology.* 1995;109(2):404–413.

8. McLeod RS, Wolff BG, Ross S, Parkes R, McKenzie M; Investigators of the CAST Trial. Recurrence of Crohn's disease after ileocolic resection is not affected by anastomotic type: results of a multicenter, randomized, controlled trial. *Dis Colon Rectum.* 2009;52(5):919–927.

9. Pallone F, Boirivant M, Stazi MA, Cosintino R, Prantera C, Torsoli A. Analysis of clinical course of postoperative recurrence in Crohn's disease of distal ileum. *Dig Dis Sci.* 1992;37(2):215–219.

10. Peyrin-Biroulet L, Deltenre P, Ardizzone S, et al. Azathioprine and 6-mercaptopurine for the prevention of postoperative recurrence in Crohn's disease: a meta-analysis. *Am J Gastroenterol.* 2009;104(8):2089–2096.

11. Regueiro M, Schraut W, Baidoo L, et al. Infliximab prevents Crohn's disease recurrence after ileal resection. *Gastroenterology.* 2009;136(2):441–50.e1; quiz 716.

12. Rigby RJ, Hunt MR, Scull BP, et al. A new animal model of post-surgical bowel inflammation and fibrosis: the effect of commensal microflora. *Gut.* 2009;58(8):1104–1112.

13. Rutgeerts P, Goboes K, Peeters M, et al. Effect of faecal stream diversion on recurrence of Crohn's disease in the neoterminal ileum. *Lancet.* 1991;338(8770):771–774.

14. Rutgeerts P, Geboes K, Vantrappen G, Beyls J, Kerremans R, Hiele M. Predictability of the postoperative course of Crohn's disease. *Gastroenterology.* 1990;99(4):956–963.

15. Sutherland LR, Ramcharan S, Bryant H, Fick G. Effect of cigarette smoking on recurrence of Crohn's disease. *Gastroenterology.* 1990;98(5 Pt 1):1123–1128.

16. Cameron JL, Hamilton SR, Coleman J, Sitzmann JV, Bayless TM. Patterns of ileal recurrence in Crohn's disease. A prospective randomized study. *Ann Surg.* 1992;215(5):546–51; discussion 551.

17. Pennington L, Hamilton SR, Bayless TM, Cameron JL. Surgical management of Crohn's disease. Influence of disease at margin of resection. *Ann Surg.* 1980;192(3):311–318.

18. Hamilton SR, Reese J, Pennington L, Boitnott JK, Bayless TM, Cameron JL. The role of resection margin frozen section in the surgical management of Crohn's disease. *Surg Gynecol Obstet.* 1985;160(1):57–62.

19. Kanof ME, Lake AM, Bayless TM. Decreased height velocity in children and adolescents before the diagnosis of Crohn's disease. *Gastroenterology.* 1988;95(6):1523–1527.

Diarrhea Following Small Bowel Resection | 137

Lawrence R. Schiller

INTRODUCTION

The gastrointestinal tract is a long tube composed of segments with varied absorptive characteristics. The end result of this arrangement is the coordinated absorption of ingested food, drink, and endogenous secretions that are added to the intestinal contents as part of the digestive process. In health, this mechanism is quite efficient. Of the 8 to 10 L of fluid passing the ligament of Treitz each day, 99% is absorbed leaving a normal stool output of approximately 80 to 100 mL of water per day.[1] Some excess capacity for absorption exists at each level of the intestine and this allows some degree of compensation for abnormalities that occur at different levels.

In intestinal diseases, like Crohn's disease and colitis, this normal orderly process is disrupted and malabsorption of fluid and electrolytes may cause diarrhea. These intestinal diseases may also result in nutrient malabsorption and the consequences of malnutrition. Intestinal resection permanently removes one or more segments of the intestine. The extent of the absorptive defect depends upon which segment has been removed, how extensive the resection has been, and the ability of other segments to compensate for the missing functions of that segment. For example, a small jejunal resection may be well tolerated, since more distal segments can compensate for the missing absorptive surface. On the other hand, distal ileal resection predictably will impair vitamin B_{12} and bile acid absorption, since no more distal segment of the intestine has the ability to compensate for these missing functions.

Table 137.1 summarizes segmental intestinal function and the dysfunction that can be expected as a result of resection of these segments.

DIFFERENTIAL DIAGNOSIS OF POSTRESECTION DIARRHEA

Diarrhea can develop shortly after recovery from surgery and refeeding or some time after recovery from surgery. The onset of diarrhea relative to the resection can be helpful in sorting through the mechanisms causing diarrhea and in developing appropriate management plans (Table 137.2).

TABLE 137.1 Segmental Intestinal Function and Dysfunction with Resection

Functions	Dysfunctions with Resection
Jejunum	
High-capacity nutrient absorption	Markedly reduced nutrient absorption
High-capacity sodium/water transport	Flooding of lower bowel with fluid
Calcium and drug absorption	Reduced absorption
Ileum	
Nutrient salvage	Reduced nutrient absorption
Absorption of sodium against gradient	Reduced sodium/water transport
Vitamin B_{12} absorption	Reduced/absent vitamin B_{12} absorption
Bile acid reabsorption	Bile acid malabsorption: cholerheic diarrhea, fat malabsorption
Ileal brake	Intestinal hurry
Colon	
Absorption of sodium against gradient	Reduced sodium/water transport
Short-chain fatty acid absorption	Osmotic diarrhea

When diarrhea develops in the immediate postoperative period as the patient is first being refed, several causes should be considered. First and foremost the loss of the absorptive surface may critically reduce the capacity for intestinal transport.[2] This is particularly true in the most common resection done for Crohn's disease, removal of the terminal ileum, ileocecal valve, and right colon. This part of the intestinal tract is specialized for absorbing sodium against a concentration gradient,

TABLE 137.2 Mechanisms of Diarrhea After Intestinal Resection

Occurring Soon After Surgery	Occurring Some Time After Surgery
Loss of absorptive surface	Recurrent Crohn's disease
Bile acid malabsorption	Partial small bowel obstruction
Fatty acid malabsorption	Gastrocolic/enterocolic fistula
Loss of ileal brake	Small bowel bacterial overgrowth
Gastric acid hypersecretion	Medication-induced diarrhea
Fecal incontinence	Irritable bowel syndrome
Partial small bowel obstruction	Other causes of chronic diarrhea
Antibiotic-associated diarrhea	
Carbohydrate malabsorption	

whereas the residual jejunum and ileum can only absorb fluid and sodium when luminal sodium concentrations are >80 to 100 mmol/L. In addition, loss of the ileocecal valve eliminates the major mechanism regulating colonic filling. This sort of resection may flood the lower part of the colon with salt and fluid beyond the absorptive capacity of the remaining colon and diarrhea then results.

Another possible mechanism for development of diarrhea after ileal resection is bile acid malabsorption and bile acid–mediated inhibition of absorption by the colon.[3] Ileal bile acid reabsorption is usually very efficient. Less than 5% of the bile acid entering the ileum enters the colon because of the brisk absorption rate of bile acid by the healthy ileum. When this area is diseased or removed, more bile acid can enter the colon. If the luminal bile acid concentration exceeds 3 to 5 mmol/L, colonic sodium and water absorption is inhibited and net secretion may develop, producing diarrhea. This is a frequent mechanism of diarrhea when less than 50 cm of terminal ileum has been resected, because, in the absence of much water malabsorption, bile acid concentrations can become high enough to be cathartic in the colon. The bile acid synthesis rate increases to offset the losses and so steatorrhea does not develop.

When longer segments of terminal ileum have been removed, water malabsorption in the small intestine dilutes bile acid concentration in the colon below the cathartic threshold. Bile acid malabsorption may be so profound that hepatic synthesis cannot compensate fully and insufficient bile acid may be present in the duodenum to permit normal fat absorption. Delivery of fatty acids to the colon increases. Fatty acid hydroxylation by colonic bacteria produces molecules that resemble ricinoleic acid, the active ingredient of castor oil, and diarrhea may result.

Additional mechanisms for diarrhea developing soon after resection include loss of the ileal brake, which ordinarily slows transit through the proximal intestine when excess nutrients enter the ileum, gastric acid hypersecretion, which complicates extensive small bowel resection, fecal incontinence, partial small bowel obstruction, and antibiotic-associated diarrhea, which may complicate the course of any patient after abdominal surgery. Carbohydrate malabsorption, such as that due to lactase deficiency, may be uncovered after intestinal resection.

When diarrhea develops weeks or months after resection, additional problems need to be considered. These include recurrent Crohn's disease, gastrocolic or enterocolic fistula, small bowel bacterial overgrowth, and medication-induced diarrhea.

Recurrent disease must be the primary consideration for late-onset postresection diarrhea. Recurrence of Crohn's disease after resective surgery occurs in roughly 50% of patients over 10 years. Although the risk of recurrence may be reduced by continuing some form of medical therapy after resection, recurrent disease still may occur. Recurrence typically develops at the anastomosis. Diarrhea also can complicate recurrent disease if the recurrence produces a gastrocolic or enterocolic fistula.

Bacterial overgrowth also may cause diarrhea after resection.[4] This is more likely to occur if the ileocecal valve has been removed or if there is an element of partial small bowel obstruction, blind loops, or diverticula that would encourage stasis and the growth of bacteria.

A perplexing group of patients are those who develop a syndrome resembling irritable bowel syndrome, characterized by abdominal pain and loose stools on an intermittent basis. This situation actually may be irritable bowel syndrome, a common functional disorder, occurring in patients who have had surgery for inflammatory bowel disease. This is a difficult diagnosis to make in the presence of a history of inflammatory bowel disease and surgery, but should be considered in this setting. Likewise, any disease producing chronic diarrhea might present after resection.

● EVALUATION OF DIARRHEA AFTER SMALL BOWEL RESECTION

The most important part of the evaluation of patients with diarrhea after resection is a careful history.[5] As mentioned in the previous section, the time of onset after surgery is an important clue to the possible cause of diarrhea. Recurrent Crohn's disease often produces the same group of symptoms that the patient originally had, particularly if the patient had systemic symptoms such as weakness, arthralgia, or uveitis. A good description of the frequency of evacuation, additional gastrointestinal symptoms such as bleeding, abdominal distention, nausea and vomiting, and weight loss and current medications are key points. Physical examination should be directed at looking for complicating features such as dehydration, malnutrition, and evidence of activity of Crohn's disease. Routine laboratory testing, including a complete blood count, serum chemistries, thyroid-stimulating hormone (TSH), and stool microbiology tests to look for infectious causes of diarrhea, may be helpful.

Every patient with postresection diarrhea should have an evaluation for structural problems. Most important is small bowel radiography or CT enterography, which can show evidence of recurrent disease or fistula, the length of the bowel remaining, and an approximate small bowel transit time. Evaluation with deep enteroscopy or colonoscopy can show evidence of mucosal recurrence or anastomotic obstruction, but may not be as helpful as radiographic studies. Capsule enteroscopy can be used to define mucosal disease, but the capsule may not pass if a stricture is present.

Analysis of stool collected as either a spot specimen or as part of a quantitative collection can be very helpful for classifying the cause of diarrhea.[5] Stool weight can give some idea of the absorptive capacity of the remaining gut and can help to distinguish conditions with low stool weight (e.g., fecal incontinence, irritable bowel syndrome) from those characterized by major water and electrolyte malabsorption. Electrolyte concentrations can be used to estimate fecal osmotic gap and allow one to categorize the diarrhea as being a secretory or osmotic process. One can also estimate electrolyte losses in the stool and more accurately replace these with intravenous fluid, if necessary. Assessment of fat excretion also is quite helpful; the presence of steatorrhea suggests the presence of bile acid deficiency in the duodenum, extensive proximal small bowel disease or resection, bacterial overgrowth, or severe intestinal hurry. Carbohydrate malabsorption can be diagnosed if there is a large calculated fecal osmotic gap and if fecal pH is <6.[6] Additional tests on stool that may be useful include a fecal occult blood test, a stained smear for fecal leucocytes, and direct measurement of bile acid excretion.

● TREATMENT

If a specific problem such as bacterial overgrowth is identified, specific treatment can be applied and may substantially improve the situation (Table 137.3). Often a specific treatable entity cannot be diagnosed and nonspecific treatment must be applied. Nonspecific treatment can provide significant improvement in symptoms and allow for utilization of the absorptive surface of the intestine in a more efficient fashion (Table 137.4).

Diet

If the patient has steatorrhea, a reduction in fat intake may help, but this is not always the case.[7] Fat is a useful source of energy calories and replacement of fat by carbohydrate can actually generate a larger load of fluid entering the colon. If possible, oral energy intake should increase to 35 to 40 kcal/kg ideal body weight.[7] In some cases, steatorrhea is caused by insufficient duodenal bile acid concentration and mealtime supplementation with exogenous bile acid (e.g., Bile Acid Factors [Jarrow Formulas, Santa Fe Springs, CA], 333 mg/tablet, 1 to 3 tablets with each meal) can improve fat absorption without necessarily inducing diarrhea.[8,9] When there is evidence of carbohydrate malabsorption, an effort should be made to identify the carbohydrate responsible. Often, it will be lactose and a lactose-free diet will be needed. Protein absorption may be inadequate and may be improved by feeding supplements containing small peptides.[10] Frequent feedings utilize the absorptive surface of the intestine on a more continuous basis and may result in better fractional absorption of fluid, electrolytes, and nutrients. In

TABLE 137.3 Treatments for Specific Conditions	
Condition	Treatment
Loss of absorptive surface	Opiate antidiarrheals, fluid/electrolyte replacement
Bile acid malabsorption	Bile acid–binding agents (e.g., cholestyramine)
Fatty acid malabsorption	Bile acid replacement, low fat diet
Loss of ileal brake	Opiate antidiarrheals
Gastric acid hypersecretion	Histamine$_2$-receptor antagonists, immediate-release proton pump inhibitor
Fecal incontinence	Assess cause and treat abnormality if possible
Partial small bowel obstruction	Surgery
Antibiotic-associated diarrhea	Metronidazole or vancomycin, if due to *Clostridium difficile*
Carbohydrate malabsorption	Identify malabsorbed carbohydrate and omit from diet
Recurrent Crohn's disease	Anti-inflammatory/immunosuppressive drugs
Gastrocolic/enterocolic fistula	Surgery, ?infliximab
Bacterial overgrowth	Antibiotics: fluoroquinolone, metronidazole
Medication-induced diarrhea	Identify agent and discontinue
Irritable bowel syndrome	Low dose tricyclic antidepressant, opiates

some cases, malabsorption may be so severe as to require nutritional support with enteral or parenteral supplements.[11] This is not routinely needed but ought to be considered in patients with postresection diarrhea who are substantially malnourished.

Antidiarrheal Medications

Opiate antidiarrheal medications can be extremely helpful in patients who have postresection diarrhea due to a loss of mucosal surface area. Slowing the progress of luminal fluid through the intestine allows more time for each of the remaining segments to reabsorb water and electrolytes, thus the total amount absorbed can increase.[12] Less potent antidiarrheals, such as diphenoxylate or loperamide, may not be sufficiently active for some patients. Deodorized tincture of opium, codeine, or morphine may be required. However, even potent opiates cannot substitute for specialized absorption defects, such as inability to absorb vitamin B$_{12}$ or bile salt.

Stool Modifying Agents

Stool modifying agents, such as fiber supplements, can improve stool consistency, but may increase total stool weight and water losses. Bile acid binding agents are of use in patients with proven

TABLE 137.4 Nonspecific Treatments for Postresection Diarrhea

Diet
Steatorrhea: low fat diet
Frequent feedings
Nutritional support: enteral or parenteral dietary supplements
Antidiarrheal medications
Diphenoxylate/atropine tablets (up to 8 daily in divided doses)
Loperamide (up to 16 mg daily in divided doses)
Codeine (up to 240 mg daily in divided doses)
Deodorized tincture of opium (up to 80 drops [40 mg morphine] daily)
Morphine (up to 40 mg daily in divided doses)
Stool modifying agents
Psyllium, methylcellulose (up to 20 g daily in divided doses)
Bile acid binding agents (up to 20 g daily in divided doses)
Adjunctive medications
Histamine$_2$-receptor antagonists (e.g., cimetidine 300 mg QID)
Anticholinergic drugs (e.g., hyoscyamine up to 0.25 mg QID)
Replacement therapy
Fluid and electrolytes (oral rehydration solution, intravenous solution)
Magnesium, calcium
Parenteral vitamin B$_{12}$, fat soluble vitamins

or suspected bile acid malabsorption and may also help some individuals with fatty acid–induced diarrhea. Bile acid binders should be given away from meal times to avoid reducing intraduodenal bile acid concentrations during the digestive period. Doses from 4 to 20 g/day can be tried and the lowest effective dose should be used. Bile acid–binding resins may bind other drugs and should be given at least 2 hours before or after other agents.

Adjunctive Medications

Several additional medicines can be of help in patients with postresection diarrhea. Histamine$_2$-receptor antagonists can be used to reduce acid secretion and the amount of fluid and electrolytes entering the upper intestine. This class of drugs is particularly useful in patients with gastric acid hypersecretion, but may help other patients by reducing fluid loads. Delayed-release proton pump inhibitors may not work as well in patients with postresection diarrhea, because there may not be sufficient time for the medication to be absorbed from the small intestine. In contrast, immediate-release proton pump inhibitors and histamine$_2$-receptor antagonists are administered in a rapidly absorbable form and can inhibit acid secretion substantially.

Anticholinergic medications can be used as anti-transit and antisecretory medications and can improve the efficiency of other antidiarrheal drugs.

Somatostatin analogue can reduce stool output acutely, but long-term results are less impressive.[13] Recombinant human growth hormone in combination with oral glutamine supplementation and a high carbohydrate, low fat diet may hasten intestinal adaptation and may reduce parenteral fluid and nutritional requirements.[14,15]

Replacement Therapy

Another important aspect of therapy is to replace malabsorbed substances.[16] These include water and electrolytes when diarrhea leads to dehydration, sodium chloride and magnesium if diarrheal losses have been too extreme, and vitamin B$_{12}$. Oral rehydration solutions may be used to replete sodium chloride, but may cause stool output to increase.[17] Repletion of magnesium is problematic, since it is a poorly absorbed ion, and efforts to replace it by giving it orally often result in worse diarrhea. Intermittent parenteral administration of magnesium may be needed in some individuals. Patients with postresection diarrhea also should be considered for parenteral vitamin B$_{12}$ administration and replenishment of fat-soluble vitamins. Since both vitamin B$_{12}$ and fat-soluble vitamins may be stored within the body, it may take some time for overt deficiencies to develop and prophylactic supplementation should be considered early in individuals who have had substantial resections.

References

1. Schiller LR, Sellin JH. Diarrhea. In: Feldman M, Friedman L, Brandt LJ, eds. *Sleisenger and Fordtran's Gastrointestinal and Hepatic Diseases. Pathophysiology, Diagnosis, Management.* 9th ed. Philadelphia, PA: Saunders Elsevier; 2010:211–232; 2006:199–219.

2. Arrambide KA, Santa Ana CA, Schiller LR, Little KH, Santangelo WC, Fordtran JS. Loss of absorptive capacity for sodium chloride as a cause of diarrhea following partial ileal and right colon resection. *Dig Dis Sci.* 1989;34(2):193–201.

3. Schiller LR, Bilhartz LE, Santa Ana CA, Fordtran JS. Comparison of endogenous and radiolabeled bile acid excretion in patients with idiopathic chronic diarrhea. *Gastroenterology.* 1990;98(4):1036–1043.

4. Vanderhoof JA, Young RJ, Murray N, Kaufman SS. Treatment strategies for small bowel bacterial overgrowth in short bowel syndrome. *J Pediatr Gastroenterol Nutr.* 1998;27(2):155–160.

5. Fine KD, Schiller LR. AGA technical review on the evaluation and management of chronic diarrhea. *Gastroenterology.* 1999;116(6):1464–1486.

6. Hammer HF, Fine KD, Santa Ana CA, Porter JL, Schiller LR, Fordtran JS. Carbohydrate malabsorption. Its measurement and its contribution to diarrhea. *J Clin Invest.* 1990;86(6):1936–1944.

7. Woolf GM, Miller C, Kurian R, Jeejeebhoy KN. Nutritional absorption in short bowel syndrome. Evaluation of fluid, calorie, and divalent cation requirements. *Dig Dis Sci.* 1987;32(1):8–15.

8. Little KH, Schiller LR, Bilhartz LE, Fordtran JS. Treatment of severe steatorrhea with ox bile in an ileectomy patient with residual colon. *Dig Dis Sci.* 1992;37(6):929–933.

9. Gruy-Kapral C, Little KH, Fordtran JS, Meziere TL, Hagey LR, Hofmann AF. Conjugated bile acid replacement therapy for short-bowel syndrome. *Gastroenterology.* 1999;116(1):15–21.

10. Cosnes J, Evard D, Beaugerie L, Gendre JP, Le Quintrec Y. Improvement in protein absorption with a small-peptide-based diet in patients with high jejunostomy. *Nutrition*. 1992;8(6): 406–411.

11. Cosnes J, Gendre JP, Evard D, Le Quintrec Y. Compensatory enteral hyperalimentation for management of patients with severe short bowel syndrome. *Am J Clin Nutr*. 1985;41(5):1002–1009.

12. Schiller LR. Review article: anti-diarrhoeal pharmacology and therapeutics. *Aliment Pharmacol Ther*. 1995;9(2):87–106.

13. Ladefoged K, Christensen KC, Hegnhøj J, Jarnum S. Effect of a long acting somatostatin analogue SMS 201–995 on jejunostomy effluents in patients with severe short bowel syndrome. *Gut*. 1989;30(7):943–949.

14. Scolapio JS, Camilleri M, Fleming CR, et al. Effect of growth hormone, glutamine, and diet on adaptation in short-bowel syndrome: a randomized, controlled study. *Gastroenterology*. 1997;113(4):1074–1081.

15. Weiming Z, Ning L, Jieshou L. Effect of recombinant human growth hormone and enteral nutrition on short bowel syndrome. *JPEN J Parenter Enteral Nutr*. 2004;28(6):377–381.

16. Jeejeebhoy KN. Short bowel syndrome: a nutritional and medical approach. *CMAJ*. 2002;166(10):1297–1302.

17. Beaugerie L, Cosnes J, Verwaerde F, et al. Isotonic high-sodium oral rehydration solution for increasing sodium absorption in patients with short-bowel syndrome. *Am J Clin Nutr*. 1991;53(3):769–772.

Clinical Management of Short Bowel Syndrome | 138

Antwan Atia and Alan L. Buchman

Short bowel syndrome (SBS) may develop in one of two fashions: congenital (bowel atresia) or acquired (bowel resection). Causes of SBS are listed in Table 138.1. Intestinal failure develops when there is insufficient absorptive surface and nutritional or fluid/electrolyte autonomy cannot be achieved. Therefore, not all patients with SBS have intestinal failure. Further, not all patients with intestinal failure have SBS. Intestinal failure may result from various malabsorptive syndromes, including refractory sprue, microvillus inclusion disease, radiation enteropathy, and chronic intestinal pseudo-obstruction, among others.

Although most of the data is derived from animal investigation, it appears that following massive resection, intestinal adaptation occurs in humans. During this process, which occurs primarily within the first 6 to 12 months postoperatively, although it may continue for up to 2 years, or even longer, the bowel hypertrophies. The intestine may lengthen to a small degree, but more importantly, the intestine increases in diameter and the density and length/depth of the villous/crypt structure increases, thereby increasing the functional absorptive surface. There may also be increased colonic fluid and electrolyte absorption. These responses appear to be hormonally mediated to a large degree, with epidermal growth factor (EGF) and glucagon-like peptide-2 (GLP-2) playing primary roles. Other growth factors, neutropic factors, and vasoactive factors may also play a role. There are a number of factors that may influence the degree of adaptation including patient age, underlying disease, oral food intake, length and anatomic location of bowel resection, and splanchnic blood flow.

SBS is defined as the presence (in adults) of less than 200 cm residual small bowel. At the time of resection, it is imperative that the surgeon measure the length of residual bowel in continuity along the antimesenteric border. That measurement is far more important than the length of resected bowel. Intraoperative measurement is most precise, but may be affected by the degree to which the intestine is stretched out. Radiologic measurement may be inaccurate due to overlying loops of bowel.

In normal individuals, virtually all nutrient digestion and absorption are completed within the first 100 to 150 cm of jejunum. The ileum is responsible for absorption of vitamin B12 and the reabsorption of bile salts. Patients who have less than 100 cm of residual jejunum often exhibit significant fluid loss with food intake. Equivalent proximal resections are much better tolerated than massive distal resections, because remaining ileum can take over much of the function of jejunum. In contrast, residual jejunum is incapable of restoring the function of vitamin B12 or bile salt absorption from the ileum. The ability to achieve nutritional autonomy is significantly affected by the presence or absence of the ileocecal valve, which may act as an intestinal "brke," mediated by peptide YY, delaying gastric emptying as well as intestinal transit. The ileocecal valve also prevents reflux and colonization of the small bowel by colonic bacteria that may increase diarrhea through competition for available nutrients. Bacteria can also deconjugate bile salts, resulting in decreased reabsorption and increased fecal losses

TABLE 138.1 Causes of Short Bowel Syndrome	
Congenital	Acquired
Jejunal atresia	Mesenteric vascular disorders
Ileal atresia	• Mesenteric venous thrombosis
Gastroschisis	• Mesenteric arterial embolism
Midgut volvulus	• Mesenteric arterial thrombosis
Meconium ileus	• Mesenteric atherosclerosis
	Crohn's disease
	Trauma
	Radiation enteritis
	Small bowel obstruction and repeated resections
	Volvulus
	Extensive aganglionosis
	Necrotizing enterocolitis

that deplete the bile salt "pool." Decreased lumenal bile salts available for micelle formation contribute to malabsorption of fat and fat-soluble vitamins in the proximal intestine.

Although the length of the residual small bowel and colon in continuity are not the only prognostic factors for nutritional autonomy, they are the most important factors. That being said, there is an imperfect correlation between residual intestinal length and fecal energy loss. In general, however, 100 cm of healthy small bowel is the minimum length necessary to avoid parenteral nutrition (PN) or fluid in the absence of an intact colon, and 60 cm with an intact colon; although there are reports in the literature of infants with an intact colon who have been able to maintain nutritional autonomy with as little as 10 cm of residual small bowel. In patients with SBS, the colon becomes an important digestive organ not only for fluid and electrolytes but also for energy by way of carbohydrate salvage. Unabsorbed carbohydrates are fermented by normal colonic bacterial flora to short-chain fatty acids (SCFAs) including butyrate, propionate, and acetate. Some studies have suggested that the presence of an intact colon can reduce energy losses by as much as 1000 kcal, or more, on a daily basis. The colon also has the ability to absorb a modest amount of amino acids and medium chain triglycerides (MCT).

● MEDICAL TREATMENT STRATEGIES

Treatment of Excessive Fluid Losses

While intestinal adaptation taking place, massive fluid and electrolyte losses occur frequently during the first week or two following an extensive small bowel resection, but may improve over the ensuing months. During the postoperative period, patients usually require parenteral fluids and nutrition. It is also important to institute enteral nutrition, preferably via the oral route, as soon as possible to hasten the intestinal adaptive response. In fact, development of hyperphagia (defined as an increase in oral energy intake equivalent of one and a half to two times—or greater—preresection oral intake) should be encouraged. Antidiarrheal medications such as loperamide, diphenoxylate, codeine, or tincture of opium (listed in order of increasing need) may be important to slow motility and increase nutrient contact time (Table 138.2). Loperamide hydrochloride, in doses up to 16 mg, or diphenoxylate may be required to control fluid losses. If not adequate, codeine sulfate (30–60 mg four times a day) or tincture of opium (10–20 drops two to four times a day) may be necessary. Clonidine, which enhances colonic chloride absorption, may also be useful (transdermal delivery or orally administered). It is important to realize that medication malabsorption may occur, just as nutrient malabsorption occurs.

Transient gastric hypersecretion, related to hypergastrinemia, also occurs for the first 6 to 12 months following a massive intestinal resection and may contribute to increased fluid and electrolyte losses. Histamine-2 (H2) antagonists and proton pump inhibitors are useful for decreasing jejunal fluid and potassium losses during this period. These medications are all absorbed in the proximal jejunum. If transit time is significantly decreased, medication absorption is correspondingly decreased, and larger doses may be necessary. High dose of calcium (2.4–3.6 g/day of elemental Ca) also may be useful

TABLE 138.2 Pharmacologic Therapy of Short Bowel Syndrome

Proton Pump Inhibitors
Nexium (esomeprazole): 40–80 mg orally or intravenously twice a day
Prilosec (omeprazole): 40–80 mg twice a day
Prevacid (lansoprazole): 30–60 mg twice a day
Protonix (pantoprazole): 40–80 mg twice a day
Higher doses of each may be required to account for malabsorption. Necessity of use generally resolves by 6 months postresection

Histamine (H2) Receptor Antagonists
Cimetidine (Tagamet): 400–800 mg orally or intravenously four times a day
Famotidine (Pepcid): 40–80 mg orally or intravenously twice a day
Ranitidine (Zantac): 300–600 mg orally or intravenously twice a day

Anti-motility Agents
Imodium (loperamide): 2–6 mg orally up to four times a day
Lomotil (diphenoxylate): 2.5–5 mg orally up to four times a day
Codeine: 15–60 mg orally up to four times a day
Morphine: 2–20 mg up to four times a day
Tincture of Opium: 0.3–1.0 mL up to four times a day
Paragoric: 5–10 mL two to four times a day

Other
Clonidine: 0.1–0.3 mg up to three times a day orally or twice weekly (transcutaneously)
Octreotide: 50–250 mcg to three to four times a day (subcutaneously)
Cholestyramine: 2–4 g up to four times a day (not if >100 cm terminal ileum resected)

for decreasing diarrhea, probably because of increased binding of fatty acids. Octreotide is rarely necessary except for some patients with high output jejunostomies. Its use should be avoided if possible because of an association with pancreatic insufficiency, malabsorption, decreased intestinal adaptation, and cholelithiasis.

The diagnosis of bacterial translocation may be difficult given that rapid intestinal transit will result in a false positive breath hydrogen test. Nevertheless, if warranted, treatment of bacterial overgrowth may be undertaken with either metronidazole or tetracycline. Unfortunately, the use of broad-spectrum antibiotics also may contribute to the worsening of diarrhea, because of either *Clostridium difficile* (which may occur in the small bowel) or non–*C. difficile*–associated diarrhea.

SBS patients with a proximal jejunostomy often secrete more water and sodium via their stoma than they consume orally; in fact, food intake may stimulate secretion. Typically, such patients have less than 100 cm of residual jejunum. Patients with high output jejunostomy should be encouraged to restrict intake of oral hypotonic fluid and to consume oral rehydration solution (ORS) that has a sodium concentration of at least 90 mmol/L, some glucose, and possibly bicarbonate. In patients with completely resected jejunum, but with remaining ileum, glucose or bicarbonate may be unnecessary. An attempt should be made to have the patient consume dry solids first, followed by isotonic liquids an hour later. However, this may be difficult in practice. Sodas and juices are hypertonic and should be avoided. If these measures are ineffective, antidiarrheal medications, H2 antagonists, proton pump inhibitors, and octreotide can be used to reduce the stomal output. These patients will require parenteral fluids, with the goal to provide the required intravenous fluid through an overnight infusion; occasionally additional parenteral fluids during waking hours are necessary.

DIETS AND SPECIFIC NUTRIENT REQUIREMENTS

One of the most important factors for the promotion of intestinal hypertrophy and optimal adaptation of the remaining segment is the provision of enteral feeding as soon as possible postoperatively. The presence of growth factors such as epidermal growth factor, produced in the salivary glands and esophagus, or GLP-2, released from intestinal L cells located in terminal ileum and right colon (although this anatomic location may have been resected in the SBS patient), makes oral feeding preferable. Patient should consume as much energy and nitrogen as possible. This may mean upward of 4000 to 6000 kcal and 150 g of nitrogen daily. Depending on the absorptive capacity of the remaining intestine (and colon), much of this may not be assimilated.

DIET COMPOSITION

Macronutrients

Dietary carbohydrate content is dependent upon whether patients have a colon in continuity with their small intestine (Table 138.3). Complex carbohydrates, soluble fibers (e.g., pectin, some gums, and to some degree soy and oats; wheat brain is an insoluble fiber), and starches are metabolized by normal anaerobic colonic flora to the SCFAs: acetate, butyrate, and propionate. These SCFAs (most notably butyrate) are the preferred fuel for colonocytes, stimulate sodium and water absorption, and may account for upward of 1000 kcal daily in energy absorption. Therefore, the residual colon and a diet containing substantial amounts of soluble fiber, complex carbohydrate, and some insoluble nonstarch polysaccharides provide an opportunity for colonic energy salvage. Patients with a colonic mucus fistula and residual small intestine should have small and large bowel reanastomosed as soon as possible. Patients without colons lack the ability to ferment complex carbohydrate to SCFA, and little difference is observed in energy absorption between a high carbohydrate and low carbohydrate diet. These patients also require more aggressive hydration due to higher stool volume. Simple carbohydrates should be avoided, as they are often osmotically active agents that will serve to increase fecal fluid losses.

Given that lactose is hydrolyzed in the proximal jejunum, lactose restriction is generally not necessary except in the very SBS patient; exclusion of lactose also serves to exclude the most significant dietary calcium source. In addition, patients should avoid consumption of caffeine-containing products and osmotically active medications or sweeteners (sorbitol for example)

TABLE 138.3 Dietary Recommendations for Patients with Short Bowel Syndrome Who Have Colon in Continuity with Their Residual Small Bowel or No Colon

Colon	No Colon
Increase carbohydrates to 40–50% of total energy using complex carbohydrates, starches, and soluble fiber	Limit simple sugars
Decrease fat but balance between decreased energy intake and increased fecal output; MCT	No value in changing fat intake
ORS, Na supplements	ORS
Limit oxalate	No oxalate limits
Induce hyperphagia and multiple meals	Induce hyperphagia and multiple meals
Unknown value of elemental or free amino acid–based nitrogen sources	Unclear value of elemental or free amino acid–based nitrogen sources

MCT, medium chain triglycerides; ORS, oral rehydration solution.

that increase fluid secretion, stimulate motility, and lead to a further decrease in intestinal transit.

Dietary fat restriction decreases steatorrhea, but given that fat contains more energy by mass than carbohydrate, net energy absorption may be diminished. Some, although not all, human studies have shown modestly enhanced nitrogen absorption with elemental diets (small peptide or free amino acid–based enteral formulas) but no effect on stool weight or energy, nitrogen, electrolyte, or mineral absorption. MCT are absorbed independently of bile salts and may provide a useful energy source for patients with significant steatorrhea, especially for patients with residual continuity of the colon. However, MCT are expensive, often unpalatable (despite modern recipes), cannot be used as a cooking oil because of a low smoke temperature, may worsen diarrhea in excessive doses (>40 g/day), and may have an adverse effect on intestinal adaptation. Dietary fat should not be completely replaced with MCT as essential fats, such as linoleic acid, are not supplied. To prevent essential fatty-acid deficiency (manifested in a rash, thrombocytopenia, and/or peripheral neuropathy), linoleic acid must constitute at least 2% to 4% of the total absorbed calories. Corn oil can be ingested or applied cutaneously, with some transcutaneous absorption occurring. It is unclear whether supplemental linolenic acid is also required. Ox bile or the investigational synthetic conjugated bile acid cholylsarcosine may be used to improve fat absorption, although there is limited supportive data, and diarrhea may be increased. Bile acid binders such as cholestyramine should be avoided in patients with a resection of more than 100 cm of terminal ileum because such medications may increase fat, fat soluble vitamin, and medication malabsorption in patients with more significant resections.

Micronutrients

Vitamins

For the patient who can be maintained without PN, regardless of the presence or absence of a colon, various vitamin and mineral supplements are often necessary. Fat-soluble vitamin (A, D, and less so E) deficiency is common in patients with SBS because of fat maldigestion, as well as malabsorption. Therefore vitamin A, vitamin D (25-OH), and vitamin E concentrations should be monitored closely to ensure adequacy of supplementation and because toxicity can result from excessive intake of any of these. Vitamin A deficiency can lead to night blindness and xerophthalmia that can progress to corneal ulceration and permanent blindness. If vitamin A deficiency is detected, therapy should be started with 8000 units daily, administered either orally or parenterally. Vitamin D deficiency leads to osteomalacia and proximal muscle weakness. Serum 25-dihydroxyvitamin D concentration should be monitored. Patients with SBS may require anywhere between 50,000 units twice weekly to 100,000 units daily of the parent vitamin D compound, depending on the degree of malabsorption. Exposure to sunlight may be very useful. Vitamin E deficiency can lead to hemolysis and various neurologic manifestations. Higher dosages of vitamin E (>400 IU/day) have been associated with increased risk of all-cause mortality in non-SBS patients, although such doses may be required in the SBS patient. In addition, vitamin E supplementation may result in an increase in bleeding risk in patients taking warfarin. Serum vitamin E concentration may vary in relation to the serum total lipid concentration. Therefore, total serum lipids should be measured simultaneously, and the ratio of vitamin E to total serum lipids actually should be used as the index of vitamin E status. Enteric bacteria synthesize much of the daily vitamin K requirement (approximately 1 mg/day); in addition to that contained in the diet, supplementation is not usually necessary in patients with a colon. Vitamin K deficiency is frequent in patients who have no residual colon and who are taking broad-spectrum antibiotics. Prothrombin time/INR should be monitored and vitamin K should be supplemented accordingly. Vitamin K deficiency may play a more important role in the development of metabolic bone disease than previously recognized. Most parenteral multivitamin formulations for both children and adults now contain vitamin K.

Water-soluble vitamins are absorbed in the proximal jejunum; therefore, deficiencies are rare in short bowel patients in the absence of a PN requirement (except in those who have proximal jejunostomies or duodenostomies). However, deficiencies may occur, and therefore it is important that patients ingest one or two B-complex vitamin supplements and 200 to 500 mg of vitamin C daily if they are not receiving daily PN. Vitamin B12 should be administered at a dose of 300 μg intramuscularly every month in patients who have had more than 60 cm terminal ileum resected, or in those who have active Crohn's disease in their remaining terminal ileum. The adequacy of vitamin B12 supplementation is best measured by following the serum methylmalonic acid concentration. Folate deficiency may develop in patients with proximal jejunal resections, and these patients should receive 1 mg folate daily. Thiamine deficiency can occur in SBS patients and it presents with beriberi and Wernicke-Korsakoff syndrome. Thiamine deficiency can be detected with measurement of the erythrocyte thiamine transketolase or serum thiamin concentration. Once diagnosis of thiamine deficiency is suspected, patients should be started on thiamine 100 mg daily parenterally. Biotin deficiency has been rarely described in SBS especially after routine supplementation of PN with biotin. Biotin deficiency can present with dermatitis and alopecia. Patients with biotin deficiency should be encouraged to stop eating raw eggs as it worsens biotin deficiency. There is a disagreement about the proper dose for biotin replacement, and a low dose of 150 to 300 μg intramuscularly daily has been suggested, although parenteral biotin is not available commercially. Pyridoxine, riboflavin, and niacin are provided in multivitamin and B-complex vitamin supplements. Although the B vitamins essentially are nontoxic, excessive vitamin C ingestion has been associated with calcium oxalate nephrolithiasis.

Minerals and Trace Metals

Adequate calcium intake is important, especially because of the adverse effects on bone of cytokines, vitamin D malabsorption, and the medications often used to treat Crohn's disease, like corticosteroids. In the absence of jejunal Crohn's disease or jejunal resections, most Caucasian patients with Crohn's disease will *not* be lactose intolerant. Unfortunately, many patients are convinced that they are and their dairy product intake is limited. This in turn may severely limit calcium intake. For the patient who is truly lactose intolerant, perhaps unrelated to Crohn's disease or their resection, additional calcium supplements are recommended. This may take the form of certain antacids, yogurt (where the lactose is already hydrolyzed), lactase-containing milk or ice cream, or hard cheeses (lactose is concentrated in the whey portion of cheese). Calcium supplementation of 1000 mg daily should be routinely provided and the dose should be increased to 1500 mg daily in patients with osteopenia or osteoporosis. Larger doses of calcium (e.g., 2–4 g/day of elemental calcium) may be associated with decreased diarrhea as the calcium binds to fatty acids in the intestinal lumen, as well as a decreased risk for calcium oxalate nephrolithiasis. Bone mineral density should be routinely followed in these patients, with consideration for biphosphonate therapy for those with increased fracture risk. This may require intravenous administration because of malabsorption.

Iron is absorbed in the duodenum and, as such, is not always required in PN patients. Iron deficiency in Crohn's disease more commonly reflects ongoing blood loss rather than iron malabsorption even in SBS. Therefore, supplementation is not routinely necessary in the absence of active Crohn's disease or gastrointestinal hemorrhage or significant duodenal resection. Serum ferritin should be monitored, although it will be elevated as an acute-phase reactant in active Crohn's disease. Hypomagnesemia is common in patients with SBS. The urinary magnesium concentration is more reliable for detecting hypomagnesemia than the serum magnesium level as the decline in urinary magnesium is a more sensitive indicator of magnesium status given that less than 1% of magnesium is present in the extracellular space, and thus measured by serum or plasma measurements. The urine magnesium should be routinely followed and values greater than 70 mg/24 hours suggest adequate magnesium stores. Oral magnesium is a cathartic and, as such, may lead to increased diarrhea and thereby increased magnesium loss. Therefore, oral magnesium replacement may be problematic, and some patients will require central venous access solely for magnesium replacement.

Zinc supplements are routinely necessary because of the significant fecal losses (12 mg/L small intestinal fluid and 16 mg/L stool). To put these losses in perspective, standard PN solutions typically provide 2 mg of zinc daily. Usually one or two 220-mg zinc sulfate tablets are sufficient. Zinc deficiency can lead to growth retardation, sexual dysfunction, delayed wound healing, and various skin lesions. Zinc deficiency also has been associated with increased diarrhea, which may be ameliorated with zinc supplementation. Plasma and leukocyte zinc concentrations are depressed in acute and chronic inflammation and they do not correlate with tissue concentration of zinc. Erythrocyte concentration of zinc may be a more useful test to assess zinc status. Zinc is bound to albumin and other proteins, although no conversion factor currently exists to adjust for decreased serum protein concentrations. Selenium status can be followed by measurement of the plasma selenium concentration. It can be supplemented (60–120 μg/day) if necessary. Deficiency has been associated with cardiomyopathy, macrocytosis, myositis, and pseudoalbinism. Copper deficiency is rare, as most excretion is biliary in origin. Deficiency has been associated with anemia, cardiomyopathy, neutropenia, neuropathy, osteoporosis, retinal degeneration, and testicular atrophy. There are few case reports of chromium deficiency in patients requiring long-term PN; however, chromium deficiency has not been reported in patients not requiring PN. Routine supplementation of chromium is not recommended because there is sufficient chromium contained as a contaminant in PN solutions and high doses have been associated with nephrotoxicity in humans.

HYPERPHAGIA AND ENTERAL TUBE FEEDINGS

Nasogastric, nasoduodenal, or nasojejunal feeding have been recommended as temporary modalities in the postoperative period to increase enteral intake. Nasogastric tube use should be limited to 6 weeks before changing nostrils. In a recently published study of 15 patients with SBS, continuous tube feeding either alone or in combination with oral feeding following the postoperative period increased the net absorption of lipids, protein, and energy compared with oral feeding alone. There is no sufficient data to recommend the usage of percutaneous gastrostomy tubes to increase enteral intake. This is due to technical difficulty in insertion of the gastrostomy tube in SBS patients because of altered anatomy and adhesions that may be present in SBS patients following surgical intestinal resection.

PARENTERAL NUTRITION

Patients are most likely to require PN and fluids initially following massive bowel resection. This continues for at least 7 to 10 days, perhaps as long as 1 to 2 years during the adaptation process, and permanently if bowel surface area and adaptation is insufficient. Patients should be provided with 30 to 33 kcal/kg/day (or use indirect calorimetry with an added activity factor) and 1.0 to 1.5 g/kg/day of amino acids. Energy is provided as dextrose (3.4 kcal/mL) and lipid emulsion (1.1 kcal/mL for the 10% and 2.0 kcal/mL for the 20% form). Requirements for young children and neonates are substantially greater per kg. Electrolytes, minerals, vitamins, and trace metals are also needed.

Baseline fluid requirements approximate 1 mL/kcal. Additional fluid to replace gastrointestinal losses usually is required. Urine output, in the absence of renal failure, is an excellent indicator of fluid status; output should be at least 1000 to 1200 mL daily. If output is less than that, additional hydrational fluid is required. Initially this replacement fluid (0.5% normal saline) should be provided intravenously. There is often, but not always, a strong correlation between fecal and urine output. When oral intake is possible, ORS and antimotility agents should be used, although some intravenous replacement fluid may be required. Histamine-2 blockers can be added directly to the PN solution. Proton pump inhibitors must be infused using a piggyback. Fluid status, weight, sodium, potassium, magnesium, and bicarbonate status should be monitored carefully. Once patients have met their prescribed goal for nutritional support, their nutritional status may be monitored by following the total lymphocyte count, visceral protein status (prealbumin; note that the half-life of albumin is approximately 20 days so short-term changes in visceral protein status would be difficult to detect), and nitrogen balance. Acid:base status can be adjusted by controlling the ratio of chloride to acetate in the PN solution, and by controlling stool losses (and therefore bicarbonate losses) to some extent.

CENTRAL CATHETER

A single-lumen, tunneled catheter should be placed with the catheter tip in either the superior or inferior vena cava in preparation for home PN once it has been determined that the patient will be unlikely to absorb sufficient energy or fluid for at least 6 weeks. In general, both single-lumen and tunneled catheters have substantially lower risk of infection compared to their nontunneled counterparts, although a properly cared for percutaneously inserted central catheter may be an exception in the short term. Because it is inserted into the basilic vein in either arm, patient catheter self-care may be impaired. Preferably, the catheter should be used only for PN and fluids. Blood draws should be obtained peripherally, and each time the catheter is used, connected or disconnected, it must be cleaned appropriately. Alcohol alone is not bactericidal. Patients should be instructed on proper catheter care and dressing changes and the prompt recognition of a catheter-related infection (e.g., fever, perhaps only during the PN infusion or chills during catheter flushing for catheter sepsis; erythema; purulence or tenderness at the exit site, indicating a cuff infection; or erythema over the site of the subcutaneous tunnel tract, indicating a tunnel infection). Absence of exit site erythema or purulent drainage only indicates lack of an exit site infection, and not catheter sepsis. The selected reading section contains information on catheter care and complications.

Home PN should be considered if oral and or oral/tube feeding cannot meet patient's nutritional requirement. Management of home PN requires a nutrition support team and, more importantly, adequate patient education. Patients should be prepared for home PN by cycling their PN and fluids so that they are received overnight. This allows maximal rehabilitation potential during the day and later enables the patient potentially to return to work. Because it may take some time for the pancreas to fully adapt to the increased insulin requirements from the infused dextrose, compression of the total volume of PN from a 24-hour infusion to a 10- to 12-hour overnight infusion should take place slowly, typically by 2-hour nightly increments. Some patients may require the addition of regular insulin to their PN (starting with 0.5–1.0 units/g of dextrose) or an increase in the percentage of lipid calories (with a decrease in the dextrose calories), at least initially. When the PN infusion for a given 24-hour period has been completed, it should be tapered off over a 30-min period. Because the half-life of insulin is longer than that of dextrose, patients with substantial amounts of insulin in their PN may require a 1-hour taper. Once the patient is stable at home, laboratory monitoring should be less frequent (as infrequently as three to four times yearly for long-term patients), and the PN volume adjusted downward as the patient's bowel adapts and normal fluid and nutritional status is maintained. Care must be taken to avoid appetite suppression by the provision of excessive energy. As oral intake increases and absorption improves, urine output and other measures of nutritional status can be used during PN reduction.

DRUG THERAPY

Recombinant Human Growth Hormone

Recombinant human growth hormone (r-hGH) is the first drug to be approved by the Food and Drug Administration (FDA) for the treatment of SBS for patients receiving PN. Nevertheless, there is still debate regarding the benefit of r-hGH in SBS patients. Some studies have shown that r-hGH increases intestinal absorption and decreases PN requirements in patients with SBS. In some of these positive studies, the effect of r-hGH on intestinal absorption did not persist after the discontinuation of r-hGH. Other studies have shown no effect of r-hGH on intestinal absorption. GH's greatest effects are on fluid retention and this actually appears more related to enhanced proximal tubular reabsorption of sodium rather than enhanced intestinal fluid absorption. During PN weaning process, it is important to provide optimal medical and dietary treatment before considering r-hGH as many patients can be weaned off PN with optimal medical and dietary treatment, alone. The effect of r-hGH may be enhanced with concomitant administration of glutamine and continuation of glutamine administration after cessation of r-hGH, although the supportive data on this is weak. Re-treatment may be necessary, although FDA approval is currently for one time (single month) dosing. Side effects are common and may include pedal edema, anasarca, and arthralgias (most likely from fluid retention in joint spaces). Treatment with r-hGH is contraindicated in patients with sepsis, new SBS diagnoses, or recurrent cancer. Patients with residual colon should be screened for colon cancer prior to starting r-hGH.

There is no data on the use of r-hGH in patients with a history of colon cancer and thus it should be used cautiously in this patient group. Further studies are needed to determine the effect of r-hGH and to determine the optimal dosage, treatment duration, and maintenance therapy.

GLP-2/TEDUGLUTIDE

GLP-2 can slow gastric emptying time, reduce gastric secretion, increase intestinal blood flow, and stimulate growth of small and large intestine. It is secreted by the L cells located primarily in the terminal ileum and colon in response to a meal. This has raised interest in the usage of GLP-2 especially in patients with end-jejunostomy who have limited meal-stimulated GLP-2 secretion. In a small trial of eight end-jejunostomy SBS patients, GLP-2 resulted in an increase in fluid absorption and a small increase in energy absorption. Teduglutide is a synthetic, long-acting GLP-2 analogue, differing by way of a single amino acid substitution from the parent compound, which is relatively resistant to degradation by dipeptidyl peptidase IV (DPP-IV). Jeppesen et al. studied the effect of teduglutide in an open-label trial of 16 SBS patients, 10 with end-jejunostomy. Teduglutide resulted in improvement in the net weight absorption that was doubled when compared with the native GLP-2, which was surprising in the six patients who had colon in continuity with small bowel. A recent multicenter, placebo-controlled study reported by O'Keefe et al indicated teduglutide was useful for the tapering of PN requirements. Additional studies have confirmed these findings.

COMPLICATIONS OF SBS

Complications of SBS include dehydration (which may result in uric acid nephrolithiasis), generalized malnutrition, electrolyte disturbances, specific nutrient deficiencies, calcium oxalate nephrolithiasis, and cholelithiasis. Patients with significant malabsorption requiring long-term PN are at additional risk for hepatic steatosis and cholestasis with potential progression to cirrhosis, either acalculous or calculous cholecystitis, metabolic bone disease, nephropathy, and central venous catheter-related problems, including infection and occlusion (thrombotic and nonthrombotic). D-lactic acidosis can develop in patients with preserved colon and can present with neurologic symptoms like slurred speech, ataxia, visual disturbances, and confusion that can progress to coma and death.

Patients with colon in continuity with the small intestine should be provided with a diet low in oxalate content as they are at increased risk for developing oxalate nephrolithiasis. The increased risk is due to calcium precipitation with fatty acids in the colon leading to more oxalate available for absorption. Bile acids can also lead to an increase in colonic permeability to oxalate directly. Foods such as chocolate, tea, cola, spinach, celery, and carrots should be avoided, as should dehydration. An increase in dietary calcium intake should be encouraged to decrease absorption of oxalate. Although some of the vitamin C in the parenteral nutrition solutions may be converted to oxalate with a resultant hyperoxaluria, patients without a colon are theoretically not at increased risk for oxalate nephrolithiasis. Enteral feeding leads to release of GLP-2 from the L cells in the distal ileum and possibly right colon helping improve gallbladder contraction and prevent sludge and biliary stone formation. Therefore, enteral feeding should be encouraged, not only to improve intestinal adaptation but also to prevent cholelithiasis.

● SURGICAL MANAGEMENT AND INTESTINAL TRANSPLANTATION

Various surgical procedures have been described in case reports and case series of patients with SBS. As a general rule, these procedures are technically difficult and should be performed in select patients only. The aim of these procedures is to slow the intestinal transit time or to increase intestinal surface area. Surgeries aimed at slowing transit time include insertion of a reversed antiperistaltic segment, colonic interposition, construction of valves, tailoring and plication, and electrical pacing of the small intestine. The Bianchi procedure and the serial transverse enteroplasty procedure (STEP) have been described to taper dilated segments of intestine and increase intestinal length, although overall surface area remains unchanged. Such procedures are not useful for patients with non-dilated intestine. In the Bianchi procedure, the small intestine is essentially divided longitudinally in the midline. The two small bowel pieces are then anastomosed end to end and the tailored bowel is half the diameter and up to double the length of the original bowel loop. Twenty percent of these patients develop postoperative complications such as necrosis of the small intestine, anastomotic leaks, fistula, or obstruction. The serial transverse enteroplasty (STEP) divides the dilated small bowel into narrower segments with a stapling device, again allowing tapering and lengthening of the small intestine. The STEP is technically less difficult than the Bianchi procedure.

Graft and patients' survival following intestinal transplantation has improved due to novel immunosuppressive agents, better surgical techniques, and better postoperative care. Intestinal transplantation should be in considered in patients who fail PN defined as intestinal failure–associated liver injury, multiple line infections, thrombosis of two of the central veins, and frequent episodes of dehydration. Although patient and graft survival have both improved substantially, transplantation is not currently an acceptable alternative to long-term PN in the absence of the aforementioned complications. Furthermore, catheter sepsis, the most common complication, is better serviced by teaching improved catheter care technique to the patient and caregivers than an intestinal transplant, but in order to avoid an intestine/liver transplant, those patients with SBS-related liver disease should be transplanted using isolated intestines, prior to development of irreversible liver disease. There are three types of transplantation: intestine alone, liver plus intestine, and multivisceral that contains stomach, duodenum, pancreas, intestine, and liver. The choice of the procedure depends on the presence of liver disease and the extent of abdominal pathology. Similar to kidney transplantation, intestinal transplantation may become cost effective within the first 2 years following surgery in some patients, but may also represent one of the most expensive procedures of any type in others. Patients with intestinal failure should receive their primary management through a center that is knowledgeable and experienced in medical intestinal rehabilitation, nontransplant bowel rehabilitation procedures, and intestinal transplantation.

Supplemental Reading

1. Buchman AL. Short bowel syndrome. In: Feldman M, Friedman LS, Brandt LJ, eds. *Gastrointestinal and Liver Disease Pathophysiology, Diagnosis, Management.* 8th ed. Philadelphia, PA: Elsevier/Saunders; 2006:2257–2276.

2. Buchman AL, Scolapio J, Fryer J. AGA technical review on short bowel syndrome and intestinal transplantation. *Gastroenterology.* 2003;124(4):1111–1134.

3. Crenn P, Morin MC, Joly F, Penven S, Thuillier F, Messing B. Net digestive absorption and adaptive hyperphagia in adult short bowel patients. *Gut.* 2004;53(9):1279–1286.

4. Jeppesen PB, Sanguinetti EL, Buchman A, et al. Teduglutide (ALX-0600), a dipeptidyl peptidase IV resistant glucagon-like peptide 2 analogue, improves intestinal function in short bowel syndrome patients. *Gut.* 2005;54(9):1224–1231.

5. Cisler JJ, Buchman AL. Intestinal adaptation in short bowel syndrome. *J Investig Med.* 2005;53(8):402–413.

6. Nightingale JM, Lennard-Jones JE, Walker ER, Farthing MJ. Oral salt supplements to compensate for jejunostomy losses: comparison of sodium chloride capsules, glucose electrolyte solution, and glucose polymer electrolyte solution. *Gut.* 1992;33(6):759–761.

7. Langnas AN, Quigley EMM, Tappenden KA, eds. *Intestinal Failure.* Oxford, UK: Blackwell; 2008.

8. Buchman AL. Dietary management of short bowel syndrome. In: Buchman AL, ed. *Clinical Nutrition in Gastrointestinal Disease.* Thorofare, NJ: Slack, Inc.;357–366.

9. Iyer K. Nontransplant surgery for short bowel syndrome. In: Buchman AL, ed. *Clinical Nutrition in Gastrointestinal Disease.* Thorofare, NJ: Slack, Inc.;367–374.

10. Fryer J. Intestinal transplantation. In: Buchman AL, ed. *Clinical Nutrition in Gastrointestinal Disease.* Thorofare, NJ: Slack, Inc.;375–382.

11. Jeppesen PK. The use of growth factors in short bowel syndrome. In: Buchman AL, ed. *Clinical Nutrition in Gastrointestinal Disease.* Thorofare, NJ: Slack, Inc.; 383–394.

12. Buchman AL, Fryer J, Wallin A, Ahn CW, Polensky S, Zaremba K. Clonidine reduces diarrhea and sodium loss in patients with proximal jejunostomy: a controlled study. *JPEN J Parenter Enteral Nutr.* 2006;30(6):487–491.

13. O'Keefe SJ, Peterson ME, Fleming CR. Octreotide as an adjunct to home parenteral nutrition in the management of permanent end-jejunostomy syndrome. *JPEN J Parenter Enteral Nutr.* 1994;18(1):26–34.

14. Nightingale JM, Lennard-Jones JE, Gertner DJ, Wood SR, Bartram CI. Colonic preservation reduces need for parenteral therapy, increases incidence of renal stones, but does not change high prevalence of gall stones in patients with a short bowel. *Gut.* 1992;33(11):1493–1497.

15. Steiger E, DiBaise JK, Messing B, Matarese LE, Blethen S. Indications and recommendations for the use of recombinant human growth hormone in adult short bowel syndrome patients dependent on parenteral nutrition. *J Clin Gastroenterol.* 2006;40(suppl 2):S99–106.

16. Buchman AL. *Practical Nutritional Support Techniques.* 2nd ed. Thorofare, NJ: Slack, Inc.; 2004.

Intestinal Transplantation | 139

Thomas M. Fishbein and Juan Francisco Guerra

The results of intestinal transplantation continue to improve, and the number of transplants performed in North America have increased threefold in the last decade.[1,2] Early outcomes were limited by technical and infectious complications leading to graft failure or death. However, recent surgical progress, better control of rejection, and decreasing infection rates have resulted in 1-year patient survival exceeding 90% at experienced centers like ours. Although long-term follow-up on large cohorts of patients receiving transplants for a single disease are still lacking, the place of intestinal transplants in the support of patients with gut failure has become clearer.

Parenteral nutrition (PN) is currently the primary maintenance therapy for patients who experience failure of intestinal absorptive function. Transplantation is currently offered to patients whose gut failure is irreversible, and who experience complications of PN. Patients who are at risk of death due to complications from diseased native gut or who cannot adapt to the limitations of PN may be candidates. Some controversy still exists regarding exactly which patients should receive a transplant, and who should remain on PN, and these judgments are best made by a team specializing in the management of intestinal failure and intestinal transplants.

● INTESTINAL FAILURE

Intestinal failure refers to the loss of nutritional autonomy due to absorptive gut dysfunction, and is initially supported through delivery of PN.[3,4] Many patients require only temporary parenteral support during which time an injured intestine may undergo adaptation, allowing eventual discontinuation of therapy. The process is unpredictable; for some patients adaptation is rapid, whereas others take years or never reach nutritional autonomy. Patients with Crohn's disease often suffer intermittent deteriorations requiring temporary dependence on parenteral therapy. Clinical factors influencing the outcome of PN treatment include jejunoileal length, patient age, underlying radiation or inflammatory injury to the mucosa, and associated motility disorders.[3,5–11] Patients who cannot regain nutritional autonomy suffer irreversible intestinal failure, and

which of these patients goes on to a transplant is determined by their success or failure with PN. One-year survival for patients treated with PN is approximately 90% in experienced centers, similar to that achieved with transplants.[4,12] However, long-term PN is associated with patient survival, at 3 and 5 years, of 70% to 63%.[4–6,8,13–15] PN-associated liver disease (PNALD) is widely recognized as the most deadly complication. It eventually develops in half of the adults and children on continuous therapy, and leads to death within a year of onset in the majority of patients in whom it is progressive.[10,16–20] Thrombosis of central catheter

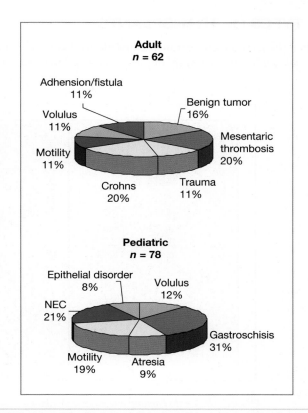

FIGURE 139.1 • Distribution of disease states among 140 recipients of intestinal transplants performed by the authors.

insertion sites, recurrent catheter sepsis episodes, dehydration, formation of renal calculi, and electrolyte disorders are other common complications.[21]

Intestinal transplants are performed in both children and adults (Fig. 139.1). The majority of children who require intestinal transplants suffer from short bowel syndrome, usually after surgical resection. It would be very rare for a child with Crohn's disease to require transplantation at such an age.[22] Rather, most children have acquired short bowel due to congenital anomalies or complications of prematurity. The majority of adult candidates also suffer from short bowel syndrome. Adults with long-standing Crohn's disease, who have decompensated after years of medical therapy, make up approximately 15% of the recipients who undergo intestinal transplantation. Such patients often have undergone multiple prior resections, and have developed secondary short bowel syndrome. However, some patients with medically refractory disease with intact jejunoileum but chronic scarring are sometimes encountered. Such patients usually suffer from rapid transit, intermittent partial obstruction, and malabsorption. Mesenteric vascular accidents, trauma, volvulus, and surgical complications account for the majority of other adult short bowel candidates, and patients with complications of obesity surgery have more recently required transplants. Exenteration and intestinal transplantation is sometimes the only treatment option for locally advanced benign mesenteric tumors. Multivisceral transplants have also been utilized for patients with portal hypertension due to extensive splanchnic venous thrombosis when liver transplantation alone cannot be performed.[23]

● TYPES OF TRANSPLANTS

When the jejunoileum is transplanted alone, it is referred to as an *isolated intestinal transplant* (Fig. 139.2A). However, other organs are commonly transplanted simultaneously from the same donor. When advanced liver disease has developed prior to transplant, the liver is replaced as well. The pancreas and duodenum are often included along with these organs to facilitate en bloc engraftment without the need for biliary reconstruction.[24] The exact degree of PNALD that indicates a liver transplant remains a matter of judgment. Early liver disease may regress after successful isolated intestinal transplant with cessation of parenteral therapy.[25,26]

Some patients require replacement of the entire gastrointestinal tract due to comorbidities in other organs. Some have undergone prior colon removal (Crohn's colitis) or stomach surgery (gastric bypass), developed chronic pancreatitis (PN), have suffered renal failure (oxalic acid stones, hypertension) or have experienced a host of other possible complications of intestinal failure or PN. In such cases, transplants that include the stomach, pancreas, small bowel, and liver are required and are referred to as *multivisceral transplants*. This requires exenteration of the entire native gastrointestinal tract to facilitate the en bloc organ graft as shown in Fig. 139.3C. The colon and or kidney[27] may also be selectively included.[28] Although technical refinements continue to occur, the operations still roughly resemble those first described by Starzl more than 40 years ago in dogs.[29–31]

A feeding tube is generally placed at the time of transplant, and allows early enteral nutrition, which is then transitioned to oral intake. An ileostomy is constructed during the transplant, to allow surveillance biopsies of intestinal mucosa to direct medical therapy. Rejection and most infections can be diagnosed by a combination of histology and serum or plasma diagnostics. Several months after transplant, when graft function is stable, the ileostomy is reversed in recipients who retain functional colon or receive it as part of the allograft.

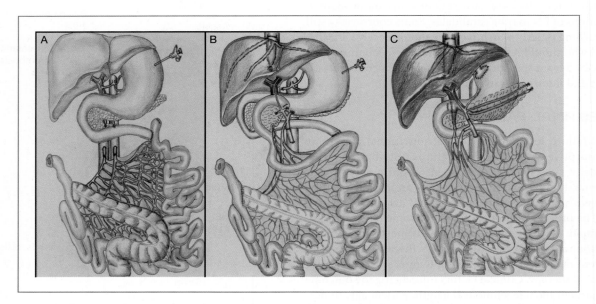

FIGURE 139.2 • (A) *Isolated intestinal transplant* with systemic drainage to vena cava. (B) *Composite liver and intestinal transplant*, which usually includes the duodenum and intact biliary system and portal circulation. With liver and intestinal transplants, the native foregut is preserved (B, gray). (C) *Multivisceral transplant* of liver, stomach, duodenum, pancreas, and small intestine, *in which* the foregut is removed and a new stomach transplanted. These transplants sometimes include the colon and/or kidney. *Preserved native* organs shown in gray and transplanted organs in color.

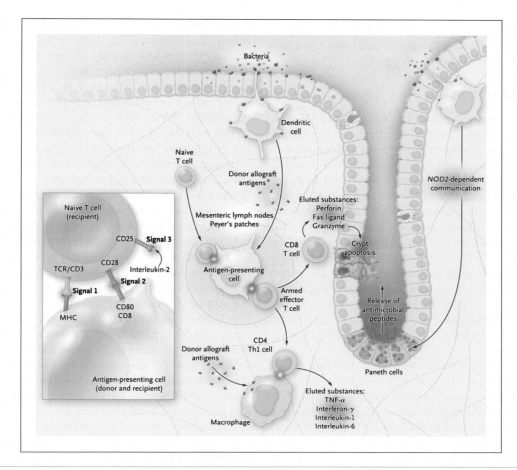

FIGURE 139.3 • (1) Naïve T cells infiltrate the allograft after transplant, undergoing priming and activation in the donor mesenteric lymph nodes and Peyer's patches. In other solid organs, this priming occurs primarily in recipient lymphoid tissues. (2) Donor antigen presenting cells (APCs) ingest "foreign" graft antigens, and display them in association with major histocompatability complex class I and II molecules. (3) APCs are stimulated to express costimulatory effectors required to "arm" naïve CD8 cytotoxic T cells and predominantly CD4 Th1 T cells. (4) Naïve T cells of the recipient are activated (inset). (5) Cytotoxic T cells attack certain donor cell targets, whereas armed Th1 T cells provoke a cytokine (interferon-γ)–driven inflammatory state. (6) The dendritic cell also maintains immune defenses of the epithelium via regulation of Paneth cell production of the antimicrobial peptide human defensin 5. Recipients with mutations in the NOD2 gene are at significantly higher risk of suffering immunologic graft loss, possibly due to inadequate antimicrobial defense resulting in epithelial damage, bacterial invasion, and a secondary inflammatory response. Reprinted with permission from the NEJM. Reprinted with permission from the Vincenti F, Larsen C, Durrbach A, et al. Costimulation blockade with belatacept in renal transplantation. *N Engl J Med.* 2005;353(8):770–781.

IMMUNOLOGY

Transplantation of the intestine is a greater immunologic challenge than other solid organs. Approximately 80% of immune cells normally reside in the gut, and are replaced after transplantation with recipient bone marrow–derived cells, while the epithelium remains donor genotype, making the organ highly chimeric and immunogenic.[32–34] Although most transplanted organs are sterile, the gut relies on mucous barrier and other immunologic mechanisms like the production of antimicrobial peptides to protect against invasion of the epithelium by huge numbers and species of commensal flora. Injury to this ileal barrier by ischemia/reperfusion injury, recipient immune cells, or defects such as impaired microbial control mechanisms result in inflammation and tissue damage increasing the likelihood of infection. This makes the augmented immunosuppression required to treat rejection particularly dangerous. In addition, Crohn's disease patients requiring intestinal transplants tend to

be those with NOD2-associated defects leading to stenotic and fistulous disease and short bowel syndrome. Early evidence suggests that the defective NOD2 sensing system contributes both to the underlying disease state as well as immunologic complications after transplantation. Fig. 139.3 summarizes our current understanding of intestinal transplant immunology.

Maintenance tacrolimus, which inhibits signal 1 activation of T lymphocytes through the inhibition of calcineurin, is the basis of current intestinal transplant immunosuppression. The recent addition of induction agents acting at signal 3, including interleukin-2 monoclonal antibodies, thymoglobulin, and sirolimus have all decreased acute cellular rejection at different centers. A new fusion protein specific for CD80 and CD86 is in current trials of renal transplantation, and would be the first approved agent for use to inhibit signal 2 activation.[35] A single regimen has yet to prove superior, and centers individualize immunosuppression. Ideally, future strategies should target mechanisms of mucosal injury specific to the ileum. The use of anti-tumor necrosis factor (TNF)-α antibodies in small studies has also been associated with healing of persistent ulceration encountered in the setting of allograft rejection.

COMPLICATIONS

Improved early outcomes reflect increasing surgical experience over the last decade. Graft thrombosis, ischemia, and technical failure have diminished, and graft losses now more commonly relate to medical and immunologic causes. This likely reflects the increased experience of several high-volume centers. Transplantation of the isolated intestine prior to the onset of liver failure improves early success, decreases hospitalizations, and allows more rapid conversion to a full enteral diet than multiorgan transplants.[36] The long-term survival advantage of single-organ transplants over multiorgan transplants has yet to be proven. However, in the case of life-threatening complications, an isolated intestine graft may be removed, and PN temporarily reinstituted while awaiting retransplantation.[37] Thus, we continue to favor earlier intervention for patients who have no chance of rehabilitation and weaning from PN.

Graft failure and death after transplant are most closely related to the development of rejection. Among 922 recipients of intestinal transplants between 2002 and 2007, an occurrence of acute rejection during the first 90 days markedly increased the risk of graft loss at 1 year (relative risk 1.96 $P < 0.002$, ITR March 2009, personal communication via Dr. David Grant). Repeated rejection is associated with the development of chronic allograft enteropathy, a state clinically similar to Crohn's disease in which waxing and waning function lead ultimately to the return to parenteral support (Fig. 139.4). Early diagnosis is critical to successful reversal of the rejection process. Endoscopic surveillance biopsy remains the gold standard with which to diagnose this problem (Fig. 139.5). Recently standardized histologic grading

of rejection has allowed more consistent early diagnosis and discrimination from viral infection.[38] Several centers have reported decreasing rates and severity of early acute rejection utilizing newer medications including monoclonal interleukin-2 antagonists, polyclonal antithymocyte antibodies, or rapamycin.[39–41] Acute cellular rejection in the first 90 days, which previously occurred in 70% to 90% of transplant recipients, currently is seen in only one-third to one-half of patients. This recent control of rejection has improved early graft survival, and can be expected to impact long-term survival with increased experience. The impact of other conditions, such as the presence of Crohn's-associated NOD2 gene mutations, are just now being recognized to increase immunologic risk as noted earlier.[42–44]

Infections remain common after transplant.[45] The medical management of intestinal transplant recipients mandates discrimination of viral or bacterial enteritis from rejection. All these states usually present to the clinician with diarrhea, and endoscopic evaluation of the graft mucosa is necessary any time after transplantation. Diarrhea may be caused by any infection, rejection, antibiotic use, or poor food choice. In the absence of known food allergy or dumping syndrome by history, histology is mandatory for accurate diagnosis. Infectious agents are evaluated with stool cultures; plasma assays for adenovirus, Epstein-Barr virus and norovirus; and immunohistochemistry of graft biopsy for cytomegalovirus, Epstein-Barr virus, norovirus, and adenovirus. Viral infection is more common in children, particularly in the first 3 months after transplantation when immunosuppression levels are still high. Judicious withdrawal of immunosuppression is coupled with antiviral medication but should be directed by the transplant center. Adenovirus, calciviruses, *Clostridium difficile,* and cytomegalovirus all may masquerade as rejection, and biopsy evaluation by a pathologist experienced with such transplants is necessary.[46,47] Bloody diarrhea is frequently a sign of severe rejection with mucosal erosion or sloughing. Ileal ulcers near an anastomotic site may also cause chronic anemia, sometimes respond to TNF antibodies, and often recur in the absence of any discernible cause, suggesting mechanisms similar to other inflammatory bowel diseases.[44] We encourage direct contact with the transplant center upon the development of any new gastrointestinal symptoms in the recipient of a transplant.

OUTCOMES

Marked improvements in survival have occurred over the last decade.[22,26,48] One-year graft survival for recipients of intestinal and multiorgan transplants in North America increased from 52% in 1997 to 75% in 2005. Similarly, 1-year patient survival improved from 57% in 1997 to 80% in 2005.[2] More recent results at centers where larger numbers of transplants are performed include survival rates exceeding 90% at 1 year and should translate to improved longer survivals.[26,48,49] Factors associated with improved success include patients who come from home to receive transplants, younger patients, first transplants, and the use of antibody therapy or maintenance rapamycin.[16,22,44,50–70] These findings collectively emphasize the importance of early referral of patients well enough to await transplantation at home, and tolerate aggressive induction immunosuppression. More than 80% of survivors attain freedom from parenteral

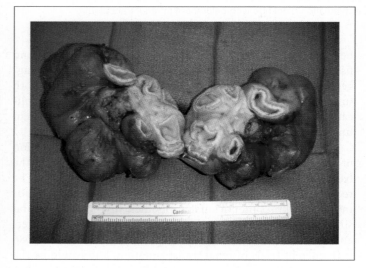

FIGURE 139.4 • Chronic rejection of the allograft, shown after removal here, leads to mesenteric fibrosis, arteriolar constriction, and muscular hypertrophy and scarring, despite the relatively normal-appearing mucosa. Figure courtesy of Cal Matsumoto, MD.

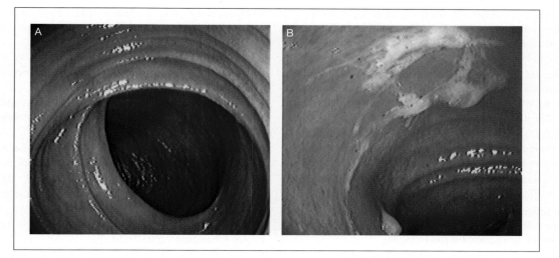

FIGURE 139.5 • (A) Endoscopy of healthy ileal allograft. (B) Acute cellular rejection of the allograft, associated with loss of mucosal folds, exudate, and ulceration. This tissue destructive process, if identified early, is reversible with alteration of immunosuppressive therapy. Figures courtesy of Stuart Kaufman, MD.

support and resume regular activities,[22] and over half of the adult survivors return to work after transplantation. Intestinal function after transplantation is usually mildly abnormal, leading to the need for some dietary restriction. Foods containing insoluble cellulose or high in simple carbohydrates may cause type 1 dumping symptoms. Thus, the diet may be modified by an individual clinician and patient according to tolerance. Patients with a longer colonic remnant or a transplanted colon may have improved function, but the use of antidiarrheal medications such as Lomotil or Imodium is common. Vitamin, mineral, and micronutrient absorption is generally good, and routine studies are not necessary. Among children, several studies have shown linear growth and development after a transition to enteral feeding,[40,71–73] but failed to demonstrate "catch up" from the depressed growth curves seen in virtually all patients prior to transplantation.

● FUTURE APPLICATIONS

Thousands of patients die from complications of inflammatory bowel disease, short bowel syndrome, or total intestinal infarction due to mesenteric ischemia annually, never having been referred to a center experienced with intestinal transplantation. The practice of aborting resection and allowing otherwise salvageable patients to expire from sepsis continues. The development of suitable life quality through the delivery of home PN, and eventual promise of a return to normal life after transplantation is altering that practice. While the numbers of intestinal transplants remain relatively small nationally, the rapid improvement in outcomes seen in the last decade presages a significant increase in volume and broadening indications to include preemptive transplantation in good-risk patients, and increased salvage of patients once thought terminal. Isolated intestinal transplants prior to the development of liver failure and the need for multiorgan transplants is likely to increase as long-term outcomes improve. The improvements seen recently in selected centers with expertise should lead to consideration of intestinal transplantation among surgeons and gastroenterologists caring for patients with inflammatory bowel disease, short bowel syndrome, and PN requirements.

Editor's note (TMB): We are indebted to Dr. Fishbein and Dr. Guerra for sharing their experience with us. Eleven percent of their adult patients had motility problems; I assume these included intestinal pseudo-obstruction although that term doesn't appear in the manuscript. I mention it here so it will be indexed.

References

1. Fishbein TM. Intestinal transplantation. *N Engl J Med.* 2009;361 (10):998–1008.

2. Hanto DW, Fishbein TM, Pinson CW, et al. Liver and intestine transplantation: summary analysis, 1994–2003. *Am J Transplant.* 2005;5(4 Pt 2):916–933.

3. Wilmore DW, Lacey JM, Soultanakis RP, Bosch RL, Byrne TA. Factors predicting a successful outcome after pharmacologic bowel compensation. *Ann Surg.* 1997;226(3):288–292; discussion 292–283.

4. Howard L, Ament M, Fleming CR, Shike M, Steiger E. Current use and clinical outcome of home parenteral and enteral nutrition therapies in the United States. *Gastroenterology.* 1995;109(2):355–365.

5. Van Gossum A, Vahedi K, Abdel-Malik, et al.; ESPEN-HAN Working Group. Clinical, social and rehabilitation status of long-term home parenteral nutrition patients: results of a European multicentre survey. *Clin Nutr.* 2001;20(3):205–210.

6. Casey L, Lee KH, Rosychuk R, Turner J, Huynh HQ. 10-year review of pediatric intestinal failure: clinical factors associated with outcome. *Nutr Clin Pract.* 2008;23(4):436–442.

7. Fishbein TM, Schiano T, LeLeiko N, et al. An integrated approach to intestinal failure: results of a new program with total parenteral nutrition, bowel rehabilitation, and transplantation. *J Gastrointest Surg.* 2002;6(4):554–562.

8. Messing B, Crenn P, Beau P, Boutron-Ruault MC, Rambaud JC, Matuchansky C. Long-term survival and parenteral nutrition dependence in adult patients with the short bowel syndrome. *Gastroenterology.* 1999;117(5):1043–1050.

9. Quirós-Tejeira RE, Ament ME, Reyen L, et al. Long-term parenteral nutritional support and intestinal adaptation in children with short bowel syndrome: a 25-year experience. *J Pediatr.* 2004;145(2):157–163.

10. Sondheimer JM, Asturias E, Cadnapaphornchai M. Infection and cholestasis in neonates with intestinal resection and long-term parenteral nutrition. *J Pediatr Gastroenterol Nutr.* 1998;27(2):131–137.

11. Carbonnel F, Cosnes J, Chevret S, et al. The role of anatomic factors in nutritional autonomy after extensive small bowel resection. *JPEN J Parenter Enteral Nutr.* 1996;20(4):275–280.

12. Howard L, Malone M. Current status of home parenteral nutrition in the United States. *Transplant Proc.* 1996;28(5):2691–2695.

13. Vargas JH, Ament ME, Berquist WE. Long-term home parenteral nutrition in pediatrics: ten years of experience in 102 patients. *J Pediatr Gastroenterol Nutr.* 1987;6(1):24–32.

14. Ricour C. Home TPN. *Nutrition.* 1989;5(5):345–346.

15. Scolapio JS, Fleming CR, Kelly DG, Wick DM, Zinsmeister AR. Survival of home parenteral nutrition-treated patients: 20 years of experience at the Mayo Clinic. *Mayo Clin Proc.* 1999;74(3):217–222.

16. Fecteau A, Atkinson P, Grant D. Early referral is essential for successful pediatric small bowel transplantation: The Canadian experience. *J Pediatr Surg.* 2001;36(5):681–684.

17. Sigalet DL. Short bowel syndrome in infants and children: an overview. *Semin Pediatr Surg.* 2001;10(2):49–55.

18. Fleming CR. Hepatobiliary complications in adults receiving nutrition support. *Dig Dis.* 1994;12(4):191–198.

19. Cavicchi M, Beau P, Crenn P, Degott C, Messing B. Prevalence of liver disease and contributing factors in patients receiving home parenteral nutrition for permanent intestinal failure. *Ann Intern Med.* 2000;132(7):525–532.

20. Chan S, McCowen KC, Bistrian BR, et al. Incidence, prognosis, and etiology of end-stage liver disease in patients receiving home total parenteral nutrition. *Surgery.* 1999;126(1):28–34.

21. Buchman AL, Scolapio J, Fryer J. AGA technical review on short bowel syndrome and intestinal transplantation. *Gastroenterology.* 2003;124(4):1111–1134.

22. Grant D, Abu-Elmagd K, Reyes J, et al. 2003 report of the intestine transplant registry: a new era has dawned. *Ann Surg.* 2005;241(4):607–613.

23. Florman SS, Fishbein TM, Schiano T, Letizia A, Fennelly E, DeSancho M. Multivisceral transplantation for portal hypertension and diffuse mesenteric thrombosis caused by protein C deficiency. *Transplantation.* 2002;74(3):406–407.

24. Sudan DL, Iyer KR, Deroover A, et al. A new technique for combined liver/small intestinal transplantation. *Transplantation.* 2001;72(11):1846–1848.

25. Fiel MI, Sauter B, Wu HS, et al. Regression of hepatic fibrosis after intestinal transplantation in total parenteral nutrition liver disease. *Clin Gastroenterol Hepatol.* 2008;6(8):926–933.

26. Fishbein TM, Kaufman SS, Florman SS, et al. Isolated intestinal transplantation: proof of clinical efficacy. *Transplantation.* 2003;76(4):636–640.

27. Todo S, Tzakis A, Reyes J, et al. Small intestinal transplantation in humans with or without the colon. *Transplantation.* 1994;57(6):840–848.

28. Kato T, Selvaggi G, Gaynor JJ, et al. Inclusion of donor colon and ileocecal valve in intestinal transplantation. *Transplantation.* 2008;86(2):293–297.

29. Matsumoto CS, Fishbein TM. Modified multivisceral transplantation with splenopancreatic preservation. *Transplantation.* 2007;83(2):234–236.

30. Starzl TE, Kaupp HA Jr, Brock DR, Butz GW Jr, Linman JW. Homotransplantation of multiple visceral organs. *Am J Surg.* 1962;103:219–229.

31. Todo S, Tzakis AG, Abu-Elmagd K, et al. Intestinal transplantation in composite visceral grafts or alone. *Ann Surg.* 1992;216(3):223–233; discussion 233–224.

32. Mayer L. Mucosal immunity and gastrointestinal antigen processing. *J Pediatr Gastroenterol Nutr.* 2000;30(suppl):S4–12.

33. Iwaki Y, Starzl TE, Yagihashi A, et al. Replacement of donor lymphoid tissue in small-bowel transplants. *Lancet.* 1991;337(8745):818–819.

34. Newell KA. Transplantation of the intestine: is it truly different? *Am J Transplant.* 2003;3(1):1–2.

35. Vincenti F, Larsen C, Durrbach A, et al.; Belatacept Study Group. Costimulation blockade with belatacept in renal transplantation. *N Engl J Med.* 2005;353(8):770–781.

36. Kato T, Mittal N, Nishida S, et al. The role of intestinal transplantation in the management of babies with extensive gut resections. *J Pediatr Surg.* 2003;38(2):145–149.

37. Fishbein TM, Matsumoto CS. Intestinal replacement therapy: timing and indications for referral of patients to an intestinal rehabilitation and transplant program. *Gastroenterology.* 2006;130(2 suppl 1):S147–S151.

38. Ruiz P, Bagni A, Brown R, et al. Histological criteria for the identification of acute cellular rejection in human small bowel allografts: results of the pathology workshop at the VIII International Small Bowel Transplant Symposium. *Transplant Proc.* 2004;36(2):335–337.

39. Tzakis AG, Kato T, Nishida S, et al. Preliminary experience with campath 1H (C1H) in intestinal and liver transplantation. *Transplantation.* 2003;75(8):1227–1231.

40. Sudan DL, Chinnakotla S, Horslen S, et al. Basiliximab decreases the incidence of acute rejection after intestinal transplantation. *Transplant Proc.* 2002;34(3):940–941.

41. Fishbein TM, Florman S, Gondolesi G, et al. Intestinal transplantation before and after the introduction of sirolimus. *Transplantation.* 2002;73(10):1538–1542.

42. Fishbein T, Novitskiy G, Mishra L, et al. NOD2-expressing bone marrow-derived cells appear to regulate epithelial innate immunity of the transplanted human small intestine. *Gut.* 2008;57(3):323–330.

43. Sarkar S, Selvaggi G, Mittal N, et al. Gastrointestinal tract ulcers in pediatric intestinal transplantation patients: etiology and management. *Pediatr Transplant.* 2006;10(2):162–167.

44. Turner D, Martin S, Ngan BY, Grant D, Sherman PM. Anastomotic ulceration following small bowel transplantation. *Am J Transplant.* 2006;6(1):236–240.

45. Guaraldi G, Cocchi S, Codeluppi M, et al. Outcome, incidence, and timing of infectious complications in small bowel and multivisceral organ transplantation patients. *Transplantation.* 2005;80(12):1742–1748.

46. Bueno J, Green M, Kocoshis S, et al. Cytomegalovirus infection after intestinal transplantation in children. *Clin Infect Dis.* 1997;25(5):1078–1083.

47. Kaufman SS, Magid MS, Tschernia A, LeLeiko NS, Fishbein TM. Discrimination between acute rejection and adenoviral enteritis in intestinal transplant recipients. *Transplant Proc.* 2002;34(3):943–945.

48. Sudan DL, Kaufman SS, Shaw BW Jr, et al. Isolated intestinal transplantation for intestinal failure. *Am J Gastroenterol.* 2000;95(6):1506–1515.

49. Reyes J, Mazariegos GV, Bond GM, et al. Pediatric intestinal transplantation: historical notes, principles and controversies. *Pediatr Transplant.* 2002;6(3):193–207.

50. Andres AM, Thompson J, Grant W, et al. Repeat surgical bowel lengthening with the STEP procedure. *Transplantation.* 2008;85(9):1294–1299.

51. Florescu DF, Hill LA, McCartan MA, Grant W. Two cases of Norwalk virus enteritis following small bowel transplantation treated with oral human serum immunoglobulin. *Pediatr Transplant.* 2008;12(3):372–375.

52. Lopushinsky SR, Fowler RA, Kulkarni GS, Fecteau AH, Grant DR, Wales PW. The optimal timing of intestinal transplantation for children with intestinal failure: a Markov analysis. *Ann Surg.* 2007;246(6):1092–1099.

53. Sudan D, Thompson J, Botha J, et al. Comparison of intestinal lengthening procedures for patients with short bowel syndrome. *Ann Surg.* 2007;246(4):593–601; discussion 601–594.

54. Torres C, Sudan D, Vanderhoof J, et al. Role of an intestinal rehabilitation program in the treatment of advanced intestinal failure. *J Pediatr Gastroenterol Nutr.* 2007;45(2):204–212.

55. Botha JF, Grant WJ, Torres C, et al. Isolated liver transplantation in infants with end-stage liver disease due to short bowel syndrome. *Liver Transpl.* 2006;12(7):1062–1066.

56. Diamond IR, Wales PW, Grant DR, Fecteau A. Isolated liver transplantation in pediatric short bowel syndrome: is there a role? *J Pediatr Surg.* 2006;41(5):955–959.

57. Sudan D, DiBaise J, Torres C, et al. A multidisciplinary approach to the treatment of intestinal failure. *J Gastrointest Surg.* 2005;9(2):165–176; discussion 176–167.

58. Chaney M. Financial considerations insurance and coverage issues in intestinal transplantation. *Prog Transplant.* 2004;14(4):312–320.

59. Sudan D, Horslen S, Botha J, et al. Quality of life after pediatric intestinal transplantation: the perception of pediatric recipients and their parents. *Am J Transplant.* 2004;4(3):407–413.

60. Kaila B, Grant D, Pettigrew N, Greenberg H, Bernstein CN. Crohn's disease recurrence in a small bowel transplant. *Am J Gastroenterol.* 2004;99(1):158–162.

61. Kellersmann R, Lazarovits A, Grant D, et al. Monoclonal antibody against beta7 integrins, but not beta7 deficiency, attenuates intestinal allograft rejection in mice. *Transplantation.* 2002;74(9):1327–1334.

62. Sudan D, Grant W, Iyer K, Shaw B, Horslen S, Langnas A. Oral beclomethasone therapy for recurrent small bowel allograft rejection and intestinal graft-versus-host disease. *Transplant Proc.* 2002;34(3):938–939.

63. Kiyochi H, Zhang Z, Jiang J, et al. Histologic comparison of small bowel, heart, and kidney xenografts in a rat to mouse model. *Transplant Proc.* 2000;32(5):964.

64. Atkison P, Chatzipetrou M, Tsaroucha A, Lehmann R, Tzakis A, Grant D. Small bowel transplantation in children. *Pediatr Transplant.* 1997;1(2):111–118.

65. Ozcay N, Fryer J, Grant D, Freeman D, Garcia B, Zhong R. Budesonide, a locally acting steroid, prevents graft rejection in a rat model of intestinal transplantation. *Transplantation.* 1997;63(9):1220–1225.

66. Zhang Z, Zhu L, Quan D, et al. Pattern of liver, kidney, heart, and intestine allograft rejection in different mouse strain combinations. *Transplantation.* 1996;62(9):1267–1272.

67. Fryer J, Jiang J, Zhong R, et al. Influence of macrophage depletion on bacterial translocation and rejection in small bowel transplantation. *Transplant Proc.* 1996;28(5):2660.

68. Zhang Z, Zhu L, Garcia B, et al. Organ-specific differences in the pattern of allograft rejection in the mouse. *Transplant Proc.* 1996;28(5):2487.

69. Quan D, Zhang Z, Zhong R, Jevnikar A, Garcia B, Grant D. Intestinal allograft rejection in lipopolysaccharide-hyporesponsive mice. *Transplant Proc.* 1996;28(5):2460–2461.

70. Fryer J, Grant D, Jiang J, et al. Influence of macrophage depletion on bacterial translocation and rejection in small bowel transplantation. *Transplantation.* 1996;62(5):553–559.

71. Ueno T, Kato T, Revas K, et al. Growth after intestinal transplant in children. *Transplant Proc.* 2006;38(6):1702–1704.

72. Nucci AM, Barksdale EM Jr, Beserock N, et al. Long-term nutritional outcome after pediatric intestinal transplantation. *J Pediatr Surg.* 2002;37(3):460–463.

73. Porubsky M, Testa G, John E, Holterman M, Tsou M, Benedetti E. Pattern of growth after pediatric living-donor small bowel transplantation. *Pediatr Transplant.* 2006;10(6):701–706.

Management of Abdominal Fistulae

140

Howard S. Kaufman and Patrizio Petrone

Abdominal fistulae in Crohn's disease may be internal or external. The most common internal fistulae include enteroenteric (including enterocolonic), enterovesical, and enterovaginal. Less common communications may develop between the intestine and ureters or intraabdominal reproductive organs. Fistulae to the hip and spine presenting with septic arthritis or osteomyeltis have also been reported. Of all enterocutaneous fistulae, approximately 25% are secondary to Crohn's disease. Fistulae may occur spontaneously or occur postoperatively following intestinal surgery. Although fistulae are found in up to one third of patients who are operated upon for Crohn's disease, they are the primary indication for surgery in only 6% of individuals. Other abdominal fistulae are clinically silent and identified at the time of surgery for other primary indications usually associated with Crohn's obstruction.[1]

INCIDENCE AND DISTRIBUTION

In population-based studies, the cumulative incidence of fistula formation in patients with Crohn's disease is 17% to 50%. One epidemiologic study showed that 35% of patients with Crohn's disease had at least one fistula. Of those fistulae, 54% were perianal, 24% were enteroenteric, 9% were rectovaginal, and 13% were classified as "other," which included enterocutaneous, enterovesical, and less common intraabdominal communications. Moreover, 33% of these patients had recurrent fistulae, which emphasizes the extent of this complication and fistulizing subtype in patients with Crohn's disease.

There is an uneven distribution of abdominal fistulae throughout the length of the gastrointestinal tract. Primary fistulae from the stomach or duodenum are exceedingly rare. When these organs are affected, it much more commonly represents secondary or "innocent bystander" involvement from either the ileum or colon. Of patients with jejunal disease (including coexisting jejunal and ileal disease), approximately 10% will have jejunal fistulae. In contrast, patients with distal ileal disease have fistulae in approximately 33% of cases.[2]

CLINICAL PRESENTATION AND TREATMENT

The treatment of fistulizing Crohn's disease requires an interdisciplinary approach between surgeons and gastroenterologists. It has evolved considerably from primarily a surgical approach to one with emphasis on pharmacological treatment (Fig. 140.1). A recent review of evidence for the surgical management of Crohn's disease by the Standards Practice Task Force of the American Society of Colon and Rectal Surgeons has been published as "Practice Parameters for the Surgical Management of Crohn's Disease."[3] There are no randomized controlled clinical trials that have addressed the surgical management of abdominal fistulae. Therefore, recommendations were derived from level III evidence. The Task Force recommended that surgery should be considered for patients with enteric fistulae who had signs of localized or systemic sepsis and had failed medical therapy. They recommended against surgery for asymptomatic patients with internal fistulae.

If the fistula secondarily involves other intraabdominal organs or the skin, most patients do not have evidence of systemic or localized sepsis. Alternatively, if a patient with an obvious fistula presents with signs of sepsis, general rules for management should be followed with the administration of systemic antibiotics and imaging to rule out a coexisting abscess. A contained abscess should be managed by percutaneous drainage, if the collection is accessible and the expertise is available. Sepsis caused by an abscess that can be drained percutaneously infrequently results in enterocutaneous fistula formation. However, abscesses that require surgical drainage are more likely to result in the development of an enterocutaneous fistula. As bowel that has contained the abscess might also need resection, the eventual development of short gut is more likely. Continued sepsis despite abscess drainage will require resection of the diseased bowel. The need for resection of the "innocent bystander" organ will depend on the degree of disease of that organ. When the secondarily affected bowel is diseased, it usually requires resection. A defect in noninflamed bowel can usually be closed

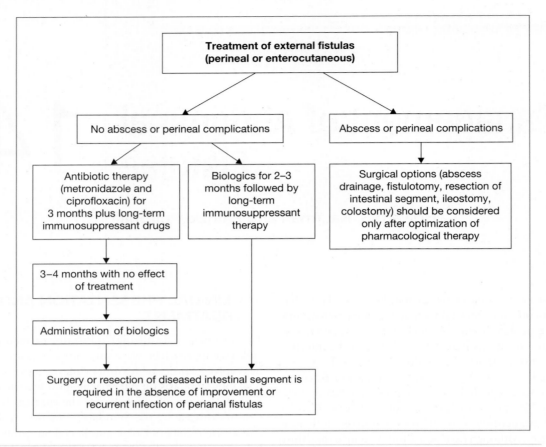

FIGURE 140.1 • Algorithm for the treatment of external fistulas in patients with Crohn's disease. Reproduced with permission from Nielsen et al.[1]

primarily. If a fistula involves the bladder of vagina, it will usually heal by secondary intention. A larger defect may require primary closure.[1]

SITE-SPECIFIC FISTULAE

Enteroenteric Fistulae

Enteroenteric fistulae may occur in 5% to 10% of individuals with Crohn's disease. They are most frequently asymptomatic and are identified either by diagnostic imaging or at the time of laparoscopy or laparotomy for otherwise symptomatic inflammatory or obstructive disease. Symptoms may occur when a significant portion of the intestine is bypassed by the fistulous communication resulting in diarrhea or when coexisting inflammation or obstruction is present. Enteroenteric fistulae are usually completely contained within the diseased segments, especially ileoileal and ileocecal fistulae, and are managed by simple resection en bloc.[4]

Ileosigmoid Fistulae

Typically, the active Crohn's disease is limited to the terminal ileum, and because of the proximity with the sigmoid colon, the sigmoid is secondarily involved by inflammatory adhesions and subsequent fistulization. Two large series have been published detailing the surgical management of ileosigmoid fistulae in Crohn's disease. Data collected from the Mayo clinic from 1975 to 1995 identified 90 patients with a nearly even distribution

between men and women and a mean age of 33.7 years (range: 14–71) at the time of surgery. The mean duration of disease was 5.8 years (range: 1 week–24 years). Common presenting symptoms included abdominal pain (34%), diarrhea (22%), fistula drainage (10%), and weight loss (9%). Other less common symptoms were small intestinal obstruction, fever, bloody stools, pneumaturia, and bloating. Only two patients were completely asymptomatic. The diagnosis was made or confirmed preoperatively by contrast imaging in 77% of patients. It was not suspected in 20 of 87 patients who were taken to surgery and was made intraoperatively. In this series, preoperative knowledge of the fistula tended to influence the surgical procedure, though the association was not statistically significant ($P < 0.07$). Patients with a preoperative diagnosis of ileosigmoid fistula underwent sigmoid resection in 42% of cases versus sigmoid repair in 45%. Alternatively, when diagnosed at surgery, 65% underwent simple repair, and 20% had a sigmoid resection. The remaining patients in both groups had more complex procedures performed. There were no significant differences in postoperative complications in patients who underwent repair or resection.[5]

Editor's note (TMB): Having this prepared preoperatively should lessen complications with resection. It is helpful to supply the surgeon with an accurate "road map" preoperatively, as described in the following.

More recently, a series of 104 patients with ileosigmoid fistulae has been reported from the Cleveland Clinic.[6] The incidence of this type of fistula was found in 7.7% of all patients who underwent major abdominal surgery for Crohn's disease between 2000 and 2007. The median age was 37 years (range: 18–78 years), and 53% were women. The combined sensitivity for preoperative diagnostic studies (including colonoscopy, CT scans, and fluoroscopic imaging) was 63%. All patients underwent ileocolic resection via laparoscopic (29 patients) or open (75 patients) approaches. The sigmoid colon was treated with primary repair (26 patients), segmental resection (71 patients), or subtotal colectomy (7 patients).

Ileovesical (Enterovesical) Fistulae

The majority of patients typically have a history of pneumaturia or fecaluria, though they may also be clinically silent. *Up to 60% of patients with enterovesical fistulae will also have ileosigmoid fistulae.* Conversely, the incidence of enterovesical fistula in patients with known ileosigmoid fistula varies between 7% and 30%. Diagnosis may be confirmed by cystoscopy, cysotography, or CT scan.

Because of the consequences of chronic urinary tract infections on renal function, most surgeons and gastroenterologists agree that the presence of an enterovesical fistula is an indication for operation. The diseased segment of intestine is resected, and the bladder is debrided and closed in layers. A Foley catheter is kept in the bladder for 5 to 10 days, depending on the operative findings, complexity of closure, and preference of the surgeon. A cystogram may be performed prior to catheter removal to confirm that the repair has healed.

Enterocutaneous Fistulae

Enterocutaneous fistulae occur in approximately 4% of patients with Crohn's disease. They result either from direct penetration of a Crohn's disease sinus through the abdominal wall or from external drainage of a Crohn's disease abscess that communicates with the diseased intestinal tract. The most common sites for spontaneous drainage of a Crohn's enterocutaneous fistula are through a previous abdominal scar or the umbilicus. Almost all primary enterocutaneous fistulae in Crohn's disease patients are the result of active intestinal disease. The remaining fistulae are usually traumatic in origin, resulting from an anastomotic leak, surgical intervention, or drainage procedures. Recurrence of Crohn's disease after complete surgical resection generally requires months to years to progress to an enterocutaneous fistula.

If the patient's underlying disease is under control and the enterocutaneous fistula has minimal output, a period of conservative management is appropriate. Nonoperative management of Crohn's disease fistulae includes clearance of sepsis, aggressive nutritional support, and appropriate medical therapy. Even with aggressive nonoperative management, Crohn's disease enterocutaneous fistulae that persist for a long time are difficult to cure, and surgical intervention is often required. Surgical treatment consists of resection of the involved intestine, extirpation of the fistula, and debridement of the tract through the abdominal wall.

Editor's note (TMB): The paper on use of inflixamab for fistula (Present et al.) was almost entirely on peritoneal disease. Those results cannot be extrapolated to enterocutaneous or enterofistula.

Enterogenital Fistulae

These types of fistulae are much less common than those involving the skin or occurring purely within the gastrointestinal tract and include enterovaginal, enterosalpingeal, and enterouterine fistulae. Enterovaginal fistulae occur in patients with previous hysterectomy, and symptoms may include a foul discharge and a passage of air per vagina. Continuous symptoms are not always present. Treatment is by resection of diseased bowel, extirpation of the fistula, and drainage of any coexisting abscess. If omentum is available, it should be placed in the cul-de-sac overlying the vaginal defect. The vaginal opening will close secondarily.

Enterosalpingeal and enterouterine fistulae are extremely rare. Treatment usually includes resection of the affected tube, drainage of the possible abscess, resection of diseased small bowel, and if necessary, hysterectomy.

Editor's note (TMB): Rectovaginal and anovaginal fistula are discussed in a separate chapter.

Surgical Approach—Open Versus Laparoscopic: Technical Considerations

The decision whether to treat the patient with fistulizing disease by laparoscopic or by open technique depends on a number of patient factors as well as surgeon's experience with complex laparoscopic surgery. A recent meta-analysis has compared these approaches from 14 studies including 881 patients with inflammatory, stricturing, and fistulizing disease.[7] The overall rate of conversion to open surgery was 11.2%, and laparoscopic procedures were associated with longer operative times by a weighted mean of 25 minutes. However, patients who had successful completion of surgery laparoscopically had more rapid recovery of bowel function, shorter hospital stay (by a weighted mean of 1.82 days), and overall lower postoperative morbidity (odds ratio = 0.57, 95% confidence interval [CI] = 0.37–0.87, $P < 0.01$). There was no difference in the rate of disease recurrence.

The presence of a fistula has been associated with a higher rate of conversion in many studies and has been a predictor of conversion in multivariate analysis in patients undergoing laparoscopic ileocecal resection. Alternatively, other studies have not suggested a higher conversion rate. From a technical perspective, mobilization of unaffected and "innocent bystander" bowel should be completed before mobilization and resection of the inflamed intestine. Division of the fistula to the healthy bowel should also be accomplished before dissection of the diseased bowel.

Whether attempted via a laparoscopic or open approach, inflamed bowel containing the origin of the fistula should be resected with 2 cm grossly disease-free margins. This margin length conserves bowel, reducing the likelihood of short gut from repeated resections, and is not associated with an increased incidence of recurrence. If deemed safe, an anastomosis is created either by a handsewn or stapled technique. There is limited evidence that a longer side-to-side stapled anastomosis may be associated with a lower incidence of recurrence. In the elective setting with an otherwise fit patient, creation of a stoma is rarely needed. However, there are a number of associated patient factors that may increase the risk of anastomotic leak, including severe malnutrition, serum albumin <3mg/dl, long-term preoperative steroid use, anemia, and urgent or emergent surgery. The presence of an abscess or fistula is also associated with a higher chance of leak. When these factors are present, the surgeon must weigh the risks and benefits of creating an anastomosis versus raising a protective stoma. *If a stoma is being considered during a preoperative consultation, referral to a wound ostomy and continence nurse (if available) is advised before the operation is undertaken.*

Postoperative Fistulae

Fistulae that develop following surgery for Crohn's disease may occur in the immediate postoperative period or in a delayed fashion. Early fistulae are most often secondary to anastomotic failure, whereas fistulae presenting later are usually due to recurrent Crohn's disease.

Early postoperative abdominal fistulae are uncommon, occurring in 0% to 4% of patients. Management in such cases is similar to a patient without Crohn's disease, though special attention must be given to immunosuppression. A septic patient should undergo appropriate fluid and electrolyte replacement. Broad-spectrum antibiotics should be started, including antifungal agents, and CT imaging should be obtained to rule out an undrained collection. If unstable or if the leak cannot be controlled, prompt return to the operating room is necessary for lavage, appropriate drainage, and usually the creation of a proximal stoma. Alternatively, a stable patient should be managed with control of the intestinal effluent to protect the skin, bowel rest, and hyperalimentation. Intrabdominal collections may need percutaneous drainage by interventional radiology techniques.

Immunosuppressants should be discontinued or appropriately weaned, and the treating team must maintain a high level of attention to the need for stress steroids, should the clinical situation not continue to improve. Cortrosyn stimulation testing may be helpful. A nasogastric tube, H_2 receptor antagonists or proton-pump inhibitors, and octreotide can decrease gastrointestinal secretions and convert high- or medium-output to low-output fistulae. However, octreotide has not been shown to decrease reoperation rates in early postoperative fistulae in Crohn's disease. With control of sepsis, protection of skin, and nutritional support, many early postoperative fistulae will heal in the first 30 days. Fistulae that do not heal in this time period are more likely to require reoperation and are often associated with the same factors that keep other non-Crohn's enterocutaneous fistulae open, such as a large abdominal wall defect, disconnection of the anastomosis, a wide and short fistula tract, proximal location of the fistula, a foreign body within the tract, previous radiation, distal obstruction, malignancy, and tract epithelialization.

The timing of reoperation is critical.[8] Early return to the operating room, especially between 2 and 6 weeks following the initial operation should be avoided. Such an early return is usually complicated by the finding of obliterative peritonitis, and the patient is placed at much higher risk for further loss of bowel that would otherwise not be affected with Crohn's disease. Longer intervals of >3 months allow for continued resolution of intraabdominal inflammation. Moreover, the abdominal wall will likely soften with more time, allowing for a greater chance of closure. More advanced strategies may still be necessary such as component separation and/or biological graft placement to obtain tension-free abdominal-wall closure and avoid intraabdominal hypertension or compartment syndrome. Consultation and reoperation with a plastic surgeon may help facilitate closure and better long-term cosmesis. In selected cases, vacuum-assisted-closure devices have been utilized with success as an adjunct with biological grafts. Synthetic materials should be avoided. With improvements in multimodality therapy for the treatment of complex enterocutaneous fistulae, ultimate closure can be achieved in 80% of patients. Although improving, mortality still remains significant at 4% to 7% in most recent large series.

Late postoperative enterocutaneous fistula formation is most often secondary to recurrent penetrating disease. Medical management should be attempted before return to the operating room. Other pharmacologic therapies have been described in detail in other chapters. When medical management is unsuccessful, management of the recurrent fistula should be undertaken with the principles described previously for primary disease.

Peristomal fistulae represent a distinct subset of patients with postoperative abdominal fistulae. Similar to enterocutaneous fistulae, they may occur in the immediate postoperative period or present themselves at a later stage. When early, peristomal fistulae are often thought to be secondary to technical factors such as tethering, tension, or ischemia. Such fistulae often create significant skin excoriation from separate leaking or undermining of the appliance. Specialized pouching appliances and frequent follow-up appointments with the surgeon and getting help from the nurse practitioner for *wound ostomy and continence may allow for healing without the need for reoperation.* However, if healing doesn't occur by 2 to 3 months, revision will most likely be necessary and can usually be accomplished via a peristomal incision. Factors that may necessitate a more extensive procedure include poor intestinal perfusion, dense adhesive disease, and active Crohn's disease at the stoma site.

Late peristomal fistulae usually occur due to recurrent Crohn's disease. Patients may present with other penetrating disease, such as peristomal or intrabdominal abscesses, and CT imaging should be obtained to rule out such processes. Endoscopy may also be necessary to rule out additional sites of recurrence. As with other recurrent fistulae, underlying septic foci should be treated, and if possible, medical therapy should be maximized before surgical therapy is undertaken. After sepsis is controlled and inflammation has settled down, patients who don't resolve with medical therapy should have stoma revision planned to include resection of the disease bowel and associated fistula tracts. Relocation of the stoma to a different abdominal quadrant may be necessary, if the peristomal soft tissue is severely diseased or if a large peristomal hernia coexists.

Editor's note (TMB): Pyoderma Gangrenosum may occur at a site of trauma, including an operative wound or stoma. Recognizing this extraintestinal manifestation, which often is independent of intestinal inflammation, is important because of the need for embarking on steroid and immunomodulator therapy. There is a chapter on pyoderma in the first book of this edition.

References

1. Nielsen OH, Rogler G, Hahnloser D, Thomsen OØ. Diagnosis and management of fistulizing Crohn's disease. *Nat Clin Pract Gastroenterol Hepatol.* 2009;6(2):92–106.

2. Marion JF, Lachman P, Greenstein AJ, Sachar DB. Rarity of fistulas in Crohn's disease of the jejunum. *Inflamm Bowel Dis.* 1995;1:34–36.

3. Strong SA, Koltun WA, Hyman NH, Buie WD. Practice parameters for the surgical management of Crohn's disease. *Dis Colon Rectum.* 2007;50(11):1735–1746.

4. Schecter WP, Hirshberg A, Chang DS, et al. Enteric fistulas: principles of management. *J Am Coll Surg.* 2009;209(4):484–491.

5. Young-Fadok TM, Wolff BG, Meagher A, Benn PL, Dozois RR. Surgical management of ileosigmoid fistulas in Crohn's disease. *Dis Colon Rectum.* 1997;40(5):558–561.

6. Melton GB, Stocchi L, Wick EC, Appau KA, Fazio VW. Contemporary surgical management for ileosigmoid fistulas in Crohn's disease. *J Gastrointest Surg.* 2009;13(5):839–845.

7. Tan JJ, Tjandra JJ. Laparoscopic surgery for Crohn's disease: a meta-analysis. *Dis Colon Rectum.* 2007;50(5):576–585.

8. Cima RR, Wolff BG. Reoperative Crohn's surgery: tricks of the trade. *Clin Colon Rectal Surg.* 2007;20(4):336–343.

Surgery for Crohn's Colitis | 141

Elizabeth Wick and Genevieve B. Melton

INTRODUCTION

Crohn's disease can affect the entire intestinal tract from the esophagus to the anus. At presentation, most patients have ileocolic disease, but approximately 25% of patients with Crohn's disease will initially present with isolated colitis. Colitis usually affects older patients and men. The disease can be contiguous from the cecum to the rectum or patchy; rarely do patients present with isolated rectal disease. Right-sided disease is most common. Disease extent is determined by a combination of colonoscopy, radiographic tests, and physical examination. Compared with isolated ileocolic or small bowel disease, colitis is frequently associated with anorectal disease. Usually, right-sided disease (terminal ileal involvement is common) is symptomatic as a result of luminal narrowing. Left-sided disease can be confused with diverticular disease and be associated with abscess, perforation, or fistula. Pancolitis can mimic ulcerative colitis. Symptoms are similar for the different disease patterns and include abdominal pain, cramping, postprandial pain, anorexia, weight loss, and diarrhea. These can be chronic and/or mild to acute and/or severe, the latter may require emergent hospitalization and surgery. Overall, patients with colitis are less likely to require operation compared with patients with small bowel or ileocolic disease. Indications for operation include medically refractory disease, intra-abdominal abscess, symptomatic fistula, dysplasia, colitis-associated cancer or severe perianal disease, toxic megacolon, or large bowel obstruction. Less commonly, surgery may be indicated for relief of extraintestinal manifestations such as pyoderma gangrenosum, uveitis, or periarteritis nodosa. In general, operation options are (1) total abdominal colectomy (if the rectum is spared) or total proctocolectomy and (2) segmental colectomy (segmental disease). Depending on the situation and bowel resection, temporary or permanent ileostomy or colostomy maybe required. Although controversial, several groups have recently reported on the use of total proctocolectomy with pelvic pouch and ileal pouch anal anastomosis in select patients with Crohn's colitis with good results. The operation must be tailored for individual patients based on disease distribution and clinical course.

GENERAL CONSIDERATIONS

Patients with Crohn's colitis need to be thoroughly evaluated to establish the correct diagnosis and determine the disease extent. Standard workup includes colonoscopy (with multiple biopsies of both inflamed and noninflamed tissue to document extent of disease and evaluate for dysplasia and/or cancer) and small bowel series or computed tomographic (CT) enterography to establish whether small bowel disease is also present. Gastrografin or barium enema should be considered if a colonic stricture is encountered during colonoscopy that prevents passage of the endoscope. History and physical examination will help establish the disease course, identify extraintestinal manifestations, and determine the extent of perianal disease. As mentioned earlier, with severe colitis, it can be challenging to differentiate Crohn's disease from ulcerative colitis. Only a minority (~25%) of patients with colitis will have granulomas on endoscopic biopsies. Clinical features that support the diagnosis of Crohn's disease include fistula (small bowel colon, colocutaneous, rectovaginal, or colovesical), skip lesions with linear ulcerations, aphthous ulcers, perianal involvement (fistula, fissures, and skin tags), or small bowel involvement.

Once the diagnosis of Crohn's colitis is established, colonoscopy should be performed periodically for surveillance and worsening symptoms. Attention should be paid to the distribution and severity of disease. Biopsies should be taken of any strictures, masses, or ulcers; random biopsies similar to techniques described for ulcerative colitis surveillance should also be performed. Similar to ulcerative colitis, the risk for dysplasia increases approximately 25% after 10 surveillance colonoscopies. If high-grade dysplasia or carcinoma is discovered on colonoscopy, surgical resection is generally indicated, given the high likelihood of discovering an occult malignancy on the surgical pathology specimen. In the event the operation is performed for dysplasia or cancer, an oncologic operation should be undertaken, including high ligation of the appropriate vasculature with adequate colonic margin. If the malignancy is in the rectum, the tumor should be staged preoperatively with either endorectal ultrasound or magnetic resonance imaging, and depending on the stage, neoadjuvant chemoradiation should be considered.

Preoperative planning will make the operation smoother. In patients with excessive inflammation in the pelvis from previous surgery or from abscess or fistula, placement of ureteric stents will aid in safe intraoperative identification and preservation of the ureters. In patients maintained on steroids for a long term, particularly in the presence of malnutrition, it may be best to stage the procedure, with the initial procedure being either a segmental or a subtotal colectomy with end ileostomy or colostomy followed by recovery and a second procedure to restore intestinal continuity. Alternatively, in these patients, primary ileocolic, colic-colic, or colorectal anastomosis can be constructed and then protected with a temporary loop ileostomy. Patients should be seen by an enterostomal therapist for counseling and identification of the stoma site. Consideration for other aspects of Crohn's colitis, such as ileosigmoid fistula, proximal disease, urinary fistula, or rectovaginal fistula, should also be made, and the appropriate assistance should be recruited (see final section).

OPERATIVE APPROACH

Surgical treatment should be carefully tailored to the length and course of disease, disease distribution, and anorectal involvement. Although an open approach is still most commonly used for these procedures, laparoscopy is being increasingly performed (see final section). Although there has been a recent trend toward bowel conservation and restorative procedures in Crohn's colitis, total proctocolectomy with end ileostomy remains a viable intervention and often the procedure of choice. The most common indication for total proctocolectomy with end ileostomy is the presence of perianal disease, rectal involvement, and/or extensive Crohn's colitis. If the left colon and rectum are involved along with perianal disease, distal proctocolectomy with colostomy may be appropriate as well. In general, proctocolectomy has the lowest recurrence rate of 10% to 20% at long-term follow-up.[1-3]

TOXIC COLITIS

Today, with advances in medical therapy, it is rare to see patients with fulminant or toxic colitis. The presentation is similar to fulminant ulcerative colitis (abdominal pain, bloody diarrhea, fevers, tachycardia, and abdominal distention). The feared complication is colonic perforation and sepsis because this carries a high mortality. Perforation may be the result of colonic dilatation, with resulting attenuation of bowel wall or full-thickness involvement of the wall with Crohn's disease. In the acute setting, the diagnosis may be impossible to distinguish from ulcerative colitis unless there are subtle signs of perianal Crohn's such as waxy skin tags or old anal fistula tracts. Abdominal radiographs and sigmoidoscopy can help guide management of toxic colitis. Stool cultures should be sent for detection of *Salmonella*, *Shigella*, *Escherichia coli*, *Campylobacter,* and *Clostridium difficile* to determine whether there is superimposed infection exacerbating the disease. Immediately, patients need to be closely monitored (vital signs, physical examination, and laboratory values) and aggressively resuscitated with intravenous fluids.

Depending on the severity of the presentation, consideration should be made for a trial of medical therapy. The operation of choice in this setting is total abdominal colectomy with end ileostomy. Usually, the rectal disease is mild in comparison to the colonic disease and will subside with fecal diversion. Pelvic dissection in the setting of sepsis is associated with significantly higher morbidity (pelvic and perineal abscesses). Furthermore, should the patient have relative rectal sparing, this operation will allow him/her to be considered for ileorectal anastomosis (IRA) (and avoid permanent stoma) when medically fit.

SUBTOTAL COLECTOMY WITH IRA

In select patients with isolated Crohn's colitis (no involvement of the rectum or perineum), total abdominal colectomy with IRA is an option. This is a particularly attractive option in young women contemplating pregnancy. Although it has not been studied, subtotal colectomy with or without IRA probably has a lower incidence of infertility because the procedures do not involve a pelvic dissection. Similarly, in men, much of the risk for sexual dysfunction is avoided with IRA. Functional results are generally satisfactory; patients can anticipate having four to five bowel movements per day. Occasionally, they may need an antidiarrhea agent. A recent study reviewed 118 patients who had undergone an IRA for Crohn's colitis and found that, at 10 years, 86% of patients had retained their rectum. Factors associated with conversion of IRA to total proctocolectomy with end ileostomy were extraintestinal manifestations of Crohn's colitis and failure to be maintained on a 5-aminosalicylic acid compound.[4] An earlier retrospective review at the Mayo Clinic identified 42 patients who had undergone an IRA for Crohn's colitis, and 11 of 42 patients (26%) required completion proctectomy and end ileostomy. Men and patients older than 36 years had a higher likelihood of retaining their rectum.[5] Overall, most patients are pleased with their bowel function and would not chose to convert to a stoma. This operation is not appropriate for patients who have significant fecal incontinence preoperatively.

SEGMENTAL COLECTOMY

Segmental colectomy has a role in the management of Crohn's colitis. If the disease is limited, that is, right-sided inflammation, sigmoid disease with abscess, and short or symptomatic stricture, segmental resection has been shown to have similar relief of symptoms as subtotal colectomy. Initially, there was concern that segmental colectomy led to more rapid recurrence of disease, but recent studies have not supported this belief. Bowel function is better with segmental colectomy than with IRA. As mentioned earlier, if there is concern for malignancy, an oncologic colon resection with high ligation of the vasculature should be performed.

TOTAL PROCTOCOLECTOMY

Total proctocolectomy has long been the definitive operation for Crohn's proctocolitis, particularly if there is significant perianal disease. This procedure entails removal of the entire colon, rectum, and anus and results in a permanent end ileostomy. Patients are still at risk for disease recurrence in the small bowel—usually, distal small bowel. Frequency of recurrence varies from series to series, with ranges from 3.3% to 46%. Thus, patients will still require monitoring after this operation. Perineal wound healing problems after proctocolectomy are common and occur in approximately 40% of patients. Healing can take up to a year in around 30% of patients, and 20% of patients may have a persistent draining sinus after 1 year. In patients with severe preoperative perianal disease, a myocutaneous flap to the perineum should be considered. Other measures to avoid wound healing problems include insertion of pelvic drains and closure of the perineal wound in multiple layers. Patients should be counseled preoperatively that they may need additional procedures (examinations under anesthesia and wound debridements) to facilitate wound healing.

● ILEAL POUCH ANAL ANASTOMOSIS

Although restorative total proctocolectomy with pelvic pouch and IPAA has become widely accepted as definitive surgical treatment for mucosal ulcerative colitis and indeterminate colitis, its use in Crohn's colitis remains controversial. Patients with known Crohn's colitis have typically not been offered IPAA. Recent reports from France[6,7] and the Cleveland Clinic[8] have demonstrated good results for highly selected patients with Crohn's colitis who undergo IPAA, with retention rates of approximately 80% at 10-year actuarial follow-up. We advocate the use of strict selection criteria in offering this procedure and only consider it for highly motivated patients with a stable period of disease (~5 years or more), rectal involvement, no perianal Crohn's disease, and no small bowel involvement. In a small subset of patients with indeterminate colitis (~10%), the diagnosis of Crohn's colitis versus mucosal ulcerative colitis is uncertain despite multiple biopsies and studies. For patients with indeterminate colitis, IPAA should be considered because these patients usually have long-term outcomes similar to patients with ulcerative colitis.[9]

● OTHER CONSIDERATIONS

Additional small bowel disease can be encountered with Crohn's colitis. Recent studies have noted that when there is significant small bowel disease and medically refractory perianal disease, resection of small bowel disease may help the perianal area to heal. In general, if there is concurrent small bowel disease and colitis, the small bowel disease, if significant, should be treated at the same time as the colonic disease; options are resection or strictureplasty depending on the pathology, extent, and location of disease.

Crohn's disease may also be associated with fistula: most common are fistulas to the bladder, bowel, or skin (i.e., enterovesical, ileosigmoid, or colocutaneous fistula). Enterovesical fistula from the colon to bladder usually occurs in men or women who have undergone previous hysterectomy. History of urinary tract infection, pneumaturia, or fecaluria suggests enterovesical fistula. Cystoscopy and cystogram may demonstrate the opening. The treatment is to resect the fistulizing segment of colon with or without primary repair of the bladder

(tailored to the size of the defect fistula) and postoperative foley catheter drainage (7–10 days).[10] Before removal of the catheter, a cystogram should be obtained to confirm that the repair is intact.

Ileosigmoid fistula can be seen in conjunction with ileocolitis. The fistula can be hard to identify on preoperative testing (colonoscopy, CT scans, small bowel series, and gastrografin enemas). The sigmoid colon has been traditionally viewed as an "innocent bystander" in this process, and some advocate primary repair of the sigmoid colon with ileocolic resection.[11,12] Results are equivalent to those reported in older studies where en-bloc sigmoid resection was advocated.

Rectovaginal fistulas are a challenge. Repair can be performed with or without proximal stomal diversion. Although diversion can be helpful for initial healing, patients frequently will experience recurrence of their fistula after closure of the stoma. In general, medical treatment or diversion alone without repair cannot heal rectovaginal fistula. Treatments for rectovaginal fistulas are tailored to the location of the fistula (low or high) and to the presence of concomitant proctitis.[13] Low fistula may be treated with a transanal approach and rectal mucosal advancement flaps. Proximal fistulas or those with significant proctitis are best treated with resection of the diseased segment of the bowel and low anterior anastomosis or coloanal anastomosis. Despite advances in medical therapy, results continue to be disappointing. Patients with proctitis and anorectal disease in the setting of rectovaginal fistula may require proctocolectomy with permanent diversion.

Laparoscopy is becoming a more widely accepted approach for colectomy in Crohn's disease. Outcomes with laparoscopy and Crohn's disease have been primarily focused on ileocolic resection. In a meta-analysis of studies comparing laparoscopy with open surgery in Crohn's disease to date (including ileocolic resection and other intra-abdominal procedures), laparoscopic procedures took longer to complete, were associated with a more rapid return of bowel function, had shorter lengths of stay, and had lower rates of morbidity. Disease recurrence was similar with both approaches.[14] In patients with severe Crohn's colitis and thickened colonic mesenteries, laparoscopy should be used with caution because the current sealing devices used for intracorporeal division of the mesentery (ligasure, harmonic scalpel, and enseal) may not be adequate to seal the larger vessels, and a hematoma may develop in the mesentery. Another option is to mobilize the bowel that is to be resected with laparoscopic techniques and then exteriorize the segment and divide the mesentery extracorporeally using standard clamps and suture.

In conclusion, Crohn's colitis is a challenging condition to treat. Meticulous preoperative evaluation in conjunction with the patient's gastroenterologist will facilitate the operation. The operation should be tailored to the patient's disease pattern, indication for operation, and long-term desires.

References

1. Fichera A, McCormack R, Rubin MA, Hurst RD, Michelassi F. Long-term outcome of surgically treated Crohn's colitis: a prospective study. *Dis Colon Rectum.* 2005;48(5):963–969.
2. Yamamoto T, Keighley MR. Fate of the rectum and ileal recurrence rates after total colectomy for Crohn's disease. *World J Surg.* 2000;24(1):125–129.

3. Yamamoto T, Allan RN, Keighley MR. Audit of single-stage proctocolectomy for Crohn's disease: postoperative complications and recurrence. *Dis Colon Rectum.* 2000;43(2):249–256.

4. Cattan P, Bonhomme N, Panis Y, et al. Fate of the rectum in patients undergoing total colectomy for Crohn's disease. *Br J Surg.* 2002;89(4):454–459.

5. Pastore RL, Wolff BG, Hodge D. Total abdominal colectomy and ileorectal anastomosis for inflammatory bowel disease. *Dis Colon Rectum.* 1997;40(12):1455–1464.

6. Regimbeau JM, Panis Y, Pocard M, et al. Long-term results of ileal pouch-anal anastomosis for colorectal Crohn's disease. *Dis Colon Rectum.* 2001;44(6):769–778.

7. Panis Y, Poupard B, Nemeth J, Lavergne A, Hautefeuille P, Valleur P. Ileal pouch/anal anastomosis for Crohn's disease. *Lancet.* 1996;347(9005):854–857.

8. Melton GB, Fazio VW, Kiran RP, et al. Long-term outcomes with ileal pouch-anal anastomosis and Crohn's disease: pouch retention and implications of delayed diagnosis. *Ann Surg.* 2008;248(4):608–616.

9. Delaney CP, Remzi FH, Gramlich T, Dadvand B, Fazio VW. Equivalent function, quality of life and pouch survival rates after ileal pouch-anal anastomosis for indeterminate and ulcerative colitis. *Ann Surg.* 2002;236(1):43–48.

10. Ferguson GG, Lee EW, Hunt SR, Ridley CH, Brandes SB. Management of the bladder during surgical treatment of enterovesical fistulas from benign bowel disease. *J Am Coll Surg.* 2008;207(4):569–572.

11. Young-Fadok TM, Wolff BG, Meagher A, Benn PL, Dozois RR. Surgical management of ileosigmoid fistulas in Crohn's disease. *Dis Colon Rectum.* 1997;40(5):558–561.

12. Melton GB, Stocchi L, Wick EC, Appau KA, Fazio VW. Contemporary surgical management for ileosigmoid fistulas in Crohn's disease. *J Gastrointest Surg.* 2009;13(5):839–845.

13. Andreani SM, Dang HH, Grondona P, Khan AZ, Edwards DP. Rectovaginal fistula in Crohn's disease. *Dis Colon Rectum.* 2007;50(12):2215–2222.

14. Tan JJ, Tjandra JJ. Laparoscopic surgery for Crohn's disease: a meta-analysis. *Dis Colon Rectum.* 2007;50(5):576–585.

Perianal Disease: Surgical Management | 142

Jason Bodzin

Crohn's disease (CD) is a chronic inflammatory bowel disease (IBD) with a tendency for full thickness inflammation leading to penetration through the bowel wall. This process results in abscesses and fistulas to many different organs and places. When this occurs around the anus, we call it Crohn's-associated perianal disease. Thirty percent of patients with CD have perianal involvement with abscess, fistula, fissure, skin tag, or stenosis. These manifestations may actually precede gastrointestinal complaints. Perianal disease is often an important factor affecting quality of life.[1] Disease factors may influence the development of perianal disease. Age at disease onset may be important with younger patients having a higher incidence often present before symptoms related to ileal or colonic inflammation.[2] Non-Caucasian race seems to be associated with perianal disease, and fistulae are definitely more common with colonic involvement. Patients who test positive for ASCA have a higher likelihood of perianal disease. Importantly, perianal manifestations, which often require aggressive therapy, appear to be a different phenotype of the disease than inflammatory fistulizing disease.[2]

The etiology of perianal fistula probably involves an interaction between genetic, microbiologic, and immunologic factors.[2] The pathophysiology usually starts with an anal crypt infection. In normal individuals, the infection is self-limiting and rarely progresses to abscess and fistula. However in CD patients, there is faulty healing, resulting in progression of the infectious process through the wall of the anus. The process continues along the path of least resistance and may form an abscess or simply tunnel out to the skin. The path it takes may be intersphincteric, transphincteric, suprasphincteric, submucosal, or some combination with branching of tracks. The process may not stop at this point. Healing may occur from the outside, and this may promote a secondary track or abscess. This process may continue with a vicious cycle and several openings may occur. Unabated, this process may produce a watercan perineum. It is important to note that nearly all of the subsequent fistula openings stem from the original fistula track. It is unusual to find more than one opening at the dentate line.

CLINICAL EVALUATION

Evaluation begins with an accurate history, which should include questions regarding the first signs of CD, appearance of perianal drainage, and whether pain was present, as well as bowel habits and the relation of perianal symptoms to the bowel function. Previous medications that have been taken should be recorded. The response to these medications is important and may help determine future therapy. The adequacy of dosage should be determined. Any difficulties with defecation may indicate anal stenosis. Incontinence should be carefully documented, especially if surgery has been performed or is being considered. Any patient with CD needs a rectal examination as part of the original evaluation. Perianal disease may be completely asymptomatic and may be missed if not looked for or asked about. Patients with perianal drainage may think the process is anal seepage and may not spontaneously volunteer this information to the physician. Once the perianal disease is discovered, workup proceeds with a careful physical examination, palpating the skin around the fistula looking for induration or secondary fistula tracks.

Irregularity at the dentate line can often be found with a rectal examination. Whereas most normal people have fistulas originating in the posterior midline, Crohn's patients may have the origin at any point along the dentate line or even removed from the dentate line. Depending on the symptomatology and physical findings, individual patients may require anal manometry, anal electromyography, nerve latency studies, or anal ultrasonography. Ultrasonography is specifically indicated in patients who have had previous surgery, sometimes years earlier, for perianal disease.[3] Under anesthesia, techniques such as methylene blue injection or hydrogen peroxide injection may further delineate fistula tracks and internal openings. Endoscopy may be helpful and should be performed on anyone with perianal disease.

Editor's note (TMB): There is a separate chapter on diagnosis of perianal disease in the first half of this edition.

CLASSIFICATION

Fistula classification may be anatomic or clinical. High fistulas originate above the dentate line, whereas low fistulas originate at or below the dentate line. Most anatomic classifications relate the course of the fistula to the anal musculature. Fistulas may be transphincteric, intersphincteric, extrasphincteric, or submucosal. Occasionally a fistula is intersphincteric involving less than one-third of the thickness of the muscle, and for surgical purposes these fistulas will behave as submucosal. Other fistulas may be complex extending into the vagina or the scrotum. In some cases, rectovaginal fistula may be the only perianal manifestation. Clinical classifications revolve around drainage, pain, number of fistula openings, significance to the overall morbidity of the disease, and other factors. I use a simplified clinical classification from 0 to 4, where 0 = no active fistula disease, 1 = a single asymptomatic opening, 2 = a single painful or symptomatic opening, 3 = multiple symptomatic openings, 4 = severe, painful, multiple symptomatic openings where diversion is being considered. This type of classification has been very useful for the comparison of pre- and postoperative evaluation. The Perianal Disease Activity Index is another subjective index that is used to evaluate the effect of a drug or procedure on perianal disease. This index assesses five categories related to fistulas: discharge, pain, restriction of sexual activity, type of perianal disease, and degree of induration. Another widely used technique is the Fistula Drainage Assessment. This instrument only assesses whether a fistula is open or closed and whether material can be expressed from it. This is the simplest assessment but probably overlooks other important aspects of the problem.

Editor's note (TMB): The chapter on classification of distal activity in the first half of this edition, contains details on these classification systems.

TREATMENT

The surgical treatment of perianal fistula disease must be individualized and related to the patient as a whole. The control of diarrhea may render a fistula much less symptomatic. When surgery is performed, the preservation of the anal sphincter muscle is mandatory. An asymptomatic fistula probably requires no treatment as long as it remains asymptomatic. If the fistula is submucosal, it should be opened with a standard fistulotomy. This obviates the need for a seton. Unfortunately, most Crohn's-related fistulas are not submucosal. Patients with troublesome drainage from a single fistula can be managed by a seton. The seton system is a process that begins with an inert small vessel loop type material, which can be placed as an outpatient procedure along with examination under anesthesia. It is pulled through the track and out the anus and tied to itself such that no ends are poking the skin. Later on in the office, this seton will be changed for three or four lengths of silk, each tied to the original seton, pulled through the track, and then tied to itself so that the patient then has three or four tiny setons in place. This is an essentially painless procedure done without any anesthesia. Silk in the fistula track stimulates granulation tissue, and the track gradually closes down over the silk. Each of these setons is removed, usually 4 to 6 weeks apart. In most cases, fistula drainage becomes minimal or none.[4] In cases where a single

symptomatic fistula persists, techniques such as fibrin glue, or the Surgisis AFP, may be used with no sacrifice of muscle. Results in CD patients have been inconsistent. Occasional patients have been treated two or three times with these techniques with eventual success.[5,6] When the fistula is branched, meaning that there is more than one opening exterior to the anus, different techniques are indicated. In cases where there are several openings in the perianal skin and buttock, it must be remembered that all of these openings can be traced to the original penetration at or near the dentate line. Frequently, there is a subcutaneous pocket or lake of purulent material that gathers and drains out of these secondary openings. These lakes are bordered by infected granulation tissue. It is most unlikely that these pockets will ever heal from antibiotic therapy or anti-tumor necrosis factor (TNF) therapy alone, as long as this infected granulation material persists. It has been shown that even if these fistulas slow down or stop draining, the tracks and pockets remain and reactivate soon after the therapy is stopped.[3]

The most successful way of eliminating the tracks and lakes in multiple perianal disease is through the technique of laser ablation.[4] Using the CO_2 laser, tracks external to the sphincter muscle are laid open and all of the infected granulation tissue is evaporated. A seton is placed in the primary fistula track around the muscle and through the anus and tied to itself as described previously. These procedures have been performed as *outpatient* care in all cases. A mixture of lidocaine ointment and Silvadene cream is used as an analgesic/antibiotic dressing. With local care and sitz baths, the tracks will heal from the inside out and be permanently eliminated in most cases. Scarring has been quite acceptable. With this process, multiple external openings are converted into a single perianal fistula containing a seton. The seton process proceeds as described earlier. After this process has been performed, the introduction of anti-TNF therapy is both palliative and curative in many cases. A diverting stoma is rarely necessary. By using this technique in my practice, a permanent stoma has not been necessary at all because of perianal disease. The algorithm of this process is described in Fig. 142.1.

PERIANAL ABSCESS

Perianal abscess is an acute process that must be addressed surgically. Simple incision and drainage is frequently all that is necessary. It is inappropriate to do fistulotomy at the initial drainage procedure because it is likely that significant perianal muscle would be sacrificed. Immediate relief of pain can be expected, and, frequently, a simple fistula will result. Additional antibiotic coverage may be utilized during this process. When a fistula develops as the result of this treatment, a seton is placed and the program continues as noted earlier.

PERIANAL SKIN TAGS

Perianal skin tags commonly occur in CD patients. Some have been preceded by anal fissure, whereas others may have occurred spontaneously without any history of previous perianal disease. They often have characteristic appearance of teardrop or elephant ear. These skin tags are sometimes symptom

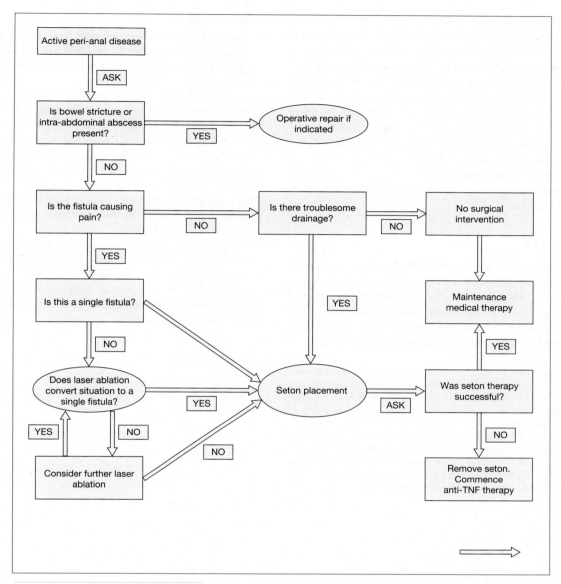

Figure 142.1. Fistula management.

ANAL FISSURE

Anal fissure can be asymptomatic or significantly painful. Patients may report that there is little or no pain between bowel movements, but significant discomfort with a bowel movement and for some period thereafter. Patients can develop a fear of having a bowel movement, and constipation with overflow diarrhea may occur. Acute anal fissure should be treated by local anesthetic and steroid creams. However, chronic anal fissure free whereas at other times they are irritating or may cause difficulty in perianal hygiene. When skin tags are significantly symptomatic, they can be removed by simple excision or laser ablation. Patients should be cautioned that they may recur. They do not involve muscle, and improvement in perianal hygiene can be gained with little sacrifice. However, they should not be removed simply because they are there.

frequently will not heal without a surgical procedure. Partial internal anal sphincterotomy is frequently performed with or without excision and primary closure of the fissure in those cases where fissures are chronic and painful. Healing may be surprisingly straightforward; however, patients should always be cautioned regarding the possibility of poor healing and of increasing urgency or incontinence.

Editor's note (TMB): Use of nifedapin and nitroglycerin petrolatum ointment, used sparingly, can be helpful. Botoxin injections are being used, especially in non-IBD patients.

ANAL STENOSIS

Anal stenosis may be the only manifestation of perianal disease. Patients may not be aware of this problem, which can go unrecognized if anal-rectal examination is not routinely done.

Anal stenosis may complicate fissure or fistula disease and may be hidden by perianal skin tags. Mild anal stenosis can be managed by self-digital dilation at home by patients receiving proper instruction. A stenosis that cannot admit the examining finger should be dilated under anesthesia with a set of sequential Hegar dilators. Dilation to 18 mm is sufficient, and patients can be supplied with a Hegar dilator that is 15 to 16 mm for their own use at home. These dilators can be purchased from medical supply houses at approximately $45 each. Self-dilation can be done as frequently as daily or in most cases, after a period of time, just two or three times per week or less frequently as needed. Lidocaine gel is used to lubricate the instrument to facilitate self-dilation.

● SUMMARY

Perianal disease may be the focus of morbidity for patients with CD. With careful examination and the judicious use of outpatient surgical intervention, the morbidity of perianal disease can be minimized or, in some cases, eliminated. The overwhelming principal is to maintain the integrity of the perianal muscle while allowing the patient to maintain the normal stool pathway.

Editor's note (TMB): There are some new insights in the pathogenesis of perianal fistulae associated with CD. Epithelial to mesenchymal transition may play a crucial role in the pathogenesis of CD fistulae (Scharl M, Weber A, Fürst A, et al. Potential role for SNAIL family transcription factors in the etiology of CD–associated fistulae. *Inflamm Bowel Dis.* 2010). These cells are near the skin surface of fistulae and are destroyed quickly by infliximab therapy. Perhaps this lead to perianal abscesses in some patients. The use of setons before initiating infliximab and then withdrawing the seton at 4 weeks, if drainage has improved, can be useful. Another approach at eliminating the cells involved in pathogenesis might be to use medication-impregnated setons.

References

1. Kasparek MS, Glatzle J, Temeltcheva T, Mueller MH, Koenigsrainer A, Kreis ME. Long-term quality of life in patients with Crohn's disease and perianal fistulas: influence of fecal diversion. *Dis Colon Rectum.* 2007;50(12):2067–2074.

2. Tozer PJ, Whelan K, Phillips RK, Hart AL. Etiology of perianal Crohn's disease: role of genetic, microbiological, and immunological factors. *Inflamm Bowel Dis.* 2009;15(10):1591–1598.

3. Losco A, Viganò C, Conte D, Cesana BM, Basilisco G. Assessing the activity of perianal Crohn's disease: comparison of clinical indices and computer-assisted anal ultrasound. *Inflamm Bowel Dis.* 2009;15(5):742–749.

4. Moy J, Bodzin J. Carbon dioxide laser ablation of perianal fistulas in patients with Crohn's disease: experience with 27 patients. *Am J Surg.* 2006;191(3):424–427.

5. van Koperen PJ, D'Hoore A, Wolthuis AM, Bemelman WA, Slors JF. Anal fistula plug for closure of difficult anorectal fistula: a prospective study. *Dis Colon Rectum.* 2007;50:2168–2172.

6. Chung W, Kazemi P, Ko D, et al. Anal fistula plug and fibrin glue versus conventional treatment in repair of complex anal fistulas. *Am J Surg.* 2009;197(5):604–608.

Rectovaginal Fistula | 143

Tracy L. Hull

In some women with perianal Crohn's disease, a fistula between the anorectum and perineum/vagina may develop. This problem can be devastating for some women, and it is difficult to eradicate. Most are true anovaginal fistula, as they arise from the anal canal/low rectum and fistulize into the vagina, perineal body, or labia. However, some are true rectovaginal fistula (RVF) from proximal disease, such as ileal disease, penetrating the upper vagina. This chapter discusses only true anovaginal fistula, referring to them as RVF, because this is the conventional misnomer.

When a woman presents with complaints consistent with RVF, a thorough history should be taken. Precise symptoms need to be clarified; they can range from infrequent gas per vagina to stool running down her leg. In addition, bowel symptomatology, comorbid conditions, associated Crohn's disease, obstetric history (delivery method, use of forceps, episiotomy, or tearing), and problems with fecal incontinence need to be defined. For instance, some women do not find their fistula symptoms distressing and they do not wish to undergo aggressive treatment, whereas other women "cannot live with the problem."

The location of the fistula is determined by physical examination. A high fistula is more difficult to treat than a low fistula. Associated anal disease, palpable induration, rectal disease, and sphincter integrity are specifically noted. If the examination is too painful for the patient to endure, examination under anesthesia may be necessary to determine the extent of disease. Painful examination may signal sepsis in the region, and drainage with a seton or mushroom catheter may be needed.

If the patient has classic RVF symptoms, but the internal opening cannot be found, a tampon can be placed in the vagina and the patient given methelene blue per rectum. If a fistula is present, the tampon will be stained in less than 15 minutes. In addition, a careful examination under anesthesia can sometimes expose a dot of granulation tissue in the vaginal area, which represents the external opening.

If the patient has not had a recent evaluation of the small bowel (small bowel series, computed tomography enterography, or magnetic resonance imaging enterography) and colon (colonoscopy or barium enema), defining any additional bowel disease may affect the RVF treatment approach. If preoperative fecal incontinence is found by history or an anterior anal sphincter muscle weakness is noted on physical examination, anal endosonography and anal physiology are considered. Incontinence that is attributable to destroyed sphincter muscle secondary to Crohn's disease may prompt different treatment goals versus incontinence and a fistula from a pure obstetric injury.

After all of the information has been gathered, realistic goals of surgery must be discussed. For instance, it would be unrealistic to discuss a curative surgical repair in a woman with severe medically refractive colorectal disease. However, a seton may palliate symptoms and delay an ileostomy for a long period. In treatment planning, the physician weighs the patient's symptoms and treatment goals against her general condition and results of the physical examination. It is generally agreed that the combination of medical and surgical therapy provides the best success in reducing symptoms.

MEDIAL TREATMENT AND DRAINAGE

All patients found to have RVF need to have complete drainage of sepsis as the first line of any treatment option.[1] This can be done with a loosely tied flexible seton or a mushroom catheter. Antibiotic treatment is considered for women with cellulitis or (fistula) sepsis that is difficult to control. Ciprofloxacin (500 mg twice a day) and metronidazole (250–500 mg thrice a day) are the most commonly chosen antibiotics. In some cases, antibiotic therapy decreases symptoms from associated Crohn's disease elsewhere and makes further treatment of the RVF unneeded. At times, extended courses of antibiotic therapy (several months) are given.

Steroids do not usually help this problem. If there are symptoms from associated disease elsewhere in the gastrointestinal tract, steroids may reduce those symptoms and make the fistula symptoms seem less severe, thus delaying further treatment.

Azathioprine and 6-mecaptopurine have been used for RVF treatment. It has been reported to close some fistula and was considered for women, especially those with few options. However, these medications seem to be used less frequently in favor of other immune-altering drugs. More recently, infliximab or other anti-tumor necrosis factor-α drugs/immunomodulators have been used to treat RVF and associated Crohn's disease. It can be considered with multiple scenarios. After sepsis is drained and a seton has been inserted, the patient is given the first and second dose of infliximab. The seton is then removed prior to the third dose. If the tract is not epithelialized, the RVF may be closed with this medication.[2,3] The second method to use infliximab is with associated anal ulcers and severe anal inflammation. Women treated with infliximab may experience improvement in the anal disease such that there is scarring in the anal canal with a persistent RVF, but no acute inflammation. In this situation, repair can go forward with the surgical repair determined by the surrounding anatomy. Typically, in this situation, I continue the infliximab right up to the repair and then restart about 4 weeks postoperatively when I am convinced there is no infection.

● SURGICAL MANAGEMENT

Fecal Diversion

Fecal diversion is considered in women who have persistent sepsis despite seton drainage. A loop ileostomy is usually done, particularly if there is any colonic involvement. Ileostomy alone does not allow the fistula to "heal." The symptoms may decrease, but when the stoma is closed, the fistula recurs. Therefore, the stoma must be combined with other treatment if fistula healing is the goal. In addition, an ileostomy can be combined with bowel resection (i.e., terminal ileal resection) and fistula repair, if needed. When doing a fistula repair, the author prefers to use a stoma for repeat surgery, when the repair did not go well technically, for complicated repairs, or for a sleeve or transabdominal repair. In some women who need a proctectomy, a laparoscopic loop ileostomy prior to colon removal gives them the opportunity to experience a stoma without the emotional finality of it. It also allows inflammation to decrease in the perineum, which may decrease the chance of an unhealed perineal wound.

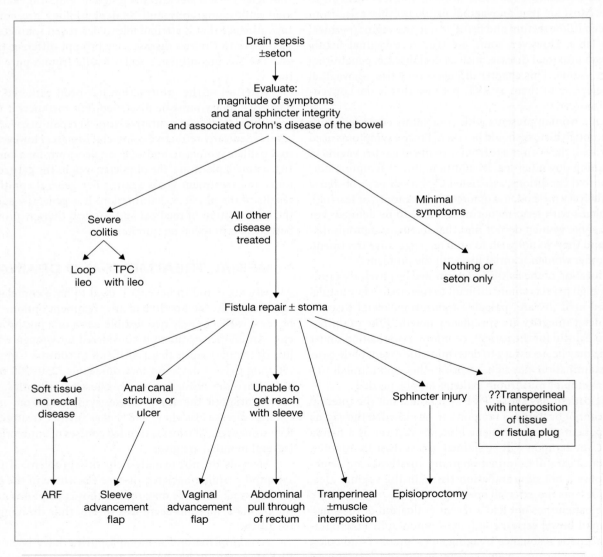

FIGURE 143.1 • Algorithm for treating rectovaginal fistula. ARF, advancement rectal flap; TPC, total proctocolectomy.

Proctectomy

At RVF presentation, some women have severe proctocolitis along with anal disease. They have few options; proctocolectomy may be the only choice.[1] Perineal wound healing may be delayed in this group of patients. It may be necessary to consider a staged operation that removes the rectum after a period of fecal diversion, either through an initial loop ileostomy or through a subtotal colectomy with ileostomy and mucous fistula.

Surgical Fistula Closure

Women who qualify for surgical closure of fistula must have all sepsis drained, and anorectal disease must be relatively quiescent. There is debate over the extent to which colonic and small bowel disease may interfere with fistula closure. Intuitively, it seems appropriate to resect severe small bowel disease and have all other Crohn's disease under good medical control before embarking on surgical RVF closure. **Fig. 143.1** shows an algorithm for treating RVF. Table 143.1 provides a comparison of treatment procedures.

Flap Repair

The *advancement rectal flap* is the most common type of flap repair performed. Approaching the fistula from the anorectum seems logical, as it represents a shunt between the high-pressure anorectum (28–85 cm H_2O) and the low-pressure vagina (atmospheric). It requires that there be minimal or no rectal disease (some mild granularity is acceptable, but ulceration is a contradiction), no anal stricture, and a pliable anal canal and rectum. I prefer that the patient undergoes a full bowel cleansing and receives intravenous antibiotics preoperatively and postoperatively. After adequate regional or general anesthesia, the patient is placed in the prone position. A semicircular incision of about 180° is made just distal to the fistula and a flap is raised. In the anal canal, the mucosa is dissected from the internal anal sphincter. Cephalad to the sphincter the full thickness of rectum is mobilized and dissected. Usually mobilization is carried at least 4 cm proximal to the fistula. The fistula is cored out and closed in layers, leaving the vaginal side open for drainage. The distal flap is trimmed and then advanced down and sewn in place. An advantage of this procedure is that it divides no sphincter muscle. Healing has been reported to be about 55%.[4,5] Use of immunomodulators has been associated with increased healing[6] or no effect on healing.[7]

Transvaginal advancement flaps are preferred by some.[4] Proponents believe that this procedure avoids manipulation of diseased rectal tissue. Most incorporate raising the flap in a manner similar to the previously described technique for the transanal approach. The anal opening is closed and the levator muscles are approximated. The flap is trimmed and closed in a manner similar to the transanal approach. Some surgeons who do this type of repair believe that the interposing of the levator

TABLE 143.1 Treatment Comparisons		
Procedure	Pros/Advantages/Indications	Cons/Disadvantages/Contraindications
Medical treatment ± drainage	Aggressive surgery not needed; drainage will decrease pain Infliximab could be curative	May not "cure" the fistula
Fecal diversion	Allows resection of diseased bowel at the same time; allows patient to "adjust to stoma"	Does not cure fistula
Proctectomy	Done with severe colonic and anorectal disease	Permanent stoma; may have problems with perineal wound healing
Advancement rectal flap	Can be done with mild to moderate rectal disease; stoma not mandatory; does not burn bridges. Unclear if immunomodulators improve success	Do not do with severe anorectal disease, anal stricture, anal sepsis
Transvaginal advancement flap	Can do with anal stricture; allows nondiseased tissue to be used; does not burn bridges or stretch sphincter muscles	Do not do with sepsis
Rectal sleeve advancement flap (transanal or transabdominal)	Can be done with anal canal ulceration and anal canal stricture; must have near normal rectum	"Big procedure"; increases sphincter stretch; if reach is not sufficient with the transanal approach—then transabdominal approach is used; do not do with perianal sepsis; avoid with fecal incontinence
Episioproctotomy	Anterior sphincter weakness with the fistula or fecal incontinence as a result of a sphincter problem; stoma not mandatory	Do not do with severe anorectal disease, high fistula, sepsis; divides the anal sphincters, which could increase problems with incontinence if healing does not occur
Use of biologic material	Plug or interposition in transperineal repair; does not burn bridges; small procedure	Long-term success is unknown; must drain all sepsis before using

muscles between the rectal wall and the vagina is the key to success with this procedure.

The *rectal sleeve advancement* is probably the most complicated of the flap repairs. This repair is indicated for certain women with anal canal ulceration or stenosis, but with minimal to no rectal disease. Again, after a full bowel preparation and intravenous antibiotics, the patient receives adequate general anesthesia and is placed in the prone position. The mucosa is stripped from the anal canal. Next, the full thickness of rectum is mobilized from the transanal approach cephalad to allow the entire circular rectal cuff to reach the dentate line with minimal tension. If the cuff of rectum does not reach, a transabdominal approach is needed. The fistula is handled as described for the advancement rectal flap. The cuff of rectum is sewn to the dentate line after the distal edge has been trimmed. Usually, this type of repair is done in conjunction with a stoma. Typically, it is also done in cases of failed previous repair of RVF.[5]

Transperineal Repair

When the sphincter muscles have a defect, with or without fecal incontinence, a transperineal repair should be considered. This repair is termed an episioproctotomy and is similar to a fourth degree obstetric injury.[6] The anal canal must be soft and pliable for success with this repair. A probe is passed through the fistula, and all tissue above the probe is divided. The sphincter ends are then dissected free and suture overlapped to repair the sphincter defect and, at the same time, close the fistula. The rectal mucosa, perineal skin, and vaginal mucosa are closed. In selected cases, this repair produces successful results.

Some surgeons perform a different type of fistula repair through the transperineal route. An incision is made transversely across the perineal body and dissected through the rectovaginal septum dividing the tract. The dissection is continued about 2 cm cephalad to the tract in the septum. Both openings are closed. The muscle, which is usually levator (but can be gracilis, if the levator is not acceptable, or even a mobilized labial fat pad[7]), is interposed between the anorectal wall and the vaginal wall. The perineal skin is then loosely approximated.

One modification of this procedure reported in the past few years is—instead of muscle—to use a biologic mesh interposed between the rectum and vagina (after the dissection described earlier).[8] The rationale of the biologic mesh is that it forms a scaffold for normal tissue to grow into and is typically resistant to infection. Although it is too early to determine success rates with widespread use of this approach, patients with Crohn's-related RVF have less success than from other causes.

Transabdominal Repair

In select cases, the rectum cannot be mobilized transanally. Sometimes, this can be anticipated from the preoperative examination of the anal area, and at other times the rectal sleeve advancement flap simply will not reach the dentate suture line during that operation. (Therefore, all patients undergoing a sleeve are told of the possibility of needing a transabdominal approach.) In these situations, rectal and sigmoid mobilization, either through an open approach or laparoscopically, are done. The mobilized rectum is advanced out the anus, trimmed, and sewn to the dentate line (after the fistula opening has been closed as described earlier). Sometimes the bowel is brought out the anus for a length of about 10 cm and left externalized for 5 to 7 days. The patient is then returned to the operating room and the extruded end is amputated and sewn to the dentate line. Delayed closure gives the external surface of the bowel a chance to adhere to the fistula and seal over the repair before sutures are placed.

Fistula Plug

Another recent addition to the surgical armamentarium is the fistula plug.[8] This consists of a tightly rolled sheet of biologic material with a button on one end. The rolled portion is pulled from the anal side through the fistula tract in a manner such that the button is then flat against the anorectal wall. The button is then sewn in place. Variable success has been reported with all published results showing a decreased closure rate comparing RVF from Crohn's disease versus obstetric etiology (at best 25% unpublished CCF data). However, this procedure does not require major disturbance of tissue in the anus and vagina. Therefore, in the event of recurrence, no bridges are burned regarding future repair choices.

● CONCLUSION

In selected patients, closure of RVF due to Crohn's disease is feasible. Individualization of approach is essential to plan the correct treatment plan. Multidisciplinary approach with medical and surgical treatment must be considered for optimal planning. It may require multiple surgical repairs for a successful result.[9,10]

References

1. Lewis RT, Maron DJ. Anorectal Crohn's disease. *Surg Clin North Am.* 2010;90(1):83–97, table of contents.

2. Sands BE, Blank MA, Patel K, van Deventer SJ; ACCENT II Study. Long-term treatment of rectovaginal fistulas in Crohn's disease: response to infliximab in the ACCENT II Study. *Clin Gastroenterol Hepatol.* 2004;2(10):912–920.

3. Parsi MA, Lashner BA, Achkar JP, Connor JT, Brzezinski A. Type of fistula determines response to infliximab in patients with fistulous Crohn's disease. *Am J Gastroenterol.* 2004;99(3):445–449.

4. Ruffolo C, Scarpa M, Bassi N, Angriman I. A systematic review on advancement flaps for rectovaginal fistula in Crohn's disease: transrectal versus transvaginal approach. *Colorecal Dis.* 2010;12(12):1183–1191.

5. Andreani SM, Dang HH, Grondona P, Khan AZ, Edwards DP. Rectovaginal fistula in Crohn's disease. *Dis Colon Rectum.* 2007;50(12):2215–2222.

6. El-Gazzaz G, Hull T, Mignanelli E, Hammel J, Gurland B, Zutshi M. Analysis of function and predictors of failure in women undergoing repair of Crohn's related rectovaginal fistula. *J Gastrointest Surg.* 2010;14(5):824–829.

7. Gaertner WB, Madoff RD, Spencer MP, Mellgren A, Goldberg SM, Lowry AC. Results of combined medical and surgical treatment of rectovaginal fistula in Crohn's disease. *Colorectal Dis.* 2010.

8. Schwandner O, Fuerst A. Preliminary results on efficacy in closure of transsphincteric and rectovaginal fistulas associated with Crohn's disease using new biomaterials. *Surg Innov.* 2009;16(2):162–168.

9. Hanaway CD, Hull TL. Current consideration in the rectovaginal fistula in Crohn's. *Colorectal Dis.* 2008;8:747–745; discussion 755–756.

10. Ruffolo C, Penninckx F, Van Assche G, et al. Outcome of surgery for rectovaginal fistula due to Crohn's disease. *Br J Surg.* 2009;96:1190–1195.

Patient Support Services

Nurse Practitioners in Gastroenterology

144

Sharon Dudley-Brown

Nurse practitioners (NPs), a type of advanced practice nurse (APN), have been around since the 1960s when the demand for primary healthcare providers in the community outpaced that of available physicians. More recently, as the healthcare delivery system has become overburdened with economic constraints, NPs have been given increasing responsibility for the provision of preventive and primary care. Although the role of the NP is well established in primary care, the role is less well established in subspecialties, such as in gastroenterology.

This chapter will describe the differences and similarities between the NP and the physician assistant (PA), the role of the NP in gastroenterology, the role of the NP specific to inflammatory bowel disease (IBD), considerations for including NPs in a GI division or practice, and the future of NPs in gastroenterology.

APNs include NPs, clinical nurse specialists, nurse midwives, and nurse anesthetists. Essentially APNs are RNs who have acquired advanced specialized clinical knowledge and skills to provide healthcare and are educated at the graduate level (masters or doctorate).[1] Core functions of the advanced practice role in the United States include clinical practice, collaboration, clinical and professional leadership, education, ethical decision making, and research.[2]

The APN in gastroenterology as defined by the Society of Gastroenterology Nurses and Associates (SGNA) is a registered nurse who has completed an advanced degree in nursing (masters or doctorate) and who, through study and supervised clinical practice, has become an expert in gastroenterology, hepatology, and/or endoscopy nursing (SGNA, 2006). The APN provides service through direct care, consultation, research, education, and collaboration with other healthcare professionals. The specific patient populations to whom direct care is provided include adults, adolescents, or children with gastrointestinal or hepatic disorders/diseases. The care provided may include but is not limited to advanced assessment, diagnosis, treatment/care planning, implementation, evaluation, and patient education. The role of the APN includes, but is not limited to the following: (1) performing a comprehensive history and physical assessments; (2) ordering and/or performing diagnostic studies; (3) establishing medical and nursing diagnoses; (4) prescribing, administering, and evaluating pharmacological and other therapeutic regimens; (5) managing follow-up care; (6) collaborating with other healthcare professionals, and (7) acting as a consultant for other providers, among other responsibilities.[3]

DIFFERENCES BETWEEN THE NP AND PA

The inclusion of the use of PAs in the specialty of gastroenterology paralleled that of the use of NPs, in the late 1980s, and has continued to grow. Terms used to describe both NPs and PAs include midlevel provider, nonphysician clinician, or physician extender. However, their background, education, and training are philosophically and inherently different.

NPs are registered nurses who are prepared, through advanced education and clinical training, to provide a wide range of preventative and acute healthcare services to individuals of all ages.[4] PAs are defined as healthcare professionals licensed to practice medicine with physician supervision.[5] The NP role developed out of a need for primary care providers in rural areas, whereas the first PA program in the United States was developed for Navy corpsmen. Educational requirements also vary. NPs are required to have a minimum of a masters degree and, by 2015, will be required to have a doctoral degree. PAs, on the other hand, frequently have a baccalaureate degree in any field and a degree or certification from an accredited PA program, depending on the state's requirements (completing either a certificate, associate, baccalaureate, or masters degree program). Although both NPs and PAs can receive national certification, it is mandatory in some but not all states. Another major difference between NPs and PAs is that PAs are licensed and practice under a physician, whereas an NP is licensed and can frequently practice independently. The scope of practice of an NP is governed by the state. As of 2005, approximately 60,000 PAs and 150,000 NPs were practicing in the United States.[6]

● EVIDENCE IN SUPPORT OF NPS

The Congressional Office of Technology Assessment (OTA) concluded that NPs can deliver as much as 80% of the health services, at equal to or better quality and at less cost. In 12 studies, OTA found that the quality of care by NPs, including communication with patients, preventive actions, and reductions in the number of patient symptoms, was higher than that for physicians.[7] The Institute of Medicine has long ago recommended eliminating restrictions on NPs that affect their ability to provide care.[8]

In a Cochrane review, patients cared for by NPs and MDs had similar short-term outcomes.[9] A randomized controlled trial[10] showed that care provided by NPs led to the same outcomes as care provided by physicians in primary care. Findings remained robust when the study was replicated.[11] Specifically on the use of preventive screening practices[12] showed that when NPs are not constrained by productivity requirements and when their patient population has more resources and more expectations, NPs perform better than their primary care (physician) counterparts, particularly with secondary prevention and assessment and counseling. In addition to studies in primary care, studies comparing NPs and physicians have been conducted in emergency care,[13-15] acute care,[16-18] long-term care,[19,20] HIV care,[21,22] and diabetes care.[23] Ohman-Strickland[23] compared care provided by NPs and PAs in family medicine practices in New Jersey and Pennsylvania through a chart audit. Those practices employing NPs were more likely to meet guidelines set by the American Diabetes Association than physician-only practices or those employing PAs.

Although there is evidence of NPs providing quality care, this issue, which has been cloaked in the guise of concern for public safety, continues to be raised, limiting the widespread use of nonphysician providers.[24]

● ROLE OF THE NP IN GASTROENTEROLOGY

The literature on the use of NPs in gastroenterology originated with the use of nurses (RNs) and NPs in the performance of flexible sigmoidoscopies for colorectal cancer screening. This was based on the premise that an increase in providers of screening for colorectal cancer would enable a greater number of patients to be screened than could be reached by physicians alone. Since that time, the data continue to suggest that nurses and NPs can perform flexible sigmoidoscopy as well as physicians and at less cost.[25-37] Despite the data, and despite the findings of Shaheen and colleagues[38] that NPs are willing and able to perform flexible sigmoidoscopies for colorectal cancer screening, it is still not commonplace in the United States.

Koornstra and colleagues[39] have recently showed that nurses can be trained and can perform colonoscopies at a similar level to a GI fellow. Although colonoscopy is still in its infancy in the United States, and despite some reluctance on the part of some gastroenterologists,[40] it is reasonable to believe that nurses and NPs can successfully perform colonoscopy, thereby increasing its uptake for colorectal cancer screening by increasing access.

More recently, upper endoscopies have been conducted safely and accurately by nurses and NPs in the United Kingdom, Europe, and Australia.[37,41-43] In addition to lower endoscopies (flexible sigmoidoscopies and colonoscopies), NPs in GI perform other procedures, such as the performance of large-volume paracentesis,[44] and assisting with placement of percutaneous endoscopic gastrostomy (PEG) tubes, with equivalent outcomes when compared to those of gastroenterologists.[45,46]

Besides procedures, the use of NPs for various aspects of GI care has been well documented,[47] transcending age (pediatric and adult) and location of services (inpatient and outpatient).[48] However, aside from procedures, other outcomes have not been measured in GI practices. Kleinpell[49] suggests examples of outcome measures used in advanced practice nursing, which include care-, patient-, and performance-related outcomes. Specific to a GI practice, these would include such outcomes as mortality and morbidity, quality of life, patient satisfaction, symptom resolution or reduction, knowledge, waiting time, adherence to practice guidelines, and quality of care.

In addition to clinical practice, another large role of GI is that of an educator, who imparts necessary knowledge in patients, families, and other healthcare professionals. Required skills as an educator include extensive clinical knowledge, knowledge of the principles of learning, effective communication skills, and the use of educational tools.[50] In addition, communication and advocacy are important roles of the NP in GI.

A survey conducted on the role of APNs in GI (specifically NPs and clinical nurse specialists) revealed that NPs were performing the majority of the procedures and had the larger number of visits for chronic disease management when compared to the clinical nurse specialist.[51] An interesting finding was that many APNs developed their own proposal for their position, highlighting the emerging role of the APN in a subspecialty of GI at that time.

Since that publication, most APNs employed in out-patient GI settings are NPs rather than CNSs, as they can directly bill for services rendered, either independently, or incident to a physician. However, in practice, much of the APN role in GI can be viewed as a blending of both the CNS and NP roles.[52] The SGNA does not specify or delineate roles within an APN practice in gastroenterology. In a subspecialty such as gastroenterology, the unique contributions of both NP and CNS roles are combined into an APN who is essentially a CNS in the specialty of gastroenterology nursing, along with the knowledge and skills in assessment, diagnosis, and treatment inherent in the NP role.

In addition to the use of NPs in gastroenterology in the United States, the role of APNs, and specifically NPs, is evident in the United Kingdom, Australia, and Canada.[53-55] Some confusion arises internationally in the terminology used to denote APNs, NPs, and nurse specialists. In the United Kingdom, in gastroenterology, specialist nurses were initially titled on the basis of specialty in IBD or as a nurse endoscopist.

The scope of practice of an NP in GI can include more than procedures. The NP can evaluate and manage outpatients (both new patients and return visits), inpatients, read capsule endoscopies, focus on nutrition support or colorectal cancer screening,[56] and focus on education, screening, and prevention. They can conduct research, conduct evidence-based and quality improvement projects, and measure outcomes. The Future Trends Committee of the American Gastroenterological Association (AGA) recommended that the integration of midlevel providers (NPs and PAs) occur to more efficiently deliver inpatient and outpatient care.[57]

Reasons for hiring NPs in a GI practice include the decrease in supply of gastroenterologists and increasing demand. On the supply side, there are fewer GI fellows, creating an increased competition for hiring. Demand has increased as a result of both the overall aging of American citizens, and the Katie Couric effect—increasing the demand for providers to provide screening colonoscopy services.

THE ROLE OF THE NP IN IBD

The role of the NP in IBD is still in its adolescence in the United States. IBD is a chronic, complex, debilitating condition, and thus patients with IBD present unique healthcare challenges, over and above other GI problems. Issues such as chronic and intermittent symptoms, altered quality of life, disability, complex medical regimens, and frequent hospitalizations are faced regularly by people with IBD and can be mitigated by a skilled NP.

In the United Kingdom, the term "nurse specialist" has been used to highlight the specialty care provided by nurses with specialized training, and more recently, further education.[58] In the United Kingdom the term "specialist nurse" has been used interchangeably with clinical nurse specialist, NPs, advanced nursing practitioner, and nurse consultant.[56] This makes comparisons among roles more difficult.

Specifically in the United Kingdom, the IBD nurse specialist has been shown to effectively develop a protocol-led service for immunomodulators,[59] implement a self-management program,[48] implement a program for administration of methotrexate,[60,61] reduce visits and inpatient length of stay,[62] hold a variety of roles,[63] improve adherence[64] and improve access to care and services.[65] Although a Cochrane review on specialist nursing interventions only found one study of low quality,[68] it is clear that the impact of specialized IBD nurses can improve outcomes.[66,67]

In addition, the use of telephone help/advice lines to provide direct access via the telephone by a nurse specialist has been shown to decrease clinic attendance, which led to directly targeting a maximum 1-week wait time for urgent visits.[58,67] In Sweden, implementing a patient- and demand-directed care through the use of an IBD nurse specialist showed an increase in efficiency and reduced waiting lists and improved quality of life.[69]

Editor's note (TMB): Chapter 149 details the experience of an NP in the role of patient advocate.

CONSIDERATIONS FOR INCLUDING AN NP IN A GI PRACTICE

According to Mayberry and Mayberry,[53] "the purpose of NPs is not and should not become: to relieve doctors of some of their workload, and to save money through lower wages" (p. 37). However, in the United States, this is already a reality. NPs (and for that matter, PAs) have been used to increase profitability of practices though the use of lower wage providers. However, though this initially allowed the gastroenterologist to spend more time doing procedures, with the recent decrease in Medicare reimbursement of procedures, this may narrow the differences in relative value units earned between the NP and gastroenterologist.

Currently, NPs in gastroenterology and hepatology practice not only in a variety of settings (inpatient and outpatient) and with a variety of ages (pediatric and adult) but also in a variety of practice patterns and roles. For example, some have their own schedule of patients, whereas others see patients from the busy physician's schedule. Some NPs have their "own" patients and others "share" patients with their physician colleagues. Whatever model is used, NPs can bring value to a practice, whether an academic or private practice.

Hiring an NP benefits patients, the physician, and the GI practice. Patients reap the benefit of improved access for both new and return appointments, thus improving outcomes. The gastroenterologist benefits by achieving greater scheduling flexibility, both for procedures and time-off; thus, the practice can benefit financially. According to *Medical Economics*, "midlevels can improve patient care and your practice's bottom line";[70] hiring midlevels makes good financial sense since hours are billable to insurance and salaries are 50% of that of a physician (p. 18). According to the Medical Group Management Association's "Physician Compensation and Production Survey: 2006 Report based on 2005 Data," PAs and NPs are able to generate practice income well above their costs.[71]

TRAINING AND THE FUTURE

There is growing demand for NP specialties in all of the healthcare disciplines, especially in gastroenterology. The forces of economics, policy, and public health are such that now is the time for NPs in gastroenterology. At present, numbers are difficult to determine because of current lack of reporting by a national organization. However, the national trend is toward specialization through a specialty organization or through residency or fellowship programs. Johns Hopkins offers such a program, a Gastroenterology Nurse Practitioner Fellowship program. Also the AGA Institute annually offers a course designed for NPs and PAs, "Principles of Gastroenterology for the Nurse Practitioner and Physician Assistant" (AGA, 2009), to help educate those new to the field of gastroenterology.

Johns Hopkins Nurse Practitioner Fellowship Program

The decreased supply of gastroenterologists, coupled with an increase in demand for gastroenterology services (e.g., colonoscopy services alone), has created significant barriers in access to care. The NP fellowship program aims to improve patient access to a provider in the field of gastroenterology. The Johns Hopkins Nurse Practitioner Fellowship program is designed to train NPs in the specialty of gastroenterology and hepatology.

The NP fellowship program integrates the IOM concepts: systems-based care, transdisciplinary team building, professional communications, and life-long practice-based learning. Applicants are NPs with a masters degree, educated and eligible for certification in adult, family, or acute care, or can be a new graduate or an experienced professional. NP fellows are integrated into the existing physician fellowship and receive clinical training comparable to that of a first-year physician fellow and also complete a postgraduate course in evidence-based practice or outcomes management. Funded by the School of Medicine, the program has both didactic and clinical components. Didactic components mirror those of the physician fellows and include daily or weekly conferences using a topical curriculum, weekly grand rounds, morbidity and mortality conferences (M & M) rounds, and journal club. Clinical components include both inpatient rotations in general GI/consultation service and hepatology, 1 month in nutrition support services, and outpatient rotations in general GI, IBD, hepatology, pancreas, and motility, as well as endoscopic procedures such as flexible sigmoidoscopy and colonoscopy training.

Editor's note (TMB): This chapter contains a wealth of well-documented information. Having Sharon Dudley-Brown, PhD, FNP. BC, as a "partner" for these past 5 years has been an enlightening and encouraging experience.

References

1. American Nurses Association (ANA). *Nursing: Scope and Standards of Practice*. Washington, DC: ANA; 2004.

2. Hamric A, Spross J, Hanson C. *Advanced Practice Nursing: An Integrative Approach, 4th ed*. St. Louis, MO: Elsevier; 2009.

3. Society of Gastroenterology Nurses and Associates (SGNA). Role delineation of the advanced practice registered nurse in gastroenterology. *Gastroenterol Nurs*. 2006:29(1);58–59.

4. American College of Nurse Practitioners (ACNP). What is a nurse practitioner? http://www.acnpweb.org/i4a/pages/index.cfm?pageid=3479. Accessed February 12, 2010.

5. American Academy of Physician Assistants (AAPA). About physician assistants. http://www.aapa.org/about-pas. Accessed February 12, 2010.

6. Simmons HJ 3rd, Rapoport DH. How will physician extenders affect our need for physicians? *Health Care Strateg Manage*. 2007;25(11):4–5.

7. US Congress, Office of Technology Assessment (OTA). *Nurse Practitioner, Physician Assistants and Certified Midwives: A Policy Analysis, Health Technology Case Study 37, OTA-HCS-37*. Washington, DC: US Government Printing Office; 1986.

8. Institute of Medicine (IOM). *Nursing Staff in Hospitals and Nursing Homes: Is It Adequate?* Washington, DC: National Academy Press; 1996.

9. Laurant M, Reeves D, Hermens R, Braspenning J, Grol R, Sibbald B. (2004). Substitution of doctors by nurses in primary care. *Cochrane Database Systematic Rev*. (4): CD001271.

10. Mundinger MO, Kane RL, Lenz ER, et al. Primary care outcomes in patients treated by nurse practitioners or physicians: a randomized trial. *JAMA*. 2000;283(1):59–68.

11. Lenz ER, Mundinger MO, Kane RL, Hopkins SC, Lin SX. Primary care outcomes in patients treated by nurse practitioners or physicians: two year follow up. *Med Care Res Rev*. 2004;61(3):332–351.

12. Hopkins SC, Lenz ER, Pontes NM, Lin SX, Mundinger MO. Context of care or provider training: the impact on preventive screening practices. *Prev Med*. 2005;40(6):718–724.

13. Cooper MA, Lindsay GM, Kinn S, Swann IJ. Evaluating Emergency Nurse Practitioner services: a randomized controlled trial. *J Adv Nurs*. 2002;40(6):721–730.

14. Sakr M, Angus J, Perrin J, Nixon C, Nicholl J, Wardrope J. Care of minor injuries by emergency nurse practitioners or junior doctors: a randomised controlled trial. *Lancet*. 1999;354(9187):1321–1326.

15. Sakr M, Kendall R, Angus J, et al. Emergency nurse practitioners: a three part study in clinical and cost effectiveness. *Emerg Med J*. 2003;20(2):158–163.

16. Hoffman LA, Happ MB, Scharfenberg C, DiVirgilio-Thomas D, Tasota FJ. Perceptions of physicians, nurses, and respiratory therapists about the role of acute care nurse practitioners. *Am J Crit Care*. 2004;13(6):480–488.

17. Hoffman LA, Tasota FJ, Zullo TG, Scharfenberg C, Donahoe MP. Outcomes of care managed by an acute care nurse practitioner/ attending physician team in a subacute medical intensive care unit. *Am J Crit Care*. 2005;14(2):121–30; quiz 131.

18. Rudy EB, Davidson LJ, Daly B, et al. Care activities and outcomes of patients cared for by acute care nurse practitioners, physician assistants, and resident physicians: a comparison. *Am J Crit Care*. 1998;7(4):267–281.

19. Aigner MJ, Drew S, Phipps J. A comparative study of nursing home resident outcomes between care provided by nurse practitioners/physicians versus physicians only. *J Am Med Dir Assoc*. 2004;5(1):16–23.

20. Lambing AY, Adams DL, Fox DH, Divine G. Nurse practitioners' and physicians' care activities and clinical outcomes with an inpatient geriatric population. *J Am Acad Nurse Pract*. 2004;16(8):343–352.

21. Hekkink CF, Wigersma L, Yzermans CJ, Bindels PJ. HIV nursing consultants: patients' preferences and experiences about the quality of care. *J Clin Nurs*. 2005;14(3):327–333.

22. Wilson IB, Landon BE, Hirschhorn LR, et al. Quality of HIV care provided by nurse practitioners, physician assistants, and physicians. *Ann Intern Med*. 2005;143(10):729–736.

23. Ohman-Strickland PA, Orzano AJ, Hudson SV, et al. Quality of diabetes care in family medicine practices: influence of nurse-practitioners and physician's assistants. *Ann Fam Med*. 2008;6(1):14–22.

24. Mullinix C, Bucholtz DP. Role and quality of nurse practitioner practice: a policy issue. *Nurs Outlook*. 2009;57(2):93–98.

25. Brotherstone H, Vance M, Edwards R, et al. Uptake of population-based flexible sigmoidoscopy screening for colorectal cancer: a nurse-led feasibility study. *J Med Screen*. 2007;14(2):76–80.

26. Dobrow MJ, Cooper MA, Gayman K, Pennington J, Matthews J, Rabeneck L. Referring patients to nurses: outcomes and evaluation of a nurse flexible sigmoidoscopy training program for colorectal cancer screening. *Can J Gastroenterol*. 2007;21(5):301–308.

27. Goodfellow PB, Fretwell IA, Simms JM. Nurse endoscopy in a district general hospital. *Ann R Coll Surg Engl*. 2003;85(3):181–184.

28. Goodfellow PB. Flexible sigmoidoscopy performed by nurses. *Endoscopy*. 2006;38(6):624–626.

29. Gruber M. Performance of flexible sigmoidoscopy by a clinical nurse specialist. *Gastroenterol Nurs*. 1996;19(3):105–108.

30. Horton K, Reffel A, Rosen K, Farraye FA. Training of nurse practitioners and physician assistants to perform screening flexible sigmoidoscopy. *J Am Acad Nurse Pract*. 2001;13(10):455–459.

31. Maruthachalam K, Stoker E, Nicholson G, Horgan AF. Nurse led flexible sigmoidoscopy in primary care—the first thousand patients. *Colorectal Dis*. 2006;8(7):557–562.

32. Sansbury LB, Klabunde CN, Mysliwiec P, Brown ML. Physicians' use of nonphysician healthcare providers for colorectal cancer screening. *Am J Prev Med*. 2003;25(3):179–186.

33. Schoenfeld P, Lipscomb S, Crook J, et al. Accuracy of polyp detection by gastroenterologists and nurse endoscopists during flexible sigmoidoscopy: a randomized trial. *Gastroenterology*. 1999;117(2):312–318.

34. Schoenfeld PS, Cash B, Kita J, Piorkowski M, Cruess D, Ransohoff D. Effectiveness and patient satisfaction with screening flexible sigmoidoscopy performed by registered nurses. *Gastrointest Endosc*. 1999;49(2):158–162.

35. Shapero TF, Hoover J, Paszat LF, et al. Colorectal cancer screening with nurse-performed flexible sigmoidoscopy: results from a Canadian community-based program. *Gastrointest Endosc.* 2007;65(4):640–645.

36. Williams J, Russell I, Durai D, et al. What are the clinical outcome and cost-effectiveness of endoscopy undertaken by nurses when compared with doctors? A multi-institution nurse endoscopy trial (MINuET). *Health Technol Assess.* 2006;10(40):iii–iv, ix-x, 1–195.

37. Williams J, Russell I, Durai D, et al. Effectiveness of nurse delivered endoscopy: findings from randomised multi-institution nurse endoscopy trial (MINuET). *BMJ.* 2009;338:b231.

38. Shaheen NJ, Crosby MA, O'Malley MS, et al. The practices and attitudes of primary care nurse practitioners and physician assistants with respect to colorectal cancer screening. *Am J Gastroenterol.* 2000;95(11):3259–3265.

39. Koornstra JJ, Corporaal S, Geizen-Beintema WM, deVries SE, van Dullemen HM. Colonoscopy training for nurse endoscopists: a feasibility study. *Gastrointest Endosc.* 2009;69(3 pt 2):696–699.

40. Ahnen DJ, Lieberman DA. Colonoscopy training for nurse endoscopists: is it possible? Is it wise? Is it worth doing? *Gastrointest Endosc.* 2009;69(3 Pt 2):696–699.

41. Basnyat PS, West J, Davies P, Davies PS, Foster ME. The nurse practitioner endoscopist. *Ann R Coll Surg Engl.* 2000;82(5):331–332.

42. Bull J, Dunn SV, Gassner L, Fraser RJ. Upper gastrointestinal endoscopy training: a retrospective audit of the first 210 examinations performed by an advanced practice nurse (APN) at a metropolitan hospital in South Australia. *J GENCA.* 2006;16(1): 5–10.

43. Smale S, Bjarnason I, Forgacs I, et al. Upper gastrointestinal endoscopy performed by nurses: scope for the future? *Gut.* 2003;52(8):1090–1094.

44. Gilani N, Patel N, Gerkin RD, Ramirez FC, Tharalson EE, Patel K. The safety and feasibility of large volume paracentesis performed by an experienced nurse practitioner. *Ann Hepatol.* 2009;8(4):359–363.

45. Patrick PG, Kirby DE, McMillion DB, DeLegge MH, Boyle RM. Evaluation of the safety of nurse-assisted percutaneous endoscopic gastrostomy. *Gastroenterol Nurs.* 1996;19(5):176–180.

46. Sturgess RP, O'Toole PA, McPhillips J, Brown J, Lombard MG. Percutaneous endoscopic gastrostomy: evaluation of insertion by an endoscopy nurse practitioner. *Eur J Gastroenterol Hepatol.* 1996;8(7):631–634.

47. Chan D, Harris S, Roderick P, Brown D, Patel P. A randomised controlled trial of structured nurse-led outpatient clinic follow-up for dyspeptic patients after direct access gastroscopy. *BMC Gastroenterol.* 2009;9:12.

48. Young R. Gastroenterology advanced practice nurse: what's in a name? *Gastroenterol Nurs.* 2008;31(6):434–435.

49. Kleinpell R. *Outcome Assessment in Advanced Practice Nursing,* 1st ed. New York: Springer Publishing.

50. Manning M. The advanced practice nurse in gastroenterology serving as patient educator. *Gastroenterol Nurs.* 2004;27(5):220–225.

51. Hiller A. The advanced practice nurse in gastroenterology: identifying and comparing care interactions of nurse practitioners and clinical nurse specialists. *Gastroenterol Nurs.* 2001;24(5):239–245.

52. Dudley-Brown S. Revisiting the blended role of the advanced practice nurse. *Gastroenterol Nurs.* 2006;29(3):249–250.

53. Mayberry MK, Mayberry JF. The status of nurse practitioners in gastroenterology. *Clin Med.* 2003;3(1):37–41.

54. McNamara S, Giguère V, St-Louis L, Boileau J. Development and implementation of the specialized nurse practitioner role: use of the PEPPA framework to achieve success. *Nurs Health Sci.* 2009;11(3):318–325.

55. Verschuur EML, Kuipers EJ, Siersema PD. Nurses working in GI and endoscopic practice: a review. *Gastrointest Endosc.* 2007;65:469–479.

56. Norton C, Kamm MA. Specialist nurses in gastroenterology. *J R Soc Med.* 2002;95(7):331–335.

57. Wang TC, Fleischer DE, Kaufman PN, et al. The best of time and the worst of times: sustaining the future of academic gastroenterology in the United States—Report of a consensus conference conducted by the AGA Institute Future Trends Committee. *Gastroenterology.* 2008;134:597–616.

58. Younge L, Norton C. Contribution of specialist nurses in managing patients with IBD. *Br J Nurs.* 2007;16(4):208–212.

59. Holbrook K. A triangulation study of the clinician and patient experiences of the use of the immunosuppressant drugs azathioprine and 6-mercaptopurine for the management of inflammatory bowel disease. *J Clin Nurs.* 2007;16(8):1427–1434.

60. Stansfield C, Robinson A. Implementation of an IBD nurse-led self-management programme. *Gastrointest Nurs.* 2008;6(3):12–18.

61. Garrick V, Atwal P, Barclay AR, McGrogan P, Russell RK. Successful implementation of a nurse-led teaching programme to independently administer subcutaneous methotrexate in the community setting to children with Crohn's disease. *Aliment Pharmacol Ther.* 2009;29(1):90–96.

62. Nightingale AJ, Middleton W, Middleton SJ, Hunter JO. Evaluation of the effectiveness of a specialist nurse in the management of inflammatory bowel disease (IBD). *Eur J Gastroenterol Hepatol.* 2000;12(9):967–973.

63. Belling R, Woods L, McLaren S. Stakeholder perceptions of specialist inflammatory bowel disease nurses' role and personal attributes. *Int J Nurs Pract.* 2008;14(1):67–73.

64. Schreiber S, Hamling J, Wedel S, et al. Efficacy of patient education in chronic inflammatory bowel disease in a prospective controlled multicentre trial. Gastroenterology. 1999;116:AB15.

65. Pearson C. Establishing an inflammatory bowel disease service. *Nursing Times Net.* 2006;102(23):27.

66. Dudley-Brown S, Fraser A. A transatlantic comparison of nurse-led, patient-centred care for ulcerative colitis. *Gastrointestinal Nursing.* 2009;7(6):38–43.

67. Miller L, Caton S, Lynch D. Telephone clinic improves quality of follow up care for chronic bowel disease. *Nursing Times.* 2002;98(31):36–38.

68. Belling R, McLaren S, Woods L. Specialist nursing interventions for inflammatory bowel disease. *Cochrane Database Syst Rev.* 2009;(4):CD006597.

69. Rejler M, Spångéus A, Tholstrup J, Andersson-Gäre B. Improved population-based care: Implementing patient-and demand-directed care for inflammatory bowel disease and evaluating the redesign with a population-based registry. *Qual Manag Health Care.* 2007;16(1):38–50.

70. Page L. Midlevels: boost or burden? *Med Econ.* 2008:18–21.

71. Medical Group Management Association (MGMA). MGMA Physician Compensation and Production Survey: 2006 Report Based on 2005 Data. http://www.mgma.com

IBD Advocacy: A Nurse's Perspective | 145

Lisa Turnbough

An advocate is "... one that supports or promotes the interests of another." (Webster)

Inflammatory bowel disease (IBD) patients, as patients with other chronic illnesses, are in need of an advocate at some point in their journey to help them navigate the healthcare system and/or deal with the chronic nature of their illness. Periods of disease exacerbation may have a profound negative effect on quality of life. Multiple medications, hospitalizations, surgery, lost time at work or school, and social embarrassment are but a few of the possible consequences of an IBD flare. These patients must learn to cope with their illness at home and in their day-to-day life. Some patients obviously find this a more daunting task than others. Factors that affect the ability to cope with chronic illness include previous life experiences, education/ability to learn, cultural values and beliefs, social support, socioeconomic standing, and the availability of the healthcare team treating them.

● IBD NURSE ADVOCATE

Nurses are natural patient advocates by way of training and job description.

It is intuitive and further proven to be beneficial to patients, to have a dedicated IBD nurse/advocate available to them. The aim of IBD patient advocacy is to assist the patient in prolonging remissions and avoiding exacerbations of their disease. In order to promote that goal, patients require clear, concise education in understandable terms; assistance in locating and making use of available resources to deal with the physical, financial, and emotional aspects of IBD; and access to their healthcare provider.

The office environment is an important and visible factor in patient advocacy. The tone of the physician/patient relationship is often set by the reception the patient gets in the office. In a patient centered practice, patients have confidence that messages are promptly delivered, that appointments are available in a reasonable time frame, and that billing is done accurately and in a timely manner. Office management is discussed in a separate chapter.

● PATIENT EDUCATION

A well-informed patient is empowered to make informed decisions about day-to-day issues such as adherence to prescribed medical therapy, lifestyle changes, and medical follow-up. Teaching is begun at the time of diagnosis and reinforced and built upon with each patient encounter. When patients feel more confident with their ability to manage at home, they tend to need fewer emergency visits.

Information is given to patients keeping in mind the individual's ability to learn at the time. Intellectual ability, age and developmental stage, emotional status, and appropriateness of the moment affect the ability to absorb and apply information. Information given during a flare may not be retained; as such stressful times are not optimal teachable moments. Further, terms commonly used by medical professionals are often foreign to the layperson. It is important to recognize miscomprehension and address educational needs respectfully.

The nonemergency office visit is an opportune time to reinforce concepts related to the disease process, rationale for prescribed therapies, and problem-solving tips. This is also the time to discuss recommendations for surveillance colonoscopies, blood work, and other testing. It can be challenging to impress the importance of surveillance testing and medical therapy when the patient is not experiencing symptoms. However, when they are not stressed by the obvious signs of IBD, they may be more able to absorb and apply the rationale for such adherence. At any point, however, attention needs to be given to avoid overwhelming the patient or family with too much information and particularly to be sure that they are not focusing on all of the possible negative outcomes.

Advocacy lends itself to outreach beyond the patient population. Educational needs exist with other healthcare providers and with the public in general. By working toward increasing awareness the IBD nurse advocates for patients. Being aware of advances in the treatment of IBD, current research studies and data collection furthers advocacy.

ACCESSIBILITY

It is during the office visit that the nurse reviews the patient's IBD history, current medications, and response to therapy. Educational needs are assessed as well as psychosocial issues and coping strategies. The need for prescriptions and diagnostic or surveillance testing is reviewed. Patients are given opportunity to pose questions and discuss their situation. Assessment data are presented to the physician so he or she approaches the patient better equipped to address needs in a prioritized and time-efficient manner. The nurse assists with the physical examination, and the treatment plan is mutually agreed upon, established, and documented. During this process the nurse becomes an accessible link to the healthcare system. Further, the patients report satisfaction with the visit as they leave with questions answered, with a clear idea of the plan and rationale, and knowing that they can contact the nurse for clarification or if problems arise between office visits.

In terms of telephone communication with patients, the IBD nurse functions as liaison between patient and physician. The nurse must be able to quickly determine the severity of the issue prompting the call in order to prioritize the urgency. Even the most articulate of patients can leave out important data needed to safely address issues related to their illness over the phone. Care must be used to sort through extraneous information, and to solicit appropriate data. The subject matter of patient phone calls can range from new onset of symptoms, failed response to therapy, adverse events, need for prescription refills, test results, insurance coverage issues, disability paperwork, or referral to other specialists. Some calls simply require an empathetic ear. The physician approves any changes in the plan of care. It is important to document phone conversations carefully for continuity of care and for legal reasons.

RESOURCES

Age, maturity level, severity of disease, coexisting medical problems, current life situation, and personal history all factor into the patient's ability to accept an IBD diagnosis. The nurse can offer hope and some sense of control by pointing out areas where they have influence on outcomes. For instance, taking medications as prescribed and compliance with medical follow-up are behaviors that impact outcomes. Further, a letter to an employer or college housing office to request that an individual be situated near bathroom facilities for easy access can relieve a tremendous amount of anxiety. Coexisting or emerging mental illness will affect an individual's ability to cope with IBD. If the stress of dealing with IBD is overwhelming, the patient should be examined and treated. The IBD nurse advocate can facilitate appropriate mental health or social work referrals when needed.

The financial burden of IBD is a concern that impacts adherence to medical therapy, and the patient's entire family. Uninsured or underinsured patients often do not have the resources to get or maintain adequate healthcare. The advocate can point such patients to state or local government agencies. Many pharmaceutical companies offer patient assistance programs.

Organizations such as the Crohn's and Colitis Foundation of America are wonderful resources. Local chapters provide meetings and events that can be enormously helpful to patients and families.

Bibliography

1. Cappell MS. Nurses make the difference. *Gastroenterol Nurs.* 2009;32(3):216–217.
2. Hunt SA. Inflammatory bowel disease nurse advocate. In: Bayless TM, Hanauer SB, eds. *Advanced Therapy of Inflammatory Bowel Disease.* Hamilton, ON: BC Decker; 2001:535–537.
3. Kane SV. Adherence issues in the patient with inflammatory bowel disease. *Practical Gastroenterology.* 2004;16–22.
4. Turnbough LH. Role of a nurse advocate. In: Bayless TM, Diehl AM, eds. *Advanced Therapy in Gastroenterology and Liver Disease.* Hamilton, ON: BC Decker; 2005:266–269.
5. Turnbough L, Wilson L. "Take your medicine": nonadherence issues in patients with ulcerative colitis. *Gastroenterol Nurs.* 2007;30(3):212–217; quiz 218.

Clinical Practice in IBD— The Role of an Experienced Medical/Administrative Assistant

146

Donna K. Rode

Now, as you are reading this chapter, take a moment, stop, and think ... when you or a family member contacted a physician's office what was your first impression of the office visit?

We all strive to receive the best care possible for ourselves and our loved ones and we therefore seek out the physician who is the best in his/her field of expertise. The physician can turn out to be everything we had read on the internet or heard that he/she was: an answer to our prayers and, in many cases, an important influence on the patient's quality of life and the difference between life and death.

No matter how good that physician is reported to be, did you or your family member decide to seek care elsewhere, due to the office staff? Or did the interaction with the support staff encourage and reassure you that you had made the correct choice?

As every surgeon knows, a truly successful practice takes team work, with he/she being the leader—setting the example and tone for the office. This is especially true with patients with inflammatory bowel diseases (IBD). Those patients are unique—not only do they have varying physical symptoms from their disease but also, socially and psychologically, they require care. Until you interact with someone who has one of the myriad of disorders that fall under "the blanket of inflammatory bowel disease," you can not truly appreciate that team work of the physicians, nurses, scheduling staff, radiologists, endoscopists, surgeons, pathologists, pediatricians, psychologists and psychiatrists, pharmaceutical companies, and scheduling staff—and along with the physician is often the physician's administrative/medical assistant at the center of this wheel (keeping the operation well greased and running smooth).

The administrative/medical assistant is usually the first contact with the patient and their families or referring physicians. One learns to recognize and respond appropriately to the sound of a frantic spouse. When one hears the frightened, almost helpless sound in a parent's voice calling about their newly diagnosed child/young adult, he or she has to empathize with the patients and their families, and provide an opportunity for them to speak unhurriedly to someone at a medical center, often miles from their home and perhaps a small town environment. One develops skills on how to convince a patient that they are not alone and, at the same time, treat them like they are unique (for no two IBD patients are exactly the same).

How can I say all of this with 100% conviction? In my 17 years at Johns Hopkins Hospital, Baltimore, Maryland, I have been fortunate to participate in the administration of the Harvey M. and Lynn P. Meyerhoff IBD Center where patients visit, seeking excellence in medical/surgical care for IBD. In addition, I've seen the "birth" of the Blaine Newman IBD Nurse Advocate position. Two people have filled that position during this time and we worked together as a team. They were both nurses, originally from oncology backgrounds, which gave them an empathetic edge. In addition, they became experts in caring for IBD patients. The preceding chapter describes their activities.

We learned to recognize the patients and/or family members' voices. We addressed them by name before they even identify themselves; which for someone with a lifetime illness can be very important. I've been told that this "gave them a precious gift—it made them "feel special"—apart from everyone else in our busy practice." This is an important part of what they needed for their feeling of well being.

I have also been taught by my physicians that patients don't want to discuss the football game or hear about my life. They call or come to see us for themselves—for their symptoms and for their illness. Because if you truly understand this disease, it is all *consuming*. They eat, breathe, and sleep with this illness, and they need the physician and his assistant to *recognize* this and *treat* them this way, "which helps restore their individuality—something this disease has robbed them of."

A good administrative assistant can run the office when her physician(s) is out. She understands, empathizes, and, when needed, gives hugs (both physically and mentally). At the nurse's or doctor's requests, they orders tests, arrange referrals, obtain prior authorizations, keep their bosses calendar, and triage calls so that the patient doesn't "get lost in the system," keeping that wheel well greased! The patients have told me over the years "how important it is that we know most of the patients and/or spouses by name. We remember births, rejoice with each "cure" either through medication or surgery, and "feel" each death. We should be our boss' right hand and anticipate the next level of his/her need in taking care of these individual patients. This is what keeps us at the "center of the team."

In summary, patients should feel welcome when they call the office, they should know without being told that they are important and each question or problem that they have is important—because they have it—and it needs to be addressed in a timely fashion with knowledge and compassion. Our IBD patients should be treated as we would want someone to treat us, our family, and/or our friends. You, as physicians, counsel them, diagnose them, and help keep them in remission. We keep them feeling like family.

Crohn's and Colitis Foundation of America: Information, Support, and Research Programs

147

Marjorie Merrick and Kimberly Frederick

Founded in 1967, the Crohn's and Colitis Foundation of America (CCFA) is a nonprofit, volunteer-driven organization dedicated to finding a cure for Crohn's disease and ulcerative colitis (collectively known as inflammatory bowel diseases [IBDs]). With more than $150 million invested in research and improved treatments, CCFA has enabled significant advances in the understanding of these devastating diseases that inflict a heavy burden on thousands of families.

CCFA's mission is to cure Crohn's disease and ulcerative colitis, and to improve the quality of life of children and adults affected by these diseases. Its vision is a future free from Crohn's and colitis.

To achieve this vision, CCFA sponsors basic and clinical research of the highest quality. The Foundation also offers a wide range of educational programs for patients and healthcare professionals, and provides supportive services to help people cope with these chronic intestinal diseases. Following are programs and services established by CCFA to educate and support patients, families, and professionals as well as to raise valuable funds toward finding a cure.

INFORMATION RESOURCE CENTER

Over the years, CCFA has distributed a wealth of patient education materials through its Information Resource Center (IRC). The IRC staff consists of master's level Information Specialists, who receive more than 1200 inquiries a month. To ensure that the most accurate, up to-date information is disseminated, the IRC manages the review and approval of CCFA materials by medical experts who participate on our National Scientific Advisory Committee.

Information specialists answer a wide variety of questions, and provide general IBD education, support, and treatment information to help patients and their families manage the disease. Patients, families, and professionals may contact the IRC in a number of ways, including a toll-free telephone number, 888. MY.GUT.PAIN (888.694.8872); e-mail (info@ccfa.org); live chat through CCFA's Web site (www.ccfa.org); and mail and fax.

PUBLICATIONS

CCFA has established a range of educational brochures, fact sheets, and programs designed to increase awareness about these digestive diseases.

The majority of our materials are free for the asking. Some materials are available for purchase through our online book store, and others are provided as a benefit of membership in CCFA. Each year, more than a million brochures and fact sheets are distributed free of charge to patients, physicians, and hospitals. These easy-to-read publications provide general information about topics of importance to patients, such as diet and nutrition, medications, flares, and surgeries.

Take Charge is CCFA's patient magazine for members, published online twice per year. Each issue is designed with patient's needs and questions in mind, and is packed with relevant and timely information, such as in-depth research articles, pediatric information, coping tips, and nutrition information and recipes.

The IBD community is intensely interested in what is happening in research. In addition to the research updates in *Take Charge*, CCFA offers *Under the Microscope*, a research newsletter published twice a year as a benefit of membership in CCFA. It includes news about new research projects, clinical trials, conference notes, and partnerships and grants.

CCFA's Annual Report details the organization's fiscal year, including information on research activities, finances, and chapters and staff.

Another important publication is *Inflammatory Bowel Diseases*, the first medical journal dedicated exclusively to IBD and one of the top 10 journals in its field.

WEB-BASED SERVICES

CCFA continues to expand its reach and influence on the Internet through its main Web site, community site, and teen site.

CCFA.ORG

CCFA's flagship site contains comprehensive, up-to-the-minute information about IBD and the Foundation's programs and services. Some of the site's sections include

- "Living with IBD"—articles on every aspect of IBD, including diagnosis and treatment, complications, coping day-to-day, and insurance issues.
- "Research"—the latest developments in basic and clinical research. There are articles on every major field of investigation.
- "Disease Information"—this section explains Crohn's and colitis, the diagnosis process, complications, and treatment and surgery options. It also houses our educational brochures, clinical trials, and our "Find-a-Doctor" directory. This directory lists all healthcare professionals who are currently members of CCFA. Although this is not a form of accreditation, it is an invaluable resource to persons who are seeking to identify a gastroenterologist with a special interest in treating IBD.
- "Chapters and Events"—lists our nationwide regions as well as our local events, educational symposia, and support groups.
- "Science & Professionals"—this section targets healthcare professionals, and includes research grant information and deadlines, professional education opportunities, and upcoming conferences.
- "Advocacy"—where members of the IBD community can support CCFA's efforts in Congress. It includes information on recent bills passed, as well as the ability to send e-mails or faxes directly to members of Congress, encouraging them to sponsor important legislation favorable to the needs of IBD patients.

CCFACOMMUNITY.ORG

CCFA has developed a free online community site, CCFACommunity.org, to provide the support individual's need in managing their condition. More than 70,000 patients, family members, and friends of those with IBD use this community to participate in discussions and share their stories with others.

UCANDCROHNS.ORG

UCandCrohns.org is a site just for teens, run by CCFA and the Starlight Children's Foundation. It is full of interactive features to help teens cope with their illness; learn to talk it out with friends, family, or teachers; and to see how other teens manage day-to-day. It includes fun polls, an "Ask an Expert" section, and a chat room.

SOCIAL MEDIA

CCFA has built a presence in the social media realm through Facebook, Twitter, and YouTube. CCFA's Facebook application, found at http://apps.facebook.com/supportccfa, allows visitors to talk with CCFA and with each other, creates awareness around education and fund-raising initiatives, and helps participants to tell their own stories. Visitors will also hear the latest news about IBD and learn about our national events. Facebook users can show their support by joining us and displaying specially designed profile badges on their own Facebook pages, furthering awareness—and, last but not least, our Facebook friends can donate directly to CCFA.

CCFA's Twitter page is located at http://www.twitter.com/ccfa. CCFA uses its Twitter page as another outlet to interact with the IBD community. We also list the latest news on research, educational resources, and programs.

The up-and-coming YouTube page is CCFA's newest venture into social media, and can be found at http://www.youtube.com/ccfa. It currently displays videos about our research efforts, as well as national events Team Challenge and Take Steps.

EDUCATION PROGRAMS

CCFA offers a variety of patient and professional education programs. These programs include national teleconferences, Web-based seminars, professional continuing education programs, and our world-renowned annual conference, "Advances in IBD."

Patient education programs are also held in local communities nationwide. These programs are developed in cooperation with CCFA's Chapter Medical Advisory Committee. Topics are presented that meet the needs of patients and families, and have included the basics of IBD, medical and surgical therapies, extraintestinal manifestations, nutrition, and coping techniques.

CCFA also provides educational opportunities for medical professionals by hosting symposia focused on the most current developments in diagnosis and treatment of IBD. This will, in turn, help to improve patient care. Most local chapters host at least one professional education symposium per year. A complete listing of chapter programs may be found in the "Chapters and Events" section on CCFA's flagship Web site, CCFA.org.

SUPPORT GROUPS

As with any chronic disease, people with IBD face psychological and social adjustments. Many people with IBD find comfort and practical information by joining a mutual support group. It is not unusual that, when first joining a support group, it may be the first time that a participant has ever met and talked with another person with Crohn's disease or ulcerative colitis. Sharing challenges, strategies for overcoming them, and personal stories can be extremely beneficial.

CCFA hosts hundreds of support groups throughout the United States. Every group has a facilitator and co-facilitator who act as moderators to ensure that discussions remain on track and everyone has an opportunity to speak. Facilitators participate in national training and adhere to support group guidelines. The structure and group schedule may be monthly, quarterly, or a few times per year depending on the needs of group members.

"Power of Two" is another supportive service offered by some of CCFA's 40 chapters. This program connects trained patient volunteers with other patients for one-on-one telephone or online peer support.

Local support groups and "Power of Two" programs are listed on CCFA's flagship site, CCFA.org, in the "Chapters & Events" section.

CAMP OASIS

CCFA Camp Oasis provides a sanctuary where kids with Crohn's disease or ulcerative colitis are not defined by their illness. All of the campers (and many of the adults) have IBD. But the focus is not on the disease—it is on having fun! This summer camp program provides activities for every interest, including swimming, hiking, and arts and crafts. Most important, Camp Oasis lets kids with IBD know that they are not alone in their struggles, and they can let their true selves shine through.

Camp Oasis provides 24-hour on-site medical supervision by physicians, nurses, and other healthcare professionals with experience treating children with IBD. There are also dedicated and understanding counselors, many of whom have IBD themselves, who are carefully screened and trained.

Camp locations are throughout the United States. Find out more online, at CCFA.org/camps.

RESEARCH

CCFA's ultimate goal is to cure and prevent Crohn's disease and ulcerative colitis by supporting the best peer-reviewed basic and clinical research available.

CCFA's commitment to IBD research has surpassed $150 million and is steadily growing. Using a rigorous peer-review process, the Foundation funds the work of both established investigators from around the world and promising young researchers training in U.S. laboratories. CCFA receives more than 250 grant applications per year and funds approximately 200 new and ongoing grants per year.

The goals of CCFA's research programs are simple:

1. Identify and fund the best peer-reviewed research in IBD
2. Provide "seed money" to allow investigators to generate enough preliminary data to be competitive at the *National Institutes of Health* level
3. Encourage outstanding young investigators to choose a career in IBD research
4. Identify and support emerging areas of research

These goals are accomplished through investigator-driven awards (both senior and training levels), research initiatives (Requests for Proposals, CCFA-driven projects), and by the creation of consortia and resources.

CCFA's research programs are guided by dynamic strategic plans known as "Challenges in IBD Research" and "Challenges in Pediatric IBD Research." Updated regularly, these plans identify the most pressing needs in IBD research, and every facet of the Foundation's research programs are geared to answer these needs. The Foundation's research investment has played a critical role in virtually every area of IBD advancement by supporting work that helped lead to the development of rodent animal models in IBD; the identification of the first IBD gene, NOD2/CARD15, which plays a role in fistulizing Crohn's disease; and early studies in tumor necrosis factor-α that played a role in the development of biologic therapies. Other areas of interest include identification of surrogate markers and understanding environmental issues and issues unique to children and adolescents such as growth retardation and skeletal health.

The Foundation's growing resources are enabling the launch of larger, more complex initiatives as well as the development of consortia and resources. A multi-million dollar effort is currently underway to better understand the human microbiome and its role in IBD, and a new initiative to study genetic aspects of IBD is expected to launch by early 2011. The Pediatric IBD Research Network, a consortium that will eventually grow to 50 centers across North America, is studying risk factors that will enable physicians to predict, at the time of diagnosis, which child is likely to develop severe disease and require surgery early in their disease. The Clinical Research Alliance has more than 40 institutional members and is studying the long-term effects of immunomodulators and biologics on more than 400 pregnant women and their newborns.

The DNA Bank offers more than 1000 carefully phenotyped and genotyped DNA samples from IBD patients, their parents (where possible), or matched controls. Open to qualified IBD researchers, this Bank offers an invaluable tool for studying the IBDs.

Further information about CCFA's research programs and grant opportunities may be found online at CCFA.org.

FUND-RAISING EFFORTS

CCFA does all of the above through contributions from individuals, foundations, and corporations. For fiscal year 2008, total contributions and revenue exceeded $42 million. Eighty cents of every dollar the Foundation raises goes directly toward its mission-critical research, education, and support programs. CCFA consistently meets the standards of an "Accredited Charity" of the Better Business Bureau, and as a reflection of the Foundation's high goals of fiscal accountability, transparency, and measurable results, the Foundation has been given an "A" rating from the American Institute of Philanthropy and a "3 Star" rating from Charity Navigator—two of the world's leading charity evaluators.

You can help—become a professional member today! Encourage your patients and their families to join and become involved with their local chapter activities. CCFA offers great nationwide events: Team Challenge, CCFA's half marathon training program, and Take Steps Walk for Crohn's & Colitis. You can also help the Foundation's future in your estate planning. Every dollar contributed, every hour volunteered, brings us closer to making IBD a disease of the past. To learn more about how you can help, please visit CCFA.org.

CONCLUSION

Over the past four decades, CCFA has become the unmistakable voice for finding answers that will one day lead to a cure for Crohn's disease and ulcerative colitis. The opportunities we can pursue today are significantly more promising than they were only 10 years ago. The Foundation will continue to provide patients and their families with the most accurate, unbiased educational material and support while continuing to help researchers in their efforts to find better therapies—and ultimately a cure.

CCFA offers everyone, lay person and professional alike, a chance to take an active part in the fight against IBD. Together, we can hasten the day when no one has to suffer with these devastating diseases.

Pediatric Patient and Family Support | 148

Maria I. Clavell, Robert D. Baker, and Susan S. Baker

Clinicians managing pediatric inflammatory bowel disease (IBD) experience a twofold challenge: understanding the effect of the diagnosis on the patient and the family unit, and understanding the role IBD plays in the physical and psychological development of children and adolescents. The role of the clinician includes (1) providing education about the medical aspects of the disease and therapy options, including drugs, nutrition, and/or surgery; (2) coordinating care by various medical providers; (3) guidance for development of coping skills to handle the disease; (4) providing education and support to the patient to allow successful transition of care to adult gastroenterologist.

Management of pediatric patients with IBD has been enhanced by advances in drug therapy, nutrition support, early diagnosis, and disease surveillance. These advances along with sources of information and support provide hope for children and families with IBD.

Data on the psychosocial functioning of patients with IBD are limited but is an area of interest for research and study. Research studies have demonstrated that psychosocial functioning is more affected in children with chronic conditions compared with healthy controls.

A combined effort of families, multidisciplinary healthcare providers, and support networks can lead children and adolescents with IBD to successfully integrate in age-appropriate activities and ensure appropriate physical and psychological development.

PEDIATRIC IBD

Except for growth delay, the signs and symptoms of IBD in children and adolescents are similar to those in older individuals. Often, IBD takes a more aggressive and severe form in young people compared with adults. Chronic diseases have the potential to negatively impact the physical and psychological development of children and adolescents. The unpredictability of IBD can be challenging for families and can result in anger and frustration often directed against the medical establishment and the physician providing care.

DIAGNOSIS

The diagnosis of IBD can produce a wide range of emotions in patients and families, including shock, fear, anxiety, guilt, relief, denial, anger, ignorance, and disbelief. As with any chronic illness, patients and families can go through several stages of grief after the initial diagnosis. Sometimes, the parents' hopes or plans for a child may be dashed by the diagnosis of IBD, and this can lead to disappointment in the child himself. The unpredictability of the clinical course, even in the face of compliance with all medical recommendations, is difficult for families to accept or understand. Because 30% of pediatric patients have a positive family history of IBD and can have affected siblings, families are often concerned that the disease will occur in other family members. From the time of the initial diagnosis, it is essential to establish a comprehensive plan for patient care; in other words, a background must be provided for the individuals to learn to live full, productive lives with their diagnosis. Achieving a better understanding of this condition will enhance therapeutic compliance and at the same time decrease levels of anxiety that are known to affect disease exacerbations. Concerns patients and families may have about genetics, malignancy, and the need for surgery are addressed in separate chapters.

EDUCATION

Physicians, nurses, nurse practitioners, and dietitians play important roles as reliable sources of information for the patient and family. The information should be complete and at the same time concise and appropriate for the level of education of the individuals. Because so many aspects of IBD and its effect on the child's life must be discussed, the initial conversations with families can be overwhelming. It is important, at least during the first several months after diagnosis, that the information be repeated in each subsequent encounter and careful efforts made to ensure that the family understands the disease, how it is treated, and how the child's life can be as normal as possible. Education is an essential step that not only helps the individuals understand and live with their disease but also assists in educating patient's contacts at home, at school, and in the community about these conditions. Currently, a variety of sources of information are available through the Internet, ranging from medical research, therapeutic trials, the North American Society for Pediatric Gastroenterology, Hepatology and Nutrition web site, and the Crohn's & Colitis Foundation of America to alternative medicine to bulletin boards for patients and families (see Resource List at the end of the chapter). The depth and topics vary from those suited for healthcare providers to those appropriate for lay people.

CAREGIVERS

A caring sympathetic doctor has a positive influence and creates a sense of confidence at a time when many families are undergoing significant stress. Patients and their families need to be taken care of and viewed as individuals. The effects of IBD go beyond the gastrointestinal tract of the patient to encompass the whole life of the patient, including nutrition, growth, and development. Helping the patient develop a positive self-image and self-confidence is important. Body image in childhood and adolescence is discussed in a separate chapter. In the case of children with IBD, particular attention must be given to maintain the sense of dignity and privacy of patients; this is vital in younger children and adolescents. Discussion of some topics, such as elimination, gas, and menses, can be difficult for the child but important so that appropriate therapy can be prescribed. They may have questions and concerns about areas of their day-to-day functions, and at times, it may be necessary to understand clues about situations they are afraid to bring up. Children and families can develop a sense of isolation when faced with the diagnosis of IBD. Occasionally, the disease may be too embarrassing for them to discuss with friends, extended families, and school contacts. The interest and concern of the caregivers foster a positive relationship that enhances the adherence of the patient to the recommended therapy. Adherence is essential for the long-term management of IBD. Patients need to be motivated to follow their medical regimens even when they begin to feel well to decrease the likelihood of a relapse; patients need to remain on therapy even if there is partial response to therapy or despite side effects of medications. A comprehensive team approach is the most successful way to treat patients diagnosed with IBD. Input from nutritionists, nursing specialists, psychologists, and social services is essential to complete the care and management of these children and their families.

COMPREHENSIVE CARE

A multidisciplinary approach is needed for the care of patients with IBD. Participation of a variety of health professionals may be needed for comprehensive patient care, including physicians, nurses, dietitians, social workers, and psychologists. It is important to educate both parents and children/teens early on regarding the physical and emotional stresses and periodically review the coping skills of patients and families to identify early maladaptive patterns.

Editor's note (TMB): For additional information, see Chapter 5: Pediatric Patient, Family and Physician Interactions and Chapter 6: Teenagers and IBD in VOLUME I and subsequent Chapter 155: Psychosocial Concomitants of Pediatric IBD.

Strategies for Children

Changes in growth and development occur rapidly in children. Interaction with children must be in the context of their cognitive and psychological development, and because they are constantly changing, their healthcare provider must be flexible and able to change as the child does. Children need a comfortable, nonjudgmental place where they can feel safe discussing the problems associated with IBD and exploring strategies they can use to cope and talk about their difficulties. Nevertheless, there are characteristics of IBD that are seen in all patients and have a profound effect on their life. For example, *fatigue* is a common problem of IBD. It can be caused by anemia, diarrhea, inflammation, fever, joint pains, or lack of sleep because of pain or diarrhea. Fatigue can also be caused by depression. Both fatigue from the chronic disease and depression may be present. Children experience a loss of control over their lives, in the larger sense, and in their immediate day-to-day functioning. Children never know when a flair will strike and they will be unable to participate in planned events. They may find school difficult because of the sudden onset of diarrhea. They may fall behind their peers. Drugs, stomas, and fistula alter body image, usually in a negative way. For older children, there is a regression to increased dependence on parents, and this can lead to rebellion and noncompliance. Helping children and parents understand these aspects of the disease can help them develop coping mechanisms and lessen feelings of guilt, helplessness, and fear that are natural and vary according to chronologic age. Children younger than about 7 years interpret their disease and all related procedures as a punishment for wrongdoing. Children between 7 and 10 years view disease as a result of germs and focus on their appearance and ability to perform activities. Impairments on any of these can profoundly affect their self-esteem. Children should be encouraged to participate in the usual age-appropriate activities and not let their disease interfere with their life. Physicians can make specific recommendations to limit activities if needed for limited time periods. Unhealthy adaptive patterns may manifest as externalizing or internalizing behaviors; school avoidance, oppositional behaviors, and depression need to be identified and addressed promptly.

ADOLESCENT EXPERIENCE

Adolescents focus on independence, sexuality, risk taking, and developing a unique identity. All these can be threatened by the constant reminders of their disease, such as intrusive symptoms, and the need to take medications. This along with rebellion that is often observed in their age group can affect their compliance with therapy. A goal for adolescent patients with IBD is a progressive transfer of responsibility for care from their parents. The process should advance under adequate but not overzealous or lax supervision. Sexuality and body image issues are discussed in another chapter.

Editor's note (TMB): For additional information, see Chapter 6: Teenagers and IBD in VOLUME I.

Role of Parents

The adjustments of the child and of the family unit are closely intermingled. The diagnosis of a chronic disease in a child causes turmoil in the family. Anxieties and fears develop and can strain relationships. Effective communication patterns and family involvement are positive factors in the mutual adjustment process. Enmeshment, rejection, and overprotectiveness are counterproductive for both families and patients; however, these behaviors commonly occur. A multidisciplinary support team can be an effective means to achieve healthy adaptive patterns for the family. It is common for parents to develop a sense of isolation that is significantly relieved once they communicate with other families affected by IBD. Unfounded feelings of guilt and helplessness should be addressed with education about the disease process and support services. Financial worries and the difficulty of dealing with third-party payers are areas of concern, frustration, and fear for families both in the short and in the long term. These worries are magnified if a parent must stop working to provide adequate care. Costs of medications, tests, hospitalizations, infusions, and office visits can mount and threaten family stability. In addition, the effect of a chronic disease on long-term insurance procurement remains a concern of many families.

● SUPPORT GROUPS

Support groups play an important role in the life of patients and families diagnosed with IBD. Families need to establish support systems beyond healthcare providers to help them cope and adjust to life with IBD, and each family should decide the type of support group that best suites their needs. There is a variety of support groups available, ranging from chat rooms and message boards on the Internet to informal groups or structured support groups.

Support groups can include individuals with IBD or family members and/or spouses of patients. Support groups provide a network of individuals who face the same experience and with whom they can share information and concerns. This also provides invaluable source of education for those newly diagnosed. Support groups can offer coping strategies and models to follow, and for many, they relate better to individuals in these groups than other peers. For children, attending camp with other patients is an excellent form of peer support.

For additional information, see Chapter 151: Pediatric Patient and Family Support.

● CONCLUSION

The diagnosis of IBD can be devastating for patients and families. They are faced with an overwhelming challenge that initially may threaten the foundations of their stability as individuals and families. Physicians play a key role in educating patients, families, and communities. Through compassion, kindness, and the use of a supporting and caring network system integrating families, healthcare providers, and community resources, patients can live normal, fulfilling lives. The ultimate goal for children with IBD is to learn to live successfully with IBD. Education and support groups, multidisciplinary interventions, and the medical developments provide a positive outlook on the quality of life of children with IBD and their families.

PEDIATRIC AND FAMILY RESOURCES

Crohn's and Colitis Foundation of America, Inc.
386 Park Avenue South, 17 th Floor
New York, NY 10016–8804
Tel: 800 932–2423 or 212 685–3440
e-mail: info@ccfa.org.
www.ccfa.org

National Digestive Diseases Information Clearinghouse
2 Information Way
Bethesda, MD 20892–3570
E-mail: nddic@info.niddk.nih.gov
Pediatric Crohn's and Colitis Association, Inc.
P.O. Box 188 Newton, mA 02168
Tel: 617 244–6678

Reach Out for Youth with Ileitis and Colitis, Inc.
15 Chemung Place
Jericho, NY 11753
Tel: 516 822–8010

United Ostomy Association, Inc.
36 Executive Park Suite 120
Irvine, CA 92714
Tel: 800 826–0826 or 714 660–8624

North American Society for Pediatric Gastroenterology, Hepatology and Nutrition
http://www.naspghan.org

Children's Digestive Health and Nutrition Foundation
http://www.cdhnf.org

References

1. Hanauer S. *Inflammatory Bowel Disease: A Guide for Patients and Their Families.* Philadelphia, PA: Lippincott Raven; 1998.
2. Kim SC, Ferry GD. Inflammatory bowel diseases in pediatric and adolescent patients: clinical, therapeutic, and psychosocial considerations. *Gastroenterology.* 2004;126(6):1550–1560.
3. Mackner LM, Crandall WV. Long-term psychosocial outcomes reported by children and adolescents with inflammatory bowel disease. *Am J Gastroenterol.* 2005;100(6):1386–1392.
4. Mackner LM, Crandall WV. Psychological factors affecting pediatric inflammatory bowel disease. *Curr Opin Pediatr.* 2007;19(5):548–552.
5. Merchant A. Inflammatory bowel disease in children: an overview for pediatric healthcare providers. *Gastroenterol Nurs.* 2007;30(4):278–82; quiz 283.

6. Northam EA. Psychosocial impact of chronic illness in children. *J Paediatr Child Health.* 1997;33(5):369–372.

7. Pidgeon V. Compliance with chronic illness regimens: school-aged children and adolescents. *J Pediatr Nurs.* 1989;4(1):36–47.

8. Polito JM 2nd, Childs B, Mellits ED, Tokayer AZ, Harris ML, Bayless TM. Crohn's disease: influence of age at diagnosis on site and clinical type of disease. *Gastroenterology.* 1996;111(3):580–586.

9. Pope A, Mc Hale S, Craighead WE. *Self-Esteem Enhancement with Children and Adolescents.* New York, NY: Pergamon; 1988.

10. Reichenberg K, Lindfred H, Saalman R. Adolescents with inflammatory bowel disease feel ambivalent towards their parents' concern for them. *Scand J Caring Sci.* 2007;21(4):476–481.

11. Thompson JR, Gustafson KE. *Adaptation to Chronic Childhood Illness.* Washington, DC: American Psychological Association; 1996.

12. Vernon D, Foley JM, Sipowicz RR, et al. *Psychological Responses of Children to Hospitalization and Illness.* Springfield, IL: Charles C. Thomas, 1965;8–58.

Insurance and Disability Advocacy Issues in IBD | 149

Douglas C. Wolf

There are approximately 1.4 million individuals with inflammatory bowel disease (IBD) in the United States of whom, historically, over 15% have been uninsured. Some of these individuals who have IBD are insured but, because of preexisting condition exclusions, do not have insurance that covers their IBD. Others, who have insurance, may have high deductibles such that the insurance is basically "catastrophic coverage" and are underinsured as a result. Unfortunately, complete disability occurs in the IBD population at a frequency that parallels disease severity. Objective criteria for disability due to IBD are delineated by the Social Security Administration. Clearly, paying for healthcare and maintaining disability options is an issue for the IBD population. The following is a summary on the subject of insurance and disability issues in the IBD population with emphasis on how physicians can be better advocates for their patients with IBD.

● VULNERABLE AGE GROUP

The peak age of onset of Crohn's disease and ulcerative colitis (18–24 years) coincides with the peak distribution of the uninsured population. Thirty percent of people between ages 19 and 24 are uninsured. Twenty six percent of people in the age group of 25 to 34 years are uninsured. Parents should understand the coverage options of their particular policy prior to their child's 18th birthday. If one has a chronic illness at age 17, insurance options should be explored to ensure continuity of coverage. Many individuals leave home at this age, and their jobs may not offer insurance or other related benefits. Once healthcare insurance lapses, it can be difficult to reestablish it. There may be a 12-month delay for coverage of preexisting conditions when establishing a new health insurance policy, though pending federal healthcare laws may eliminate this issue. If one takes out a new individual health insurance policy, there is no guarantee of acceptance, and no limit established on the policy premium.

Individuals aged 18 to 23 + may continue on their parent's health insurance if they are true dependents (i.e., living in their home), if they maintain full-time student (college) status, or if they are medically disabled. This can vary depending on the wording of the particular plan. In some states, the upper age limit has been extended, and current healthcare reform includes a proposal for a nationwide upper age limit of 26 years with no restrictions on dependency or student status (Affordable Care Act). Effective October 2009, the "Michelle's Law" allows a seriously ill or injured full-time college student to take up to a year off from school or reduce classes to a part-time load and continue to be covered by their parent's medical insurance.

● CHANGING EMPLOYMENT

An individual with IBD may be turned down when they apply for coverage with a new individual health insurance policy. Key to the insurability determination is the status of the individual's disease. An individual with no hospitalizations over the prior 3 years may qualify but pay a higher rate. An individual with multiple hospitalizations within the past year or so likely would be denied individual coverage, though he or she would likely be included in most large group plans. When individual coverage is obtained, the risk-adjusted premium may amount to several multiples of a standard policy rate. Insurance companies want to avoid any situation in which they will lose money. An insurance agent or broker can help a patient find the best rate. Although insurance consultants are available to make recommendations, these individuals may charge an hourly rate or other fee.

● NEW HEALTH INSURANCE POLICIES

When an individual has an active or chronic medical condition, it is best to be employed by a company that provides health insurance coverage, ideally a company with more than 20 employees, as then most healthcare protections are mandated by law. It would seem acceptable to work for a lower wage, if otherwise unavailable benefits became available as part of the compensation package. Self-employed individuals should contact trade groups, associations, the local Chamber of Commerce, or other groups that may offer group health programs.

Employees change jobs and do not stay with the same employer "for life." Due to economic conditions, 6 million jobs were lost in the year leading up to September 2009, and ongoing job losses are expected. Furthermore, 53% of those newly unemployed are without health insurance. As a result, transitional insurance programs are needed. Such short-term health policies and conversion options exist, and they can be engaged for periods up to 6 months, possibly with one renewal option. Preexisting conditions may be excluded, but the policy may be costly. If one is leaving employment and there is a lapse prior to reemployment, a group medical plan can be converted to an individual plan, for which the full premium is paid.

The Consolidated Omnibus Budget Reconciliation Act (COBRA) of 1985 represented the first national employer mandate to address the portability problems associated with the loss of employment-related health insurance. Any company with a group insurance plan and 20 or more full-time or part-time employees during 50% of the business days in the preceding year must offer COBRA coverage. Under COBRA, continuation of coverage for a period of 18 months can be exercised if coverage is lost due to a "qualifying event," which includes voluntary or involuntary employment termination. If the qualifying event is family related, such as the divorce, legal separation, or death of an insured worker, then coverage is offered for 36 months. The COBRA option, which allows the individual to continue group coverage for the period between jobs, must be exercised within 60 days of the qualifying event, so one must act quickly with a job loss or change. The premium is 102% of the basic coverage cost.

In August 1996, the Kassenbaum-Kennedy Health Insurance Reform Bill was passed and became known as the Health Insurance Portability and Accountability Act (HIPAA). HIPPA's major provision is to prevent gaps in coverage that could expose individuals to preexisting condition exclusions when they change, leave, or lose their job. It has no impact on the uninsured, the unemployed, or on health insurance cost. Although HIPAA applies to those in both group and individual healthcare plans, individual coverage requirements are more stringent than coverage requirements for the group market. Under HIPAA, if one loses or leaves a job but has been continuously insured for the previous 12 months, one can purchase an individual insurance policy. Every insurer must offer two policy options, and exclusions for preexisting conditions are severely curtailed. Key HIPAA provisions include no ineligibility for health-related status, continuity for preexisting conditions, and same rates for those with and without medical problems. Whereas the details of HIPAA may seem complicated, the general message is simple. Individuals changing jobs should obtain details about how HIPAA may apply to them and their families. A certificate of coverage needs to be obtained from the previous employer. This hopefully will lessen the occurrence of "job lock," where one is afraid to change jobs because of fear of losing healthcare coverage and also lessen the problems associated with job loss and job change. The portability of a healthcare plan when one changes, leaves, or loses his or her job is an important benefit for anyone with a chronic illness, such as an individual with IBD.

Managed Care

The majority of health plans currently offered are managed care plans. These plans, offered by most major insurers, attempt to manage cost of care by restricting access. Plans may restrict access to care, particularly subspecialty access, by limiting covered services such as procedures, lab testing, preventive care such as vaccines, and certain prescription drug coverage. Choice of physician is often restricted, as is choice of hospital. The restrictions can have a significant impact on the patient with IBD. Whereas prescription drug coverage often is provided, a particular brand may not be on the managed care formulary. A telephone call or letter to the medical director may be needed to obtain approval for the use of nonformulary medication, and at times, these attempts are repeatedly unsuccessful. Directing one's efforts to the highest level individual accessible is best; direct letters and calls to the Medical Director of the Plan, and if they are not accessible, contact the Pharmacy Director of the plan. In one case that exemplifies others, a month of repeated calls and letters to the Medical and Pharmacy Directors finally led to approval of high-dose anti-TNF therapy for ulcerative colitis (not a covered service). Some prescription assistance programs are listed in Table 149.1.

Table 149.1 Prescription Assistance Programs	
Web Sites	Program
www.together-rx.com	Link to multiple US and Canadian discount pharmacies
www.rxhope.com	Link to 1000 medications, including IBD medications
www.pparx.org	Link to 2500 medications, via patient assistance programs, which include several FDA approved oral mesalamine medications
www.HUMIRAhelp.com	Link to patient assistance program for adalimumab (Humira)
www.cimzia.com/cimpay	Link to patient assistance program for certolizumab pegol (Cimzia)
www.centocoraccessone.com	Link to Centocor (infliximab/Remicade) patient assistance programs
www.pentasaus.com	Link to patient assistance program for mesalamine (Pentasa)
www.lialda.com	Link to patient assistance program for mesalamine (Lialda)
www.asacol.com	Link to patient assistance program for mesalamine (Asacol)
www.salix.com	Link to Salix (balsalazide disodium/Colazal & rifaximin/Xifaxan) patient assistance programs

Table 149.2 Medicare Coverage of IBD Medications	
Part B	Part D
Certolizumab pegol (lyophilized)	Certolizumab pegol (prefilled syringe)
Infliximab	Adalimumab
Natalizumab	Orally administered IBD medications

Benefits Programs

Medicare

Individuals who are 65 years of age or older, or those who have received Social Security Disability Insurance (SSDI) benefits for 2 years, are eligible for Medicare. Medicare is made up of part A, which covers inpatient care or other facility care, and part B, which covers physician care, health worker–administered treatments and several other services, and some supplies that part A does not cover. Medicare D is the category for nearly all Medicare self-administered prescription benefits.

In a standard Medicare policy, medications are not covered services on an outpatient basis, with the exception of health worker–administered medications. *Approved infusion biologics include infliximab, which is approved for both Crohn's disease and ulcerative colitis, and natalizumab, which is approved for Crohn's disease. Adalimumab is a subcutaneously self-administered anti-TNF agent that is covered under part D. Certolizumab is covered under part B for the nurse-administered lyophilized product and under part D for the self-administered prefilled syringe. Virtually all other IBD medications are covered under part D (Table 149.2).*

Medicaid

Medicaid is a state-run program for patients with low income and limited resources. Medicaid programs often service the pediatric population with chronic illnesses such as IBD. For information about Medicaid eligibility in your state, contact the welfare office, which may have a specific name, such as Department of Family and Children Services. Many states also are funding insurance coverage for children through the Children Health Insurance Program (CHIP) legislation. This insurance provides coverage for children of low-income parents who do not qualify for Medicaid.

High-Risk Insurance

High-risk insurance pools provide coverage to people who are unable to obtain private health insurance because of a preexisting condition, such as Crohn's disease or ulcerative colitis. People who do not have insurance available through their place of employment typically use this. Not all states offer high-risk insurance pools. Every state has its own criteria for eligibility and these vary from state to state. The following are usual requirements:

- proof of ineligibility for Medicare or Medicaid
- proof that you were rejected by a private insurer
- proof of your inability to obtain coverage comparable to that offered by the state plan

To determine whether this is available in your state, one should call the State Department of Insurance or the National Association for Insurance Commissioners at 816-842-3600.

Family and Medical Leave

Patients and family members of patients with IBD should be aware of the Family and Medical Leave Act (FMLA). Employers covered by the FMLA must, pursuant to a written company policy, give an eligible employee the right to take unpaid leave for up to 12 work weeks in a year if his own medical condition or that of a family member makes him unable to perform his job. To be eligible, the employee must

- have worked for this employer for at least 12 months
- have completed at least 1250 hours of service during the previous year
- work at a site within a 75-mile radius of 50 employees of the company.

The following are qualifying criteria for a patient with a chronic condition such as IBD that

- requires periodic hospital visits for treatment
- continues over an extended period of time
- causes episodic rather than continuous incapacity.

The law protects any employee from being disciplined or discharged for requesting or using FMLA leave. A patient who is experiencing a flare-up or a family member who is providing support or comfort to a patient may take leave. If the leave is foreseeable, 30 days notice must be given. If the leave is unforeseeable, then 2 working days notice is needed. The employee may be responsible for paying 100% of his or her medical insurance premiums while on leave, depending on an employer's written FMLA policy. Although FMLA protects most employees, "key employees," who are exempt from overtime laws and are among the highest paid, may be subject to certain qualifications at the time of their job restoration.

Disability Programs

Social Security Disability Benefits

If an individual's IBD has progressed to the point that the individual is not able to continue to work or function for a sustained period, then an application to the Social Security Administration is appropriate. Individuals can obtain applications and assistance for Social Security Disability from the local Social Security Office. Social Security offers a toll-free number (800–772-1213) for information, including the location of the nearest Social Security Office. The Web site is www.ssa.gov (Table 149.3). The treating physician must submit a report to Social Security, documenting the nature and features of the disability. Reapplication is part of the process. The greatest frequency of approvals occurs upon repeated reapplication, when the case is presented at a hearing before a Social Security Administrative law judge. The initial application may be initiated by the patient or family, but reapplications are most successful if the assistance of a disability attorney or related professional is sought.

Table 149.3 Helpful Web Sites for Assisting the IBD Patient

Web Sites	Organization
www.ccfa.org	Crohn's and Colitis Foundation (CCFA)
www.MyIBD.org	The Foundation for Clinical Research in IBD
www.advocacy for patients.org	Advocacy for Patients with Chronic Illness, Inc.
www.ada.gov	Americans with Disabilities Act (provisions)
www.ssa.gov	Social Security Administration
www.hhs.gov	Department of Health and Human Resources (HIPPA, Civil Rights)

Table 149.4 Listing of Impairments

Inflammatory bowel disease (IBD [5.06]) documented by endoscopy, biopsy, appropriate medically acceptable imaging, or operative findings with:

A. Obstruction of stenotic areas (not adhesions) in the small intestine or colon with proximal dilatation, confirmed by appropriate medically acceptable imaging or in surgery, requiring hospitalization for intestinal decompression or for surgery, and occurring on at least two occasions at least 60 days apart within a consecutive 6-month period.

OR

B. Two of the following despite continuing treatment as prescribed and occurring within the same consecutive 6-month period:

　1. Anemia with hemoglobin of less than 10.0 g/dL, present on at least two evaluations at least 60 days apart.

　2. Serum albumin of 3.0 g/dL or less, present on at least two evaluations at least 60 days apart;

　3. Clinically documented tender abdominal mass palpable on physical examination with abdominal pain or cramping that is not completely controlled by prescribed narcotic medication, present on at least two evaluations at least 60 days apart.

　4. Perineal disease with a draining abscess or fistula, with pain that is not completely controlled by prescribed narcotic medication, present on at least two evaluations at least 60 days apart.

　5. Involuntary weight loss of at least 10% from baseline, as computed in pounds, kilograms, or BMI, present on at least two evaluations at least 60 days apart.

　6. Need for supplemental daily enteral nutrition via a gastrostomy or daily parenteral nutrition via a central venous catheter.

Short bowel syndrome (SBS [5.07]) due to surgical resection of more than one-half of the small intestine, with dependence on daily parenteral nutrition via a central venous catheter (see 5.00F).

Weight loss due to any digestive disorder [5.08] despite continuing treatment as prescribed, with BMI of less than 17.50 calculated on at least two evaluations at least 60 days apart within a consecutive 6-month period.

There are two ways in which the application of an individual with IBD may be approved. The first way is when criteria are met or exceeded in the "Listing of Impairments" in Table 149.4. The second way disability can be justified is by demonstrating that the symptoms, such as diarrhea, pain, or fatigue, preclude full-time employment. There are no specific criteria for this, and a thorough description of the nature of the symptoms and their ramifications is needed. Proper documentation in the medical record is important because the entire medical record will be reviewed multiple times. A thorough summary letter is necessary as part of the disability application. It should reflect the level of symptoms and disability contained in the medical record (see section on "Disability Letters").

Returning to Work After Social Security Disability

Individuals who recover from their disability can try to return to work or train for a new career. Increasingly, individual clinical responses to immunotherapy (e.g., azathioprine or 6-mercaptopurine), biologic therapy (e.g., antitumor necrosis factor/anti-TNF), and surgery are restoring the health of patients with IBD. The Social Security Administration offers work incentives that allow the patient to continue to receive monthly benefits for a set period of time while returning to work or while entering a vocational training program. These programs allow a patient to attempt work reentry and to determine whether they are able to work on a regular basis, without risking or reapplying for benefits. Work incentives differ with Social Security Insurance and SSDI. Detailed information is available from the Social Security Administration.

Americans with Disabilities Act

The American Disabilities Act (ADA) was enacted in 1991 and revised with major amendments in 1995 and 2008. The ADA Amendment Act of 2008 broadened the definition of disability, thereby benefiting many individuals with chronic illness. This federal legislation has implications during the hiring process and throughout employment. The ADA prohibits discrimination on the basis of disability in employment, state and local government, public accommodation, commercial facilities, transportation, and telecommunications. To be protected by the ADA, one must have a disability or have a relationship or association with an individual with a disability. To get a thorough overview of the provisions of the ADA, go to the Web site www.ada.gov. Employers may not base their decisions to hire an individual on the basis of his or her disabilities.

Once an employer has knowledge that an employee is disabled, the employer is required under the ADA to provide reasonable accommodations to the affected employee. For an individual with IBD, the accommodations may be relatively simple: more time for necessary visits to the restroom and flexible time schedules for diet or rest. Extra time off may be needed for exacerbations or hospitalizations. Each case depends on a set of variables, and the employee's needs must be balanced by the ability of the employer to provide the requested accommodations.

Education for the Disabled Patient with IBD

The All Handicapped Children's Act of 1975 guarantees a free public education for all children with disabilities. If a child is unable to attend school because of a disabling chronic illness, home schooling or in-hospital instruction must be provided. This usually is needed for limited periods of time. It is best if students and parents work together with teachers and the school system to help provide this benefit. The Crohn's & Colitis Foundation of America (CCFA) brochure, "A Teacher's Guide to Crohn's Disease and Ulcerative Colitis," is helpful in this dialogue.

The 1973 Rehabilitation Act, Section 504, addresses discrimination in higher education. This ruling covers any program or activity that receives financial assistance from the US Department of Education, and this includes public school districts, institutions of higher education, and other state and local education agencies. Medical information can be requested only after the student has been accepted to a school and, once obtained, cannot be used to exclude a student from school activities. Additional information can be obtained from the Office for Civil Rights, US Department of Health and Human Services, 200 Independence Ave., Washington, DC 20201 or www.hhs.gov/ocr.

Disability Letters

Physicians are periodically asked to write letters on behalf of patients to justify their disability or accommodation. It is a physician's responsibility to write these letters so patients obtain the benefits that they are entitled to under the law. It is important to explain how the symptoms of the medical condition (e.g., Crohn's disease or ulcerative colitis) qualify for disability under the law. Try to use key terms that will justify a favorable decision. If abdominal pain is a symptom and it is frequent or chronic, explain that the patient is unable to concentrate or work for any substantial period of time because of the degree and duration of the pain or the need to take (e.g., narcotic) medications to control the pain. If diarrhea is a symptom, and it is frequent, explain that the diarrhea (and perhaps, the associated cramping), frequently leads to interruptions in work and focus, as well as fatigue and need for rest. One might suggest that the fluid and electrolyte losses likely contribute to fatigue or weakness. In addition, if there has been 10% loss of body weight, a Hgb <10 and/or albumin <3.0, these are additional objective parameters that will strengthen or "clinch" the disability claim. Criteria in Table 149.4 can be used and expanded on to support the need for disability. Although not specifically listed in the table from the Social Security Administration, extraintestinal manifestations or secondary emotional considerations (e.g., depression) in the context of IBD may constitute justification for disability. There are newly added "sample" disability and related letters available to physicians on the CCFA Web site (Table 149.3).

Accommodations are needed for individuals when the typical work day or work situation is too difficult for them. An employee or a student with IBD may need accommodation for extra "breaks" to go to the bathroom, without penalty. Many schools require bathroom passes or have other rules. It is best if the parent and/or student address the potential need early, at the beginning of the year, or upon return to school, so that there is a clear understanding of the real need for the accommodation. Employees or students with active disease may need extra time off, more frequent absences or time off for infusions, doctors' visits, and lab testing. It is better to overestimate rather than underestimate these potential needs. The criteria for Social Security Disability have been modified since the last edition of this book and further refinements of the criteria are expected. Updates can be viewed at www.ssa.gov.

DISABILITY INSURANCE

Individual disability insurance is difficult to obtain once a diagnosis of IBD has been made. If insurance is available, a significant surcharge may apply. Group disability insurance is often part of the benefits package of large companies. If one has disability insurance, it is best to maintain it, and this may be possible even when one changes jobs. However, HIPAA and other related legislation applies to health insurance and not to disability or other insurance.

SUMMARY

It is important for the treating physician to be knowledgeable about health insurance and disability issues to provide the best guidance and information for patients with IBD. Evolving federal disability and health insurance reforms can be followed at www.healthcare.gov.

Special Tips Regarding Health Insurance and Disability Rights

1. Keep health insurance coverage current—do not allow insurance policy to lapse.
2. If you do NOT have health insurance coverage, research options for obtaining it.
3. Be sure to visit your physician for periodic/regular visits because insurers look favorably on patients who do so and are involved in their own care. Regular visits also help keep you well.
4. Taking medication as prescribed is extremely important! IBD rarely improves without medication. Continue to take medication as prescribed even if taking medication temporarily disallows eligibility for an insurance plan.
5. If possible, choose a job with group insurance coverage and portable benefits.
6. For parents of children with IBD, anticipate their need for modified coverage prior to their 18th birthday. Consult with your insurance agent or benefits representative well in advance of reaching age of 18 to determine the best options for continuing coverage after 18.

Editor's note (TMB): We are grateful for Dr. Wolf's researching this important area and providing guidance for us to help our patients get the benefits they deserve.

References

1. Ananthakrishnan AN, Weber LR, Knox JF, et al. Permanent work disability in Crohn's disease. *Am J Gastroenterol.* 2008;103(1):154–161.
2. Feagan BG, Bala M, Yan S, Olson A, Hanauer S. Unemployment and disability in patients with moderately to severely active Crohn's disease. *J Clin Gastroenterol.* 2005;39(5):390–395.
3. Fuller A. Young adults swelling ranks of uninsured. *The New York Times.* September 5, 2009: p.A10.
4. Jaffe JC. *Know Your Rights: A Handbook for Patients with Chronic Illness.* Advocacy for Patients with Chronic Illnesses, Inc. 2008.
5. Loftus EV, Guerin A, Yu AP. Direct and indirect economic burdens and impact on salary growth of moderate to severe Crohn's disease. *Gastroenterol Hepatol.* 2009;5(8) (suppl 17):15.
6. Longobardi T, Jacobs P, Bernstein CN. Work losses related to inflammatory bowel disease in the United States: results from the National Health Interview Survey. *Am J Gastroenterol.* 2003;98:1064–1072.
7. March, Bill. Jobless, sleepless, hopeless. *The New York Time Week in Review.* September 6, 2009: p.4.
8. Procaccini NJ, Bickston SJ. Disability in inflammatory bowel diseases: impact of awareness of the Americans with Disabilities Act. *Practical Gastroenterol.* 2007:16–23.
9. Crohn's & Colitis Foundation of America, Inc. www.ccfa.org. Accessed September 4, 2009.
10. Social Security Administration. Disability Evaluation Under Social Security, Blue Book. September 2008. www.ssa.gov/disability/professionals/bluebook/5.00-digestive-adult.htm. Accessed October 10, 2009.

Sexual Adjustments and Body Image | 150

Paula Erwin-Toth

The effect of inflammatory bowel disease (IBD) on body image, sexuality, and sexual functioning ranges from minor to profound. Physical and psychosexual adjustments depend on the extent and progress of the disease, side effects of medications, and individual variables. No one responds to a chronic illness in exactly the same way; however, there are some interventions that the physicians and healthcare professionals caring for these patients can implement to assist patients facing difficulties with body image and sexual adjustments. Detailed interventions and therapies relating to sexual counseling are beyond the scope of this chapter. Persons with persistent or severe sexual adjustment difficulties or a history of sexual trauma should be referred to a licensed sex therapist specializing in sexuality and chronic illness.

DISCUSSION OPPORTUNITIES

The most important intervention is to give the patient permission and encouragement to discuss matters related to body image and sexuality in a supportive, unhurried manner. In a busy clinical practice, this is often easier said than done. The benefits to patients in their overall adjustment to IBD as well as adherence to the medical regime can be enhanced by attention to this important topic. A brief statement relating to coping, body image, and sexuality as it relates to IBD can open the door to discussion. The age, gender, and sexual orientation of the patient are important considerations. Whether they are or have been sexually active, married or single, divorced or widowed can provide helpful baseline information. Some authors suggest that this type of data can be gathered from a brief questionnaire, but others claim that this type of personal disclosure is best obtained on a one-to-one basis.

BODY IMAGE

Body image is defined as the way in which we view ourselves within the context of our physical being. Body image is a component of self-concept, but the sense of self has an even more all-encompassing presence in an individual. For example, children born with birth defects have no inborn knowledge that they are different from other children; despite profound problems, many can be raised with a good self-concept that enables them to cope with the fact of their physical challenges and to feel positive about themselves and their bodies. Conversely, the literature is filled with evidence of body-image and self-concept disorders in persons with no outward physical challenges—indeed, many with what others consider highly attractive physical characteristics. It is important for the clinician to ascertain the patient's pre-illness and present body-image and self-concept patterns. This information can provide clues as to the duration and extent of the problem.

COPING MECHANISMS

Gaining insight into successful and unsuccessful coping mechanisms that the patient has developed can assist in developing a plan of care. Locus of control, a concept frequently applied in studies of patients with diabetes mellitus, has applicability to persons living with IBD. Determining an individual's locus of control in life and management of disease can provide valuable information as well. Does the person view himself or herself as helpless over fate? These individuals demonstrate a sense of little to no control and no desire or perceived ability to exert control over their lives, disease, or therapies. They are said to have an external locus of control and may need specific advice and exercises to address their issues regarding body image and sexual adjustment.

Individuals with an internal locus of control demonstrate a sense of mastery over self and events. When IBD does not respond the way they want it to, such patients may need to undertake some general coping and relaxation strategies to enhance adjustment to the unpredictable nature of the disease. Events beyond their direct control can pose coping difficulties for these patients in all aspects of their lives.

SEXUAL ADJUSTMENT PROBLEMS

Sexual adjustment problems and IBD can be related to three key areas: the disease process itself, side effects of medications, and psychosexual or psychosocial influences. The duration and extent of the disease has a direct impact on sexual adjustment. Frequent stools, abdominal pain, fatigue, and perianal skin problems ranging from irritation to fistulae are some of the most common problems related to body image and sexual adjustment. Problems with extraintestinal manifestations of IBD, pelvic floor dysfunction, dyspareunia, and tenesmus can interfere with normal sexual functioning. Patients who require abdominal stomas or who experience enterocutaneous fistulae or other skin problems benefit from the interventions of an enterostomal therapy nurse for physical and psychological rehabilitation. There is a separate chapter on enterostomal therapy.

The myriad of medications used to treat the condition can alleviate or control many of the symptoms of IBD. Unfortunately, the side effects of these same medications can create a whole new set of difficulties for the patient. Mood swings, loss of libido, impotence, vaginal dryness, and weight gain are only a few of the complications patients may experience as a result of medications used to treat IBD. Concerns regarding sexual activity and reproduction are common in relation to both the disease and the treatments. Use of budesonide, a rapidly metabolized steroid with less side effects, is discussed in two separate chapters.

● STAGES OF LIFE

Individual psychosexual and psychosocial characteristics determine how a patient is able to adjust to the progress of the disease and therapies. Erikson's Theory of Psychosocial Development can provide some insight into developmental crises and tasks people face at various stages of their lives. Because IBD can occur at almost any time across the life span, it is important for the clinician to consider the potential effects of IBD in patients of all ages. Even those with longstanding disease will face new challenges as they age and the progress of their disease changes. These challenges will, in turn, have an impact on body image and sexual adjustment.

Infancy and Childhood

A sense of trust versus mistrust is being established in infancy. Although diagnosis of IBD in this age group is relatively rare, parents have reported that children diagnosed with IBD demonstrated gastrointestinal difficulties in infancy. Separations and discomfort caused by physical symptoms and medical tests may interfere with an infant's ability to trust and potentially threaten parent-child bonding.

Toddlers are said to be developing a sense of autonomy versus shame. At this stage, IBD presents particular challenges, as the child attempts to gain mastery over himself and his environment, especially toilet training. A sense of self and burgeoning body image can be at odds with the symptoms and management of IBD.

Preschoolers are developing initiative versus guilt. A diagnosis of IBD at this stage could lead a child to believe his efforts at increased independence and inventiveness are being thwarted or punished. As children enter the school-age years, the developmental crisis experienced is industry versus inferiority.

These years are instrumental, as a child develops a sense of pride and accomplishment, an emphasis on peer relationships, and a heightened self-concept and body image. During these years, IBD can disrupt education and recreational activities critical to normal development. The chapter on the pediatric patient and family support addresses some of these issues.

Adolescence

During the teen years, IBD is particularly challenging for the young person establishing a sense of identity versus identity diffusion. Efforts to establish greater independence from parents and strong peer relationships and a strong emphasis on body image, sexual attractiveness, and potential sexual activity can be thwarted by the disease and associated therapies. Young adults face further issues relating to establishing a sense of intimacy versus isolation. The presence of IBD could potentially interfere with their ability to establish a meaningful relationship with another, establish a career, and further their independence from their parents. A protracted illness may leave a young adult with conflicting emotions and desires.

Middle Years

During the middle years, IBD occurs at a time when adults are establishing generativity versus stagnation. This is generally a time of maximum earning potential, launching of offspring to adulthood, and caring for aging parents, combined with the onset of menopause and perceived loss of youth and vitality. At this stage of life, IBD can present with particular difficulties, as patients are coping with multiple challenges. Concerns over sexual attractiveness and sexual function can be of special significance during midlife.

Older Adults

Older adults said to be undergoing ego integrity versus despair can be especially vulnerable to the physical, sexual, and financial aspects of living with IBD. The need to maintain social contacts, including intimate relationships, can be adversely affected by IBD. Potential loss of self-esteem and social isolation can be devastating to seniors coping with IBD.

● RISK FACTORS FOR ADJUSTMENT DIFFICULTIES

High-risk indicators for sexual adjustment difficulties in patients with IBD include lack of social support, family or relationship dysfunction, history of alcohol or drug abuse or eating disorders, and history of coping difficulties. On an intrapersonal level, persons with low self-esteem or other self-concept disturbances, including expressions of powerlessness or hopelessness, high or mild anxiety, anger or depression, are at high risk. The socioeconomic impact of IBD cannot be overlooked. Financial worries related to employment and insurance difficulties can combine to erode self-esteem and have a negative impact on intimate relationships.

● COMMUNICATION PATTERNS

Establishing and maintaining effective communication patterns are essential to overall coping with IBD and enable the patient to make successful sexual adjustments as they live with the disease. Active listening is the cornerstone of successful two-way communication. The permission, limited information, specific suggestions, intensive therapy model can be a useful guide to the clinician providing sexual counseling and rehabilitation.

The first step, permission, opens the door to frank discussion of the patient's sexual concerns. In the second step, limited information, the clinician provides factual information related to the patient's current condition. The third phase, specific suggestions, focuses on interventions tailored for the patient's specific needs and concerns. Finally, if the clinician determines deep-seated or complex sexual problems, the fourth phase, intensive therapy, should be considered. Intensive therapy will require the interventions of a licensed sex therapist, psychologist, psychiatrist, or, in the case of some conditions such as a rectovaginal fistula, a surgical consultation.

Sexual adjustments to IBD are as varied as the symptoms and patients themselves. It is the responsibility of the clinician to address patient concerns regarding body image and sexual adjustments in an open, individualized manner. Changes in the patient's physical, developmental, intrapersonal, or socioeconomic status will signal the need for the clinician to modify the plan of care to optimize the patient's body image and sexual functioning.

Editor's note (TMB): The concept of an IBD nurse advocate is discussed in a separate chapter. The issues in this chapter on sexuality and body image could be addressed by nursing personnel as well as, if not better than, by the physicians.

Further Reading

1. Annon JS. The PLISSIT model: a proposed conceptual scheme for the behavioral treatment of sexual problems. *Sex Educ Ther.* 1972;2:1.

2. Benirschke R. *Alive and Kicking.* San Diego, CA: Firefly Press; 1996.

3. Engström I. Family interaction and locus of control in children and adolescents with inflammatory bowel disease. *J Am Acad Child Adolesc Psychiatry.* 1991;30(6):913–920.

4. Erikson E. *Childhood and Society.* 2nd ed. New York: WW Norton; 1993.

5. Erwin-Toth P. Enterostomal therapy. In: Corman M, ed. *Colon and Rectal Surgery.* 4th ed. Philadelphia, PA: Lippincott-Raven; 1998.

6. Erwin-Toth P. The effect of ostomy surgery between the ages of 6 and 12 years on psychosocial development during childhood, adolescence, and young adulthood. *J Wound Ostomy Continence Nurs.* 1999;26(2):77–85.

7. Kane S. Women's issues in inflammatory bowel disease. Foundation Focus. Magazine of the Crohn's & Colitis Foundation of America. 1999; Summer:16–18.

8. Konen JC, Summerson JH, Dignan MB. Family function, stress, and locus of control. Relationships to glycemia in adults with diabetes mellitus. *Arch Fam Med.* 1993;2(4):393–402.

Behavioral Therapy

Psychiatric Disorders in IBD

151

Glenn J. Treisman

INTRODUCTION

There is a longstanding acknowledgment of the complex inter-active relationship between psychologic states and gastrointestinal (GI) dysfunction. The psychiatric conditions associated with bowel diseases include complex changes in cognition, mood, sensory processing, behavior, and psychologic function. Psychiatric conditions occur both as a result of GI disorders and as a risk factor for GI disorders. Historically, GI disorders have been ascribed to underlying psychiatric conditions, and psychologic symptoms ascribed to a variety of GI disorders. Psychoanalysis, which dominated psychiatric thought through the 1930s to 1960s, was thought to be an effective treatment for bowel conditions of nearly every sort. Orgel reported complete cure of ulcer disease in 10 out of 15 patients treated with psychoanalysis.[1] The 10 patients who were cured all completed their analysis (deep analysis 5 times a week for 3 to 5 years with a range of 592–942 sessions, 50-minute analytic sessions), whereas the 5 who failed to complete their analysis all had ulcer recurrence. The origins of "psychosomatic medicine" are rooted in the relationship between GI disorders and psychiatry. Terms like "rumination" are used to describe both psychologic and digestive phenomena, and phrases like "follow your gut" allude to the relationship between emotion and visceral sensation.

PSYCHOLOGIC ISSUES IN PATIENTS WITH IBD

The first category of psychiatric problems includes conditions traditionally associated with psychologic understanding of the individual patient. These include the disorders related to inadequate parenting, trauma, negative experiences, and deprivation. In the GI clinic, patients present with symptoms that represent being "overmastered" as described by Jerome Frank in the 1960s. They have difficulty managing relationships, their disorder, and their lives. They may come because of family conflict, sexual or physical misuse, or because they simply feel incapable of managing their GI condition. Again, these patients often have comorbidity and vulnerability caused by the conditions described previously, but it is critical to recognize the role of the experience of the individual for treatment to be successful.

The concept that adverse life experiences can result in mental disorders has become unfashionable in a world that is driven by *DSM* (*Diagnostic and Statistical Manual of Mental Disorders*) codes. Life experience is difficult to subject to randomized clinical trials and does not fit well into "evidence-based medicine" but is an important way to understand human behavior. Behavior develops out of the assumptions one makes about the world. A patient with limited resources and chronic bowel disease may have had a very negative experience with institutional medicine and may, therefore, be hostile and irritable on initial contact. This in turn generates behavior that may cause staff and physicians to become defensive and uncomfortable. Emotionally provoked staff members will behave in ways that only further confirm the patient's expectation that they will receive bad treatment. This cycle can be interrupted at any point in its evolution. The clinician can behave as if the patient is very important despite the patient's misbehavior. This often leads to a change in the patient's experience. The clinician might point out the meaning of the patient's behavior leading to altered assumptions about the clinical experience. The clinician might confront some of the assumptions the patient has made and, with cognitive therapy, he or she can change those assumptions. Finally, behavioral interventions will alter the patient's behavior, and this may lead to a positive experience in the office.

Good clinicians recognize the need to change this cycle instinctively and use variations of this method in a manner that becomes reflexive. The difficulty is that they are not systematically supported for doing so. There is no reimbursable *DSM* code that allows them to bill for the time they spend working on this element of patient care, yet they must spend the time to succeed with difficult patients. Moreover, confrontation about behavior, behavioral requirements, and directive treatments are not valued in the era of patient (customer) satisfaction. The current politically correct climate that requires clinicians to accept any goal a patient brings, even an unhealthy goal, undermines the need for guidance and direction from the clinician for these patients. Sadly, the term "patient-centered care" has become synonymous with "patient-directed care," much to the detriment of this group of patients. Patients require an understanding of the psychologic precedents that shape their behavior and need a clinician willing to intervene in their behavior and shape it toward more adaptive and successful function.

● PSYCHIATRIC DISEASES IN PATIENTS WITH IBD

The psychiatric conditions that we see in the GI clinic can be categorized as described by Dr. Edwin in chapter 151.

Some disorders in psychiatry can be thought of as diseases; that is, they represent dysfunction produced by a broken part, or lesion in an area of the brain. These are conditions that are best modeled by lesions of the CNS and have a syndromal nature with categorical features. These conditions make the most sense to gastroenterologists, as they fit our logic when considering diagnosis. These conditions include depression, schizophrenia, bipolar disorder, and Alzheimer's dementia. The most important one for our discussion is major depression, as it has the greatest comorbidity with GI conditions.

Depression

"Major depression" is the term currently used to describe a syndrome recognized since the time of the ancient Greeks. The features include an abrupt decline in function in a previously healthy person accompanied by a decline in mood, sense of wellness and energy (vital sense), and sense of being a good, useful, and valuable (self-attitude). There is also a profound loss of the ability to experience pleasure (anhedonia) that some think is the core feature of the condition. The condition also often involves anxiety, excessive rumination, sleep disruption, loss of appetite, impaired cognition, and in extreme cases, hallucinations and delusions. The term "depression" can also be used to describe the psychologic state of decreased mood that accompanies a psychologic loss or disruption. The DSM uses the term "adjustment disorder" but we prefer the term favored by Jerome Frank, "demoralization." In the diagram in Fig. 151.1 there is a third category shown, which is labeled "dysthymia." Dysthymia is used to describe chronic depression, pessimistic and negative personality style, and mild (subsyndromal) major depression. As is shown in the figure, there is overlap, and patients can suffer from both or even all three conditions.

In medically ill patients with bowel disease it can be hard to distinguish demoralization from major depression, but both are seen at higher rates in patients with inflammatory bowel disease. The criteria in *DSM* were developed out of observations made in general populations of people presenting for psychiatric treatment. Vital sense is diminished by illness, and mood is lowered by the burdens imposed by illness. Anhedonia, associated with such signs as loss of pleasure, satiation, or satisfaction associated with appetite-directed behaviors (food, sex, and sleep) or daily functions (work, hobbies, and exercise), is probably the most sensitive and specific diagnostic finding in our experience. Patients will say that they no longer feel they can go on with treatment or that they have become isolated or just that they feel ill, but a careful interview will reveal that things that they ordinarily enjoy or find diverting have lost their savor.

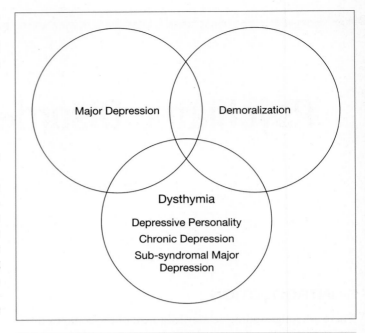

FIGURE 151.1 • Depression, demoralization, and dysthymia in a Venn diagram.

Demoralization responds to support, encouragement, therapeutic optimism, and the "tincture of time." Most of these are familiar and tools for gastroenterologists. Major depression responds to antidepressants (and some types of psychotherapy, though this is a contentious issue).

There is increasing evidence that many inflammatory conditions cause or trigger mood disorders, in part through the actions of cytokines and the hypothalamic-pituitary-adrenal stress axis. Patients with a variety of psychiatric disorders are at higher risk for several GI conditions, and there is often debate about which came first, as the symptoms of many psychiatric disorders and GI disorders are overlapping. This is not surprising given the fact that the GI tract has a nervous system with great complexity that is derived from the same embryonic tissue as the central nervous system.

There is a complex relationship between inflammatory diseases and major depression. It is clear that depression is often an underlying driver of GI complaints, particularly in functional bowel disease such as irritable bowel disease. Major depression has many physiologic manifestations, including autonomic changes and bowel dysfunction. Depression has also been associated directly with many inflammatory conditions, and cytokines have been shown to produce a variety of depression-like syndromes in animal models. There is increasing evidence that the stress axis and the immune system are integrally involved in major depression. One question that has arisen is whether depression exacerbates inflammatory bowel disease or whether inflammatory bowel disease causes depression.

Studies have shown that there is a relationship between depression and a worsened course of IBD. There is some evidence for an increased risk of developing depression in patients with IBD, and some evidence that depression exacerbates IBD.

In a meta-analytic review of the area, depression or stress-related symptoms correlated with more relapse or a worsened course in populations of either UC or Crohn's disease, but not in mixed populations.[2] Furthermore, Maunder et al. reported that in pANCA-negative UC, disease activity was correlated with depression and stress whereas in pANCA-positive UC patients no correlation was seen.[3] The degree of association between depression and IBD is less than that observed with IBS, but the increasing evidence for a link between depression and autoimmune inflammatory disorders has made this an area of increasing interest.

Treatment of Depression

Slide 1 shows a categorical list of the currently available antidepressants. There are many methodological issues in comparing the drugs, but all of the drugs have been shown to be effective in about two thirds of patients with major depression. The choice of drug is directed at which side effects will be helpful rather than harmful when considering the underlying GI problems faced by the patient. It is unclear why some drugs seem to be more beneficial in some patients and poses intriguing basic science questions as well. For instance, one report showed differential effects of antidepressants on TNF-alpha, though the significance of the finding remains unclear.[4]

Tricyclic Antidepressants

Tricyclic antidepressants vary in the degree of anticholinergic effects that they produce, but these effects can be helpful in some patients. They promote weight gain, decrease GI motility, ameliorate chronic pain, promote sleep, and decrease anxiety. They have therapeutic ranges that are meaningful but have a narrow therapeutic index, so levels must be monitored. They cause varying degrees of alpha-adrenergic blockade and, thus, may cause orthostatic blood pressure changes. They have quinidine-like effects on cardiac function and can produce fatal arrhythmias at toxic levels. Patients complain of dry mouth, urinary retention, constipation, weight gain, dizziness, blurred vision, and even confusion. Despite these issues, we have found these to be very useful in the treatment of depressed patients with inflammatory bowel disease.

SSRI and SNRI Antidepressants

Fluoxetine (originally marketed as Prozac) was the first SSRI drug approved in the United States (it was citalopram elsewhere) and introduced a revolution in the treatment. These drugs were (and are) fairly easy to use, have a broad therapeutic index, are simple to dose, and are mostly well tolerated. They have little anticholinergic activity (paroxetine has the most and has anticholinergic activity that can be of clinical significance), do not produce orthostatic changes, and are far less toxic than tricyclic antidepressants. SSRIs are all somewhat GI activating, which can produce diarrhea (sertraline seems to cause the most), but this can be useful in patients with slowed gut function. All can produce a very unpleasant sense of restlessness in some patients. All can produce apathy in some patients. All can produce decreased sexual drive and anorgasmia (they are used for premature ejaculation), but this effect occurs in a minority of patients. One

admonition is that higher doses of the drug are needed for full clinical effect than the doses commonly used in general practice. Although this can be debated, the doses used in registration trials are usually too low to get maximal benefit in patients.

The SNRI drugs are have noradrenergic effects that sometimes make them effective when SSRI drugs fail. They may produce less apathy and are more useful for chronic pain. In patients with chronic GI pain we have found these drugs more useful. The same issue for dosing is true here as well.

Other Agents

The other agents frequently used are listed in Table 151.1. Trazodone is a heterocyclic agent, much safer than TCAs, and usually used for sleep because it is so sedating rather than as an antidepressant. A much less sedating drug, nefazodone, has similar properties and would probably be widely used if it were not for the rare but serious hepatotoxicity that can occur. Both are useful for chronic pain, have relatively less anticholinergic effects than TCAs, but have enough to be therapeutic in patients

TABLE 151.1 Commonly Used Antidepressants

	Distinction
Tricyclic Antidepressants	
Protriptyline	Most potent, least alpha block and least anticholinergic, least sedating
Desipramine	Slightly more anticholinergic and alpha blocking, slightly more sedation
Nortriptyline	Slightly more anticholinergic and alpha blocking, slightly more sedation (this is the TCA I use most in GI patients)
Doxepin	Most sedating second-generation tricyclic-good for sleep and antihistaminic
Imipramine	More anticholinergic and sedating
Clomipramine	Similar to imipramine but best TCA for OCD patients
Amitriptyline	More anticholinergic and sedating
SSRIs	
Citalopram	Relatively balanced profile
Escitalopram	S-isomer of citalopram
Fluoxetine	Longest half-life, a little more motor activation
Fluvoxamine	Approved for OCD, profile between citalopram and fluoxetine
Paroxetine	Most anti-cholinergic (still modest effect for most), most sedation, most weight gain
Sertraline	Most GI activating (I use this first in gastroparesis)

Continued

TABLE 151.1 *Continued*

SNRIs	Better for chronic pain than SSRIs and more adrenergic activity
Duloxetine	Balanced activity
Desvenlafaxine	Metabolite of and slightly less activation than venlafaxine
Milnacipran	Probably least activating, newest agent and therefore least experience using it
Venlafaxine	Most activating SNRI and probably better as a twice a day drug, use XR formulation, better tolerated
Atypical agents	
Trazodone	Heterocyclic antidepressant with much less toxicity than TCAs. Good for sleep but most patients cannot tolerate a therapeutic dose (400–600 mg)
Nefazodone	Heterocyclic antidepressant with much less toxicity than TCAs and much less sedation than trazodone. Unpopular due to rare but serious hepatotoxicity. Safer alternative to TCAs with some of their advantages.
Miratzepine	Sedating and good for sleep, much apetite stimulation and weight gain. Safer alternative to TCAs with some of their advantages.
Bupropion	Least sedating antidepressant, least sexual side effects. Use slow release formulation. Lowers seizure threshold.
Monoamine oxidase inhibitors	Important but rarely used class of agents, usually reserved for expert use in refractory cases.

GI, gastrointestinal.

who benefit from a mild anticholinergic action. Mirtazepine is also an alternative to the TCAs with less anticholinergic activity. It is great for circumstances where weight gain is needed, but it is quite appetite stimulating and can cause excessive weight gain if used incautiously. It is sleep promoting and tends to be sedating when patients initiate treatment. Bupropion is the most activating antidepressant and has the least sexual side effects (some patients report improved function). The activation does NOT include GI activation as occurs with SSRIs and, in terms of GI side effects, is well tolerated. It can produce bruxism in some patients. Monoamine oxidase inhibitors are shown but are rarely used except in special circumstances.

● PERSONALITY DISORDERS

This set of conditions can be seen as derived from an over- or under-endowment of normal traits. These are best modeled by measuring traits in populations and looking at the difficulties that are associated with them. Intelligence, warmth, risk-taking, sensitivity, and other normal traits, which when over- or under-represented, make people "vulnerable" to problems. For gastroenterologists, problems occur when patients are overly sensitive to internal sensations, excessively emotionally expressive, or excessively worried or ruminative (a great GI word in psychiatry). Personality disorders fit this category.

William Osler said, "It is much more important to know what sort of patient has a disease than what sort of disease a patient has." The "kind" of patient describes the characteristic response of the patient to a stimulus. The whole area of personality and temperament is confounded by entrenched psychologic theories and dogma about the developmental influences of certain kinds of trauma. The concept of *borderline personality* originates in psychoanalytic ideas of the early 20th century that have become doctrinaire. For the sake of this chapter, we will focus on the branch of psychology that has attempted to measure temperament or disposition, as this allows us to skirt the issue of who is right in the analytic understanding of character. In the simplest terms, character can be seen as the outcome of underlying temperament or disposition interacting with learning and environment. The methods used to measure traits of personality have been reliable over time[5] and seem to have predictive validity. We will focus on two traits of personality for our discussion, introversion-extraversion and instability-stability.[6,7] These traits are normally distributed in a Gaussian manner in the population. Most psychologists see these traits as neutral; that is, extremes of these traits make one specialized for a particular environment but vulnerable in another environment. Average endowment (the middle of the curve) of a trait creates a temperament that can adapt to multiple environments but does not help the individual thrive in a particular one. Fig. 151.2 is a diagram depicting the distribution of introversion and extraversion.

The most straightforward description of this axis of personality is that introverts react to stimulation with inhibition, whereas extraverts react with excitation.

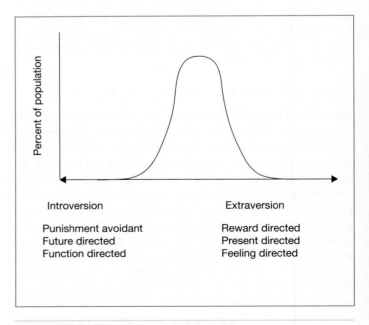

FIGURE 151.2 ● Simplified model of disposition.

As shown in the diagram, introverts are consequence-avoidant, future-directed, and function-directed individuals. They avoid circumstances likely to lead to negative outcomes rather than seeking circumstances that will lead to positive outcomes. Their behavior is more likely to be shaped by consequences, and they are less sensitive to rewards. They are concerned about illness, physical sensations, their own internal milieu, and avoiding negative consequences. They are, therefore, concerned about side effects of treatments, the correctness of diagnosis, the effects of their illness, and, when faced with decisions, tend to hesitate rather than act in error.

These patients are "ruminative" (note the origin of the term) and may worry obsessively about symptoms. They are often acutely aware of body sensations and may amplify those sensations to a great extent. They often present to GI specialists, but it may be hard to evaluate the seriousness of their complaints because of their elaborate and overly inclusive descriptions. A focus on control of bowel function and vivid descriptions of consistency, quality, frequency, and quantity of their stool may lead clinicians to dismiss them as hypochondriacal without a complete work-up. On the other hand, many of them continue to have test after test and see many specialists trying to reassure themselves about their symptoms.

Extraverts are reward-sensitive, present-focused and feeling-focused individuals. They actively seek positive feelings and desired emotional states, pursuing circumstances likely to provide a positive emotional outcome. They tend to want relief from discomfort immediately, and their behavior is reinforced strongly by rewards, particularly those associated with positive emotions. They are concerned about comfort, appearance, and obtaining the medication or treatment they have chosen. They will pursue a particular diagnosis or status from clinicians if it will get them what they desire.[8]

Introverts are at their best when analyzing situations that require thought and consideration before action. They are good at accounting, law, and medicine, and thinking about safety, prevention, and right and wrong. They are at a disadvantage in situations requiring action when all choices have potential negative consequences, such as embarking on treatment or accepting diagnostic labels. Ruminating patients can get trapped in endless lists of side effects, adverse outcomes, dangers related to tests and procedures, and about the consequences of a particular diagnostic label. The "What if you are wrong?" type of question can paralyze them and obstruct their treatment. They are particularly sensitive to the social meaning of certain diagnoses, such as psychiatric conditions. Physicians tend to be introverted; therefore, they often have an easier time relating to the obsessive introvert who ruminates endlessly about their illness and the decisions in treatment. Nonetheless, physicians can eventually lose patience and become frustrated by the patient's relentless need for reassurance. They often struggle with the recapitulating patient and need to learn ways to encourage the patient forward.

Fortunately, clinical medicine has an endless list of terrible consequences that can be used to help shape the behavior of introverts. Introverts usually respond well to advice and direction to avoid "bad" decisions, negative consequences, and missed opportunities. They can usually be directed to good

decisions by clear clinical analysis of pros and cons of a decision in terms of risks and benefits. They can get bogged down in worries about side effects and ruminative doubts about wrong diagnoses and the need for further tests. Physicians are familiar with these type of behaviors and can usually lead the introvert patient to the best choice and course of action. Physician's clear descriptions of the "bad things that will happen if you miss your medications" are a powerful motivator for introverts.

Extravert patients present a different paradigm for introverted doctors and need different strategies in managing their healthcare. They focus on feelings, rewards, and the present and often demand instant relief, have an predetermined agenda, and believe they can direct their own care better than the doctor. The statement, "I know what helps me," particularly when delivered in an impatient or irritated tone of voice, is nearly pathognomonic of the difficult extraverted patient. These patients almost always demand specific tests, treatments, and medications and have fixed ideas about their diagnoses. They want to be made comfortable and associate comfort with wellness, whereas doctors usually associate improved physical function with wellness. In the words of Dr. King (my wife, who is a primary care physician), "our therapeutic goals are not aligned." The patient's goal of feeling comfortable and without pain often leads to excessive use of benzodiazepines for anxiety, opiates for pain, sedative hypnotics for sleep, and stimulants for the inevitable accompanying sedation. Their attitude that this problem can be "fixed" leads to excessive surgery and tests.

Physicians are often frustrated by the extravert patient's emotional landscape of forceful responses and focus on getting what *they want right now*. They love you when they get what they want and hate you when they do not. This leads to their changeable nature. Because they are so present focused and seem to forget what you have done for them in the past, there is nothing "in the emotional bank" in terms of trust, patience, and previous positive physician-patient experiences. They see themselves as a victim of events that "happen to them." They do not see their own responsibility and role in helping to improve and get better. They follow the trends of our current culture of victimization and tendency to blame others or "the system" for difficult circumstances.

As we mentioned earlier, there is also a stability-instability axis (instability is called neuroticism by many), which is orthogonal to the extraversion-introversion axis (**Fig. 151.3**). Stable patients have emotions that are slow to change, have a small emotional response to a large emotional stimulus, and have a very consistent emotional response to a given stimulus. Unstable patients have emotions that change quickly, have a large emotional response to a small stimulus, and have an inconsistent emotional response to a given stimulus. When this axis is combined with the extraversion-introversion axis, one gets the four Greek Humors of temperament that physicians have described from the dawn of time.

Research into the relationship between personality features and IBD has suggested a role for personality in the manifestation of IBD.[9] It is far too early to tell whether having the condition contributes to the expression of particular traits or whether

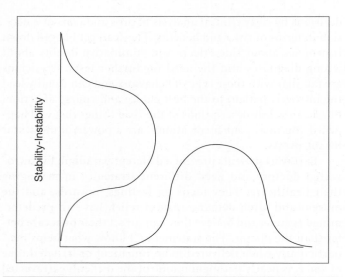

FIGURE 151.3 • The stability-instability axis superimposed on the introversion-extraversion axis.

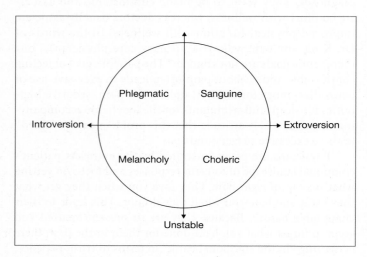

FIGURE 151.4 • The 4 humors of the ancient Greeks related to the dimensions of personality.

having a set of traits influences the manifestations of the disease (Fig. 151.4).

In working with patients with personality disorders, many clinicians use treatment contracts to help delineate the limits and expectations for treatment. Our experience has been that such contracts may be very useful and can also serve as the way to "get rid" of patients who have overwhelmed the system. We have begun to advocate discharging uncooperative patients early with a smile and much encouragement to return if they decide our approach might be useful to them. This does not mean that we think that any patient who is not completely cooperative should be discharged; rather the decision to discharge targets only those patients who are exhausting resources and who are either not benefiting or, more commonly, actually being harmed by the treatments that they end up getting. This approach also gets rid of patients who are uncooperative, using resources without gaining benefit, and demoralizing their doctors, but it allows them time to rethink their behavior and return to treatment when they are confronted with the need to change.

ABNORMAL BEHAVIORS AND ADDICTIONS

This category includes disorders that are the result of behavioral conditioning. These are conditions that are best modeled with behavioral research and include addictions, abnormal illness behaviors, and eating disorders. These are disorders that usually involve learning a behavior and being reinforced by complex physical and psychologic factors. We see them in our clinics as patients who have been conditioned to be disabled and to exacerbate their symptoms. They include "medication-seeking" and "procedure-seeking" patients. They also include those who have developed internal patterns of pathologic reinforcement, such as addicted patients, eating disordered patients, and even a group of patients with unusual practices that include self-disimpaction, laxative abuse, and pica. These patients often have other psychiatric conditions that make them more vulnerable to behavioral disorders such as OCD, schizophrenia, or personality disorders, but behavioral disorders can develop in the absence of comorbidity as well.

A comprehensive discussion of addictions is beyond the scope of this chapter, but patients suffering from addictions frequently have GI sequelae related to their drug use. This is particularly true of opiates and alcohol. Alcohol is GI toxic in many ways, having a role in pancreatitis and liver disease, but a more subtle role in exacerbating inflammatory bowel conditions. Opiates relieve pain acutely, but often cause a rebound increase in spasm and pain. Clinicians often initiate opiates to help patients with acute pain, but as use becomes chronic, the situation is confounded as the patient gets into alternating patterns of overuse and withdrawal.

The issues of alcohol and opiate use are complicated by the fact that patients are seldom forthcoming about this element of their condition. Talking to outside informants and other clinicians may be essential to accurately diagnose substance dependence and clarify the role of opiates and alcohol in GI conditions.

The behavioral models of thinking about reinforcement and conditioning have been productive ways to approach addiction. Patient's behavior is shaped by the rewarding nature of the drugs they use until the behavior becomes a loop of positive reinforcement that gradually excludes all other activities.

Addicted patients inevitably seek to maintain their addiction. This frequently results in surreptitious manipulation of doctors and medical resources. Patients who are abusing illicit substances or misusing prescribed controlled substances present to their physicians in confusing ways and are often perceived as difficult. The initial problem is usually one of missed diagnosis. The physician is puzzled by why his or her best efforts with a patient are repeatedly thwarted or why he or she always has a nagging sense that something about the interaction was "off." Behaviors associated with substance use include manipulation, coercion, and lying. In addition, the loss of employment and disruptions in family relationships caused by substance use remove the supports most often sought by physicians caring for the addicted patient. These patients drain the resources of the office staff with requests for early refills of controlled substances, miss or turn up late for appointments, and indulge in antisocial behaviors that disrupt office flow and orderly function. A high level of suspicion must be entertained for substance abuse in difficult patient encounters, in order not to miss signs of addictions, as they are associated with high morbidity and mortality and are eminently treatable.

Patients with chronic pain often become addicted to the pain medications that they are prescribed. This is more likely in patients already suffering from addictions, but it is also much more likely in those vulnerable for other reasons, such as extraversion, depression, or chronic medical illness.

A thorough discussion of addiction treatment is beyond the scope of this chapter, but the essentials can be described in five steps.[10] The first step is to get patients to recognize the addiction as a disorder that needs treatment. Some patients must lose nearly everything in their life before they can "hit bottom" and see the severity of their condition. Others can heed the properly presented warning of a good clinician. "Motivational interviewing"[11] and "confrontation with a smile" are two descriptors of ways to achieve this. Essentially, in this step patients accept the diagnosis of an addictive disorder and decide that they are ready to get better. This step is sometimes referred to as "conversion."[12] The second step is detoxification. Patients who are actively in the loop of using and craving are usually unable to break out of that loop without an intervention to detoxify them. The third step is rehabilitation. As patients are progressively more addicted, their lives become focused entirely on the behaviors involved in obtaining and using drugs and gradually exclude all other activities. They become socially, occupationally, and recreationally disconnected. As they recover there is little to fill their time other than craving drugs and little to distract them from negative feelings. The activities that result in positive reinforcement of behavior in life and give life a sense of pleasure and satisfaction usually involve activities in these life domains. Rehabilitation means filling up these domains with meaningful life activities, but these must be rebuilt (or built) over time. This is often the most time-consuming element of recovery. It is not uncommon to hear people who have successfully recovered describe this phase in months and years. The fourth step occurs simultaneously with the third and consists of the treatment of comorbid conditions, both medical and psychiatric. Depression, personality disorders, HIV, hepatitis C, and chronic pain all act as triggers and interfere with recovery. The last step is relapse prevention. This is a long-term (indefinite) plan to prevent the elements that combined to allow the addiction to develop in the first place from allowing it to recur. Twelve-step programs, physician monitoring, and constant reminders of the danger of recurrence of addiction are needed in a long-term systematic way.

CHRONIC GI PAIN

Although discussed elsewhere, the issue of the management of chronic pain is central to the role of dealing with difficult patients. Patients with acute pain are usually relatively straightforward to manage, whereas those with chronic pain are far more difficult. Chronic pain is not usually the result of ongoing tissue damage but rather the result of altered sensory and sympathetic nervous function. Patients are often given opiates at ever-increasing doses to try to combat their pain, and though some may benefit, many become increasingly intoxicated and exhibit more dysfunction as the dose increases. Unfortunately, the efforts to make pain a vital sign and to ensure that all pain is relieved have led to a massive overuse of narcotics and escalated the problem of iatrogenic addiction. Nonmalignant chronic pain is often not relieved with chronic opiates and can be made worse by chronic opiate use.[13] Although some patients benefit from chronic opiate administration, it is increasingly clear that many do not. Alternative methods of pain management may be more useful for chronic pain.[14]

Pain has two components, a sensory element and an affective element. It is the affective element that produces the distress associated with pain. As described earlier, patients with depression have an increased sensitivity to pain, particularly the affective component. Patients with significant extraversion or instability are more reactive to the distress associated with pain and will tolerate a lower level of function in their effort to eliminate pain. They are at increased risk for addiction and medication overuse.

Patients with chronic pain often are in the "difficult patient" category and are often focused entirely on the goal of pain relief to the detriment of getting better and improving function. They arrive demanding escalating doses of opiates and often are given comfort-directed pharmacologic interventions such as benzodiazepines and other sedative-hypnotics. In what follows, we discuss a behavioral approach to the management of chronic pain and related conditions.

A BEHAVIORAL APPROACH TO GI REHABILITATION

In the early 1900s, Ivan Pavlov described the ability to change behavior in animals by association with a particular stimulus. He was able to measure salivation in dogs in response to food, but then by pairing the food with a tuning fork, he was able to elicit salivation in response to the tuning fork. This has been described as classical conditioning and occurs passively. This type of conditioning has been observed with patients in many settings. Patients who have had several exposures to chemotherapy will often develop nausea and may even vomit when arriving at the infusion center.[15] It is possible to condition changes in immune function,[16] condition asthma attacks,[17] and to condition neutral stimuli to cause pain.[18] Classical conditioning (or Pavlovian conditioning) occurs when a patient associates a behavior with a desirable or undesirable stimulus or experience.

Operant conditioning, described later by B.F. Skinner, occurs when a behavior performed by the patient is associated with a specific consequence. This type of conditioning increases or decreases the likelihood of the associated behavior. As an example, a pigeon pecks a key and receives a food reward. This results in more frequent and faster key-pecking behavior. Skinner described "shaping," where successive rewards could result in more complex behaviors. Pigeons can be "shaped" to peck a ball into a slot for food by first shaping it to peck the ball and then rewarding it only when it pecks the ball in a specific direction.

Patients are positively reinforced by opiate and sedative hypnotic medications, attention from doctors, disability payments, and by permission to express prohibited feelings. They are negatively reinforced by the relief from pain that opiates provide, relief from insomnia from sedative hypnotics, and relief from expectations and demands at work and at home. This will increase medication seeking, doctor seeking, and pain-related behavior. This will also shape patients to be less committed to recovery.

Fortunately, these same behavioral tools can be used to shape recovery-related and function-related behaviors. Izzy Pilowsky described illness-related behaviors in the absence of ongoing pathology, with the term "abnormal illness behavior."[19] Many of these behaviors are conditioned to occur as described previously. Ignoring abnormal illness behaviors will help result in their extinction. Rewarding healthy behaviors such as rehabilitation, function, and coping will encourage patients to develop themselves. Examples of this include the use of letters, forms, attention, and personal approval as positive reinforcers of specific behavior. Patients on chronic opiate treatment for pain might be required to demonstrate 40 hours of structured activity a week to stay on opiates. Rehabilitation of chronic pain using these techniques was described by William Fordyce in 1968,[20] and the operant conditioning approach has been a standard (though, sadly, underrecognized) approach to chronic pain.[21,22] It is also important to recognize that patients condition their physicians as much as we condition them. In a seminal study of prescription writing behavior, Turk showed that non-verbal pain behaviors have a potent influence on the prescription writing–behavior of doctors.[21,22]

Patient often want to engage in a debate as to whether or not the doctors thinks their disease is real or "all in their head." Directing focus on the fact that the patient is not functioning well and that the condition is chronic and not "curable" at this time is useful. The deliberate application of behavioral techniques to treatment of patients with chronic GI pain and dysfunction takes much of the emotional element out of the picture. We emphasize that we will focus on what the patient is doing and not on what they are feeling. The steps for successful treatment can be described as occurring in five steps, similar to those for addictions. Prior to beginning treatment, a full evaluation for medical and psychiatric conditions must be completed. It is critical to know the case when starting treatment with difficult patients.

Treatment begins with a role induction. This consists of describing the entire formulation to the patient of what the doctor thinks is wrong. We include medical and psychiatric elements in the discussion. We allow ample time for the patient to ask questions about is the nature of each condition, why we think they have it, and how it affects them, but we do not allow patients to derail the discussion or argue about the diagnosis. When patients argue about the diagnosis, we tell them that if they disagree after we explain things fully, we will arrange for them to get a second opinion. It is important not to allow the patient to short-circuit the discussion of diagnosis by leaping to treatment. The discussion of treatment begins after the patient has heard the diagnostic formulation completely. Typical formulations describe the medical problems first, then the way they are complicated by the lack of reward in major depression, the amplification of sensation due to temperament, and the lack of coping skills and aversive experiences that have made it hard to get good treatment. We finally discuss the way in which conditioning has systematically incapacitated the patient's GI

function. We offer an optimistic discussion of treatments that are often contrary to the patient's requested treatments but explain how they will result in better outcome. We stress the losses and indignities the patient has suffered from their illness and how important it is to try to recover their lives. We finish the role induction by pointing out that we could be wrong and that the patient will need to decide whether they want to seek treatment elsewhere or engage in the treatment we have prescribed. Although this approach is paternalistic, it establishes the critical core of the doctor-patient relationship. The patient can fire you and go elsewhere, but they cannot prescribe his or her own treatment.

The next step involves detoxification, if needed, and the development of a set of behavioral goals with associated rewards and consequences. This is the equivalent of the detoxification step in addictions treatment, in which the rewards that maintain abnormal illness behavior are removed.

The initiation of medical and psychiatric treatments (equivalent to the treatment of comorbid conditions in addictions) is critical to the success of the overall treatment. This is done in concert with the initiation of behaviorally based rehabilitation. Treatment often includes an opiate taper, physical therapy, and comprehensive rehabilitation for chronic pain and chronic bowel dysfunction (and any other chronically deconditioned organ system). Finally, relapse prevention must take place in the form of a program to prevent the recrudescence of the pathologic response to the underlying illness. Almost all patients will continue to need attention and treatment. Without ongoing care, the pattern of behavioral reinforcement for disability and deconditioning is likely to recur.

● SUMMARY

The most difficult patients usually present with underlying illness that has been made worse not only by psychiatric conditions that exacerbate the illness and lead to disability but also by a system that rewards poor medical care, focuses on symptoms rather than on diagnoses, and directs treatment at comfort rather than function. A comprehensive diagnostic formulation that includes comorbid psychiatric conditions allows clinicians to develop treatment plans that overcome the barriers to successful medical treatment. The route to success is to focus on the patient's medical treatment and their behavior and to pay less attention to their feelings, emotional provocations and manipulations, and comfort. Unfortunately, these patients require more time, are less satisfied, use more resources, and are less able to pay for their treatment. The current medical care system does not adequately reward clinicians for their time, nor does it provide an incentive for successful treatment. The growing emphasis on customer satisfaction, financial efficiency, and allowing patients to prescribe their own treatment has been a disservice to these patients. It is tragic to watch such patients flail against those who want to help them and exploit weaknesses in the system to ensure their own demise.[23] Clinicians are discouraged from engaging with difficult patients by a system that can actually penalize clinicians for caring for them appropriately.[24] Because these patients are often conditioned to engage in self-defeating behavior, they may sabotage their own care to hurt a clinician when they are angry about something, even though, it defeats their purpose.

It has become politically popular to see difficult patients in terms of their rights,[25] but a patient who is difficult may be suffering from impaired autonomy and is not making decisions in an autonomous fashion. There is also growing literature that explain the characteristics of physicians who have difficulty with patients[26,27] and how to improve physician skills,[28] suggesting that difficult patients are a product of clinician failure. Certainly, better skills are helpful in managing difficult patients, but mastery of treating the underlying problem is necessary to rehabilitate patients to full function. "Understanding" how the patient feels may be comforting but no more therapeutic than the orthopedic surgeon "understanding" a fracture. Ultimately, the best way to manage a difficult patient is to help him or her get better, but many patients need to hear the same message repeatedly before they are ready to accept the treatment plan most likely to succeed. Patient advocacy, oddly enough, sometimes involves advocating for something that the patient does not want, but certainly needs.

References

1. Orgel SZ. Effect of psychoanalysis on the course of peptic ulcer. *Psychosom Med.* 1958;20(2):117–123.

2. Maunder RG, Levenstein S. The role of stress in the development and clinical course of inflammatory bowel disease: epidemiological evidence. *Curr Mol Med.* 2008;8(4):247–252.

3. Maunder RG, Greenberg GR, Hunter JJ, Lancee WJ, Steinhart AH, Silverberg MS. Psychobiological subtypes of ulcerative colitis: pANCA status moderates the relationship between disease activity and psychological distress. *Am J Gastroenterol.* 2006;101(11):2546–2551.

4. Kast RE. Anti- and pro-inflammatory considerations in antidepressant use during medical illness: bupropion lowers and mirtazapine increases circulating tumor necrosis factor-alpha levels. *Gen Hosp Psychiatry.* 2003;25(6):495–496.

5. Lucas RE, Diener E, Grob A, Suh EM, Shao L. Cross-cultural evidence for the fundamental features of extraversion. *J Pers Soc Psychol.* 2000;79(3):452–468.

6. Costa PT Jr, Widiger TA. *Personality Disorders and the Five-Factor Model of Personality.* Washington, DC: American Psychological Association; 1994.

7. Eysenck HJ. Genetic and environmental contributions to individual differences: the three major dimensions of personality. *J Personality.* 1990;58:245–261.

8. Eysenck HJ, Eysenck SBG. *Eysenck Personality Questionnaire.* San Diego, CA: Edit TS/Educational and Industrial Testing Service; 1975.

9. Barrett SM, Standen PJ, Lee AS, Hawkey CJ, Logan RF. Personality, smoking and inflammatory bowel disease. *Eur J Gastroenterol Hepatol.* 1996;8(7):651–655.

10. Treisman GJ, Angelino A. *The Psychiatry of AIDS: A Guide to Diagnosis and Treatment.* Baltimore: Johns Hopkins Press; 2004.

11. Prochaska JO, DiClemente CC, Norcross JC. In search of how people change. Applications to addictive behaviors. *Am Psychol.* 1992;47(9):1102–1114.

12. Tiebout, H. Therapeutic mechanisms in alcoholics anonymous. *Am J Psychiatry.* 1944;100:468–473.

13. Ossipov MH, Lai J, King T, Vanderah TW, Porreca F. Underlying mechanisms of pronociceptive consequences of prolonged morphine exposure. *Biopolymers.* 2005;80(2–3):319–324.

14. Clark MR. Psychiatric issues in chronic pain. *Curr Psychiatry Rep.* 2009;11(3):243–250.

15. Stockhorst U, Steingrueber HJ, Enck P, Klosterhalfen S. Pavlovian conditioning of nausea and vomiting. *Auton Neurosci.* 2006;129(1–2):50–57.

16. Exton MS, von Auer AK, Buske-Kirschbaum A, Stockhorst U, Göbel U, Schedlowski M. Pavlovian conditioning of immune function: animal investigation and the challenge of human application. *Behav Brain Res.* 2000;110(1–2):129–141.

17. Bouhuys A, Justesen DR. Allergic and classically conditioned asthma in guinea pigs. *Science.* 1971;173(991):82.

18. Greeley J. Pavlovian conditioning of pain regulation: insights from pharmacological conditioning with morphine and naloxone. *Biol Psychol.* 1989;28(1):41–65.

19. Pilowsky I. Abnormal illness behaviour. *Br J Med Psychol.* 1969;42(4):347–351.

20. Fordyce WE, Fowler RS, DeLateur B. An application of behavior modification technique to a problem of chronic pain. *Behav Res Ther.* 1968;6(1):105–107.

21. Turk DC, Swanson KS, Tunks ER. Psychological approaches in the treatment of chronic pain patients–when pills, scalpels, and needles are not enough. *Can J Psychiatry.* 2008;53(4):213–223.

22. Turk DC, Okifuji A. What factors affect physicians' decisions to prescribe opioids for chronic noncancer pain patients? *Clin J Pain.* 1997;13(4):330–336.

23. Fee C. Death of a difficult patient. *Ann Emerg Med.* 2001;37(3):354–355.

24. Sonnenberg A. Personal view: passing the buck and taking a free ride – a game-theoretical approach to evasive management strategies in gastroenterology. *Aliment Pharmacol Ther.* 2005;22(6):513–518.

25. Reeves RR, Douglas SP, Garner RT, Reynolds MD, Silvers A. The individual rights of the difficult patient. *Hastings Cent Rep.* 2007;37(2):13; discussion 13–13; discussion 15.

26. Krebs EE, Garrett JM, Konrad TR. The difficult doctor? Characteristics of physicians who report frustration with patients: an analysis of survey data. *BMC Health Serv Res.* 2006;6:128.

27. Batchelor J, Freeman MS. Spectrum: the clinician and the "difficult" patient. *S D J Med.* 2001;54(11):453–456.

28. Haas LJ, Leiser JP, Magill MK, Sanyer ON. Management of the difficult patient. *Am Fam Physician.* 2005;72(10):2063–2068.

Psychosocial Concomitants of Pediatric IBD | 152

Stanley A. Cohen and Sobha P. Fritz

Inflammatory bowel disease becomes insinuated like a constant shadow, allowing a normal childhood one minute and then humbling everyone as they flare, engendering havoc for the entire family and rampaging through with an ominous, often unspoken fear left in their wake. It has to be more than difficult for a child to wonder if he or she is going to die or to wonder if he or she is going to have much of a life. They seem at times isolated and fearful, worrying whether other children know of their problems and will accept or tease them, worrying that yet another procedure will have to be performed. It has to be disheartening to make sure that the location of every bathroom is known, that every activity and meal have to be thought through, that medicine schedules are always met, that sometimes they actually want to see their doctors, that a cure and disease control are almost always further away than anyone would like.[1]

In individuals with inflammatory bowel disease (IBD), the complexity of the relationship between behavioral/social functioning and the physical/medical component is now becoming more widely recognized. This was not always true. Initially, IBD was characterized as a psychosomatic illness by some and then disputed. The pendulum then swung to an approach that if IBD was effectively treated, the psychological manifestations would then dissipate. We now understand that there seems to be a bidirectional feedback loop that influences both processes almost reciprocally (as often alluded to, a mind-body connection). This comorbidity is perhaps even more pronounced in pediatric IBD.

● ANTECEDENTS

Childhood and adolescence can be a challenge for even healthy individuals as they attempt to establish their independence, emotional maturity, and self-esteem. The additional factors (Table 152.1) and complications frequently seen in pediatric IBD, such as short stature and delayed puberty, expand the issues that teens and preteens must deal with as they navigate their way with peers. Frequent school absences and the inability to participate with friends in activities often exacerbate the

TABLE 152.1 Factors Contributing to Psychosocial Issues in Children and Teens with IBD

Normal challenges
Establishing independence
Physical and emotional maturity
Developing self-esteem
Comprehending body image and function
Healthy sexuality
Family and peer relationships
Recognizing authority and priorities
Possible challenges exacerbated by IBD
Short stature
Delayed puberty
Fatigue
Pain, diarrhea and/or seeing blood in bowel movements
Limited participation in sports because of reduced size and strength
Explaining school absences to peers, teachers, and staff
Academic make-up work
Inability to participate in activities
Embarrassment
Frequent, urgent visits to the bathroom.
Lack of a stable course
Laboratory draws and IVs
Procedures and preparations
Adherence to medical regimen (diet, medication, lifestyle)
Steroid side effects
Immunomodulatory side effects and risks
Surgery or its potential
Having an ostomy

IBD, inflammatory bowel disease.

problem as they attempt to catch up on school work and keep up with their peers in various skill sets. Moreover, the fatigue they may face and adolescent size may impact their ability to participate on an equal playing field with other peers.

Children and adolescents can be embarrassed by having frequent, urgent visits to the bathroom. Many determine their activities and participate in those that allow them immediate access to a bathroom, if needed. The lack of a stable course, the need for frequent physician visits, and procedures/laboratory draws can interrupt peer participation and quotidian, school and family responsibilities that can be challenging enough at this age. The responsibility of taking medications and adhering to diets is often burdensome for patient and parent alike, with reminders creating a focal point for family disagreements and outright struggles. In addition, the relapsing and remitting course and the unpredictable nature of the illness make this an even greater challenge, at a time when adolescents and children are still on the path to emotional maturity, when they have limited resources to adapt and develop positive strategies, and when they are still dependent on their parents for their coping skills. Often, parents are perplexed by these problems and unsure of how to address IBD-related issues with their children.

Compounding these problems are the superimposed issues of intermittent dependence on corticosteroids for treatment with its attendant emotional lability and additionally embarrassing side effects of "moon facies" and acne as well as psychiatric disorders, with as many as 52% of patients on more than 20 mg of daily prednisone developing psychiatric symptoms and 12% severe enough to have hospitalization for severe depression or mania in the adult population.[2]

When children have undergone surgery, or where that possibility has been discussed, another level of fear and concern is added. For those living with an ostomy, the issues are multiplied by the impact the illness has had on their body image, especially as that young body is still being formed. Moreover, many of these children take special care to conceal their stoma and supplies from their friends, with even some going to the extent of not revealing the presence of an ostomy to roommates at college. But body image is of concern to most teens and, in those with IBD, dietary adherence is correlated with greater satisfaction with body image.[3]

While these antecedent emotional factors are plentiful and difficult to fully comprehend, their pain and its psychological effects are shared by others of their age. Daily abdominal pain is reported in 3.2% of adolescents, with an additional 14% reporting abdominal pain as moderate in frequency. Sixteen percent of all adolescents are at risk for depression, with the risk of depression increasing from 16% to 45% when that pain is daily, with those having daily pain much more likely to miss more school and express loneliness.[4] Other comparable groups include children with functional gastrointestinal (GI) disorders, because they may describe more pain when having a colonoscopy than children with IBD, although they express less anxiety than children with other chronic illnesses.[5]

Depression is significantly higher in children with IBD than in children with cystic fibrosis, as reported in an earlier study by Burke et al.,[6] with a higher lifetime prevalence of depression in IBD. Comparison to adult populations is exceedingly different

and perhaps not even relevant, because psychological issues are in part age dependent, and the life events that occur in each age group are different qualitatively.

APPRECIATING CHALLENGES

Although a large portion of patients with IBD believe that stress influences their disease activity,[7] causality of specific life events or how stressors create an exacerbation of the disease has not been well researched.[8] As reviewed elsewhere in this book, a number of psychological mechanisms are reputed to be pathophysiologically involved in stress-induced intestinal damage.

The recognition that stress may be impacting the immunologic and physiologic pathophysiology is a relatively new concept in IBD, although it has been well studied in cardiac disease, other GI diseases, and even the common cold. Applying the appropriate methodology in terms of psychosocial research has only recently allowed a better understanding of the relationship. However, few studies have been done in pediatrics. In large populations, reliable administration of structured interviews has been a problem.[9] In addition, the instruments that are often used to assess these issues on a consistent basis, such as the Revised Children's Manifest Anxiety Scale[10] and the Children's Depression Inventory,[11] raise numerous questions within such that the tools may either measure physiologic anxiety or symptomatology related directly to IBD. Conversely, it is difficult to distinguish whether IBD or its attendant psychosocial components cause changes in health-related quality of life (QOL). Although it may seem unimportant to make that distinction, little within the literature guides us to predict which children are more likely to experience significant psychological issues and need further attention; though even suicide has been reported in the pediatric population of patients with IBD.

ANXIETY AND DEPRESSION

The rates of psychological impairment or dysfunction reported by parents or children on self-reporting questionnaires demonstrate that children with IBD had more emotional or internalizing symptoms than healthy children. This includes anxiety and depression, generally following the pattern seen in other chronic illnesses. The variability in the rates of psychiatric disorders in part depend on methodological issues, particularly sample size. Those with larger samples reported lower rates, 4% to 28%, whereas those with smaller samples and less optimal methodology have higher rates, 59% to 73%.[12] Our experience with 84 patients younger than 18 in our IBD clinic demonstrated a 2% rate of depression documented by the Children's Depression Inventory and 8% with anxiety using the revised Children's Manifest Anxiety Scale (11% when eliminating all physiologic symptoms).[13] A number of studies have shown no significant relationship to any disease factor, activity scores, growth delay, and/or frequency of relapse, though anxiety in our population did correlate with physician global assessment and active disease demonstrated by the Pediatric Crohn's Disease Activity Index. Similarly specific symptoms of depression have been correlated by others with some disease severity indicators.

The concurrence of functional GI disorders in children and adolescents with quiescent Crohn's disease have been studied by rectal barostat demonstrating that protracted abdominal pain in a small sample of children with quiescent Crohn's disease may be related to visceral hypersensitivity and anxiety.[14]

Editor's note (TMB): There are separate chapters on the coexistence of IBS and IBD.

Depression and problems with memory have been prevalent in children with IBD on steroids than those who were not. There has been no correlation with age of diagnosis; however, in other chronic disease states, family functioning and coping skills are strategies that are predictors of behavioral functioning.

In IBD, 65 adolescents with an expectation about the disease and less use of depressive reaction patterns are associated with better health-related QOL, suggesting that coping styles relate not only to depression but also to health-related QOL, as might be assumed.[15] Anhedonia, fatigue, and decreased appetite as expressions of depression have been selectively correlated with IBD severity. Of note, children with IBD have lower sleep subscales than healthy controls on the PedsQL Fatigue Scale—and, although there is little information on children with IBD, frequent sleep interruption and sleep disturbance may be a possible contributor to fatigue/depression/anxiety in adults with IBD.[16]

Patients on steroids are more likely to have depression index scores that are significant, demonstrating as well that depressed children with new onset pediatric IBD had less severe illnesses but were more likely to have maternal history of depression, families characterized by less cohesion and more conflict, and more stressful life events in their history.[17] These mood disorders and anxiety, though inconsistently related to measures of disease, are manifested by school truancies, social isolation, and behavioral problems.[18]

● FAMILY AND SOCIAL INTERACTIONS

These multilayered, rapid psychosocial transitions of dealing with IBD, in addition to the normal turmoil of adolescent years, both impact the family and are impacted by them (and are further reviewed elsewhere in this volume). Marital difficulties and medical severity are often correlated with the life events of the children with IBD, with insecure attachments suggesting at-risk relationships.[19] On the other hand, the family often functions as the child's or teen's primary resource and a major mechanism for coping with feelings of vulnerability, diminished control, and the perceptions of differences from healthy peers and siblings.

When family dysfunction has been present, it is often related to more severe disease, increased pain and fatigue in the child, children with more bowel movements, and a greater number of behavioral and emotional symptoms.[12] Despite this, adolescents with IBD often felt ambivalence as they described how they felt about their parents' responses to the disease. This was categorized as an oscillation between seeking close contact with parents or staving them off—anxiously seeking them for protection and support, then trying to achieve a more distant dialogue with them, expressing very conflicting attitudes, reactions, and emotions among the 17 patients studied.[20]

Parents frequently report that their children with IBD often have worse social confidence than healthy children in establishing peer relationships and participating in organized activities.[12] Almost surprisingly, siblings of children with IBD often tend to function well, at the mean or higher, in behavioral and emotional functioning.[21]

● ADJUSTMENT AND COPING STRATEGIES

Adolescents with inflammatory disease are reported to show more clinically significant social problems compared to an adult population, including their social and family functioning.[22] This may be difficult to assess, as adolescents might withhold information from their healthcare practitioners seemingly because of a lack of trust.[23] Yet, there are subsets of children with good mental health despite bad somatic conditions[24] with normal psychosocial functioning similar to that of healthy children in those with currently mild IBD of greater than a year's duration.[25] With this variance, it appears that some patients cope adequately where others are unable to accept their diagnosis and seem unable to adjust to their lives.[23]

A number of coping strategies have been suggested (Table 152.2). In the adult population, low-intensity exercise seemed to decrease Crohn's disease activity and reduce psychological stress improving QOL.[26] Disease-specific summer camps are now accessible to children with IBD. There is now a specific one for those children with ostomies. Statistically significant improvements in bowel symptoms, social functioning, and treatment intervention scores as well as total QOL scores occurred immediately post-camp. However, it is uncertain as to whether those measures are sustained over the remainder of the year.[27] Of note, as well, is that yoga in adolescents with IBS reduced functional disability, GI symptoms, and maladaptive coping strategies.[28]

TABLE 152.2 Coping Strategies and Interventions
Support groups
Internet Web sites
Chat rooms and social media
Camps specifically designed for IBD and ostomy
Summer camps with healthy children
Extracurricular activities
Yoga and exercise
Relaxation strategies
CCFA-focused activities
Spiritual support and guidance
Art therapy
Cognitive-behavioral therapy
When necessary: Individual psychotherapy and psychopharmacologic agents

IBD, inflammatory bowel disease.

Psychologically based interventions for IBD have been used both in individual and group settings. With art therapy projects, the hope has been that allowing children to express their feelings about IBD has been successful in allowing children and adolescents to vent their frustrations, concerns, and hopes Fig. 152.1A and 152.1B. These interventions have included having the children simply directed at drawing pictures of their own experiences with the disease and making masks that express the

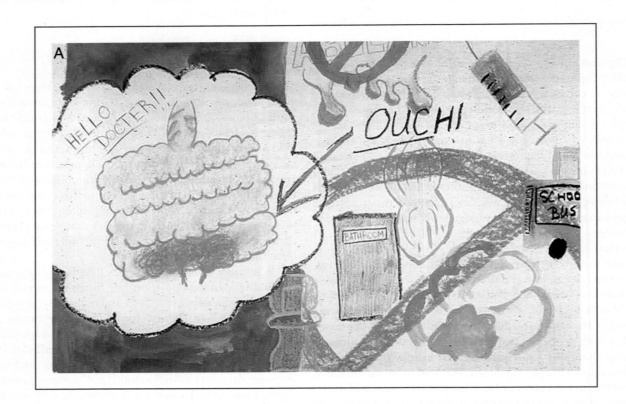

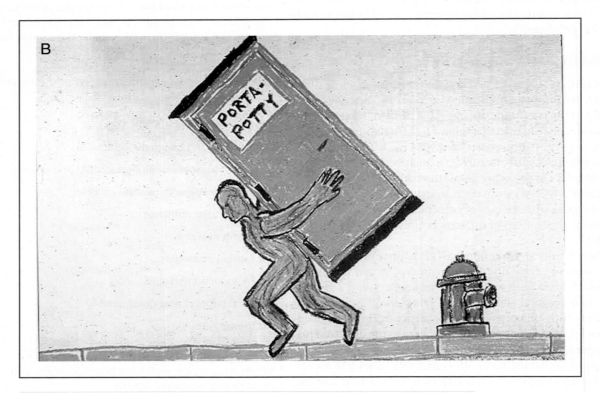

FIGURE 152.2 • A and B Samples of artwork created by children, during art therapy sessions.

face they show to the world versus the face they show internally. Projects have also been done and recorded where they created puppets that could speak about their disease for the children. Similarly, the IBD quilt project has crafted drawings by children with IBD into quilts that travel the country, helping the children who are creating the project to be expressive and then encouraging broader understanding and compassion by those who view them. A writing project collected the expressions of 40 children who not only wrote of their own experiences but also answered specific questions such as, "how do you handle missing school when you don't feel well, making up for school work when you are sick, when you have an accident, dating, acne, and issues with 'the bathroom.'"[29]

Support groups established for teenagers as well as their parents have allowed the sharing of information and feelings of support among preteens, teens, and their parents. Web sites, comic books, peer chat rooms, and other social media are readily accessible and are being used by many patients with Crohn's disease, not only to access information but also to seek support and interaction with other children who are similarly suffering. Although these are useful, they are also of significant concern, because misinformation, promiscuous behaviors, and breaches of confidentiality have the potential to be damaging. Of some concern as well is that parents of children with IBD are turning more frequently to alternative and complementary sources of their care, relying on anecdotes from acquaintances and the Internet to guide them.

● FUTURE DIRECTIONS

Though various interventions have been studied in adults, the results of these in the pediatric population have been less well documented. Cognitive-behavioral therapy employing skills-based psychological intervention for adolescent females has been studied recently using parent/child dyads with interval and single-day interventions.[30,31] Results showed significant changes in the therapeutic direction for adolescent somatic symptoms, adaptive coping strategy, and diminishing catastrophizing cognitions from pre- to postintervention. Another similar trial based solely on adolescents demonstrated significant reductions in depression diagnoses and depressive symptoms with improvement in global psychological and social functioning.[32] Psychotherapy and relaxation techniques were used in addition to standard medical therapy. In the adolescent population, depression, anxiety, global functioning, and physical health perception improved upon completion of cognitive-behavioral therapy and those improvements were maintained over a 12-month treatment period, though nearly half of the youth required psychopharmacologic support.[33] Over a 6-month follow-up period, patients undergoing coping skills training illustrated somatic reductions of symptoms as well as a decrease in the parent's protective responses allowing them to effect better limit-setting and change from a coddling behavior to a coaching behavior and be grateful for that change.[30] The benefit can be seen at least in adults, with hospital days and sick leave days decreasing in those receiving psychological therapy over a 1-year period.[34]

Translating these findings and strategies into clinical impact requires larger scale studies that can validate these findings and can determine the best clinical practices. Also, it requires improved treatment design, cost benefit analysis, and, most importantly, application by medical healthcare providers as part of a support team. Our own experience has shown that providing care in a comprehensive program involving psychologists and therapists, child life interventions, and a physician will increase understanding of the psychological and psychosocial impacts affecting, and affected by, IBD in children and adolescents, leading, hopefully, to better outcomes with patients becoming more independent and better skilled at their coping strategies during their childhood and adolescent years as well as when they transition their care as young adults.

References

1. Cohen SA. Forward for parents and friends. In Doyle J, ed. *Hand to Hand, Voice to Voice to Voice: Young Journeys of Courage Living with Crohn's & Colitis.* Conover, WI: D&S Publications; 2001:15–16.

2. Fardet L, Flashault A, Kettaneh A, et al. Copricosteroid-induced clinical adverse events: frequency, risk factors, and patient's opinion. *Br J Dermatol.* 2007;157:142–148.

3. Vlahou CH, Cohen LL, Woods AM, Lewis JD, Gold BD. Age and body satisfaction predict diet adherence in adolescents with Inflammatory Bowel Disease. *J Clin Psychol Med Settings.* 2008;15(4):278–286.

4. Youssef NN, Atienza K, Langseder AL, Strauss RS. Chronic abdominal pain and depressive symptoms: analysis of the national longitudinal study of adolescent health. *Clin Gastroenterol Hepatol.* 2008;6(3):329–332.

5. Crandall WV, Halterman TE, Mackner LM. Anxiety and pain symptoms in children with inflammatory bowel disease and functional gastrointestinal disorders undergoing colonoscopy. *J Pediatr Gastroenterol Nutr.* 2007;44(1):63–67.

6. Burke P, Meyer V, Kocoshis S, et al. Depression and anxiety in pediatric inflammatory bowel disease and cystic fibrosis. *J Am Acad Child Adolesc Psychiatry.* 1989;28(6):948–951.

7. Moser G, Maeir-Dobersberger T, Vogelsang H, et al. Inflammatory bowel disease: Patent's beliefs about the etiology of their disease—A controlled study. *Psychosom Med.* 1993;55:131.

8. Bernstein CN, Walker JR, Graff LA. On studying the connection between stress and IBD. *Am J Gastroenterol.* 2006;101(4):782–785.

9. Mackner LM, Crandall WV, Szigethy EM. Psychosocial functioning in pediatric inflammatory bowel disease. *Inflamm Bowel Dis.* 2006;12(3):239–244.

10. Reynolds CR, Richmond BO. *Revised Children's Manifest Anxiety Scale (RCMAS).* Los Angeles, CA: Western Psychological Services.

11. Kovacs M. *Children's Depression Inventory (CDI).* North Tonawanda, NY: Multi-Health Systems; 2003.

12. Mackner LM, Crandall WV. Psychological factors affecting pediatric inflammatory bowel disease. *Curr Opin Pediatr.* 2007;19(5):548–552.

13. Cohen SA, Fritz S, Coleman S, et al. A comprehensive care model for pediatric inflammatory bowel disease (IBD): initial findings. JPGN in press.

14. Faure C, Giguère L. Functional gastrointestinal disorders and visceral hypersensitivity in children and adolescents suffering from Crohn's disease. *Inflamm Bowel Dis.* 2008;14(11):1569–1574.

15. van der Zaag-Loonen HJ, Grootenhuis MA, Last BF, Derkx HH. Coping strategies and quality of life of adolescents with inflammatory bowel disease. *Qual Life Res.* 2004;13(5):1011–1019.

16. Marcus SB, Strople JA, Neighbors K, et al. Fatigue and health-related quality of life in pediatric inflammatory bowel disease. *Clin Gastroenterol Hepatol.* 2009;7(5):554–561.

17. Burke PM, Neigut D, Kocoshis S, Chandra R, Sauer J. Correlates of depression in new onset pediatric inflammatory bowel disease. *Child Psychiatry Hum Dev.* 1994;24(4):275–283.

18. Yi MS, Britto MT, Sherman SN, et al. Health values in adolescents with or without inflammatory bowel disease. *J Pediatr.* 2009;154(4):527–534.

19. Szajnberg N, Krall V, Davis P, Treem W, Hyams J. Psychopathology and relationship measures in children with inflammatory bowel disease and their parents. *Child Psychiatry Hum Dev.* 1993;23(3):215–232.

20. Reichenberg K, Lindfred H, Saalman R. Adolescents with inflammatory bowel disease feel ambivalent towards their parents' concern for them. *Scand J Caring Sci.* 2007;21(4):476–481.

21. Wood B, Watkins JB, Boyle JT, Nogueira J, Zimand E, Carroll L. Psychological functioning in children with Crohn's disease and ulcerative colitis: implications for models of psychobiological interaction. *J Am Acad Child Adolesc Psychiatry.* 1987;26(5):774–781.

22. Mackner LM, Crandall WV. Brief report: psychosocial adjustment in adolescents with inflammatory bowel disease. *J Pediatr Psychol.* 2006;31(3):281–285.

23. Lynch T, Spence D. A qualitative study of youth living with Crohn disease. *Gastroenterol Nurs.* 2008;31(3):224–230; quiz 231.

24. Engstrom I. Inflammatory bowel disease in children and adolescents: mental health and family functioning. *J Pediatr Gastroenterol Nutr.* 1999;28(4):S28–S33.

25. Mackner LM, Crandall WV. Long-term psychosocial outcomes reported by children and adolescents with inflammatory bowel disease. *Am J Gastroenterol.* 2005;100(6):1386–1392.

26. Ng V, Millard W, Lebrun C, Howard J. Exercise and Crohn's disease: speculations on potential benefits. *Can J Gastroenterol.* 2006;20(10):657–660.

27. Shepanski MA, Hurd LB, Culton K, Markowitz JE, Mamula P, Baldassano RN. Health-related quality of life improves in children and adolescents with inflammatory bowel disease after attending a camp sponsored by the Crohn's and Colitis Foundation of America. *Inflamm Bowel Dis.* 2005;11(2):164–170.

28. Kuttner L, Chambers CT, Hardial J, Israel DM, Jacobson K, Evans K. A randomized trial of yoga for adolescents with irritable bowel syndrome. *Pain Res Manag.* 2006;11(4):217–223.

29. Doyle J, ed. *Hand to Hand, Voice to Voice to Voice: Young Journeys of Courage Living with Crohn's & Colitis.* Conover, WI: D&S Publications; 2001.

30. Hayutin LG, Blount RL, Lewis J, Simons LE, McCormick ML. Skills-based group intervention for adolescent girls with inflammatory bowel disease. *Clin Case Studies.* 2009;8(5):355–365.

31. McCormick M, Reed-Knight B, Blount R, Lewis J. Development and evaluation of a coping skills training program for adolescents with inflammatory bowel disease. In preparation.

32. Szigethy E, Levy-Warren A, Whitton S, et al. Depressive symptoms and inflammatory bowel disease in children and adolescents: a cross-sectional study. *J Pediatr Gastroenterol Nutr.* 2004;39(4):395–403.

33. Szigethy E, Carpenter J, Baum E, et al. Case study: longitudinal treatment of adolescents with depression and inflammatory bowel disease. *J Am Acad Child Adolesc Psychiatry.* 2006;45(4):396–400.

34. Deter HC, Keller W, von Wietersheim J, Jantschek G, Duchmann R, Zeitz M; German Study Group on Psychosocial Intervention in Crohn's Disease. Psychological treatment may reduce the need for healthcare in patients with Crohn's disease. *Inflamm Bowel Dis.* 2007;13(6):745–752.

Exaggerated and Factitious Disease | 153

David Edwin

Gastrointestinal (GI) problems of one sort or another plague all of us throughout our lives, from our childhood bellyaches to the dyspepsia of old age. Obviously our survival depends upon maintaining adequate nutrition, and any significant disruption of that process at any stage—from food choice and swallowing through elimination—can have serious implications. At the same time, the act of eating lies at the center of our lives and our relationships with others—from nursing to courting, from the family dining room to the formal banquet hall. *As* a result, disruptions in eating and nutrition reverberate in many other arenas of life, and disruptions in important activities and relationships may impact dramatically on eating and nutritional behavior. This is the context in which digestive symptoms develop and persist, and its interplay of biological and psychosocial influences provides opportunities for serious problems to arise.

● ABNORMAL ILLNESS BEHAVIOR

Pilowski[1] coined the term "abnormal illness behavior" to encompass a variety of problems that arise out of the way patients relate to their doctors about their healthcare. Physicians are the authorities who formally sanction the sick role for patients, and this certification brings with it both rewards (attention, remuneration) and relief from tiresome obligations (work, school). Indeed, some of the most vexing conflicts that arise in medical care involve disputes over the entitlement of individuals to the sick role. Some patients get caught up in abnormal "illness denying" behavior, and we are hard put to persuade them that they are really ill and need to behave accordingly. We think about these patients using concepts like denial, flight into health, and, sometimes, psychotic illness. Other patients become caught up in "illness affirming" behavior; they seem to suffer from (or even *aspire to)* illnesses they do not have or have only in mild form. A substantial, somewhat unsatisfying part of the psychiatric nomenclature is devoted to a classification of such patients; this classification describes the great diversity of problems, but its categories are neither exhaustive nor mutually exclusive and do not necessarily discriminate among cases or

link them to rational interventions. It is to these persistently troubling patients that we turn our attention now.

Consider four views of patients and their symptoms that may guide responses.[2,3] The viewpoint of *disease* assumes that the patient's complaints are caused by a "broken" body part or system; this may imply either a disease of peripheral organs (inflammatory bowel disease or pancreatitis), a disease of brain (delusional depression, schizophrenia, and dementing illnesses), or their interaction (metabolic encephalopathy). This is the arena in which physicians are most comfortable and effective, and in which referral or disposition becomes straightforward. The *trait* method focuses on temperamental attributes (like intelligence or dependency) that render individuals vulnerable to exaggerating, enhancing, or otherwise distorting the problems and symptoms of illness. The viewpoint of *behavior* focuses attention on voluntary choices—to sustain hunger or to eat, to remain sober or to drink—and the intended and unintended consequences of these decisions. It becomes apparent that many of these problems are first and foremost behaviors, actions taken voluntarily in the service of goals that are not always obvious. The *narrative* method focuses on understanding the meanings of symptoms and illnesses, and the behaviors they engender, in the context of the patient's autobiography or subjective life story. Clinical and general life experiences often provide accurate intuitions across these methods, even when the behaviors themselves seem to defy understanding.

● CLASSIC SYNDROMES
Primary Psychiatric Illness

First, dramatic, unlikely, or even impossible physical complaints may of course be symptomatic of *primary psychiatric illness.* Somatic preoccupations are common in both schizophrenia and major depression, and may range from a chronic sense of unwellness to the fixed conviction of a dread disease (acquired immunodeficiency syndrome, cancer), to bizarre ideas of infestation, or to deliberate implantation of foreign bodies or devices. The true *anorexia* of depression, as well as the odd and rigid eating patterns seen in schizophrenia, obsessive compulsive disorder, and eating disorders, may lead to weight loss and delayed transit times suggestive of primary medical illness. Indeed, some such patients may deliberately injure themselves in direct response to hallucinated commands or delusional convictions. Drawing out patients' beliefs about their illnesses may reveal these processes, but formal psychiatric consultation, including personal and family history, mental state examination, and corroborative interviews, are necessary to establish the diagnosis and institute treatment.

Somatization Disorder

Somatization disorder (or Briquet's syndrome) describes a chronic pattern of behavior—dating at least to early adulthood—of complaints about many symptoms across multiple body systems that result in medical consultation, work interruption, or self-medication, and do not lead to evidence of medical illness sufficient to justify those complaints. This behavior pattern is not uncommon; epidemiologically, it is observed in 0.1% to 2.0% of the general population, perhaps 5% of medical outpatients, and 9% of medical inpatients. These patients by definition do not have major psychiatric illness, and pursuit of physical causes for each of their symptoms may lead to repeated invasive procedures and the surgical removal of a great deal of healthy tissue. Recourse to physicians and pursuit of investigations indeed become habituated as a constant feature rather than a troubling interruption of normal life. There is a high proportion of *personality disorder,* including antisocial disorder, among these patients. Characteristically, they have both extraverted and obsessive traits of personality—they may be very suggestible about physical sensations and, once so impressed, they may be hard put to "let go" of their uneasy feelings even when they are reassured. Their life stories are often organized around themes of the losing struggle against encroaching illness, and family histories reveal that these dramas are often multigenerational.

Hypochondriasis

Hypochondriasis describes an attitude—a more focused preoccupation with the *conviction* or the *fear* of having a particular disease even when confronted with evidence or reassurance of its absence or mild nature. Hypochondriacal patients may be exquisitely sensitive to common normal or trivially deviant body sensations; they may enhance or distort these sensations and misinterpret them as evidence of dreaded diseases. A distinction may be drawn between individuals who have no physical disease at all and those who have a mild or manageable disease that becomes unnecessarily disabling because of the patient's preoccupation with it (e.g., cardiac neurosis). Often very anxious by nature or by virtue of clinical syndromes (generalized anxiety disorder), these patients are usually resistant to reassurance and may in fact become angry or dismissive when offered reassurance.

Conversion Disorder

Conversion disorder (hysteria) describes symptoms or deficits, usually affecting sensation or voluntary motor performance, without underlying physiologic or anatomic abnormality. These symptoms suggest a disease that thorough investigation fails to reveal or substantiate. Often, they are inconsistent over time and may fail to map onto anatomically or physiologically coherent patterns. These symptoms are *by definition not* voluntarily produced or consciously feigned, but seem to arise in the context of a psychosocial stressor or to resolve some psychosocial dilemma confronting the patient. Suspicion is aroused when patients display personalities described as extraverted, attention-seeking, seductive, immature, and/or dependent.[4] These stereotypical characteristics are, in fact, *not* of much diagnostic value; they produce numerous false-positive and false-negative assessments, and play into the prejudice that the concept of hysteria merely reflects "a parody of femininity." And, the history of medicine is replete with reports of patients diagnosed with hysteria succumbing to undiagnosed illnesses.[5]

Editor's note: Neurotics are not immortal.

Malingering or Factitious Behavior

The *deliberate* production of physical or psychological symptoms for an identifiable goal that makes intuitive sense (time off from work, disability compensation, or financial settlement) is referred to as *malingering* and is regarded as criminal behavior rather than evidence of psychological disorder. On the other hand, the same behaviors, when they seem to serve no other purpose than to compel medical attention or treatment, are diagnosed as a *factitious disorder*. The most notorious factitious variant is "Munchausen syndrome"[6] (related terms include *pseudologia phantastica* and *hospital hobo);* these patients wander from hospital to hospital, making up elaborate histories and presenting utterly imaginary or self-inflicted symptoms, often soliciting admission and invasive investigation. They are predominantly male, socially marginal individuals many of whom have chronic psychiatric illness or profound personality disorder. Much more common are more socially integrated but personally troubled patients, more often women and frequently employed in health-related professions, who are referred to specialists by conscientious primary providers who are baffled or overwhelmed by complaints that defy diagnosis or rational treatment. This is typically a fairly chronic behavior pattern, although there are individuals who will present with problems like laxative abuse as a way of coping with situations they feel are unbearable. In retrospective reviews, as many as 40% of these patients are found on GI services.[7]

It is important to appreciate that malingered or factitious symptoms are distinguished from conversion or hypochondriacal symptoms only by the patient's awareness or self-consciousness, which is ultimately a private experience that clinicians can only infer from behavior and self-report. Similarly, the only factor that discriminates malingering from factitious disorder is the presumed goal of the behavior, which is of course equally private and also available to others only by inference. Moreover, we are all aware that self-awareness cane be a *dimension* rather that an all-or-none attribute of behavior and that intentions are very often mixed. Many patients experience genuine symptoms with exaggerated intensity in the (ultimately futile) attempt to have their lives "made whole" by litigation, and some may exacerbate such symptoms deliberately in order to compel attention to illnesses they "know" are real and threatening but unrecognized or unappreciated by physicians.

THE CONTEXT AND MANAGEMENT OF ABNORMAL ILLNESS BEHAVIOR

Many factors determine the intensity with which an individual experiences and responds to physical symptoms.[8] Certainly, the magnitude of the stimulus is important, as is its duration. Its perceived seriousness, the degree to which it disrupts normal activity, and the knowledge, beliefs, and past experiences, of the patient are important determinants as well. Perhaps as a function of personal temperamental vulnerabilities, other contemporaneous factors in the patient's life, particularly aversive demands, current or anticipated stressors, and perceived sources of available support, may more or less powerfully influence the relative weight accorded these symptoms in proportion to other life concerns. In most cases, the symptoms themselves determine the patient's presentation to the physician (and the collaboration that follows) much more than the other factors. The physician's experience and intuition often guides inquiry as the other factors come into play, but when they begin to predominate, more specialized methods are needed.

Maintaining the Therapeutic Relationship

A first principle of management is so fundamental that it merits attention *only* because these patients can render it so difficult: even as doubts grow, it is crucial to maintain the patient's confidence that you are his or her doctor and that you will continue to care for him or her. At times, these symptom-enhancing and symptom-creating patients make it very difficult to sustain compassion and doctorly commitment. They consume precious time and resources over "nothing" in an era of encroaching scarcity. We have undertaken to care for them, and they violate their one simple and essential obligation: to tell us the truth as they know it. In this sense, they refuse to be patients, and yet they (and everyone else) expect us to continue to be their doctors. Indeed, this is the essence of abnormal illness behavior.

Psychiatric consultation should be undertaken as early as possible when such a behavioral component is suspected, especially in this era when outpatient visits may be rationed and hospital stays are brief. At this point, some of theses patients may become increasingly vocal about what they will and will not do. Some may become hurt or indignant at the introduction of a psychiatrist or psychologist. Some will refuse psychiatric referral, insisting that the problem is in their bodies and not in their heads. Some may respond positively to euphemisms about their being "under stress," but others will see this approach as a ruse. Some will have declined this recommendation in the past, and others may have accepted it with disappointing results for a variety of reasons. In all cases, it is crucial to provide firm assurance that you will do what is necessary to care for them and consultation is an essential part of that care.

Psychiatric Illness

When the experience of bodily symptoms or the conviction of illness seems to result from neuropsychiatric illness, patients may require a shift of focus to the treatment of that illness; they may become the primary responsibility of the psychiatrist and even need admission to a psychiatric service. Even in these cases, however, their presenting medical problems may still require investigation or management by the medical specialist, and this, too, may be facilitated by the medical specialist's reassurance of continued interest in the patient's condition. Patients with primary depressive or schizophrenic illnesses will typically become less preoccupied with their medical complaints *as* their affective and ideational symptoms are resolved, but these resolutions may come over a period of many weeks and may often be incomplete.

Abnormal Illness Behavior

The same principle applies to the management of illness behavior that is *not* produced by major psychiatric illness. Patients who are obsessively concerned about relatively minor problems will need continued medical care and support as they are helped to become reabsorbed into their work and family lives. In the absence of true psychiatric illnesses like depression, some personality traits may place patients at high risk for somatic symptoms and the conviction of illness. Extraverted persons tend to be vulnerable to suggestion and influence, and may report frustratingly protean symptoms. Individuals with *obsessive traits* have great difficulty accepting reassurance once a notion has taken root, and may defend the notion with endless new observations and "what ifs." Indeed, it has been observed that patients with somatization disorder often manifest both kinds of traits—extraverted dispositions that render them vulnerable to sensation and ideas about them, and obsessive traits that make it difficult to abandon these experiences. Modest intelligence and impoverished behavioral repertoires (and even very substantial resources may be taxed by some levels of challenge) may leave some individuals with few alternatives to the sick role in coping with demands the fear they cannot meet. It is rarely helpful to try to persuade patients that their symptoms are not real. The physician must first persuade the patient that he or she fully understands that a psychological diagnosis provides no immunity to other medical conditions, and that he or she has not lost interest in the patient's health and treatment. Such patients tend to do better if they are approached from a "rehabilitation" rather than a curative perspective and supported for their courage and determination in returning to their lives despite their health concerns *rather* than encouraged to relinquish those concerns altogether. It is usually much more helpful to *focus on overcoming barriers to* that reabsorption rather than on historical problems that may appear to have caused or maintained their medical preoccupations.

In some instances, conversion symptoms and even some factitious symptoms (e.g., laxative abuse) may respond rapidly when the complaints are met with *studious inattention* and the patient is redirected and supported in addressing the conflicts or demands underlying their appearance. Family and other intimates may be engaged in supporting "rehabilitation" without anyone being confronted with the hypothesized "psychogenic" nature of the complaints. In most cases of somatization disorder and hypochondriasis, however, where illness has become a way of life[9] management becomes more a matter of long-term support and "damage control" than of cure or resolution. The most effective element of treatment is the doctor-patient relationship, and it is often the doctor closest to the patient—the family or primary care physician—who carries most of the burden. It is often helpful for the primary care physician to see the patient at regular intervals, even—or especially—in the absence of new complaints, so that new symptoms do not become necessary as tickets of admission to the doctor's office. The *subspecialist* then serves as a *support* and a "backup," offering occasional supplementary specialty examinations while echoing and underscoring the primary doctor's sympathetic encouragement. The importance of this support in avoiding expensive and potentially injurious reexaminations and procedures cannot be overestimated.

Editor's note: This means not doing another endoscopic retrograde cholangiography or another colonoscopy just to "reassure" the patients.

● FACTITIOUS ILLNESS

Clinical Suspicion

The outright manufacture of symptoms by a nonpsychotic patient is a rare but serious and potentially life-threatening pattern of behavior, and the most dramatic violation of the doctor-patient relationship. One of its most difficult features is that it places the physician in the role of detective as much as doctor, a very uncomfortable turn of events for most caretakers. Moreover, factitious disorder may coexist with other significant medical illnesses, and, in fact, may make them more difficult to detect and diagnose. Nonetheless, a number of features may serve as warning indicators when patients are referred for consultation.[10] A history of complaints in times of personal stress may be difficult to elicit. However, when multiple physicians have been baffled or suspicious, or when the patient has felt disappointed, abandoned, or betrayed by several doctors, concern is appropriate. Symptoms that fail to respond to appropriate treatments, or that worsen when they should have improved—especially when the patient knew they would worsen—should also arouse concern. A history of "bad luck" from an early age, or of repeated treatment complications should also serve as a warning. The disproportionate representation of healthcare workers among factitious disorder patients is also a clue in many cases.

Psychiatric Collaboration

Based on these and other indicators, the possibility of factitious disorder should be evaluated as early as possible. Psychiatric collaboration should be engaged at the earliest point possible; euphemisms are less helpful in overcoming resistance than firm insistence along with equally firm reassurance that you are and will remain the patient's doctor. A two-track workup is crucial: the patient should be aware that the systematic evaluation of alternative *medical* diagnoses progresses along with the search for a psychological appreciation of the patient's experience. It is extremely helpful to find the "smoking gun" of contradictory or unlikely medical findings or evidence that is consistent only with factitious illness (e.g., enteric organisms in the blood, contaminated syringes, or phlebotomy equipment among that patient's possessions in the hospital).

Discussing Factitious Behavior

When the time comes to acknowledge explicitly the concern about self-inflicted symptoms, patients may be hurt or indignant. I have found it useful to make several points. First, factitious behavior is in fact a phenomenon that doctors encounter with some regularity. Second, certain clinical presentations (e.g., recurrent fevers of unknown etiology) make it necessary and prudent to evaluate factitious behavior, and the failure to do is negligent. Third, there is no specific constellation of personal traits that is associated with factitious disorder—patients with this behavior are most often not "crazy" or bizarre in their behavior. I have found it helpful to say that I am strongly inclined to believe the patient's denials, and that I usually believe what patients tell me. However, I have learned that I make mistakes in this regard, and that it would be irresponsible of me to wager patients on an uncertain intuition. It may also be helpful to tell the patient, if possible, about other medical explanations that remain under investigation.

Confrontation

If you are persuaded that the patient has been producing the symptoms, and if you have ruled out all of the other reasonable possibilities, it is usually best to engage the patient in a compassionate and nonjudgmental discussion of the evidence together with the psychiatric consultant as well others who have been consistently involved in the patient's care (nurses and even family members) and who have observations to contribute. This is always a difficult and often a painful process. There is a widely circulated idea that confrontation of factitious behavior precipitates suicide; however, although patients may leave the hospital or fire their doctors when challenged or confronted with evidence, instances of suicide have not been reported.

Psychiatric Admission

Following this confrontation, our practice is to admit the patient to an inpatient psychiatric service if at all possible. I have never regretted admitting a patient to a psychiatric service but I have on several occasions sorely regretted failing to do so. Given the potential life-threatening nature of the behavior, involuntary admission is certainly a viable option if the patient cannot otherwise be persuaded. Voluntary or involuntary, psychiatric admission accomplishes several goals. It makes clear the reality and the importance of the psychiatric diagnosis in the context of the patient's ongoing medical care. It formalizes the shift of primary responsibility for the behavior to the psychiatry service while allowing the medical subspecialist to remain an active consultant about the medical issues, and thus to address the patient's fear of being medically abandoned. A common explanation offered by patients for this behavior is that they know they have an illness and they have been doing what was necessary to *maintain* their doctors' interest and involvement. Psychiatric care should not be identified with the withdrawal of that care and involvement.

Involving Family

Perhaps the most important consequence of psychiatric admission is that it becomes impossible for the patient to maintain the capsule of secrecy that has allowed the behavior to persist. Secrecy is simply incompatible with the effective management of factitious behavior. This tends to be a recurring behavior, so it is crucial for the treatment team to mobilize the patient's family and other resources to support him or her in *not* succumbing to this behavior again when stress or provocations occur, as they inevitably must. Patients are often resistant to their families being informed of their diagnosis, and it is all too easy to empathize and identify with humiliation involved in sharing this kind of information with others. It is crucial, however, that these patients continue to have the support—and sometimes the surveillance—of those who care most about them. It is awkward to negotiate such a requirement with a patient, especially in the present context of acute vigilance about confidentiality; but once a patient is safely on a psychiatric service, the staff can often help the patient and the family come to terms with the behavior and develop a plan to avoid its recurrence.

● CONCLUDING COMMENTS

Even in the best of circumstances, it is difficult for most of us to understand the motivations of individuals who choose to organize their lives around illnesses from which they do not *need* to suffer. In this era when physicians must cope with increasing demands and diminishing resources, patients who exaggerate or even manufacture medical problems pose a frustrating challenge to our skills and our time. Nonetheless, these are patients in pain and in peril, and a careful and collaborative approach can make their care an interesting and rewarding process.

References

1. Pilowski I. Abnormal illness behavior. *Br J Med Psychol.* 1969;42:347–351.

2. McHugh PR, Slavney PR. *The Perspectives of Psychiatry.* Baltimore, MD: Johns Hopkins University Press; 1998.

3. Edwin D. Psychological perspectives on patients with inflammatory bowel disease. In: Bayless T, Hanauer SB, ed. *Advanced Therapy of Inflammatory Bowel Disease.* Toronto: CV Mosby Co; 2001:555–582.

4. Slavney PR. *Perspectives on Hysteria.* Baltimore, MD: Johns Hopkins; 1990.

5. Shorter E. *From Paralysis to Fatigue: A History of Psychosomatic Medicine in the Modern Era.* New York: Free Press; 1992.

6. Asher R. Munchausen's syndrome. *Lancet.* 1951;1(6650):339–341.

7. Reich P, Gottfried LA. Factitious disorders in a teaching hospital. *Ann Intern Med.* 1983;99(2):240–247.

8. Mechanic D. The concept of illness behavior. *J Chronic Dis.* 1975;17:189–194.

9. Ford CV. *The Somatizing Disorders: Illness as a Way of Life.* New York: Elsevier; 1983.

10. Eisendrath SJ. When Munchausen becomes malingering: factitious disorders that penetrate the legal system. *Bull Am Acad Psychiatry Law.* 1996;24(4):471–481.

Stress Management and Relaxation Training | 154

H. Richard Waranch

Stress represents one of the greatest threats to our physical and emotional well-being. However, living a stress-free life is unrealistic because stress is a normal part of life. When stress is mild to moderate, it may motivate a person to try harder and perform better. It is when stress is severe and prolonged that physical and emotional problems are more likely to develop. Today, with the widespread use and portability of cell phones, voice mail, computers, e-mail, and so on we have 24/7 access to work, investments, news, family, and friends. As a result, we often work longer hours and feel obligated to respond immediately to e-mail and voice mail. The dramatic rise in physical and psychological disorders such as headaches, chronic pain, irritable bowel disorder, hypertension, insomnia, depression, and anxiety can unquestionably be attributed in part to increased stress and reduced time for recreation and relaxation. Since stress cannot be completely eliminated, a more practical goal is to learn to deal actively and effectively with stress. Stress management is not a single treatment technique applied to an illness called "stress." Rather, stress management refers to a general treatment approach that may combine many techniques to help improve a broad category of health and behavioral problems.

Five steps are recommended in designing an appropriate stress management program for an individual:

1. Assess the individual's problem(s)
2. Educate
3. Increase healthy behaviors
4. Increase healthy thinking
5. Teach relaxation techniques

● ASSESSMENT

Each person with symptoms or behaviors that appear to be stress related (e.g., headaches, insomnia, anxiety) presents with a different history and set of circumstances that must be assessed before treatment can begin. For example, Joe is a 40-year-old married man, who was referred by his neurologist for biofeedback and relaxation training. His presenting symptoms were chronic left-sided facial pain and low back pain. Medical records from the neurologist and the patient's internist summarized his medical history in scrupulous detail and his lack of response to multiple medications as well as acupuncture, chiropractic treatment, and treatment by a dentist specializing in temporomandibular joint dysfunction. Magnetic resonance imaging, blood work, and physical examinations were all essentially normal. Notably absent from the medical reports was information about Joe's lifestyle. An interview revealed that Joe worked in a family construction business. He typically worked 7 days a week and 14 to 16 hours per day. He rarely took a day off, and he had taken only one 4-day vacation in 11 years of marriage. He believed that he personally had to supervise every job and employee or something would go wrong. Joe had always been a hard worker and somewhat of a perfectionist about work, but he became even worse after his father died a year earlier. His father was the founder of his company and after his father's death, Joe felt even more responsibility for all aspects of the business. Also, he now assumed responsibility for taking care of his elderly mother. Joe was about 25 pounds overweight, did not exercise, and often ate fast food on the run. Given his history and lifestyle, it was not surprising to me that Joe's symptoms did not improve with conventional medical treatment. My recommendation to Joe was that he needed to make some lifestyle changes rather than pursue biofeedback treatment.

● EDUCATION

Most people who present to me with stress-related symptoms are given a brief overview of the basic stress mechanism as described by Walter B. Cannon, 1953. Cannon introduced the theory that humans react to stressful events (stressors) with physical preparation to fight or flee. He proposed that our prehistoric ancestors developed a nervous system that responded to life-threatening events by preparing the body to do battle or to run away. He called this mechanism the "fight-flight" response (Fig. 154.1). When faced with perceived danger, heart rate and blood pressure skyrocket, the liver pours out glucose to be converted into energy, breathing becomes deeper and more rapid, and blood is diverted from nonessential functions to the brain and muscles. This is precisely what our prehistoric ancestors needed to survive when faced with acute, relatively short-term, physical threats.

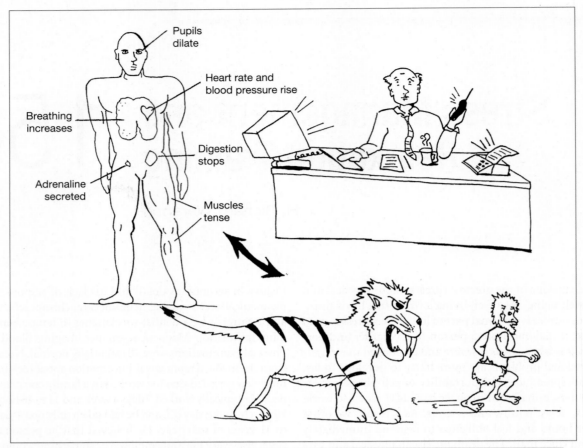

FIGURE 154.1 • Cannon's fight-flight response. Note: Cannon's fight-flight mechanism comparing prehistoric with modern man. I keep a copy of this picture in my office and I show it to patients in explaining how stress can play a significant role in contributing to their specific problem(s).

Civilization, by contrast, presents a host of everyday events that may be perceived as stressors. For example, traffic jams, commuting, household and car repairs, unexpected bills, and long work hours may elicit the same response in us as the sight of a saber-toothed tiger did in our prehistoric ancestors. Human beings are equipped to deal with such stressors, even if they do not happen too often. However, our bodies were not meant to deal with prolonged chronic stress. When stressful events happen repeatedly over a lifetime, the effects multiply and compound. Unfortunately, the implied promise that technology would somehow increase leisure time and make people more relaxed has certainly not materialized. If anything, technology has added to our stress level and eaten away at leisure activities. My patient, Joe, complained that whenever he misses a day at work, he returns to dozens of e-mails, faxes, and voice mails waiting for his immediate response.

● INCREASING HEALTHY BEHAVIORS

It is well known that it is unhealthy to abuse alcohol, drugs, and nicotine; to have an unhealthy diet; to be overweight; to constantly work for long hours; to rush and to lose one's temper. At the same time, everyone knows that it is healthy to exercise, to get an adequate amount of sleep, and to schedule time for relaxation and recreation. Once the physician determines that

a problem exists for a particular patient, practical and realistic recommendations must be presented. Merely telling a patient to "quit smoking" or "lose weight" is unlikely to result in behavioral changes. Rather, if appropriate, the patient should be referred to an appropriate program to help them lose weight or stop smoking. Specific recommendations should be made whenever possible and handouts and recommendations for articles or books may be suggested. Asking patients to agree to take a particular action to begin a program of more healthy behavior is a good way to start. Then, a follow-up phone call and scheduling follow-up appointments is critical in letting patients know that they have a serious problem and that you will partner with them in helping them change their behavior. Changing behavior is not easy, must be done gradually and in small steps and is facilitated by positive reinforcement.

● INCREASING HEALTHY THINKING

The following example provides an illustration of how a person's negative thinking can affect their behavior. When I first saw Joe, he was about 10 minutes late for his appointment, which he stated was fairly typical of him. On leaving his office, he was left with barely enough time to make our appointment as long as there was no traffic. However, there was traffic and he admitted getting very tense and frustrated and driving somewhat recklessly in an attempt to get to the appointment on time. He also admitted to such thoughts as "I should have left earlier," "I shouldn't be taking time away from my office anyway," "I know something will go wrong while I'm gone," and "I know this will be a waste of time anyway." Joe's self-talk is meant to illustrate that how we think or talk to ourselves can determine how we feel and what actions we decide to take.

Some explanations that we give ourselves are positive and empowering. Others arouse anger, feed our frustration, or lead to feelings of depression or anxiety. Shakespeare's Hamlet put it succinctly in saying, "There is nothing either good or bad but thinking makes it so." Our internal dialogue has been called "self-talk" by rational emotive theorist Albert Ellis, 2001, and "automatic thoughts" by cognitive theorist Aaron Beck, 1979. Most people talk to themselves quite differently than they talk to others. In talking to others, we are usually rational and objective and able to describe events as cause and effect relations. However, in talking to ourselves, we can be subjective and irrational. We are usually unaware of the continuing chatter in our heads, so we do not connect our negative feelings with our negative thoughts. Learning to change self-talk is the focus of cognitive therapy, and classic self-help books, such as *Feeling Good* and *The Feeling Good Handbook*, by David Burns, can help a person learn to increase healthy thinking.

● LEARNING RELAXATION TECHNIQUES

People learn to be tense and anxious and they can learn to relax. Learning to relax is like learning any new skill, learning takes place gradually and only after regular practice. However, once relaxation skills are learned, maintaining the skill typically requires much less effort. Learning different ways to relax can counteract the unhealthy effects of the body's fight-or-flight response. Relaxation can be achieved through a number of different approaches. For patients with more severe problems, there are psychologists and social workers who work with individuals, using a variety of relaxation techniques. For patients with mild to moderate problems, there are formal classes in meditation and yoga. For patients with milder problems, there are self-help books and CDs. Merely making a referral to a psychologist or a recommendation to enroll in a yoga course is not likely to be effective without some type of follow-up from the physician. Again, follow-up telephone calls or scheduled appointments are important to let the patient know that their problem is serious. One relaxation technique that can usually be taught in 5 to 10 minutes is diaphragmatic breathing. The exercise outlined below can easily be demonstrated in the office and most people will learn it quickly. A copy of the steps described below should then be given to the patient.

The following section can be copied and given to patients to practice on their own.

Diaphragmatic Breathing

Diaphragmatic breathing involves learning to use the diaphragm, rather than the shoulders and chest muscles, to draw air into the lungs. This allows more efficient breathing with less muscular work. It allows you to relax the neck and shoulder muscles while breathing.

Training Procedures for Relaxation and Diaphragmatic Breathing

Use a Recliner

A recliner or high-backed chair with arms is ideal initially because the entire body is supported and musculature tension is reduced. Once learned, diaphragmatic breathing can be used in a variety of settings and with different postures to help you relax.

Hand Placement

Place your right hand on your stomach, between the bottom of your rib cage and your navel. Place your left hand on your chest, just below your collar bone.

Loosen Restrictive Clothing

Unbutton your pants and loosen your belt. Research has demonstrated that people take in less oxygen when they are wearing restrictive clothing around the abdomen.

Baseline Breathing

Begin by breathing regularly and pay attention in a passive manner to your breathing. Notice the air passing through your nostrils and, at the same time, notice the rise and fall of your hands as you inhale and exhale. Do NOT try to control your breath, but simply sustain your awareness through the entire inhalation and exhalation cycle. For now, all other thoughts apart from the sensations of breathing are distractions. If your mind begins to wander or you feel distracted by other thoughts, sounds, or sensations—return your focus to your breathing.

Diaphragmatic Breathing Practice

As you inhale, imagine your stomach to be a balloon that inflates, lifting your right hand. As you exhale, the balloon deflates and your right hand falls. Your left hand remains still as your right hand rises and falls.

Feedback

Do not try to force it. Just attend to the motion of your hands and the feelings in your chest. Allow your right hand to rise and fall while your left hand remains still.

Slow Breathing

Next, slow your breathing by pausing very briefly at the top and bottom of each breath for just a second or so. Do not hold your breath or pause too much so that you become uncomfortable. Aim for one breath about every 6 or 7 seconds.

Tension Release

Each time you exhale, let your whole body become limp all over and allow it to sink deep in your chair.

Repeat the Word "Calm"

Some people find it helpful to anchor their mind on the breath by silently repeating a word with each exhalation. I like the word "calm," but any word that is personally meaningful (e.g., "peace," "one," or "uhm") could be used. If you use a word along with the breath, try to keep the actual sensation of breathing in the foreground of your awareness, and the word itself in the background, a quiet whisper in the mind.

Placement of Hands at Sides

After one or two sessions with the hands on your chest and abdomen, the hands can usually be placed on the arms of the chair or in your lap.

Some Difficulties

For most people, diaphragmatic breathing is awkward and uncomfortable initially. As in learning any new skill, with consistent practice, most people can become proficient and comfortable with this new style of breathing.

Practice

Try to practice at least 5 to 10 minutes once or twice a day to become familiar with the technique. Most people find that a convenient time to practice is in bed just prior to going to sleep. However, the goal of relaxed breathing is a state of relaxed alertness and if you are too drowsy you might fall asleep. So perhaps practicing at the end of the work day or before dinner might be better. Once you have mastered the technique and can do it rather quickly, you can begin using it whenever feeling stressed. Regular practice in nonstressful situations should be done first or diaphragmatic breathing is not likely to be very helpful when using it when you feel stressed.

When Feeling Stressed

Diaphragmatic breathing will be most useful if you notice the symptoms early and begin diaphragmatic breathing. Once in the midst of a full-blown anxiety attack or a severe migraine, it is not likely to help. Taking 5 to 10 minutes to practice breathing at the onset of such symptoms may serve to actually abort the symptoms or delay their occurrence.

Other Relaxation Training Techniques

There are many other techniques that patients can learn to help them relax. For example, progressive muscle relaxation is a set of exercises where patients are instructed to contract and relax major muscle groups in sequence while attending to the opposing feelings of tension and relaxation, and imagery is a technique where patients learn to imagine themselves in a safe and stress-free place like the beach or a mountain meadow. For my own patients, I have developed a Relaxation Training Program CD that contains four different relaxation techniques that comes with instructions on how to use each of the four exercises. This CD is available through the two sources listed below and both sources offer many other books, CDs, DVDs on various aspects of stress management and relaxation training.

Sources for Relaxation Materials
Biofeedback Instruments, Inc.
1-800-521-4630
BiofeedBack Resources International
1-877-669-6463

Supplemental Reading

Beck A. *Cognitive Therapy and the Emotional Disorders.* New York: Penguin Books; 1979

Burns DD. *Feeling Good: The New Mood Therapy.* New York: William Morrow; 1980.

Burns DD. *The Feeling Good Handbook.* New York: Penguin; 1989.

Cannon WB. *Bodily Changes in Pain, Hunger, Fear and Rage.* 2nd ed. Boston: Charles T. Branford Co.; 1953.

Davis M, McKay M, Eshelman E. *The Relaxation and Stress Reduction Workbook.* Oakland: New Harbinger Publications; 2006.

Ellis AT. *Overcoming Destructive Beliefs, Feelings and Behavior.* New York: Prometheus Books; 2001.

Chronic Abdominal Pain | 155

Willemijntje (Sandra) Hoogerwerf and P. Jay Pasricha

All of us have experienced acute pain, an unpleasant sensory and emotional experience that is associated with actual or potential tissue damage and which tells us that something is wrong with our body. This pain has a function because it allows for rapid identification of the site of origin of the underlying disease or injury and it allows for initiation of targeted therapy. On the contrary, *chronic* pain, one of the most common gastrointestinal (GI) conditions seen by primary care physicians and gastroenterologists, usually does not allow for rapid diagnosis of an underlying organic problem and is even less likely to lead to satisfactory therapy. Patients with chronic abdominal pain often have a track record of frequent emergency room visits and multiple physician examinations and of having been through a variety of diagnostic studies.

Pain is a subjective experience; there are no diagnostic tests that can determine the quality or intensity of an individual's pain. Regardless of whether there is an apparent so-called "organic" cause of the pain or not, the physician should bear in mind that pain often dominates the lives of patients in a negative fashion. Unfortunately, the patient with chronic abdominal pain is increasingly perceived as a clinical "liability" by the busy practitioner, with his or her symptoms either trivialized or, perhaps worse, dismissed as representative of either "malingering," "psychosomatic," or "drug-seeking" behavior. These and various other, rather unscientific euphemisms of a similar nature are reflective of the physician's lack of understanding of the biological basis, as well as the psychosocial dimensions, of chronic pain and the consequent frustration of not being able to place the symptom in a conceptually familiar frame of reference (as compared with a symptom such as hematochezia). This has led to a set of physician behaviors, which are often rather irrational, toward these patients, which include multiple diagnostic testing ("furor medicus"), referrals to various other specialists, and a pervasive fear of prescribing anything more than the mildest of analgesics. Ultimately, however, such behaviors do a disservice to both the medical community as well as the patients whom it serves. The truth is that most patients with chronic abdominal pain are neither hypochondriacs nor drug addicts and their suffering is real and considerable. It therefore behooves the careful

and compassionate gastroenterologist to remain engaged in the management of chronic abdominal pain; indeed the care of this condition can be both rewarding and relatively simple to perform, provided some basic principles are adhered to. Our purpose, in this chapter, is to review some of these principles and provide our own personal approach to these patients.

THE BIOLOGY AND PSYCHOLOGY OF CHRONIC PAIN

Neural Pathways

A proper understanding of the application and limitations of these approaches requires a good knowledge of the neuroanatomic pathway serving visceral pain. As with other organs, this pathway involves at least three levels of neurons. Peripheral nerve endings of the first-order neuron (the "primary nociceptor") exit from the target organ to travel along with the sympathetic nerves (but are not part of the sympathetic nervous system), passing without interruption through one of several prevertebral autonomic plexi associated with the corresponding visceral artery (e.g., celiac, hepatic, superior mesenteric) on their way to the dorsal root ganglia where their cell bodies lie. From here, the primary nociceptors send out shorter central branches to the dorsal horn of the spinal cord where they make contact with neurons in the gray matter. Postsynaptic (i.e., second-order) neurons then travel cephalad within ascending pathways to synapse in several thalamic and reticular formation nuclei of the pons and medulla, which in turn project to other parts of the brain, including the limbic system, somatosensory, and frontal cortices.

Sensitization

In the context of clinically important pain, it is also important to understand the concept of sensitization. This refers to a phenomenon in which the "gain" of the entire nociceptive system is reset upward by neuronal changes in either the periphery or within the central nervous system (CNS). Some form of sensitization invariably accompanies any kind of chronic pain, such

945

as that seen with persistent inflammation. The net result is that noxious stimuli now elicit a pain response that is much greater when compared with the normal state, a phenomenon termed *hyperalgesia.*

A further characteristic of the sensitized state is called *allodynia,* a phenomenon in which innocuous or physiologic stimuli are perceived as painful. As an example of mechanical allodynia, patients with chronic pancreatitis may experience pain in response to physiologic changes in intraductal pressure, which would be insensate in normal subjects. Similarly, subsequent minor flare-ups of inflammation in such patients could also cause the associated pain to be felt as far more severe than if being experienced for the first time (hyperalgesia).

Referred Pain: A Key Characteristic of Visceral Pain

A patient with "pure" visceral pain is seldom seen in the clinic, as this phase usually lasts only a few hours. Instead, most clinically significant forms of visceral pain are referred to somatic areas. Although the physiologic basis for referred pain is incompletely understood, it is generally believed to result from the fact that nerve signals from several areas of the body may "feed" the same nerve pathway leading to the spinal cord and brain. *Visceral pain* by itself is typically felt in the midline in the epigastric, periumblical, or hypogastric regions, reflecting the ontogenic origin of the involved organ from the fore-, mid-, or hind-gut, respectively, and is perceived as a *deep* and *dull discomfort* instead. *Referred pain,* which sets in soon after and comes to dominate the clinical picture, is perceived in overlying or remote superficial somatic structures such as skin or abdominal wall muscle, with the site varying according to the involved visceral organ. Further, referred pain is now *sharper* and assumes several of the characteristics of pain of somatic origin and indeed may dominate or even mask any underlying visceral pain.

If carefully questioned, many patients with chronic abdominal pain of visceral origin will indeed describe two types of pain, not always occurring simultaneously. However, physicians often make the mistake of lumping these together into a single pain; the result is that the disparate descriptions (e.g., *one diffuse and dull,* the other *localized and sharp*) are now perceived as paradoxical and serve to reinforce the perception that the complaints are not "organic" in nature. *Referred pain* is therefore more helpful in determining the site of the underlying disorder than the original pure visceral pain, which tends to be perceived in the midline regardless of the organ involved.

Pain, Suffering, and Illness Behavior

Nociception, or the process by which the nervous system detects tissue damage, is not synonymous with pain; increased afferent signaling to the CNS by itself does not always make a patient with chronic pain seek medical attention. However, nociception can, and often does, lead to suffering, a negative response to the perceived threat to the physical and psychological integrity of the individual and made up of a combination of *cognitive* and *emotional factors* such as *anxiety, fear,* and *stress.* This in turn can lead to certain patterns of *illness behavior,* which in turn determines the clinical presentation. Such behavior is a complex mixture of physiologic (e.g., pain intensity/severity or

associated features), psychological (mental state, stress, mood, coping style, prior memories or experiences with pain, etc), and social factors (concurrent negative life events, attitudes, and behavior of family and friends; perceived benefits such as avoidance of unpleasant duties, etc). Thus individual attitudes, beliefs, and personalities, as well as the social and cultural environment, strongly affect the pain experience. Although the biological basis of these interactions is poorly understood, it is important to understand that the clinical presentation of chronic pain represents a dysfunction of a system that is formed by the *convergence* of biological, social, and psychological factors (the so-called *biopsychosocial continuum*). These factors not only modulate each other but also, together, are responsible for an individual's sense of well being. In a given patient or at a given time in the same patient, the primary disturbance may disproportionately affect one component of the spectrum. An example would include intense nociceptive activity associated with an inflammatory flare-up in a patient with chronic pancreatitis; this is expected to dominate the clinical picture while the episode lasts, and the physician should concentrate on suppressing pain with strong analgesics. In between such episodes, when nociceptive activity is low, the spectrum may shift toward the psychosocial end and the wise physician may focus more on counseling and behavior modification. However, in either case, the patients' suffering is equally valid.

Indeed, most patients with chronic pain, regardless of etiology (somatic or visceral, "organic" or "functional") frequently suffer from depression, anxiety, sleep disturbances, withdrawal, decreased activity, fatigue, loss of libido, and morbid preoccupation with their symptoms, suggesting that these features may actually be secondary to the pain and not the other way around.

● APPROACH TO THE PATIENT WITH CHRONIC ABDOMINAL PAIN

It is not the purpose of this chapter to describe a comprehensive differential diagnosis to abdominal pain. Most experienced gastroenterologists will have no difficulty in readily identifying the underlying cause in the presence of typical clinical and laboratory features. Instead, we would like to focus on the approach to the *difficult* patient with chronic abdominal pain. These patients fall into the following three categories, as discussed in greater detail in the following sections: (1) the patient with unfamiliar or rare causes of abdominal pain, (2) the patient with a known cause of abdominal pain but one that is not easily brought under control, or (3) the patient with no apparent cause of abdominal pain.

The Patient with Unfamiliar or Rare Causes of Abdominal Pain

When a careful history and examination and routine laboratory tests fail to reveal a cause of abdominal pain, consideration must be given to rare syndromes. These include disorders that primarily affect *visceral nerves* rather than the organs themselves, such as *acute intermittent porphyria,* chronic poisoning with *lead* or *arsenic,* or *diabetic radiculopathy.* Women on *oral contraceptives* may experience mysterious attacks of abdominal pain that in some cases can be related to *mesenteric venous thrombosis.*

A clinical suspicion of "adhesions" is also often entertained by both physicians and patients with chronic abdominal pain even though the literature suggests that such a diagnosis is seldom validated. Adhesions are very common in women, even in the absence of prior surgery and are found in equal proportion in patients complaining of pelvic pain and those with other complaints. Indeed, laparoscopy for chronic pain seldom leads to a specific diagnosis and even less often to a change in management.

In contrast to the aforementioned disorders, our experience suggests that it is far more fruitful to carefully examine the abdominal wall in patients with chronic pain. This is an aspect that is frequently overlooked by gastroenterologists. Pain arising primarily in the abdominal wall can result from a poorly defined group of conditions whose pathophysiology remains obscure. The diagnosis is suggested when the pain is superficial, localized to a small area that is usually significantly tender, associated with dysesthesia in the involved region, and a positive Carnett's sign (if a tender spot is identified, the patient is asked to raise his or her head, thus tensing the abdominal musculature; greater tenderness on repeat palpation is considered positive). It is postulated that such tender spots are often due to entrapment neuropathy or a neuroma; however, we speculate that they could also represent an extreme manifestation of referred pain (see earlier section), particularly in the absence of a surgical scar or history of trauma, when they have been referred to as a "*myofascial trigger points.*" Regardless of etiology, it is important to make this diagnosis because such pain can often be managed in a relatively simple manner.

The Patient with a Known Cause of Abdominal Pain That Is Not Easily Brought Under Control

This type of pain is exemplified by the patient with *chronic pancreatitis*. Pain is not only the most important symptom of chronic pancreatitis but also the most difficult to treat. Pharmacologic, surgical, and endoscopic approaches have been tried in this condition for many decades, with inconsistent and often less than satisfactory results. The care of these patients remains challenging and imposes a significant burden on society with the attendant problems of disability, unemployment, and ongoing alcohol or drug dependence. Pain can also be a prominent and sometimes intractable feature of other syndromes, such as gastroparesis. Although often dismissed as functional, it is quite possible that the pain in this condition can be neuropathic in origin, reflecting the underlying pathophysiology (e.g., diabetes). The management of these pain syndromes is considered in greater detail later.

The Patient with No Apparent Cause of Abdominal Pain

In many patients with chronic abdominal pain, no definite abdominal pathology will be found to account for the symptoms. Indeed in the absence of obvious clinical or laboratory clues, it is relatively unusual for specialists to uncover a new pathophysiologic basis for pain in patients who have already been evaluated by their primary care physician. Although minor abnormalities in test results may be found, they may be more a reflection of statistical laws than true pathophysiology and often have questionable relevance to the pain. Eventually, many of these patients will be classified as having a "functional" pain syndrome such as noncardiac chest pain, nonulcer dyspepsia, and irritable bowel syndrome (IBS), depending principally on the location of the pain and association with physiologic GI events, such as eating or defecation. In some of these patients, there is increasing evidence to support the concept of *visceral hyperalgesia*, a manifestation of *neuronal sensitization* possibly resulting from previous and remote inflammation (e.g., a bout of infectious gastroenteritis). As discussed earlier, neuronal sensitization in these patients may not only exaggerate pain perception in response to noxious stimuli (*hyperalgesia*) but also lead to normal or physiologic events (such as gut contractions) being perceived as painful (*allodynia*). The chapter on IBS can be helpful (see Chapter 39, "Irritable Bowel Syndrome").

In a minority of patients, the pain does not seem to be connected to any overt GI function such as eating or bowel movement and has been termed *functional abdominal pain syndrome (FAPS)*. This and the more well-studied syndromes described in the previous paragraph have much in common including a predominance of women; heavy use of medical resources; psychological disturbances and personality disorders; and dysfunctional relationships at work, with family, and in other social settings. Conceptually, some of these patients can be perceived as occupying an extreme end of the biopsychosocial continuum of chronic pain discussed earlier. Thus, if patients with painful pancreatitis represent an example of a disturbance primarily (but not exclusively) affecting nociceptive signaling, then patients with FAPS can be viewed as representing a dysfunction of perception, coping, or response strategies. In either case, the net result is a patient with a hard-to-manage illness behavior.

● MANAGEMENT

A readily identifiable and treatable cause of chronic abdominal pain, although uncommonly found at a tertiary care setting, is of course a straightforward problem to address. More often, however, the gastroenterologist is left dealing with a patient who falls into one of the categories discussed in the previous section. In this regard, it is important to carefully examine the patient for an abdominal wall source as this may show a gratifying response to *local neural blockade*. Our approach is to identify a trigger point by digital examination, and inject a small amount of *lidocaine* or *bupivacaine* at the site of greatest tenderness elicited by the tip of the needle. Although the response may be short lived, it can provide valuable information as a therapeutic trial. Further, many patients get long-lasting relief after one or two injections alone. In those patients in whom relief is temporary, a 1:1 mixture of *lidocaine* and steroids (e.g., *triamcinolone*) can be used. More ablative chemicals (e.g., *phenol*) are best left to the *anesthesiologist* to administer.

Patients with chronic pancreatitis are increasingly being approached as problems in "plumbing" with various endoscopic or surgical interventions designed to decompress what is thought to be a partially obstructive ductal system. This is discussed in greater detail elsewhere in the pancreatic and biliary sections of this book, but many of these patients remain in pain after these procedures. Other patients of chronic abdominal pain with no obvious cause are also rarely substantially pain free after 1 or more years of follow-up. In most of these cases, a presumed cause of pain will have been diagnosed and treated, only to see the pain remain or a new type of pain manifest itself elsewhere.

Palliation is therefore an appropriate goal, and, in most patients, it is achievable. In the following sections, we will describe the basic principles of our therapeutic approach common to both these categories of patients, realizing that some "tailoring" is appropriate depending upon the suspected underlying problem. In general, the therapeutic approach to functional forms of pain is similar to the multifactorial approach to other forms of chronic pain described later, with perhaps greater emphasis on the psychosocial dimensions. As with any chronic illness, it is essential to have a robust patient-physician relationship based on patient education, realistic goal, and clarification of mutual expectations.

Pharmacologic Therapy of Chronic Pain

Narcotics

Although narcotics are arguably the most effective of available analgesic agents, their use is commonly perceived to lead to addiction, leading to a reluctance on the part of most gastroenterologists to use these agents. We agree that such agents should be *avoided* as far as possible in patients *with the functional bowel syndromes*. However, many, if not most, other patients with chronic abdominal pain will at some point in time require their use, and the compassionate physician is often faced with no other alternative to relieve suffering. The key elements that make for comfortable and judicious use of these drugs is a solid patient-physician relationship, careful patient selection, and the adherence to a fairly rigid protocol for prescription that also includes certain expectations from the patient (e.g., restriction of analgesic prescribing to a single physician, return to work, etc). When *mild chronic pain* necessitates analgesic use, weak opioids such as *propoxyphene* or *codeine* are often used, even though they are probably no more potent than simple analgesics, such as acetaminophen alone. *More severe pain* requires stronger analgesics; for short-term use *meperidine* or *morphine* can be used. For patients requiring long-term analgesics, sustained release preparations, such as *transdermal fentanyl* (Durgesic), are probably more useful. Agents with mixed agonist-antagonist profiles, such as *methadone* and *buprenorphine,* have been advocated by some to avoid addiction, although their use in chronic abdominal pain is not well substantiated.

Opioid analgesics have an *adverse effect* on GI motility and, in addition, can induce or exaggerate nausea. *Tramadol* (Ultram) is a good agent to use in patients with underlying dysmotility, such as gastroparesis, because it is reported to cause less GI disturbance. *Meperidine* (Demerol) is generally felt to be the drug of choice for patients with pancreatitis because of its lesser tendency to cause sphincter of Oddi spasm; however, this has only been shown to be true at *subanalgesic doses*. Because it is more likely to produce other side effects, however, it is seldom used for chronic pain management.

Antidepressant Agents as Analgesics

The class of agents that we prescribe most often for chronic abdominal pain is *tricyclic antidepressants (TCAs)*. The efficacy of these drugs has been best validated in patients with somatic neuropathic pain syndromes. Effective analgesic doses are significantly lower than those required to treat depression, and there is reasonable evidence to conclude that the beneficial effects of antidepressants on pain occurs independently of changes in mood. However, in this regard, diminution of anxiety and restoration of mood and sleep patterns should be considered desirable even if they represent primary neuropsychiatric effects of the drug. There are details on psychotropic medications in a separate chapter on functional GI disorders (see Chapter 43, "Psychotropic Drugs and Management of Patients with Functional Gastrointestinal Disorders").

Selective serotonin reuptake inhibitors (SSRIs), such as *paroxetine* (Paxil), *sertraline* (Zoloff), and *fluoxetine* (Prozac), which are currently the mainstay in the treatment of depression, have fewer side effects and have also been advocated for patients with chronic abdominal pain, particularly for patients with functional constipation as they can increase bowel movements and even cause diarrhea. However, they have been less well evaluated in the management of pain per se than TCAs; at present, the literature suggests that the efficacy of these agents for chronic pain is *equivocal* at best. Newer antidepressants, the *serotonin/norepinephrine reuptake inhibitors* such as *venlafaxine* (Effexor), hold more promise in this regard but have not been subjected to extensive testing in this setting. An older agent in the same class, *trazadone* (Desyrel), has been used with good effect in patients with noncardiac chest pain; although it does not have the usual side effects of the TCAs, it is more sedating and can cause priapism in males.

Before beginning antidepressants, it is important to assess the psychological profile of the patient, as this may be important in determining the choice of therapy. If the patient is not depressed, it is critical to spend some time explaining the scientific rationale for the use of antidepressants, with an attempt to clearly separate the analgesic effects from the antidepressant ones. We usually begin with *nortryptiline* (Pamelor) at a dose of 10 to 25 mg/day and progress as required (and tolerated) to no more than 75 to 100 mg/day. This is given at night and will almost immediately begin helping with disturbed sleep pattern that often accompanies chronic pain. Daytime sedation may occur but tolerance develops rapidly. Tolerance to the antimuscarinic effects may take longer and it is important to advise the patients about this. In the absence of significant side effects, the dose of the antidepressant is gradually increased until adequate benefit is achieved or the upper limit of the recommended dose is reached. It is also important to tell the patient that the analgesic effect may take several days to weeks to develop and that, unlike conventional analgesics, the drug is not to be taken on a "as needed basis" but on a fixed schedule. A trial of at least 4 to 6 weeks at a stable maximum dose is recommended before discontinuation. At that time, one may consider switching to another class of antidepressants such as *nefazadone* (Serzone), *mirtazepine* (Remcron), or *venlafaxine* (Effexor). *Venflaxine* may also be substituted for a TCA if excessive sedation is observed with the latter.

If the patient is *depressed,* it may be more appropriate to use *full antidepressant doses* of a drug that also has analgesic properties. This could be either a TCA with a low side-effect profile or perhaps one of the newer agents discussed earlier (not an SSRI). If the patient is already on an antidepressant, but this does not have proven analgesic activity (such as an SSRI), consideration should be given to switch to one that does, or to use small doses of a TCA, if tolerated. Such decisions should be made in conjunction with the psychiatrist taking care of the patient.

Other Drugs

A variety of drugs including neuroleptics (*fluphenazine* [Prolixin], *haloperidol* [Haldol]) and antiepileptics (*phenytoin* [Dilantin], *carmazepine*) have been used in chronic somatic pain with equivocal evidence of efficacy and a significant risk of adverse effects. However, we frequently use *gabapentin* (Neurontin), a drug with considerably more promise and safety that is widely used for neuropathic pain syndromes. Although admittedly anecdotal, our experience suggests that it may be useful in patients with functional bowel pain syndromes, especially in patients with *diabetic gastroparesis.* It can also be used in patients with chronic pancreatitis, in an attempt to "spare" narcotic use. Finally, mention must be made of the use of *benzodiazepines,* which are frequently used by patients with chronic pain including insomnia, anxiety, and muscle spasm. Although useful in these settings for short-term use, there is a significant risk for dependence on these drugs and there is little, if any, evidence that they have any real analgesic effect.

Behavioral and Psychological Approaches

Although pharmacologic therapy has a valuable role in these patients, it is also clear that a successful outcome requires taking into consideration several, equally important, factors. As explained previously, chronic pain cannot be viewed as a purely neurophysiologic phenomenon and has many other facets, the most important of which is the psychological dimension, consisting of cognitive, emotional, and behavioral processes. The combination of these factors results in *functional disability,* a third dimension of chronic pain that is often ignored. Several psychological techniques have been used with good effect in the management of a variety of chronic pain syndromes, although specific evidence for their efficacy in chronic abdominal pain syndromes is generally lacking. *Operant interventions* focus on altering maladaptive pain behaviors, such as reduced activity levels, verbal pain behaviors, and excessive use of medications. *Cognitive behavioral therapy* extends beyond this to also include cognitions or thought processes, based on the premise that these closely interact with behavior, emotions, and eventually physiologic sensations (i.e., the biopsychosocial continuum); altering one of these components can therefore result in changes in the others. Positive cognitions include ignoring pain, using coping self-statements, and indicating acceptance of pain. Negative processes include catastrophizing (i.e., viewing the pain as the worst thing in the world and believing it will never get better). *Biofeedback and relaxation* techniques teach patients to use control physiologic parameters and decrease sympathetic nervous system arousal. *Hypnosis* attempts to bring about changes in sensation, perception, or cognition by structured suggestions and has recently shown promise for patients with IBS. *Group therapy* exposes patients to others with similar problems and allows them to feel less isolated. *Dynamic (interpersonal) psychotherapy* attempts to reduce the physical and psychological distress caused by difficulties in interpersonal relationships.

It is, therefore, highly desirable, and probably necessary in some cases, to involve a clinical psychologist in the care of these patients. Indeed, as with somatic pain clinics, one can make a case for a broader team approach to chronic abdominal pain, involving other specialists such as anesthesiologists, occupational therapists, and pharmacists. However, in the absence of such an infrastructure, the gastroenterologist needs to assume some key responsibilities in this regard particularly in the form of ongoing patient education about the relationship of their symptoms to both underlying pathophysiology as well as to psychosocial factors. There is a chapter on exaggerated and factitious disease (see Chapter 42, "Factitious or Exaggerated Disease").

Neurolytic Blockade and Miscellaneous Approaches

The value of local blockade in abdominal wall syndromes has been described before. Theoretically, interruption of the pain pathways should provide relief of other forms of abdominal pain as well. This has led to the development of various techniques, both for diagnostic and therapeutic purposes. Neurolytic techniques are valuable for certain subsets of patients, such as those with cancer. By contrast, their use for pain relief in non-neoplastic pain, such as chronic pancreatitis, is not routinely recommended because of low efficacy (50%) and the short duration of relief (around 2 months), even in those patients who initially respond. Anecdotal experience suggests a similar disappointing outcome with the use of these techniques in functional bowel pain.

Indwelling epidural and *intrathecal access systems* have been effectively used for some patients with intractable chronic pain and to deliver opiates and other drugs, such as clonidine and baclofen. A variety of *electrical stimulation techniques,* including peripheral (transcutaneous electrical nerve stimulation), spinal, and cerebral stimulations have been used for various somatic pain conditions, as well as for angina pectoris, with encouraging results. *Acupressure* is another alternative medicine technique that has been widely used for pain, with results that are mixed. However, none of these techniques have been well studied, if at all, in patients with abdominal pain.

● CONCLUSION

The diagnosis and management of abdominal pain, particularly when chronic, is one of the most challenging clinical problems that a gastroenterologist encounters. Significant progress has been made in our understanding of the pathogenesis of somatic sensitization and it is hoped that this will lead to similar advances in visceral pain. Although there is a clear role for pharmacotherapy, the successful management of pain requires an intensely engaged physician who can interpret this symptom along with the psychosocial context of the patient.

Supplemental Reading

1. Cervero F, Laird JM. Visceral pain. *Lancet.* 1999;353(9170):2145–2148.

2. Hyams JS, Hyman PE. Recurrent abdominal pain and the biopsychosocial model of medical practice. *J Pediatr.* 1998;133(4):473–478.

3. Jackson JL, O'Malley PG, Tomkins G, Balden E, Santoro J, Kroenke K. Treatment of functional gastrointestinal disorders with antidepressant medications: a meta-analysis. *Am J Med.* 2000;108(1):65–72.

4. Mayer EA, Gebhart GF. Basic and clinical aspects of visceral hyperalgesia. *Gastroenterology.* 1994;107(1):271–293.

5. Pasricha PJ. Approach to the patient with abdominal pain. In: Yamada T, ed. *Textbook of Gastroenterology.* 4th ed. Philadelphia, PA: Lippincott Williams and Wilkins; 2003:781.

6. Suleiman S, Johnston DE. The abdominal wall: an overlooked source of pain. *Am Fam Physician.* 2001;64(3):431–438.

7. Wilcox G. Pharmacology of pain and analgesia. In: Committee ISP, eds. *Pain 1999—An Updated Review.* Seattle, WA: IASP Press; 1999:573–592.

8. Drossman DA. Chronic functional abdominal pain. *Am J Gastroenterol.* 1996;91(11):2270–2281.

9. Hunt SP, Mantyh PW. The molecular dynamics of pain control. *Nat Rev Neurosci.* 2001;2(2):83–91.

Diet, Fitness, and Attitude— A Patient's Perspective

156

Peter Nielsen

Editor's note (TMB): We have included this chapter so that the health care professional is aware of some of the information that IBD patients receive. Although the chapter has been edited, the opinions expressed are those of the author.

Very little was known about Crohn's disease in 1977 when Nielsen was diagnosed and doctors knew little about how to tell him to fend off the crippling symptoms of the disease—abdominal pain and bleeding and malnutrition. He began to study nutrition and exercise and worked with doctors to develop a personal package of health and fitness. He dedicated himself to keeping healthy and went on to compete as a body builder earning more than 50 titles including Mr. International Universe and Mr. World. He is now a fitness and health expert and trainer with fitness centers in the Detroit area, has written several books, and hosts his own nationally syndicated television show, Peter's Principles. He is also a speaker for the Crohn's and Colitis Foundation.

We know how critical medical interventions and family support are when facing this chronic struggle with inflammatory bowel disease (IBD), and those factors are somewhat beyond our control. But one area you can control is your lifestyle—your diet and exercise habits and how you feel about yourself. These are very powerful factors and critical elements in helping overcome symptoms of IBD. In life, I believe there is always opportunity, no matter what disappointments or challenges we face. These challenges, the disappointments and even failures, can be opportunities to make something more and better of ourselves.

I learned this after being diagnosed with Crohn's disease at the age of 15. That Christmas in 1977, I found myself in the hospital for a series of tests to see what was wrong with me. I woke up in the morning with tubes connected to me and a pouch on my side. They had removed 2.5 feet of my intestine, and my family was told I had Crohn's disease, a debilitating and chronic gastrointestinal disease that included these crippling bouts of abdominal pain and bleeding that I had been having. The disease can also cause tremendous weight loss and malnutrition from poor nutrient absorption. At first I felt overwhelmed, depressed, and afraid—fearful that I would never be able to have a "normal" life.

● ADVERSITY TURNED INTO OPPORTUNITY

For me, my response to this physical adversity of trying to overcome the symptoms of Crohn's disease took the form of building a healthier lifestyle for myself.

When I was first diagnosed, I went from 145 pounds to 86 pounds and felt so terrible about my body and how bad I looked. For a teenager in high school, when most of your peers first judge you by appearance, this was pretty depressing.

Soon I realized that feeling depressed wasn't getting me any better, so I started to take my mind off the negatives of this disease and to focus on something positive, something I could do to feel better about my body—and I began to appreciate and use the gifts that God had given me. I stopped the self-pity and started to concentrate on diet and fitness.

I studied nutrition and exercise and worked with my doctors to create an overall package of health and fitness for me. There were many days when I could barely move. But I concentrated on my diet and adhered to a steady fitness plan, which included cardiovascular activity and weight lifting.

Keeping my exercise program consistent helped me tremendously to get through flare-ups, relieve pain, and keep a positive attitude. Now, working out is a part of my daily routine and I feel better than ever. Everyday I appreciate my ability to move and exercise. I love exercising and developed it into a career. I am determined to make the most of my body, and now I'm trying to help others do the same. Many people helped me along my journey to become confident and healthy, and now everyday in my career as a health and fitness expert and on my TV show, I am involved in helping others to develop that same desire to overcome illness—the desire that saved my life!

● WHEN AND HOW MUCH TO EXERCISE?

Fitness has given me a better quality of life, self-love, and appreciation of my body and health. It is an incredible vehicle, especially for someone with Crohn's disease. But those with IBD need a specific program and special attention in many areas. I recommend getting personal training with an exercise physiologist who can recommend a program tailor-made for your specific circumstances. For example, they can recommend specific exercises appropriate for a vertical or a horizontal surgical scar.

Some forms of exercise that are good for everyone include

- Resistance/weight training, which increases bone density and lean tissue
- Walking as opposed to running, which is easier on your abdomen
- Swimming, which is a great form of exercise that puts no stress on joints

Not every day is great when you face a chronic disease and flare-ups, but we must be realistic knowing some days you feel great and others not so good. Some days you might have a fissure, or blood in the stool and can't work out. But I know that this will happen from time to time and I must expect it. You must be in tune with how your body feels and what's going on each day, and know your limitations! When you feel good, you should take every advantage and get moving. But don't feel upset or defeated if you have to miss a day or two—that's OK. That is part of living with Crohn's disease or any other chronic illness.

● MEDICATIONS AND FITNESS

Fitness training and exercise is wonderful when fighting Crohn's disease because it builds up the immune system. Some medications taken to battle the disease are catabolic steroids that tear down muscle and bone density in the process. So it is so important when your doctor permits; you should start exercising in order to build back the muscle and bone density you lost from the steroids. I know that my exercise and fitness regimen makes me strong enough to endure the flare-ups that are going to come. Also taking your medications can make you feel nauseous, so my doctors helped me find a solution: work out early in the morning and take medications at night—so that problem was solved.

Although there is no known cure at this time, variable drug therapies may be prescribed for these diseases, and new drugs are constantly being tested. If a drug is prescribed for you, research it and ask for a list of all the drugs that are available based on your individual needs. Find out which new drugs will be coming out in the near future. Ask for referrals to websites that will help to keep you informed on any new information.

Editor's note (TMB): Yes, although it is important for our patients to be well informed, physicians and other health professions should consider patient education one of their duties. This is discussed in chapters 5, 6, 8, and 144–150. There is a well-researched discussion on balancing benefits and risks of biologic therapy in Chapter 115. Yes, it is also important to listen to the patient, who may have first hand memories of benefits or of adverse events that are not clearly delineated in the chart or medical record. The current fragmentation of care makes it even more important to let the patient tell his or her story. The health care professionals specializing in IBD care will use their knowledge of the field along with an individual patient's situation and concerns to make recommendations.

● EXERCISE AND ATTITUDE

Exercise and fitness training also helps you mentally, and it gives self-confidence and strength to fight Crohn's disease. Crohn's disease affects people often in their late teens and 20s, when self-esteem and confidence are so important. Exercise is the best way to help you feel good. It is a natural antidepressant because, when exercising, your body secretes endorphins, which help boost your mood. I tell everyone around me that if I am not working out, I am not feeling good. If I feel well, then I am exercising!

The human body was designed to move around and not sit still for hours on end. Many of us spend too much time sitting, either in work-related jobs, computer time, or relaxation in front of the television. Sometimes you're stuck sitting somewhere, whether you want to be or not. You don't need to be standing to get some exercise. An energy break, even while seated, can make a big difference in your productivity, your ability to handle stress, and your overall well-being. Whether you're at home or at the office, or you just find yourself sitting in a chair too long, these simple, easy-to-do exercises will help you destress, stretch and strengthen muscles, improve your circulation and mobility, burn a few more calories, and probably improve or boost your energy and mood.

Especially when you're at the office, make sure that every hour or even half hour, if you can, get up and move around. Your body will thank you! Incorporating these simple exercises into your daily routine will quickly become a habit and you'll become a little more active every day. You will soon notice increased energy and pain relief caused by sitting for hours.

Exercises Anyone Can Do, Anywhere

Each of the following can be performed sitting in a chair or on a couch and takes only a minute to do. You can complete all the exercises in mini 10-minute workouts, or you may prefer to select only two or three to perform during your break.

Sit/Stand Exercise

Purpose: Increases circulation and mobility, strengthens legs, buttocks, and core muscles.

- Stand with your back to a sturdy chair with your feet about 6 inches in front of the chair seat. Separate your feet hip-width apart, legs straight.
- Bend knees, sitting back on your heels until your buttocks or back of your thighs touches the edge of the chair seat without sitting down. As you squat, extend arms out in front of you at chest height, palms facing the floor.
- Straighten legs and stand up.
- Repeat 10 to 16 times and progress to 20.

Seated Crunches

Purpose: Strengthens abdominals.

- Sit tall in a chair with your hips touching the chair back, feet flat on the floor, knees bent and aligned over ankles.
- Cross your arms, placing hands on opposite shoulders, elbows lifted to shoulder height.
- Exhale and contract your abdominals, drawing them in, bringing your elbows toward your thighs. Keep your midback to your tailbone against the chair back; this is a small motion; only use your abdominals.
- Inhale and sit up tall. Repeat 10 to 16 times and progress to 20

Leg Toners

Purpose: Strengthens front of thighs and abdominals, increases hamstring flexibility, improves circulation.

- Sit tall in a chair with your hips touching the chair back, feet flat on the floor, knees bent and aligned over ankles.
- With hands holding the sides of the chair, arms straight, lift both feet off the floor, knees bent (for an easier version, keep feet on the floor).
- Straighten one leg out in front of you. Bend knee, then straighten the other leg.
- Continue to alternately straighten and bend legs. Repeat 10 to 16 times and progress to 20.

Bun Burner

Purpose: Helps develop firm buttocks and shape them.

- Sit tall in a chair with your hips touching the chair back, feet flat on the floor, knees bent and aligned over ankles, hands on your thighs.
- Tighten and squeeze your buttocks. Hold for 2 seconds and release.
- Repeat 15 to 20 times, progress to 25.

● NUTRITION AWARENESS—WHAT YOU EAT DOES EFFECT HOW YOU FEEL

Controlling your eating habits and what goes into your body is so important in helping you to feel your best. This is true for everyone, but especially for those who have inflammatory bowel disease (IBD) or other chronic illness. We should learn to view food through two lenses: one lens looking at food as appetizing and appealing, like when I look at my favorites, a plate of shrimp scampi or linguine with clam sauce and another viewing it in the sense of nutrition and what foods provide your body with energy. You don't have to lose the pleasure or the enjoyment of eating. But you do need to begin to think about your eating habits and what you eat from day to day.

Food is the fuel that drives your body and allows you to perform and engage in activity. We need to make sure our body is getting enough nutrients and protein to sustain important body functions. This is even more important for someone fighting a chronic disease such as Crohn's or cancer because disease puts additional stressors on the body and raises more demands on our health. This is especially true for athletes.

Knowledge is power when it comes to dealing with digestive diseases. If you can learn to help make foods work for you instead of against you, that is half the battle. A balanced and healthy diet is crucial for us. I believe you need to know the quantity of nutrients and the protein you take in. Because I am a bodybuilder and this is my profession, I count every gram of protein and carbohydrates that go into my body. You don't need to watch it as closely as I do, but you do need to have a knowledge of basic diet and nutrition guidelines. You should structure a healthy dietary regimen to fit your tastes and your life style.

● WHAT CAN I EAT?

Generally, the patient is advised to eat a well-balanced diet with adequate protein and calories. There are books that can help you create healthy meals. Just be sure that they are approved for your particular condition. The physician may recommend a multivitamin and iron supplement, but I use and highly recommend Daily Body Restore Digestive Care Products (see resource list).

Nutrition Tips

- Take precautions and learn what you can and cannot tolerate. If a certain meal makes you sick, write down exactly what you ate and try to pinpoint which foods caused it and avoid those foods in the future.
- Easy foods to digest include grilled skinless chicken, grilled salmon without butter, egg white omelets, potatoes without butter, and oatmeal.
- Avoid foods with shells, fruit skin, food high in fat, spices, and sugar alcohols.
- Avoid chewing gum, which releases enzymes in the stomach that may cause acid that can bother you. Sugar-free gums may contain sorbitor, a cause of gassiness, as described in chapters 40 and 42 on carbohydrate intolerance.
- Many people with digestive diseases find they become lactose intolerant and dairy products may cause bloating or a laxative effect.
- During an acute phase, it is a good idea to avoid bulky foods, such as bran cereal and milk and milk products, which may increase diarrhea and cramping.

Editor's note (TMB): There is additional detailed information on nutrition, food-induced symptoms, and food allergy in chapters 30, 42, 53, 117, and 120.

Importance of probiotics and digestive enzymes: Although a healthy diet and exercise are essential to good health, eating healthy foods is only the first step. In order to stay healthy, our bodies must assimilate the nutrients from our food. No matter how healthy your diet is, if the vitamins, nutrients, and minerals in your meals are not being properly absorbed, your health will suffer. Some of the factors in my digestive health plan are probiotics and digestive enzymes.

Poor digestion can contribute to many serious conditions including heartburn, constipation, gas, bloating, inflammation, irritable bowel syndrome, gastric reflux, fatigue, lower immune responses, and malnutrition. It can also contribute to serious illnesses such as osteoporosis, cardiovascular disease, digestive diseases, autoimmune diseases, cancer, and other serious health issues. When the digestive tract is not functioning properly, critical body systems do not receive adequate nutrient supply.

In order to benefit from eating the foods that you eat, your body has to properly digest and absorb the nutrients. As food enters the mouth and we start to chew, our teeth help to make the food pieces smaller, and saliva adds moisture that allows food to travel down into our stomach where digestion begins. The stomach and pancreatic juices contain several enzymes that work together to partially break down food substances. These **digestive enzymes** break down the food into nutrients that are then absorbed through the small intestine. When you lack these digestive enzymes, your body doesn't digest food properly, and as a result, the body does not absorb the valuable nutrients it needs.

It may surprise you that there isn't just one enzyme or molecule that breaks down all the food we eat. The process of digestion is very complex and involves several enzymes, each with a specific function. The human body alone produces 22 different enzymes. Other sources of enzymes are raw vegetables, fruits, grains, and meat. Eating lots of raw fruits and vegetables and whole grains can provide appropriate amounts of digestive enzymes, but the truth is that most Americans eat too much processed food, which has very little nutritional benefit.

Also, as we get older, our bodies naturally produce less digestive enzymes. This isn't just a problem for the older folks, it might shock you to know that the production of enzymes in the digestive tract (stomach, intestines, and pancreas) starts to decline at the **age of 35**! It can even happen at a younger age, so everyone should be concerned about having a healthy diet and ensuring you have the proper amount of digestive enzymes and probiotics in your system.

Probiotics are "friendly" bacteria that naturally occur in our digestive tracts. They too are essential for normal digestive function. One must make sure to keep the digestive tract balanced with the natural level of friendly bacteria. There is a wide range of research and clinical studies focusing on the role of probiotics or "friendly bacteria" in heart disease, cancer, and even chronic systemic inflammation.

Making sure you have the appropriate balance of probiotics and digestive enzymes in your diet to ensure proper digestion and absorption of nutrients is essential to one's overall health. Probiotics may help relieve chronic constipation and may help restore beneficial bacteria in the digestive tract to healthy levels. Probiotic supplementation may help the body cope with numerous health conditions that deplete your natural probiotics. Health care specialists may recommend probiotic supplementation as a part of any daily health regimen because they understand the importance of maintaining the balance of intestinal flora.

Editor's note (TMB): Probiotics are discussed in detail and in an objective fashion in chapters 48 and 76.

● STRESS AND IBD

Editor's note (TMB): Chapters 8, 33, and 44 are about IBD and stress.

Be aware that certain conditions can trigger a flare-up or aggravate your symptoms. The following is a list of things that are known to trigger flare-ups and should be avoided:

- Stress
- Caffeine (a stimulant)
- Alcohol (a depressant)
- Lack of sleep
- Too much sun

Table 156.1 lists some foods and products that I believe help to naturally reduce stress and promote overall health.

● WATER—THE FORGOTTEN NUTRIENT

Water is really the "forgotten" nutrient. Many people are dehydrated and do not even know it. Being tired, moody, and fatigued are the symptoms of dehydration—not having enough water in your body. Technically, water is not a nutrient at all. But it is crucial to virtually every basic body function from temperature regulation to blood circulation, metabolism, immune system function, and waste elimination.

Everybody, thin or fat, needs plenty of water every day. Be grateful to your kidneys, nature's filtering department. Without them, you would need to drink 2500 gallons of water every day just to flush out the system. How much water do we really need every day? The average person should be drinking at least 6 to 8 cups of

TABLE 156.1 Food Sources of Nutrients

	What it does
Holy basil	
	Decreases cortisol levels
	Promotes clarity during times of physical/emotional stress
	Support healthy adrenals
Foods with vitamin B6	What it does
Sweet Potatoes	Helps manufacture serotonin (necessary for coping with stress)
Asparagus	Boosts autoimmune system
Avocados	
Spinach	
Chick peas	
Foods with folic acid	What it does
Asparagus	Member of B vitamin family
Avocados	Crucial when coping with stress
Spinach	May ease depression
Foods with vitamin C	What it does
Citrus fruit	Boosts autoimmune syatem
Peppers	
Foods with calcium	What it does
Broccoli	Needed for communication among nerve cells
Salmon	
Yogurt	
Foods with magnesium	What it does
Spinach	Helps relax muscles
Pumpkin	
Foods with carbohydrates	What it does
Potatoes	Excellent source of energy during stress
Brown rice	Complex carbohydrates replenish serotonin
Pasta	
Bread	

water each day. To be more specific, divide your body weight by two. That gives you the number of ounces of water you should be drinking. Divide that by eight to get the number of cups.

The average person loses about two cups daily through perspiration (temperature control), even without unusual physical exertion. Another two cups disappear in the respiration process. The intestines and kidneys together use about six cups a day. That is about 10 cups total, not counting water loss through perspiration during any heavy exercise. Some of the water loss is replaced through the food we eat—liquid or solid.

Editor's note (TMB): Importantly, patients with ileostomies or ileoanal pouches are at increased risk of dehydration because they have lost the fluid sensing and control system that originates in the colon.

The fact is millions of Americans do not come close to drinking their daily need for water. Their rationale that consuming lots of soda, coffee, beer, or wine is considered liquid and that will satisfy intake of fluid is NOT true, quite the opposite. Alcohol and caffeine or caffeine drinks, besides depleting the body of vitamins and minerals, are natural diuretics, meaning they actually lead to fluid elimination and dehydration.

Dehydration occurs when one does not take in enough water to replace all that is lost through breathing, urination, and exercise. There are many degrees of dehydration, of course, but depending on our lifestyle many of us could be dehydrating ourselves on a regular basis. So there are many factors that affect the amount of water in your body. Working all day in a stuffy house or office building, or spending 3 to 4 hours on an airplane, you lose large amounts of fluid invisibly. Stress, as well as alcohol and caffeine, acts as a diuretic. You need to drink more water if you have any of the factors listed in Table 156.2.

Here's another interesting fact about water intake and weight loss. Drinking water suppresses appetite, and naturally helps the body metabolize stored fat. If you are overweight or if you have fluid retention problems, you should be drinking **more water**. Overweight people with a larger metabolic load need more water than thin people. If you keep your body adequately supplied with water, it actually speeds up your metabolism and makes you burn more calories. If the body is not being given enough water, your body reacts as if it is a threat to survival and like a camel, begins to hold on to every drop. If you drink more water, the body will release the excess.

TABLE 156.2 Dehydrating Factors
Where you live and work—no ventilation all day
Hot weather
Airline travel (more than 3 hours)
Stress
Caffeine intake
Alcohol intake
Amount of exercise and exertion levels
Various medications such as diuretics

Dehydration Affects Muscles and Physical Performance

Seventy-five percent of muscle tissue is water. If a muscle loses 3% of its water, you lose 10% of contractual strength and 8% of speed. Dehydration also increases blood viscosity, making blood thicker and more concentrated, and this stresses the heart. Your arteries become less able to provide muscles with nutrients and oxygen and to eliminate accumulated wastes. So you do not need to be a scientist, rocket or otherwise, to figure out that dehydration is a common cause of poor athletic performance.

Dehydration Affects the Brain

Dehydration can produce a minuscule but crucial shrinkage of the brain. Deprive yourself of enough water and your concentration and coordination will be affected. In other words, you need those 6 to 8 cups a day whether you are pumping iron in a gym or crunching numbers at a desk.

● WHEN AND HOW TO DRINK WATER

People often tell me, "No problem; I drink tons of water with my meals." Well, that is exactly the wrong way to consume water. It dilutes your food and blocks the efficient absorption of nutrients. Milk is an acceptable drink with meals, because milk becomes a semisolid in the stomach. But avoid drinking water beginning 15 minutes before a meal and for 30 to 60 minutes after a meal. This allows your stomach time to begin an efficient digestive process.

Feeling thirsty is a poor indication that you need water. You need to make drinking water a habit. Ninety percent of achieving the battle with any new dietary/exercise regimen is nothing but habit—getting used to doing it day after day, so give it a try and start carrying a squirt bottle with you and drink water throughout the day. Nowadays, seeing people with water bottles is quite common and socially acceptable.

● TIPS ON CHOOSING YOUR DOCTOR AND LEARNING ABOUT YOUR DISEASE

Find a list of doctors in your area. Interview at least two or three before selecting the person with whom you want to work. You'll want a general practitioner, a surgeon, and a GI specialist. Ask a lot of questions. Here are a few to get started with.

- Are you Board certified? Are you a member of the Crohn's and Colitis Foundation of America?
- What is your educational background?
- How many surgeries have you performed?
- What is your success rate?
- Have you had any malpractice suits?

There are numerous problems associated with these diseases, so you need to educate yourself about yours and then learn to practice moderation in everything you do. While we all experience stress, learn to avoid the situations that produce it. The same goes for the other possible triggers. Nutrition is extremely important as you have read and you need to learn what foods you should and should not eat and ways to supplement your diet.

ATTITUDE IS EVERYTHING

During my early struggles with this disease I did not realize it, but now I look back and realize that I was blessed with this opportunity to be a vehicle to touch the lives of many people—people of every sort from persons with physical handicaps or serious challenges to top-ranking athletes who have attained the pinnacle of performance in their fields. It has always been my desire to help people learn from my experience, not only the good things I did, but my mistakes as well.

One important lesson I learned through my struggle with Crohn's disease **is that opportunity is adversity turned upside down.** We can use whatever challenges and disappointments we face, to turn it upside down into something beneficial. But it is our attitude toward it that permits us, as William Faulkner said, not only to endure but also to prevail.

Having a positive "can-do" attitude is so important. The last thought I leave with you is to keep an attitude of H.O.P.E., which stands for "Having Optimum Positive Emotions." Believe in yourself, stay focused and never give up. Find your faith and enjoy each day to the fullest. If you believe you can work through the pain, the depression, and the disease, then you will!! I am living proof of it.

RECOMMENDED RESOURCES/ WEBSITES

www.petersprinciples.com Peter Nielsen's website and newsletter
www.ccfa.org Crohn's and Colitis Foundation of America
www.dailybodyrestore.com

Editor's note: These products are personal recommendations of Peter Nielsen, not those of the editors nor publisher.

Complementary and Alternative Medicine in IBD

157

Robert J. Hilsden and Marja J. Verhoef

Gastroenterologists frequently encounter patients who are using or want to use an alternative therapy to treat their inflammatory bowel disease (IBD). The patient may have known about the therapy through friends or family, books, media, or the Internet or may have seen a complementary practitioner. Managing these situations can be difficult for gastroenterologists because they may not be knowledgeable about the therapy and are likely hesitant to support a therapy without strong scientific evidence for its efficacy and safety. In this chapter, we provide a brief overview of what is currently known about the use of complementary and alternative medicine (CAM) by patients with IBD and then focus on practical guidelines for informing and counseling patients about the use of CAM. Finally, we will recommend some useful sources of information on complementary therapies.

COMPLEMENTARY AND ALTERNATIVE MEDICINE

The term CAM is commonly used to refer to the diverse collection of health systems and diagnostic and therapeutic modalities that are not part of the conventional Western medical system. The National Institutes of Health's National Centre for Complementary and Alternative Medicine (NCCAM; nccam. nih.gov) groups CAM practices into five main categories, that can often overlap: (1) whole medical systems (e.g., homeopathic medicine, naturopathic medicine, traditional Chinese medicine, and ayurveda), (2) mind-body medicine (e.g., meditation, prayer, and mental healing), (3) biologically based practices (herbal products, dietary supplements, and other natural products), (4) manipulative and body-based practices (e.g., chiropractic or osteopathic manipulation), and (5) energy medicine (e.g., therapeutic touch and Reiki).

These therapies may be used in three ways. A complementary therapy is used in conjunction with a conventional therapy, whereas an alternative therapy is used instead of a conventional therapy. Mostly, it is the patient who seeks out the complementary therapy and might use the therapy without the knowledge of his/her IBD physician. Those using CAM as an alternative may not regularly see their physician. Finally, *integrative medicine* intentionally combines evidence-based treatments from conventional medicine and CAM (see chapter 123). It is likely that this practice is currently uncommon in the management of IBD.

Editor's note (TMB): There is an earlier chapter on integrated medicine in IBD. This includes discussion of curcumin.

CAM practitioners often have a different view of disease and its treatment than conventional physicians.[1-3] They usually place a strong emphasis on holism, vital forces, and naturalism. An holistic approach is characterized by an emphasis on diagnosing and treating illness through an understanding of the whole person (body, mind, and spirit) and how the individual interacts with the world around him/her. Furthermore, disease may be seen as the result of a blockage or disruption of the vital energy or an imbalance between two opposing forces, and treatments are directed at restoring a healthy balance and flow between these forces and stimulating the self-healing potential of the body. Naturalism emphasizes people's intimate relationship with the natural world and relies on detoxification (often through fasting) and natural remedies (herbs and vitamins) to improve and maintain health. These philosophies often lead to highly individualized treatment packages, which are highly valued by CAM users. Patients choosing CAM often want to play a more active role in their treatment, and they may be seen as the primary agent of healing helped by the guidance of the practitioner. The patient-centered focus of CAM along with the common emphasis on health and well-being, rather than on disease, may be particularly appealing to patients.

USE OF COMPLEMENTARY THERAPIES BY PATIENTS WITH IBD

CAM use by the general population is common. Approximately, 40% of US adults used some form of CAM in 2007.[4] Therefore, it is not surprising that adult and pediatric patients with IBD commonly use CAM. Studies have reported that approximately 40% to 50% of patients with IBD have used or are using some form of CAM.[5-7] These studies have found that patients with IBD use many different therapies, including herbs (aloe vera, cat's claw, and ginseng), chiropractic manipulation, diets (gluten-free diet and carbohydrate-specific diet), homeopathy, naturopathy, prayer, and exercise.[5,8-11] The therapies that are most commonly used vary among countries, suggesting that the patients' cultural background and local availability are likely important determinants of the therapy chosen by a patient. A complementary practitioner may provide these therapies, but more commonly, patients self-treat with any of the therapies that are readily obtainable from health food stores or drug stores, by mail order, or over the Internet.

Patients with IBD use CAM for their IBD and for concomitant medical conditions and/or general well-being. *Important factors that lead patients to use CAM for their IBD are dissatisfaction with their conventional medical treatments, especially a lack of effect or side effects of medical treatments, and a desire to avoid surgery.*[5] However, factors related to patients' health beliefs, culture, knowledge, and their previous experiences with CAM are also important. Some patients' health beliefs may be more compatible with CAM philosophies, and therefore, they may use them early during the course of their disease.[12] Others may be comfortable with conventional medicine and only seek out CAM when they believe they have seen the limitations of conventional medicine.

In general, patients do not abandon conventional medicine in favor of complementary therapies. Instead, *they tend to use both*, often hoping for a synergistic effect or that the complementary therapy will ameliorate or prevent side effects from the conventional medicine. We found that many patients reported using conventional medicine when their disease was more active and used complementary therapies to try to maintain remission or when they had chronically but moderately active disease that was not responding to conventional treatments.

Several studies have found that past CAM use is substantially higher than current use by patients with IBD. However, the reasons why many patients have used CAM in the past but do not continue to do so are poorly understood. Most studies do not report reasons for CAM discontinuation, and therefore, whether a therapy is discontinued because of adverse events, lack of effect, or resolution of IBD symptoms is unknown.

Patients report obtaining a number of benefits through the use of CAM.[13] *One of the most common benefits is a greater sense of being in control of the management of their disease.* Often such benefits overshadow any improvement in their symptoms resulting from the use of CAM. A patient may not perceive any improvement in his/her disease but still be satisfied with the use of CAM because of his/her increased sense of control or with receiving treatment that fits with his/her beliefs. It is important for the gastroenterologist to understand this because it helps explain why rational patients demonstrate, what is from the gastroenterologist's perspective, an irrational health behavior—the use of an unproven therapy. Understanding patients' use of CAM requires looking beyond symptoms to the effect the disease and its treatment has on every aspect of patients' lives and their beliefs and motivations.

Patients frequently exclude their gastroenterologist when deciding to use a CAM and then often do not inform them about using it out of fear that their physician will reject their use of CAM or because they do not see their physician as being knowledgeable about these therapies, and they frequently do not include their physician in the decision-making process.

EFFICACY AND SAFETY OF ALTERNATIVE IBD TREATMENTS

One of the main problems facing both patients and physicians is the lack of information about the safety and efficacy of CAM. In fact, we found that many patients rated CAM as one of their most important information needs. In general, there are no major safety concerns with the common forms of therapy (herbs and nutritional supplements) used by patients with IBD. Potential risks include allergic reactions, contamination or mislabeling of herbal products, nutritional deficiencies resulting from restrictive diets, and neck and spine injury resulting from spinal manipulation. However, physicians and patients should be aware that some therapies are associated with the risk for serious side effects because of the therapy's chemical constituents (e.g., hepatic veno-occlusive disease from herbs such as comfrey that contain pyrrolizidine alkaloids), contamination with heavy metals (reported with some medicines prepared in Asia), and the potential risk for toxicity to the fetus.

The potential for interactions between complementary and conventional medicines exists but is poorly documented for most therapies.[14-16] Many herbs can affect the absorption or metabolism of conventional medicines. Patients on immunosuppressants, biologics, or other medications with a narrow therapeutic window should be especially careful.

There is even less information on the efficacy of common forms of CAM used by patients with IBD (see also chapter 123).[17] Many CAMs based on traditional healing practices have a rich folk history supporting their use; however, there is little, if any, direct scientific evidence supporting the benefits of most forms of CAM. Much of the evidence that patients and physicians have access to is anecdotal. Some controlled trials of specific therapies have been conducted, but these are often reported in journals unfamiliar to practicing physicians, are flawed, and examine treatments not widely used or available. There is a body of ethnopharmacology and basic science research on some herbal products that support a possible role in the treatment of IBD.

APPROACH TO THE PATIENT USING OR WISHING TO USE A COMPLEMENTARY THERAPY

Counseling patients about CAM use is important and can help the patient make a more informed choice. To be effective, it must be done in a sensitive and nonjudgmental fashion, and gastroenterologists should avoid an authoritative "advice-giving" or direct persuasion approach because this can push the patient into a more resistant and defensive position. This is not to say that physicians must agree with their patients' use of CAM. In my experience, patients often recognize that they are obtaining only one side of the story from those promoting a complementary therapy. However, they want more than just a "No, don't use it" from their gastroenterologist. They value their gastroenterologist as an information source and want an open discussion of the potential value or risks associated with a therapy, even if ultimately the gastroenterologist disagrees with the use of CAM.

Dr. David Eisenberg has written a valuable article on advising patients who seek alternative medical therapies.[18] It is directed toward the patient who is seeking care from a complementary practitioner. Even though I find that most patients with IBD self-treat with complementary therapies rather than see a complementary practitioner, Eisenberg's guidelines are still appropriate. Below are the steps that I use when counseling a patient.

Documenting CAM Use

Determining current and past use of CAM should be part of the routine medical history for all patients. There are several reasons for doing so. First, use of a CAM may be an indication that the patient is dissatisfied with his/her current treatment either because he/she is not achieving the benefits he/she desires or because he/she is suffering from side effects. Second, the use of potentially dangerous therapies can be discovered. Third, potential drug–CAM interactions can be anticipated. Finally, the effects of CAM, either good or bad, will not be misconstrued as resulting from a conventional treatment.

Patients, however, are reluctant to reveal their use of CAM, especially if they view their gastroenterologist as being intolerant or uninformed. Therefore, it is not wise to use terms such as quackery, fraudulent, or unconventional therapies. I routinely ask the patients whether they (1) use herbal or natural therapies, (2) have made any dietary changes, and (3) use any other therapies for their IBD. There is no evidence that inquiring about CAM use will lead a nonuser to begin using one of these therapies.

Determine Reasons for Seeking CAM

A patient who is using or considering using a complementary therapy should be asked about his/her reasons for doing so. This is important because determining specific areas of dissatisfaction with the patient's conventional treatment could allow modifications to be made. Again, careful questioning is required because patients may be reticent to reveal issues that they feel may be perceived as criticism by their gastroenterologist. Open-ended questions such as "What do you see as the potential benefits of using this therapy?" and "Do you have any concerns about your current treatment for your IBD that is leading you to consider this new therapy?" allow patients to openly discuss their perspective on their treatment. It is also valuable to obtain some sense of the patient's health beliefs.

If the patient is a firm believer in the principles of complementary medicine, it is unlikely that they will be convinced not to use one. If, on the other hand, the patient is more comfortable with conventional medicine but is seeking alternatives because he/she is experiencing problems, then he/she may be willing to first try a modification in his/her conventional medical treatment.

Explore the Patients' Knowledge and Source of Information About CAM

Many sources of information available to the patient, for example books and Internet sites, provide an overly optimistic and one-sided account of the effectiveness of a therapy and are often based only on testimonials. Often information about safety is not provided. The patient's understanding of how the therapy works and its potential benefits and harms should be determined. Some patients have realistic expectations. They may understand that their chance of obtaining some benefit is low, but they are willing to try it on the off chance that they do benefit. However, many patients have unrealistic expectations and expect a quick cure. In the short time available for counseling a patient, it is impossible and impractical to teach him/her the principles of scientific medicine and the randomized controlled trial. However, patients should be encouraged to define realistic treatment goals and to reevaluate their use of a therapy after a set period of time.

Many patients believe that CAM is without risk, often because they are "natural" therapies. This belief is often promoted by advertisements for the therapy. Therefore, the patient may not have considered the possibility of side effects. Physicians should ask patients whether they know the possible side effects of a therapy and should warn patients about the possibility of interactions with alcohol or other drugs. Patients should be encouraged to think of any therapy in terms of a trade-off between potential benefits and potential risks. Often patients think more about the potential benefits and neglect to consider whether they are willing to incur the risks of a CAM, including its cost.

Determine How the Patient Will Obtain and Use the Therapy

If the patient is seeing or will be seeing an alternative practitioner, the gastroenterologist can provide the patient with questions they should ask the practitioner. These would include (1) is the practitioner licensed and what was their training, (2) how experienced are they in treating patients with IBD, (3) what can the patient expect from the treatment in terms of benefits and side effects, (4) what is the basis for these expectations, and (5) what will be the cost of the treatment.

Patients should not start a number of different therapies, especially a combination of conventional and complementary therapies, at the same time. If this is done, it will be impossible to determine which therapy resulted in any benefits or side effects.

Finally, some method for monitoring for side effects should be agreed upon. This will depend on the potential risks associated with a therapy.

● INFORMATION SOURCES ABOUT COMPLEMENTARY THERAPIES

There are a variety of valuable information sources available for physicians, although none of them are specifically focused on IBD. Patients should be advised NOT to rely heavily on the advice or recommendations provided by employees of health food stores or other stores selling herbal and nutritional supplements because they are often not qualified to provide such advice. Often, only the owner or the manager of the store has much experience and knowledge about the therapies.

Below are listed several useful sources of information on CAM. We have chosen these because they critically review therapies and provide supporting evidence for any claims made.

- National Center for Complementary and Alternative Medicine Web site (nccam.nih.gov)
- This Web site includes a wealth of information about CAM, including brief fact sheets on many therapies and health conditions. The site also provides information on research studies found by the NCCAM.
- *Oxford Handbook of Complementary Medicine* (Authors: M.H. Pittler, E. Ernst, B, Wider, and K. Boddy. Oxford University Press, 2008).
- This comprehensive book provides evidence-based information on CAM. The book is targeted at physicians and other healthcare providers and includes sections on various diseases and conditions, with only a few pages on Crohn's disease and ulcerative colitis.
- *The Desktop Guide to Complementary and Alternative Medicine*, 2nd Edition (Authors: E. Ernst, M. Pittler, and B. Wider). Same authors and similar format to above.
- *Professionals Handbook of Complementary and Alternative Medicines*, 3rd Edition year? (Authors: C.W. Feltrow and J.R. Avila. Lippincott Williams & Wilkins).
- This book describes the chemical components, actions, reported uses, and suggested doses of many herbs and alternative medicines. The authors also list potential adverse events and drug interactions. The book is less critical of claims made about the efficacy of the treatments than the above two books.
- *Herb Contraindications and Drug Interactions*, 3rd Edition (F. Brinker. Eclectic Medical Publications). This book describes known and speculated side effects, contraindications, and drug interactions of herbs. The book is well referenced and indexed.

References

1. Fulder S. The basic concepts of alternative medicine and their impact on our views of health. *J Altern Complement Med.* 1998;4(2):147–158.

2. Verhoef MJ, Rapchuk I, Liew T, Weir V, Hilsden RJ. Complementary practitioners' views of treatment for inflammatory bowel disease. *Can J Gastroenterol.* 2002;16(2):95–100.

3. Aakster CW. Concepts in alternative medicine. *Soc Sci Med.* 1986;22(2):265–273.

4. Barnes PM, Bloom B, Nahin R. *Complementary and Alternative Medicine use Among Adults and Children: United States 2007.* Hyattsville, MD: National Center for Health Statistics; 2008. CDC National Health Statistics Report #12.

5. Hilsden RJ, Scott CM, Verhoef MJ. Complementary medicine use by patients with inflammatory bowel disease. *Am J Gastroenterol.* 1998;93(5):697–701.

6. Kong SC, Hurlstone DP, Pocock CY, et al. The Incidence of self-prescribed oral complementary and alternative medicine use by patients with gastrointestinal diseases. *J Clin Gastroenterol.* 2005;39(2):138–141.

7. Langhorst J, Anthonisen IB, Steder-Neukamm U, et al. Patterns of complementary and alternative medicine (CAM) use in patients with inflammatory bowel disease: perceived stress is a potential indicator for CAM use. *Complement Ther Med.* 2007;15(1):30–37.

8. Moser G, Tillinger W, Sachs G, et al. Disease-related worries and concerns: a study on out-patients with inflammatory bowel disease. *Eur J Gastroenterol Hepatol.* 1995;7(9):853–858.

9. Rawsthorne P, Shanahan F, Cronin NC, et al. An international survey of the use and attitudes regarding alternative medicine by patients with inflammatory bowel disease. *Am J Gastroenterol.* 1999;94(5):1298–1303.

10. Bensoussan M, Jovenin N, Garcia B, et al. Complementary and alternative medicine use by patients with inflammatory bowel disease: results from a postal survey. *Gastroenterol Clin Biol.* 2006;30(1):14–23.

11. Joos S, Rosemann T, Szecsenyi J, Hahn EG, Willich SN, Brinkhaus B. Use of complementary and alternative medicine in Germany—a survey of patients with inflammatory bowel disease. *BMC Complement Altern Med.* 2006;6:19.

12. Li FX, Verhoef MJ, Best A, Otley A, Hilsden RJ. Why patients with inflammatory bowel disease use or do not use complementary and alternative medicine: a Canadian national survey. *Can J Gastroenterol.* 2005;19(9):567–573.

13. Hilsden RJ, Verhoef MJ, Best A, Pocobelli G. Complementary and alternative medicine use by Canadian patients with inflammatory bowel disease: results from a national survey. *Am J Gastroenterol.* 2003;98(7):1563–1568.

14. Crone CC, Wise TN. Use of herbal medicines among consultation-liaison populations. A review of current information regarding risks, interactions, and efficacy. *Psychosomatics.* 1998;39(1):3–13.

15. Manns MP, McHutchison JG, Gordon SC, et al. Peginterferon alfa-2b plus ribavirin compared with interferon alfa-2b plus ribavirin for initial treatment of chronic hepatitis C: a randomised trial. *Lancet.* 2001;358(9286):958–965.

16. Fugh-Berman A. Herb-drug interactions. *Lancet.* 2000;355(9198):134–138.

17. Hilsden RJ, Verhoef MJ. Complementary and alternative medicine: evaluating its effectiveness in inflammatory bowel disease. *Inflamm Bowel Dis.* 1998;4(4):318–323.

18. Eisenberg DM. Advising patients who seek alternative medical therapies. *Ann Intern Med.* 1997;127(1):61–69.

Fertility and Pregnancy in IBD 158

Uma Mahadevan

Inflammatory bowel disease (IBD) often affects women during their peak reproductive years. As medical therapy for IBD advances, more patients will be in a position to consider pregnancy; however, striking the balance between optimal medical therapy and fetal health has become increasingly complex. This chapter will review questions that a patient considering pregnancy frequently asks during his/her consultation. These questions are summarized in Table 158.1.

⬤ WILL MY CHILD DEVELOP IBD?

Perhaps. Family history is the strongest predictor for developing IBD. If one parent is affected, the risks of the offspring developing IBD are 2 to 13 times higher than in the general population. One study estimated that the risk for IBD in first-degree relatives of probands with ulcerative colitis (UC) and Crohn's disease (CD) was 1.6% and 5.2%, respectively, numbers that were even higher in the Jewish population.[1]

⬤ WHAT ARE MY CHANCES OF GETTING PREGNANT?

As good as anyone else of your age if you have not had surgery. Infertility is defined in specific terms as the failure to conceive after a year of regular intercourse without contraception. In general, women with CD seem to have similar fertility rates to the general population. Community-based and population-based studies suggest infertility rates (5–14%) similar to the general population. Surgery for CD may decrease fertility compared with medical therapy alone.[2]

Surgery

Women with UC have fertility rates similar to the general population before surgery. A study by Olsen et al.[3] of 290 women with UC versus 661 non-IBD controls found that women with UC had fecundability ratios (FR; the ability to conceive per menstrual cycle with unprotected intercourse) equal to the general population (FR = 1.01). However, after surgery for an ileal pouch anal anastomosis (IPAA), the FR decreased to 0.20

($P < 0.001$). The reduction in fertility may be due to surgery in the pelvis and the consequent adhesions and damage to the reproductive organs.

The risk of infertility should be discussed with the patient before surgery as part of the potential risks of the operation. It is unclear whether techniques such as laparoscopic IPAA or a subtotal colectomy with rectal stump and ileostomy during the childbearing years are helpful in reducing infertility and sexual dysfunction rates. The drawbacks of the latter procedure include rare ileostomy complications during pregnancy such as obstruction and stoma-related problems, technical difficulties in creating a functioning pouch several years after the initial surgery, and the patient's reluctance to have a long-term stoma.

⬤ WILL I BE ABLE TO HAVE A SUCCESSFUL PREGNANCY?

Yes, but you have a higher risk of adverse outcomes compared with the general population and therefore should be followed up by a high-risk obstetrician. Women with IBD have an increased risk for preterm birth, low birth weight (LBW) and small for gestational age (SGA) infants, and higher rates of cesarean sections. Overall, the risk of congenital anomalies does not seem to be increased compared with the general population. A population representative cohort study of women with IBD in the Northern California Kaiser population[4] compared women with IBD ($n = 461$) matched to controls ($n = 495$) by age and hospital of delivery. Women with IBD were more likely to have a spontaneous abortion, odds ratio (OR) = 1.65 (95% confidence interval (CI), 1.09–2.48), an adverse pregnancy outcome (stillbirth, preterm birth, or SGA infant), OR = 1.54 (95% CI, 1.00–2.38), or a complication of labor, OR = 1.78 (95% CI, 1.13–2.81). However, there was no difference in the rate of congenital malformations in patients with IBD versus controls or individually among patients with CD and those with UC. Independent predictors of an adverse outcome included a diagnosis of IBD, a history of surgery for IBD, and non-white ethnicity. Severity of disease and medical treatments were not associated with an adverse outcome, suggesting that even women in remission with

TABLE 158.1 Common Patient Questions and Answers

1. Will my child get IBD?
a. 1.6% if mother has UC; 5.2% if mother has CD
b. 36% if both spouses are affected
2. What are my chances of getting pregnant?
a. Fertility is similar to the general population for presurgical UC and CD
b. IPAA reduces fertility by 50–80%
c. Surgery for Crohn's may also slightly reduce fertility
3. Do women with IBD have higher rates of sexual dysfunction?
a. Yes. Depression and surgery are predictors
4. What are my expected pregnancy outcomes?
a. Increased spontaneous abortion and stillbirth
b. Increased preterm birth, low birth weight, small for gestational age infants
c. Increased complications of labor and delivery
d. Congenital anomalies—data mixed, but no clear increased risk
e. Even if disease is under good control, increased risk of adverse outcomes compared with the general population
f. All women with IBD should be followed as high risk obstetric patients
5. What will pregnancy do to my IBD?
a. The risk of flaring is the same as if not pregnant—34% at one year
6. What medications can I use? (FDA category)
a. Mesalamine (B): conception, pregnancy, lactation
i. Sulfasalazine—increase folic acid to 2 mg daily
ii. Asacol (R) and olsalazine are category C
b. Corticosteroids (C) and budesonide (C):
i. Use if needed, but avoid use in first trimester
1. increased risk of cleft palate
ii. Increased risk of gestational diabetes
c. Azathioprine/6Mercaptopurine (D)
i. Low risk. Benefits of maintaining remission outweigh risk
ii. Compatible with use in conception, pregnancy and lactation
iii. Wait 4 h after taking dose to breastfeed
d. Infliximab and Adalimumab (B)
i. Low risk. Compatible with use in conception, pregnancy, lactation
ii. Transfers across placenta. Avoid use in late third trimester
iii. Consider holding rotavirus vaccination in infant (live virus)
e. Certolizumab (B)
i. Low risk. Compatible with use in conception, pregnancy, lactation
ii. Limited transfer across placenta in third trimester so dose on schedule
f. Natalizumab (C)
i. Limited data. No reports of congenital anomalies
g. Methotrexate (X)
i. Contraindicated. Discontinue 6 months before conception

IBD were more likely to have complications of pregnancy than their general population counterparts.

WILL MY IBD FLARE DURING PREGNANCY?

You are as likely to flare during pregnancy, as when not pregnant. Nielsen et al.[5] reported an exacerbation rate of 34% per year during pregnancy and 32% per year when not pregnant in women with UC. Pregnant women with CD also had similar rates of disease exacerbation. In the Kaiser population,[4] the majority of patients had inactive disease throughout their pregnancy with no sudden increase in the postpartum. Although breastfeeding has anecdotally been associated with an increase in disease activity in the postpartum, this has not been shown to be a contributing factor independent of medication cessation to facilitate breastfeeding.

WILL DISEASE ACTIVITY AFFECT MY PREGNANCY?

Yes. Although it was initially thought that the increased disease activity led to higher rates of spontaneous abortion, preterm birth, and LBW infants, in the Kaiser population,[4] disease activity was not predictive of an adverse outcome in any category. Even when limited to the presence of moderate to severe disease activity, there was still no association with an adverse outcome. The majority of patients with both UC and CD, however, did have inactive or mild disease throughout pregnancy. Similarly, a population-based study from Denmark[6] reported that women with active disease had adjusted risks for LBW, LBW at term, preterm birth, and congenital anomalies of 0.2 (0.0–2.6), 0.4 (0.0–3.7), 2.4 (0.6–9.5), and 0.8 (0.2–3.8), respectively. The crude risk for preterm birth was 3.4 (1.1–10.6) in those with moderate to high disease activity. Overall, these two population-based studies suggest that patients with IBD have higher rates of adverse pregnancy outcomes regardless of disease activity. However, it makes sense that severe disease activity with its effect on maternal nutrition, levels of inflammation, and need for increased medical therapy will negatively impact pregnancy outcome. The population-based studies may not have had enough sick patients to differentiate this from the already increased level of adverse outcomes with IBD in general.

CAN I HAVE A VAGINAL DELIVERY?

Yes, with two exceptions. There is an increased rate of cesarean sections in women with IBD. In general, the decision to have a cesarean section should be made on purely obstetric grounds. The two exceptions are active perianal disease and the presence of an ileoanal pouch. If a patient has inactive perianal disease or no history of perianal disease, he/she is not at increased risk for perianal disease after a vaginal delivery.[7] However, if the patient has active perianal disease, he/she can risk aggravating his/her injury with a vaginal delivery.

Patients who have an *IPAA* can have a normal vaginal delivery without fears of damaging the pouch.[8] However, the concern with vaginal delivery is for damage to the anal sphincter. Although pouch function may deteriorate during pregnancy, after pregnancy, it reverts to the prepregnancy state.[8] However, over time, damage to the anal sphincter may be compounded by aging, and the effects on the pouch will not be seen for several years when incontinence and number of bowel movements may increase significantly. The patient, his/her obstetrician, and his/her surgeon should discuss the theoretical risk to long-term pouch function before making a decision on mode of delivery.

SHOULD I CONTINUE MY IBD MEDICATIONS WHEN I AM PREGNANT?

Yes, with a few exceptions! Overall, the majority of medications used for the treatment of IBD are not associated with significant adverse effects, and maintaining the health of the mother remains a priority in the management of these patients. Patients should discuss their medications with their physician *before* considering conception. The US Food and Drug Administration (FDA) classification of drugs offers a guide to the use of medications during pregnancy. The FDA categories are listed in Table 158.2 and are noted for each drug discussed.

TABLE 158.2 FDA Categories for the Use of Medications in Pregnancy

FDA category	Definition
A	Controlled studies in animals and women have shown no risk in the first trimester, and possible fetal harm is remote.
B	Either animal studies have not demonstrated a fetal risk but there are no controlled studies in pregnant women, or animal studies have shown an adverse effect that was not confirmed in controlled studies in women in the first trimester.
C	No controlled studies in humans have been performed, and animal studies have shown adverse events, or studies in humans and animals not available; give if potential benefit outweighs the risk.
D	Positive evidence of fetal risk is available, but the benefits may outweigh the risk if life-threatening or serious disease.
X	Studies in animals or humans show fetal abnormalities; drug contraindicated

FDA, Food and Drug Administration.
[a]From Administration FDA.[9]

TABLE 158.3 Medications Used in the Treatment of IBD[a]

DRUG	FDA Category	Recommendations for Pregnancy	Breast Feeding[11]
Adalimumab	B	Limited human data: low risk Likely cross placenta	No human data: probably compatible
Alendronate	C	Limited human data; long half life: Animal data suggest risk.	No human data: probably compatible
Azathioprine/6-mercaptopurine	D	Data on IBD, transplant literature suggest some risk, but low	Limited transfer. Likely compatible
Balsalazide	B	Low risk	No human data: potential diarrhea
Budesonide	C	Data with inhaled drug low risk. Limited human data for oral drug	No human data
Certolizumab	B	Limited human data: low risk Limited transfer across placenta	No evidence of transfer. Likely compatible
Ciprofloxacin	C	Avoid: Potential toxicity to cartilage	Limited human data: probably compatible
Corticosteroids	C	Low risk: possible small risk of cleft palate, adrenal insufficiency, premature rupture of membranes	Compatible
Cyclosporine	C	Low risk	Limited human data: potential toxicity
Fish Oil Supplements	–	Low risk. Possibly beneficial	No human data
Infliximab	B	Low risk: limited human data: crosses placenta and detectable in infant after birth	No evidence of transfer. likely compatible
Mesalamine Asacol (C)	B	Low risk	Limited human data: potential diarrhea
Methotrexate	X	Contraindicated: Teratogenic	Contraindicated
Metronidazole	B	Given limited efficacy in IBD, would avoid in first trimester	Limited human data: potential toxicity
Olsalazine	C	Low risk	Limited human data: potential diarrhea
Risedronate	C	Limited human data. Long half life	Safety unknown
Rifaximin	C	No human data. Animal data report some risk	Safety unknown
Sulfasalazine	B	Low risk. Give folate 2 mg daily	Limited human data: potential diarrhea
Tacrolimus	C	Low risk	Limited human data: potential toxicity
Thalidomide	X	Contraindicated: Teratogenic	No human data: potential toxicity

[a]Low risk is defined as "the human pregnancy data does not suggest a significant risk of embryo or fetal harm"[10]
IBD, inflammatory bowel disease; FDA, Food and Drug Administration.

Table 158.3 summarizes the safety of IBD medications for pregnancy and breastfeeding. As each drug has multiple safety studies, please refer to American Gastroenterological Association guidelines for the use of medications during pregnancy for a full list of references.

Aminosalicylates

All aminosalicylates (sulfasalazine, mesalamine, and balsalazide) are pregnancy category B drugs, except olsalazine, which is a pregnancy category C drug. Asacol recently was changed to category C due to the presence of dibutyl phthalate in the coating. However, no increase in birth defects has been reported. Sulfasalazine has not been shown to increase congenital malformations in multiple studies. However, given the concern over potential antifolate effects of the drug, it is recommended that women take folic acid 2 mg daily in the prenatal period and throughout pregnancy. Breastfeeding is also considered low risk with sulfasalazine. Unlike other sulfonamides, bilirubin displacement, and therefore kernicterus, does not occur in the infant.

Multiple studies on the use of mesalamine in pregnancy also do not suggest an increased risk to the fetus. Breastfeeding while on aminosalicylates has been rarely associated with diarrhea in the infant. Women can breastfeed while being treated with 5-aminosalicylates, but infants should be observed for a persistent change in stool frequency.

Antibiotics

Metronidazole is a pregnancy category B drug. It should be avoided in the first trimester because of a small risk of cleft lip with or without cleft palate. However, overall, multiple studies have suggested that prenatal use of metronidazole is not associated with birth defects. Metronidazole is excreted in breast milk. If a single dose of metronidazole is given, the American Academy of Pediatrics (AAP) recommends that breastfeeding should be suspended for 12 to 24 h. Potential toxicity exists for longer-term use of metronidazole, and it is not compatible with breastfeeding.

Quinolones (e.g., ciprofloxacin, levofloxacin, and norfloxacin) are pregnancy category C drugs. Quinolones have a high affinity for bone tissue and cartilage and may cause arthropathies in children. The manufacturer reports damage to cartilage in weight-bearing joints after quinolone exposure in immature rats and dogs. However, studies have not found an increased risk of congenital malformations. Overall, the risk is believed to be minimal, but given safer alternatives, the drug should be avoided in pregnancy. The data on breastfeeding are limited, but quinolones are probably compatible with use.

Rifaximin is a pregnancy category C drug. This is a new agent, and little information exists on safety in pregnancy. Rifaximin has been found to cause teratogenicity in rats and rabbits, including cleft palate and incomplete ossification. Safety in breastfeeding is unknown.

In general, given the limited evidence of benefit of these agents in IBD and the extended duration of use in the treatment of CD and UC, they should be avoided during pregnancy. Short courses for the treatment of pouchitis can be considered based on the safety data presented previously. An alternative antibiotic for pouchitis is amoxicillin/clavulanic acid, a pregnancy category B drug compatible with breastfeeding.

Editor's note (TMB): I do not know if there is information in the use of topical metronidazole (troches) for pouchitis.

Corticosteroids

Corticosteroids are pregnancy category C drugs. Use in the first trimester should be limited given the findings of an increased risk for oral clefts in the newborn and in later trimesters given the theoretical risks for gestational diabetes and adrenal suppression in the newborn. However, if the mother is ill and needs

it, it should be used because overall safety data are good. Oral budesonide (category C) is also considered low risk in pregnancy. Safety in lactation is not known.

Bisphosphonates

The bisphosphonates alendronate and risedronate are pregnancy category C drugs, and the safety in breastfeeding is unknown. Many patients with IBD are started on these medications in conjunction with corticosteroids for prevention of bone loss. Both agents should be avoided in pregnancy because animal studies have shown that alendronate does cross the placenta and gets stored in fetal bone, causing anatomic changes. Both agents have half lives up to 10 years. The concern in giving this agent to a woman of childbearing potential is that the drug is slowly released from bone and may result in a low level of continuous exposure to the fetus throughout gestation.

Immunomodulators

Immunomodulators are the most controversial agents used in the treatment of pregnant women with IBD.

Methotrexate

Methotrexate, a pregnancy category X drug, is clearly teratogenic and should not be used in women considering conception. It should be discontinued at least 6 months before attempting conception. It is contraindicated in breastfeeding.

Azathioprine/6-Mercaptopurine

6-Mercaptopurine (6-MP) and its prodrug azathioprine (AZA) are pregnancy category D drugs. Animal studies have demonstrated teratogenicity. Transplacental and transamniotic transmission of AZA and its metabolites from the mother to the fetus can occur. The oral bioavailability of AZA (47%) and 6-MP (16%) is low,[12] and the early fetal liver lacks the enzyme inosinate pyrophosphorylase needed to convert AZA to 6-MP. Both features may protect the fetus from toxic drug exposure during the crucial period of organogenesis.

The largest evidence on safety comes from transplantation studies where rates of anomalies ranged from 0.0% to 11.8% and no evidence of recurrent patterns of congenital anomalies emerged. In IBD, multiple case series have not noted an increase in congenital anomalies. However, a Danish nationwide cohort study[13] found that women with CD exposed to corticosteroids and AZA/6-MP were more likely to have preterm birth (12.3% and 25%, respectively) compared with non-IBD controls (6.5%). Congenital anomalies were also more prevalent among AZA/6-MP–exposed cases compared with the reference group (15.4% vs. 5.7%) with an OR of 2.9 (95% CI, 0.9–8.9). However, only 26 women were exposed to AZA/6-MP during conception versus 628 patients in the reference group, and the authors controlled for "disease activity," which they defined as > or < 2 admissions for disease exacerbation, accounting for only the most severe patients. Finally, the largest single study to date[14] studied 189 women who called a teratogen information service after exposure to AZA during pregnancy and compared them with 230 women who did not take any teratogenic medications during pregnancy. The rate of major malformations did not differ between groups with six neonates in each; for AZA, the rate was 3.5%, and for the control group, it was 3.0% ($P = 0.775$; OR 1.17; 95% CI, 0.37–3.69).

Breastfeeding, initially discouraged, may now be compatible with AZA use because multiple small studies show low to minimal transfer to the infant. An elegant study[15] of eight lactating women on AZA obtained milk and plasma samples at 30 and 60 min after drug administration and hourly for the following 5 h. The variation in the bioavailability of the drug was reflected in a wide range of peak plasma values of 6-MP within the first 3 h. A similar curve, but with an hour's delay and at significantly lower concentrations varying from 2 to 50 µg/L, was seen in maternal milk. The majority of 6-MP in breast milk was excreted within the first 4 h after drug intake. On the basis of maximum concentration measured, the infant ingested 6-MP of <0.008 mg/kg bodyweight/24 h. The risks and benefits of breastfeeding must be considered carefully; however, at this time, there does not seem to be an absolute contraindication to breastfeeding while on AZA/6-MP, and mothers should be advised to wait 4 h after dosing to feed.

Cyclosporine and Tacrolimus

Cyclosporine is a pregnancy category C drug and does not seem to be a major human teratogen. There are several case reports of successful cyclosporine use during pregnancy to control UC and complete the pregnancy. In the setting of severe, corticosteroid-refractory UC, cyclosporine may be a better option than colectomy, given the substantial risk to the mother and fetus of surgery during this time.

Cyclosporine is excreted into breast milk in high concentrations. Therefore, the AAP considers cyclosporine contraindicated during breastfeeding because of the potential for immune suppression and neutropenia.

Tacrolimus is also a pregnancy category C drug. There is no clear increase in birth defects in the transplant experience, although mothers suffered from other complications such as preterm birth—which may be due to their underlying medical condition, versus the effect of the drug itself. A single case report of a patient with UC who had a successful pregnancy on maintenance tacrolimus was recently published. No other data on IBD are published at this time. Tacrolimus is contraindicated in breastfeeding because of the high concentrations found in breast milk.

Thalidomide

Thalidomide, a pregnancy category X drug, has some anti-tumor necrosis factor (anti-TNF) effects and has been used successfully for the treatment of CD. However, its teratogenicity has been extensively documented and includes limb defects, central nervous system effects, and abnormalities of the respiratory, cardiovascular, gastrointestinal, and genitourinary system. Thalidomide is contraindicated during pregnancy and in women of childbearing age who are not using two reliable methods of contraception for 1 month before starting therapy, during therapy, and for 1 month after stopping therapy. There are no human data on breastfeeding, but it is not advised given the potential toxicity.

● BIOLOGIC THERAPY

Infliximab

Infliximab (INF), a pregnancy category B drug, is an IgG1 antibody, which does not actively cross the placenta in the first trimester but efficiently crosses in the second and third trimester.[16] Although this protects the infant from exposure during the crucial period of organogenesis, INF crosses the placenta efficiently in the third trimester and is present in the infant for several months from birth.

There is a growing body of evidence that suggests INF is low risk in pregnancy. The two largest studies are from the TREAT Registry[17] and the INF Safety Database[18] maintained by Centocor (Malvern, PA). The TREAT Registry is a prospective registry of patients with CD.[17] Patients may or may not be treated with INF. Of the >6200 patients enrolled, 168 pregnancies were reported, 117 with INF exposure. The rates of miscarriage (10% vs. 6.7%) and neonatal complications (6.9% vs. 10%) were not significantly different between INF-treated and INF-naïve patients, respectively. The INF Safety Database is a retrospective data collection instrument. Pregnancy outcome data are available for 96 women with direct exposure to INF.[18] This was primarily exposure during conception and the first trimester. When patients found that they were pregnant, the treatment was often stopped. The 96 pregnancies resulted in 100 births. The expected versus observed outcomes among women exposed to INF were not different from those of the general population. A series of 10 women with maintenance INF use throughout pregnancy was also reported.[19] All 10 pregnancies ended in live births, with no reported congenital malformations.

INF crosses the placenta and is detectable in the infant for several months after birth. In a case series[20] of eight patients receiving INF during pregnancy, all eight patients delivered a healthy infant. The mothers were receiving INF 5 mg/kg every 8 weeks, and the mean time between delivery and the last infusion was 66 days (range, 2–120 days). The INF level at birth was always higher in the infant and cord blood than in the mother, and it took anywhere from 2 to 7 months for the infant to have undetectable INF levels. These findings support the fact that IgG1 antibodies are efficiently transported across the placenta in the third trimester, but the infant's reticuloendothelial system is too immature to effectively clear the antibody rapidly. INF has not been detected in breast milk.[21]

So far, there has been no reported adverse event associated with increased INF levels in the newborns. In our experience, infants exposed to INF in utero have appropriate response to standard early vaccinations.[22] In adults receiving a similar agent, adalimumab (ADA), pneumococcal and influenza vaccinations were given safely and effectively. However, live vaccinations such as varicella, small pox, etc are contraindicated in immunosuppressed patients—such as those on anti-TNF therapy. Traditionally, the first live virus encountered by an infant was at 1 year of age (varicella, measles-mumps-rubella) when INF levels would be undetectable. However, now, rotavirus live vaccine is given at 2 months of age. Although it is given orally and is significantly attenuated, its safety in this setting is not known, and the mother and the pediatrician should be cautioned against its use if INF or ADA levels may be present.

Adalimumab

ADA, a pregnancy category B drug, is also an IgG1 antibody. Multiple case series have not documented an increase in adverse events, including congenital malformations, when used during pregnancy. ADA would be expected to cross the placenta in the third trimester as INF does. However, because ADA levels cannot be checked commercially, this has not been confirmed. ADA is considered compatible with breastfeeding, although there is no human data.

Certolizumab Pegol

Certolizumab pegol (CZP) is a PEGylated Fab' fragment of a humanized anti-TNFα monoclonal antibody. Because it does not have an Fc portion, it should not be actively transported across the placenta as INF and ADA. This theory was confirmed in two patients with CD receiving CZP during pregnancy.[23] Both patients received drug during the 2 weeks before delivery. The mothers' CZP levels were high (19, 60), but CZP levels in the infant (1.02) and cord blood (1.65) were low on the day of birth. However, one concern may be that in theory the Fab' fragment (and the IgG1 antibodies) may cross the placenta passively in low levels in the first trimester during the period of organogenesis.

Natalizumab

Natalizumab, a pregnancy category C drug, is an IgG4 antibody. Review of the clinical trials data and postmarketing surveillance has not documented an increase in adverse outcomes in 164 women exposed to the drug during pregnancy.

Summary on Anti-TNF therapy

If a pregnant woman is on infliximab, I will continue it during pregnancy and give the last dose around 30 weeks of gestation to minimize placental transfer. The next dose is given immediately after delivery, and the mother can breastfeed if desired. If the child's infliximab level is undetectable at the last possible time to give rotavirus vaccine, the vaccine can be given; if not, this and other live virus vaccines should be held. For ADA, I give the last dose 6 to 8 weeks before delivery, give the next dose immediately after delivery and do not recommend rotavirus vaccine for the child because we cannot confirm levels. If at any time the mother flares, I will give the scheduled dose; however, most do well during this time period. If the scheduled dose is due close to the delivery date—such as within 2 weeks, I will consider a short course of steroids to minimize transfer to the infant. Certolizumab is continued throughout pregnancy without interruption, and the infant receives all scheduled vaccines given the low transfer rate. At 7 months of age, all infants exposed to anti-TNFs *in utero* should get assessed for response to *Haemophilus influenzae* and tetanus toxoid to confirm appropriate immune response.

Fish Oil Supplements

Many patients with IBD use fish oil supplements as an adjunct to standard medical therapy. Because this is a supplement and not a drug, it is not rated by the FDA. A randomized controlled trial of fish oil supplementation demonstrated a prolongation of pregnancy without detrimental effects on the growth of the fetus or on the course of labor. Fish oil supplementation may also play a role in preventing miscarriage associated with the antiphospholipid antibody syndrome. In women with IBD who may be at increased risk for preterm birth and miscarriage, fish oil supplementation is not harmful and may be of some benefit.

● SUMMARY

The use of IBD medication during conception and pregnancy is generally low risk. For a drug to clearly be associated with congenital anomalies, the same defect must be seen repeatedly, a phenomenon not demonstrated with any IBD medication, except methotrexate and thalidomide, both of which are contraindicated. The risk of an adverse fetal event must be weighed against the benefit to the health of the mother from continuing the medication and controlling the underlying disease.

On the basis of the available evidence, a woman with IBD contemplating pregnancy should be in optimal health and remission. Methotrexate and thalidomide should be discontinued 6 months before attempting conception. Aminosalicylates, AZA/6-MP, and anti-TNF agents are continued during conception and pregnancy. Two potential nuances to this policy: a patient on sulfasalazine may be switched to a mesalamine agent, if tolerated, to minimize antifolate effects, and a stable patient on combination AZA/6-MP and an anti-TNF agent may consider discontinuing AZA/6-MP before conception to minimize risk to the fetus. Although this may seem inconsistent because data suggest continuing AZA/6-MP during pregnancy is low risk, at every opportunity, we want to maintain the mother's health and minimize risk to the fetus. Discontinuing AZA/6-MP in a patient stable on INF has not been associated with an increase in adverse events.[24] Corticosteroids and antibiotics should be avoided in the first trimester to avoid the small risk of congenital malformations. However, if a patient is flaring, steroids may need to be used at any point in pregnancy. A patient naïve to AZA/6-MP should not get it for the first time during pregnancy because the risk of leucopenia and pancreatitis is unpredictable. Anti-TNFs can be started in a naïve patient during pregnancy. Use of INF and ADA should be minimized in the third trimester (we stop dosing of INF at week 30 and ADA 6 to 8 weeks from the due date if tolerated), given the high rates of placental transfer. If an anti-TNF is to be given for the first time during pregnancy, CZP may be the ideal choice, given the low rate of placental transfer.

References

1. Yang H, McElree C, Roth MP, Shanahan F, Targan SR, Rotter JI. Familial empirical risks for inflammatory bowel disease: differences between Jews and non-Jews. *Gut.* 1993;34(4):517–524.

2. Hudson M, Flett G, Sinclair TS, Brunt PW, Templeton A, Mowat NA. Fertility and pregnancy in inflammatory bowel disease. *Int J Gynaecol Obstet.* 1997;58(2):229–237.

3. Ørding Olsen K, Juul S, Berndtsson I, Oresland T, Laurberg S. Ulcerative colitis: female fecundity before diagnosis, during disease, and after surgery compared with a population sample. *Gastroenterology.* 2002;122(1):15–19.

4. Mahadevan U, Sandborn WJ, Li DK, Hakimian S, Kane S, Corley DA. Pregnancy outcomes in women with inflammatory bowel disease: a large community-based study from Northern California. *Gastroenterology.* 2007;133(4):1106–1112.

5. Nielsen OH, Andreasson B, Bondesen S, Jarnum S. Pregnancy in ulcerative colitis. *Scand J Gastroenterol.* 1983;18(6):735–742.

6. Norgard B, Hundborg HH, Jacobsen BA, Nielsen GL, Fonager K. Disease activity in pregnant women with crohn's disease and birth outcomes: a regional danish cohort study. *Am J Gastroenterol.* 2007;102(9):1947–1954.

7. Ilnyckyji A, Blanchard JF, Rawsthorne P, Bernstein CN. Perianal Crohn's disease and pregnancy: role of the mode of delivery. *Am J Gastroenterol.* 1999;94(11):3274–3278.

8. Hahnloser D, Pemberton JH, Wolff BG, et al. Pregnancy and delivery before and after ileal pouch-anal anastomosis for inflammatory bowel disease: immediate and long-term consequences and outcomes. *Dis Colon Rectum.* 2004;47(7):1127–1135.

9. Administration FDA. Regulations. 1980;44:37434–37467.

10. Mahadevan U, Kane S. American gastroenterological association institute medical position statement on the use of gastrointestinal medications in pregnancy. *Gastroenterology.* 2006;131(1):278–282.

11. Briggs GG, Freeman RK, Yaffe SJ. *Drugs in Pregnancy and Lactation.* 7th ed. Philadelphia, PA: Lippincott, Williams, Wilkins; 2005.

12. Polifka JE, Friedman JM. Teratogen update: azathioprine and 6-mercaptopurine. *Teratology.* 2002;65(5):240–261.

13. Nørgård B, Pedersen L, Christensen LA, Sørensen HT. Therapeutic drug use in women with Crohn's disease and birth outcomes: a Danish nationwide cohort study. *Am J Gastroenterol.* 2007;102(7):1406–1413.

14. Goldstein LH, Dolinsky G, Greenberg R, et al. Pregnancy outcome of women exposed to azathioprine during pregnancy. *Birth Defects Res Part A Clin Mol Teratol.* 2007;79(10):696–701.

15. Christensen LA, Dahlerup JF, Nielsen MJ, Fallingborg JF, Schmiegelow K. Azathioprine treatment during lactation. *Aliment Pharmacol Ther.* 2008;28(10):1209–1213.

16. Simister NE. Placental transport of immunoglobulin G. *Vaccine.* 2003;21(24):3365–3369.

17. Lichtenstein G, Cohen RD, Feagan BG, et al. Safety of infliximab in Crohn's disease: data from the 5000-patient TREAT registry. *Gastroenterology.* 2004;126(suppl 1):A54.

18. Katz JA, Antoni C, Keenan GF, Smith DE, Jacobs SJ, Lichtenstein GR. Outcome of pregnancy in women receiving infliximab for the treatment of Crohn's disease and rheumatoid arthritis. *Am J Gastroenterol.* 2004;99(12):2385–2392.

19. Mahadevan U, Kane S, Sandborn WJ, et al. Intentional infliximab use during pregnancy for induction or maintenance of remission in Crohn's disease. *Aliment Pharmacol Ther.* 2005;21(6):733–738.

20. Mahadevan U, Terdiman JP, Church J, et al. Infliximab levels in infants born to women with inflammatory bowel disease. *Gastroenterology.* 2007;132(suppl 2):A-144.

21. Kane S, Ford J, Cohen R, Wagner C. Absence of infliximab in infants and breast milk from nursing mothers receiving therapy for Crohn's disease before and after delivery. *J Clin Gastroenterol.* 2009;43(7):613–616.

22. Mahadevan U, Kane SV, Church J, Vasiliauskas E, Sandborn W, Dubinsky M. The effect of maternal peripartum infliximab use on neonatal immune response [abstract]. *Gastroenterology.* 2008;134(suppl 1):A-69.

23. Mahadevan U, Siegel C, Abreu M. Certolizumab use in pregnancy: low levels detected in cord blood. *Gastroenterology.* 2009;136(5): abstr 960.

24. Van Assche G, Magdelaine-Beuzelin C, D'Haens G, et al. Withdrawal of immunosuppression in Crohn's disease treated with scheduled infliximab maintenance: a randomized trial. *Gastroenterology.* 2008;134(7):1861–1868.

IBD Medications in Pregnancy | 159

Sharon Dudley-Brown

Inflammatory bowel disease (IBD) is a disease that affects women of childbearing age because peak onset is between 15 and 30 years. Medications for IBD in pregnancy need to be considered in all women of childbearing age with IBD because 50% of pregnancies are unplanned. Although risk–benefit ratio of using a drug versus untreated disease needs to be considered, it has been shown that untreated disease during pregnancy is more likely to result in adverse outcomes for the mother and fetus, rather than the drugs used to treat IBD.[1,2] In addition, the rate of relapse in pregnant women on medications was 9.7% versus 34% in patients with IBD not taking any medications during pregnancy.[3]

The US Food and Drug Administration (FDA) has classified the safety of drugs used in pregnancy (Table 159.1). Tables 159.2 and 159.3 summarize the safety of IBD medications for pregnancy. However, despite such classifications, the statements are often difficult to interpret and use in practice for both in counseling the patient and as a guide for the healthcare provider.[4] Not all the medications used to treat IBD are approved by the FDA to treat IBD, but the following classes are used in practice. Because drug treatment trials almost always exclude pregnant women, data are mainly from retrospective and case–control studies.

5-AMINOSALICYLATE ACID PREPARATIONS

This class includes sulfasalazine, mesalamine, olsalazine, and balsalazide. All of these are pregnancy category B, except for olsalazine, which is category C. Use of 5-aminosalicylate acid (5-ASA) products during pregnancy in patients with IBD is generally considered safe, based on several studies.[5–7] A recent meta-analysis, including seven studies, suggested no association among 5-ASA drugs and congenital abnormalities, stillbirths, spontaneous abortions, preterm deliveries, and low birth weight.[8] Both aminosalicylates and sulfasalazine are poorly systemically absorbed, and there is little placental transfer. High-dose aminosalicylates should be avoided during pregnancy because of reported fetal nephrotoxicity,[9] and because studies have been universally performed on the dose of 2.4 g/day. In addition, the use of topical (rectal) preparations has also been shown to be safe for use during pregnancy.[10]

Although sulfasalazine has not been shown to increase congenital malformation in studies, it works by interfering with normal folate metabolism. It is known that folic acid is critical to normal fetal development and to prevent neural tube defects. Thus, women with IBD who are taking sulfasalazine, should be on folic acid supplements to 2 mg/day during conception and throughout pregnancy.[11]

CORTICOSTEROIDS

Corticosteroids include parenteral, oral, and topical agents. Parenteral agents include hydrocortisone, adrenocorticotropic hormone, and methylprednisolone. Oral agents include

TABLE 159.1 US Food and Drug Administration Categories for the Use of Medications in Pregnancy

FDA Pregnancy Category	Definition/Interpretation
A	Controlled studies show no risk
B	No evidence of risk in humans
	Animal findings show risk but human studies do not
	OR
	Animal studies are negative but there are no adequate human studies
C	Risk cannot be ruled out
	Animal studies positive or lacking, human studies lacking
D	Positive evidence of fetal risk
	Can still use if benefit outweighs risk
X	Contraindicated during pregnancy

FDA, US Food and Drug Administration.

TABLE 159.2 Medications Use in the Treatment of IBD[a]

Medication	FDA Category	Recommendations for Pregnancy
5-Aminosalicylate		
Sulfasalazine	B	Low risk. Add folic acid 2 mg daily
Mesalamine	B	Low risk
Balsalazide	B	Low Risk
Antibiotics		
Metronidazole	B	Avoid first trimester
Quinolones	C	Avoid: potential toxicity to cartilage
Steroids		
Corticosteroids	C	Low risk: possible small risk of cleft palate, adrenal insufficiency, premature rupture of membranes
Budesonide	C	Limited human data for oral drug. Low risk with inhaled drug.
Purine analogs		
6-MP/Azathioprine	D	Data (IBD and transplant) suggest some risk, but low
TNF-alpha Inhibitors		
Infliximab	B	Limited human data: low risk
		Crosses placenta and detectable in infant after birth
Adalimumab	B	Limited human data: low risk
		Likely crosses placenta
Certolizumab	B	Limited human data: low risk
		Limited transfer across placenta
Thalidomide	X	Contraindicated: Teratogenic
Integrin Receptor Antagonist		
Natalizumab	C	No human data
Immunosuppressives		
Cyclosporine	C	Low risk
Tacrolimus	C	Low risk
Antimetabolites		
Methotrexate	X	Contraindicated: Teratogenic

[a] Adapted from Gilbert, 2009.

prednisolone, prednisone, and budesonide. Topical agents, suppositories, and enemas are effective in treating proctitis and left-sided colonic disease.

Prednisone has been used extensively in pregnancy without teratogenesis or fetal adrenocortical insufficiency, despite theoretical concern.[12,13] Corticosteroids do cross the placental barrier, and animal studies report an increase of cleft palate and stillbirth. Placental 11-hydroxygenase metabolizes prednisone, thus the fetus is exposed to only 10% of the maternal dose. Although immune deficiency in the newborn is theoretically possible, it is rare in clinical practice.[12]

Although fetal risks are negligible with corticosteroid use in pregnancy, maternal risks are similar to those of a nonpregnant patient. These risks are of the side effects of hypertension, glucose intolerance, and preeclampsia. It is important to use corticosteroids in women with moderate to severe disease activity in pregnancy in the same way as in a nonpregnant patient.

Although there are no data on oral budesonide in pregnancy (warranting a category C), inhaled or intranasal budesonide poses no risk to the fetus. Rectal preparations may be used until the third trimester, unless miscarriage or premature delivery is a concern.[14]

November, 2008, there have been 64 women enrolled prospectively in the pregnancy registry, and 25 have delivered 27 healthy infants with no birth defects attributed to natalizumab.[36]

NUTRITIONAL THERAPIES

Both total parenteral nutrition and supplemental enteral nutrition have been used safely in pregnant patients with IBD.[15]

Although both probiotics and fish oil supplements are not regulated by the FDA, there have been no reports of adverse effects to the mother or fetus. Fish oil supplementation may be useful in those at increased risk for preterm delivery and miscarriage.[37]

SYMPTOMATIC THERAPIES

Loperamide, pregnancy category B, is considered safe to use in pregnancy,[38] however with caution.[14] However, diphenoxylate with atropine, pregnancy category C, is teratogenic in animals, and malformations have been observed in infants exposed to it during the first trimester.[39] Its use should be avoided in pregnancy. Kaolin and pectin preparations are safe, as are fiber supplements.[40,41] Cholestyramine is effective in treating diarrhea, especially those with ileal disease or resection.[14]

SUMMARY AND RECOMMENDATIONS

Because the incidence of IBD is highest during the reproductive years, the safety and choice of medications during pregnancy is a concern for all involved. In addition, as one half of all pregnancies are unplanned, preconception counseling on medication use is imperative for this population. The risk of pregnancy-related complications seems to be linked to active disease at the time of conception rather than medication use per se, and any flare of disease during pregnancy may negatively impact fetal outcome more than any risk from the medications used.[20] Despite previous recommendations to avoid pregnancy or avoid potentially toxic medication use in pregnancy, there is a growing safety record, which has not demonstrated reproducible patterns of fetal malformation.[17] Thus, the imperative to obtain and maintain remission in this population using all available therapies. However, consideration of a switch to a medication that may be safer in pregnancy is advised.[42]

Once a pregnancy is established in a patient with IBD, the goal is to maintain remission and aggressively treat any flares. Partnerships among the gastroenterologist, obstetrician, and patient are essential to this goal. The use of any medications in pregnancy for IBD seem to be safe, balanced against the well established fact that disease activity has been found to poorly affect pregnancy outcomes. The first-line therapies, 5-ASA preparations, selected antibiotics, and symptomatic drugs can safely be used for maintaining remission and managing symptoms.[42] The use of steroids to manage a flare up in pregnancy also seems to be safe. In addition, data from registries suggest that the use of immunomodulators and biologic agents may safely control disease flare and severity during pregnancy of those with moderate to severe disease,[17] and that their use to maintain maternal health outweighs any potential risk to the fetus. Gisbert[32] suggests caution when interpreting much of the data on pregnancy outcomes and medications, citing multiple limitations, including the lack of data on human trials, the lack of data specifically on patients with IBD, the observational and retrospective nature of the data collected, small sample sizes, lack of a truly normal (nonrelated) control group, and lack of information regarding disease activity and comorbidities. Thus, it is clear that further data are necessary on the use of IBD medications during pregnancy.[43,44]

References

1. Sachar D. Exposure to mesalamine during pregnancy increased preterm deliveries (but not birth defects) and decreased birth weight. *Gut*. 1998;43(3):316.

2. Mahadevan U, Sandborn WJ, Li DK, Hakimian S, Kane S, Corley DA. Pregnancy outcomes in women with inflammatory bowel disease: a large community-based study from Northern California. *Gastroenterology*. 2007;133(4):1106–1112.

3. Connell W, Miller A. Treating inflammatory bowel disease during pregnancy: risks and safety of drug therapy. *Drug Saf*. 1999;21(4):311–323.

4. Koren G, Pastuszak A, Ito S. Drugs in pregnancy. *N Engl J Med*. 1998;338(16):1128–1137.

5. Diav-Citrin O, Park YH, Veerasuntharam G, et al. The safety of mesalamine in human pregnancy: a prospective controlled cohort study. *Gastroenterology*. 1998;114(1):23–28.

6. Habal FM, Hui G, Greenberg GR. Oral 5-aminosalicylic acid for inflammatory bowel disease in pregnancy: safety and clinical course. *Gastroenterology*. 1993;105(4):1057–1060.

7. Marteau P, Tennenbaum R, Elefant E, Lémann M, Cosnes J. Foetal outcome in women with inflammatory bowel disease treated during pregnancy with oral mesalazine microgranules. *Aliment Pharmacol Ther*. 1998;12(11):1101–1108.

8. Rahimi R, Nikfar S, Rezaie A, Abdollahi M. Pregnancy outcome in women with inflammatory bowel disease following exposure to 5-aminosalicylic acid drugs: a meta-analysis. *Reprod Toxicol*. 2008;25(2):271–275.

9. Colombel JF, Brabant G, Gubler MC, et al. Renal insufficiency in infant: side-effect of prenatal exposure to mesalazine? *Lancet*. 1994;344(8922):620–621.

10. Bell CM, Habal FM. Safety of topical 5-aminosalicylic acid in pregnancy. *Am J Gastroenterol*. 1997;92(12):2201–2202.

11. Moscandrew M, Kane S. Inflammatory bowel diseases and management considerations: fertility and pregnancy. *Curr Gastroenterol Rep*. 2009;11(5):395–399.

12. Alstead E. Fertility and pregnancy in inflammatory bowel disease. *World J Gastroenterol*. 2001;7(4):455–459.

13. Fraser FS. (1995). Teratogenic potential of corticosteroids in humans. *Teratology*. 1995;51:45–46.

14. Steinlauf AF, Present DH. Medical management of the pregnant patient with inflammatory bowel disease. *Gastroenterol Clin North Am*. 2004;33(2):361–85, xi.

15. Kroser J, Srinivasan R. Drug therapy of inflammatory bowel disease in fertile women. *Am J Gastroenterol*. 2006;101(12 Suppl): S633–S639.

16. Moskovitz DN, Bodian C, Chapman ML, et al. The effect on the fetus of medications used to treat pregnant inflammatory bowel-disease patients. *Am J Gastroenterol*. 2004;99(4):656–661.

17. El Mourabet M, El-Hachem S, Harrison JR, Binion DG. Anti-TNF antibody therapy for inflammatory bowel disease during pregnancy: a clinical review. *Curr Drug Targets.* 2010;11(2):234–241.

18. Roubenoff R, Hoyt J, Petri M, Hochberg MC, Hellmann DB. Effects of antiinflammatory and immunosuppressive drugs on pregnancy and fertility. *Semin Arthritis Rheum.* 1988;18(2):88–110.

19. Goldstein LH, Dolinsky G, Greenberg R, et al. Pregnancy outcome of women exposed to azathioprine during pregnancy. *Birth Defects Res Part A Clin Mol Teratol.* 2007;79(10):696–701.

20. Mahadevan U, Kane S. American gastroenterological association institute technical review on the use of gastrointestinal medications in pregnancy. *Gastroenterology.* 2006;131(1):283–311.

21. Pearson DC, May GR, Fick G, Sutherland LR. Azathioprine for maintaining remission of Crohn's disease. *Cochrane Database Syst Rev.* 2000;(2):CD000067.

22. Treton X, Bouhnik Y, Mary JY, et al. Azathioprine withdrawal in patients with Crohn's disease maintained on prolonged remission: a high risk of relapse. *Clin Gastroenterol Hepatol.* 2009; 7(1):80–85.

23. Coelho J, Beaugerie L, Colombel JF, et al. Pregnancy outcome in inflammatory bowel disease for women treated with thiopurine: cohort from the CESAME Study. Abstract (#141) presented at Digestive Disease Week, Chicago, IL, 2009.

24. Caprilli R, Gassull MA, Escher JC, et al. European evidence based consensus on the diagnosis and management of Crohn's disease: special situations. *Gut.* 2006;55(suppl 1):i36–i58.

25. Dignass AU, Hartmann F, Sturm A, Stein J. Management of inflammatory bowel diseases during pregnancy. *Dig Dis.* 2009;27(3):341–346.

26. Bar Oz B, Hackman R, Einarson T, Koren G. Pregnancy outcome after cyclosporine therapy during pregnancy: a meta-analysis. *Transplantation.* 2001;71(8):1051–1055.

27. Simister NE. Placental transport of immunoglobulin G. *Vaccine.* 2003;21(24):3365–3369.

28. Lichtenstein G, Cohen RD, Feagan BG, et al. Safety of infliximab in Crohn's disease: data from the 5000-patient TREAT registry. *Gastroenterology.* 2004;126(4 suppl):A54.

29. Katz JA, Antoni C, Keenan GF, Smith DE, Jacobs SJ, Lichtenstein GR. Outcome of pregnancy in women receiving infliximab for the treatment of Crohn's disease and rheumatoid arthritis. *Am J Gastroenterol.* 2004;99(12):2385–2392.

30. Mahadevan U, Kane S, Sandborn WJ, et al. Intentional infliximab use during pregnancy for induction or maintenance of remission in Crohn's disease. *Aliment Pharmacol Ther.* 2005;21(6):733–738.

31. Mahadevan U, Terdiman J, Church J, et al. Infliximab levels in infants born to women with inflammatory bowel disease. *Gastroenterology.* 2007; 132(4 suppl):A144.

32. Gisbert J. (2009). Safety of immunomodulators and biologics for the treatment of inflammatory bowel disease during pregnancy and breastfeeding. *Inflamm Bowel Dis.* 2010;16(5):881–895.

33. Kane SV, Acquah LA. Placental transport of immunoglobulins: a clinical review for gastroenterologists who prescribe therapeutic monoclonal antibodies to women during conception and pregnancy. *Am J Gastroenterol.* 2009;104(1):228–233.

34. Johnson DL, Jones KL, Chambers CD, Salas E. Pregnancy outcomes in women exposed to adalimumab: the OTIS autoimmune diseases in pregnancy project. Abstract (142) presented at Digestive Disease Week, Chicago, IL, 2009.

35. Mahadevan U, Abreu MT. Certolizumab use in pregnancy: low levels detected in cord blood. Abstract (960) presented at Digestive Disease Week, Chicago, IL, 2009.

36. Mahadevan U, Martin CF, Sandler RS, et al. A multi-center national prospective study of pregnancy and neonatal outcomes in women with inflammatory bowel disease exposed to immunomodulators and biologic therapy. Abstract (#562) presented at Digestive Disease Week, Chicago, IL, 2009.

37. Sands B, Kooijmans M, Bozic C, Hamdy A, Kouchakji E, Hogge G. Natalizumab use in patients with Crohn's disease and relapsing multiple sclerosis: updated utilization safety results from the Touch™ prescribing program, the pregnancy registry, and the Inform and Tygris studies. Abstract (S1044) presented at Digestive Disease Week, Chicago, IL, 2009.

38. Dubinsky M, Abraham B, Mahadevan U. Management of the pregnant IBD patient. *Inflamm Bowel Dis.* 2008;14(12):1736–1750.

39. Einarson A, Mastroiacovo P, Arnon J, et al. Prospective, controlled, multicentre study of loperamide in pregnancy. *Can J Gastroenterol.* 2000;14(3):185–187.

40. Bonapace ES Jr, Fisher RS. Constipation and diarrhea in pregnancy. *Gastroenterol Clin North Am.* 1998;27(1):197–211.

41. Black RA, Hill DA. Over-the-counter medications in pregnancy. *Am Fam Physician.* 2003;67(12):2517–2524.

42. Katz JA. Pregnancy and inflammatory bowel disease. *Curr Opin Gastroenterol.* 2004;20(4):328–332.

43. Cassina M, Fabris L, Okolicsanyi L, et al. Therapy of inflammatory bowel diseases in pregnancy and lactation. *Expert Opin Drug Saf.* 2009;8(6):695–707.

44. Okoro NI, Kane SV. Gender-related issues in the female inflammatory bowel disease patient. *Expert Rev Gastroenterol Hepatol.* 2009;3(2):145–154.

Special Situations

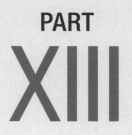

Discrepancies in Delivery of Care in IBD | 160

Smita Halder and Geoffrey C. Nguyen

Inflammatory bowel disease (IBD) is characterized by a constellation of chronic symptoms that remit and relapse throughout the lifetime of an affected individual. The main goals of a gastroenterologist are to accurately diagnose the disease, to treat the symptoms adequately, and to induce and maintain remission using medical therapy. Patients with ulcerative colitis (UC) and Crohn's disease (CD) may have individual experiences of their disease course, which is influenced by several factors. These can range from patient- and physician-specific factors to issues surrounding the availability of treatment and societal barriers to receiving appropriate care. Despite many advances worldwide in the management of IBD from the development of effective medications and the dissemination of treatment guidelines to improve clinical practice, there still remain wide discrepancies in the delivery of care for affected patients.[1] This chapter will examine why and how these discrepancies can occur and will explore ways to minimize them to achieve a standardized level of care across all patient groups.

PATIENT FACTORS

Healthcare Accessibility

Access to health care is not equitable across societies. There are underprivileged communities for whom even the provision of comprehensive primary care cannot be taken for granted. Access to timely care is most vital during the onset of symptoms and at the time of an IBD flare. Delays in diagnosis and initiation of appropriate therapy can affect the course of disease detrimentally. It is estimated that on average, a patient with UC suffers symptoms for more than 2 months before correctly diagnosed,[2] and this delay increases to more than 5 months in older age groups because, presumably, alternative diagnoses are excluded first. For patients with CD, older age at presentation also seems to be a disadvantage because an incorrect preliminary diagnosis is made in up to 60% of elderly patients compared with up to 15% of young adults.[3]

Patients with IBD from low-income families generally have the poorest access to health care.[4] Primary care services may be less comprehensive in inner cities, and as the gatekeepers to specialty care, primary care providers can make a significant difference to the diagnosis and ongoing management of IBD.[5] There is evidence that certain minorities, especially blacks and Hispanics, have less access to specialty care in various medical conditions, including IBD, simply because they were not referred to specialists. Thus, it is important for primary care providers to be vigilant of the presenting symptoms of IBD to refer to a gastroenterologist for both diagnosis and long-term management.[6]

Lack of health insurance and drug plans are additional factors that may contribute to delays in the diagnosis and treatment of symptoms. As many as 7% of patients with IBD in the United States may be uninsured, and even a higher number of patients are underinsured. Under these circumstances, concerns over costly bills may deter a patient with insufficient coverage to seek medical help early. Therapies for IBD such as 5-aminosalicylic acid and particularly biologics can be expensive. As a consequence, individuals may choose not to continue such medications especially for maintenance of remission when they are feeling well.

The timely diagnosis of IBD and effective management of a flare may require time-consuming procedures and tests. For economically disadvantaged individuals for whom time off work may be financially detrimental, attending appointments for clinic visits and tests may become low priority. Such individuals may delay seeking care until they become severely ill or require urgent treatment in an emergency department. For these individuals, offering alternative after-hour or weekend clinics may facilitate access to care. In addition, it is important to provide low-income or uninsured patients access to social workers who may be able to help them secure financial assistance through state and federal programs.

Side Effects of Fatigue and Depression

IBD may have systemic manifestations leading to general fatigue, lack of energy, and depression. These symptoms may themselves prevent or hinder patients from seeking medical care. Furthermore, treatment of generalized fatigue in IBD may be difficult and lead to frustration and loss of confidence in the physician. A resulting rift in the physician-patient relationship may therefore impede overall care. In managing a patient with IBD, it is thus important to adopt an integrative approach that addresses fatigue and sorts out any contributing role of depression in addition to treating gastrointestinal symptoms. Access to patient support groups and psychiatrists and psychologists may help patients cope with some of these more difficult-to-treat symptoms.

Complementary and Alternative Medical Therapies

Dissatisfaction and frustration with conventional IBD medical therapy may lead patients to seek alternative treatment options that adopt a more holistic approach. A more traditional medical approach typically starts with less toxic treatments early and progressing to more efficacious, but more harmful, drugs as the disease becomes more severe. Patients may sometimes want to turn to other therapeutic options for symptom control or explore "safer and natural" comparable treatments with less frequent monitoring required. The use of complementary and alternative medicines (CAM) in patients with IBD is increasing and may be as high as 50%.[7] Such therapies can take the form of herbal preparations, vitamins, dietary manipulations, homeopathy, relaxation, and acupuncture. It is believed that in the majority, the use of CAM is in conjunction with conventional medicines,[8,9] but in a proportion, there may be a conscious decision to steer away from chemical treatments (drugs) perceived to have known potentially harmful side effects.

Important factors that influence the use of CAM include overall disease experience, illness attitudes, and behaviors.[10] CAM use tends to be more likely as an individual's disease course becomes more severe and confidence on his/her physician wanes.[10] Common reasons cited by patients with IBD for using CAM include "wanting greater control over my life and disease" and a belief that "complementary therapies would be more effective." Patients may believe that CAM provides a holistic approach to managing their disease and addresses more than just the physical aspects of IBD. Understanding the reasons behind CAM use would facilitate joint decision making between the patient with IBD and the physician. In this modern era, patient autonomy and preferences toward alternative therapies should be respected and considered a natural adjunct to conventional therapy. However, it is the responsibility of the physician to educate patients as to the relative risks and benefits of medical therapy and the consequences of not taking IBD medications, so that they can make informed decisions.

Editor's note (TMB): There are two other chapters dedicated to complementary therapies.

● PHYSICIAN FACTORS

Physician-Patient Relationship and Communication

The physician-patient relationship is fundamental for providing and receiving effective health care. A healthy patient-doctor relationship is nurtured by mutual respect, open and honest communication, compassion, and trust. Trust between the two parties is possibly of the greatest importance and is a predictor of adherence to medical advice, treatment, and follow-up in chronic diseases, including IBD.[11–14,15]

Physician-related factors may become impediments to a successful physician-patient interaction. It has been shown that the level of discordance between physician and patient has a direct influence on adherence, especially in patients who are psychologically nondistressed.[16] Discordance is a measure of the difference between a physician's and patient's evaluation of clinical information and expectations after a consultation. For example, a patient may perceive his/her symptoms as disabling, but his/her physician may rate them as manageable; a patient may expect further investigations, whereas a physician may view them unnecessary. A mismatch in such perceptions and expectations can lead to frustration and poor cooperation on the part of the patient. In these instances, poor communication can be partly to blame. Good communication skills are an essential requirement for any physician, but not always implemented well. In addition, given time constraints, office appointments may be perceived by patients as rushed and their medical needs and questions not adequately addressed.

Physician Gender and Ethnicity

Gender and ethnic discordance may be additional factors that may hinder an effective physician-patient relationship. This would most probably arise in the case of a female patient and male doctor. An IBD consultation often involves intimate questioning and examination. A female patient who has cultural sensitivities may find a consultation with a male physician especially difficult and awkward. A thorough examination may not be possible, and a full assessment is compromised. This situation could be avoided if any concerns are raised in advance of the appointment, and if there are additional female staff available; unfortunately, this is not always the case. Along the same lines, one study has shown that patients who are of the same race as their physician rate their providers as more participatory in decision making.

Another study suggests that racial concordance between physician and patient results in longer patient visits, more positive patient effect, and greater patient satisfaction. Although this issue is not one that is easily addressed, it underscores the importance of striving to achieve an ethnically and culturally diverse physician workforce in gastroenterology.

Adherence to Clinical Guidelines

Although the management of patients with IBD is tailored to the individual, clinical guidelines serve as a framework for managing patients using good practices to optimize outcomes. These clinical guidelines are usually developed by expert panels and driven by evidence-based research and cover topics from medical management with immunomodulators and biologics to screening and management of complications such as osteoporosis and IBD-associated neoplasia. However, adherence to these guidelines is often suboptimal and variable. It remains unclear as to how much of this is due to inadequate dissemination of published clinical guidelines or physician or patient unwillingness to comply.

THE ROLE OF MULTIDISCIPLINARY CARE

Management of IBD can become complex, especially in patients who develop severe disease and may require surgery or nutritional support. With respect to diagnostic testing, it is critical for the physician to have access to radiologists and pathologists who have extensive experience in interpreting radiologic imaging and pathology specimens in patients with IBD. Such access may be difficult in the community setting. In addition, for patients contemplating bowel surgery, it is important to be able to refer them to experienced colorectal surgeons and high-volume centers because these factors may influence short- and long-term outcomes. High-volume centers may also have other ancillary services such as nursing support for stoma care and nutritionists. As we have previously alluded to, managing the mental health aspects of an individual with chronically relapsing IBD may be particularly challenging but crucial to the patient's overall well-being. Psychiatrists and psychologists who are familiar with the effect of IBD on psychological well-being are invaluable resources in attaining this goal. Many of these specialist services may be more readily accessible at tertiary centers, and consideration should be given for early referral of a complication to an IBD center of excellence.

CONCLUSION

Despite the rapidly paced progress in the medical treatment of the IBDs, not all patients with IBD will reap these benefits equally. There are social inequities in health insurance and household income that may directly or indirectly limit access to optimal medical care. These socioeconomic issues will not likely be resolved in the near future. For gastroenterologists and primary care providers, nurturing the patient-physician relationship can make the most impact on an individual. Over the past half century, this intricate relationship has been jeopardized because physicians are pressed to see more and more patients during increasingly shorter clinic visits. In this current environment, a model of health care that includes IBD nurse specialists may help restore the mutual trust and respect between patients and their health providers. IBD nurse specialists can serve both as patient advocates and as educators, and provide a crucial bridge to physicians.

As Internet-savvy patients become increasingly more knowledgeable about their IBD and treatment options, gastroenterologists will need to learn to respect patient preference in the decision-making process—even if this means not accepting treatment recommendations. At the same time, it is the responsibility of an IBD physician provider to keep abreast of clinical guidelines and adhere to them under the appropriate clinical context.

Editor's note (TMB): This is an excellent thought-provoking chapter. See additional information in the other chapters on compliance, nurse practioners, IBD nurse advocates, complementary medicine, and psychic social support systems.

References

1. Reddy SI, Friedman S, Telford JJ, Strate L, Ookubo R, Banks PA. Are patients with inflammatory bowel disease receiving optimal care? *Am J Gastroenterol.* 2005;100(6):1357–1361.

2. Zimmerman J, Gavish D, Rachmilewitz D. Early and late onset ulcerative colitis: distinct clinical features. *J Clin Gastroenterol.* 1985;7(6):492–428.

3. Foxworthy DM, Wilson JA. Crohn's disease in the elderly. Prolonged delay in diagnosis. *J Am Geriatr Soc.* 1985;33(7):492–495.

4. Blendon RJ, Schoen C, DesRoches CM, Osborn R, Scoles KL, Zapert K. Inequities in health care: a five-country survey. *Health Aff (Millwood).* 2002;21(3):182–191.

5. Wilson K, Rosenberg MW. Accessibility and the Canadian health care system: squaring perceptions and realities. *Health Policy.* 2004;67(2):137–148.

6. Nguyen GC, Torres EA, Regueiro M, et al. Inflammatory bowel disease characteristics among African Americans, Hispanics, and non-Hispanic Whites: characterization of a large North American cohort. *Am J Gastroenterol.* 2006;101(5):1012–1023.

7. Rawsthorne P, Shanahan F, Cronin NC, et al. An international survey of the use and attitudes regarding alternative medicine by patients with inflammatory bowel disease. *Am J Gastroenterol.* 1999;94(5):1298–1303.

8. Hilsden RJ, Verhoef MJ, Best A, Pocobelli G. Complementary and alternative medicine use by Canadian patients with inflammatory bowel disease: results from a national survey. *Am J Gastroenterol.* 2003;98(7):1563–1568.

9. Moser G, Tillinger W, Sachs G, et al. Relationship between the use of unconventional therapies and disease-related concerns: a study of patients with inflammatory bowel disease. *J Psychosom Res.* 1996;40(5):503–509.

10. Li FX, Verhoef MJ, Best A, Otley A, Hilsden RJ. Why patients with inflammatory bowel disease use or do not use complementary and alternative medicine: a Canadian national survey. *Can J Gastroenterol.* 2005;19(9):567–573.

11. Thom DH, Ribisl KM, Stewart AL, Luke DA. Further validation and reliability testing of the Trust in Physician Scale. The Stanford Trust Study Physicians. *Med Care.* 1999;37(5):510–517.

12. Piette JD, Heisler M, Krein S, Kerr EA. The role of patient-physician trust in moderating medication nonadherence due to cost pressures. *Arch Intern Med.* 2005;165(15):1749–1755.

13. Schneider J, Kaplan SH, Greenfield S, Li W, Wilson IB. Better physician-patient relationships are associated with higher reported adherence to antiretroviral therapy in patients with HIV infection. *J Gen Intern Med.* 2004;19(11):1096–1103.

14. O'Malley AS, Sheppard VB, Schwartz M, Mandelblatt J. The role of trust in use of preventive services among low-income African-American women. *Prev Med.* 2004;38(6):777–785.

15. Nguyen GC, LaVeist TA, Harris ML, Datta LW, Bayless TM, Brant SR. Patient trust-in-physician and race are predictors of adherence to medical management in inflammatory bowel disease. *Inflamm Bowel Dis.* 2009;15(8):1233–1239.

16. Sewitch MJ, Abrahamowicz M, Barkun A, et al. Patient non-adherence to medication in inflammatory bowel disease. *Am J Gastroenterol.* 2003;98(7):1535–1544.

Colitis in the Elderly

161

Anne Silverman

A discussion of colitis in the elderly requires an understanding of the terms "colitis" and "elderly." Colitis implies any inflammation of the colon, including, but not limited to, inflammatory bowel disease (IBD). "Elderly" previously referred to individuals older than 65 years; however, the fastest growing segment of the current population is individuals older than 85 years. Colitis may present clinically with symptoms of diarrhea, hematochezia, fever, leukocytosis, volume depletion, and weight loss or atypically with constipation or megacolon. Only recently it has been recognized that both Crohn's disease and ulcerative colitis may present for the first time in older patients. Other forms of colitis that may present similarly include infectious colitis, diverticular colitis, ischemic colitis, microscopic colitis, radiation colitis, nonsteroidal inflammatory drugs (NSAIDs)–induced colitis, and colorectal cancer.[1]

● INFECTIOUS COLITIS

Infectious colitis is the most important cause of colonic inflammation in the elderly, particularly because this population of patients often have underlying chronic diseases, may have a weakened immune system, are more likely to have acquired or iatrogenic hypochlorhydria, and are more likely to be on polypharmacy. In addition, elderly women are more likely to have been treated with antibiotics for urinary tract infections. Most cases of acute self-limited infectious diarrhea result from viruses such as Norwalk, sapovirus, and Norwalk-like viruses. Inflammation of the colon secondary to infectious bacteria is attributable to *Clostridium difficile, Salmonella* (with a recent nationwide outbreak from infected peanuts and eggs), *Shigella, Campylobacter,* and *Escherichia coli* O157:H7. Immunocompromised hosts are at risk for cytomegalovirus (CMV) infection manifesting as colitis or systemic disease with nonspecific symptoms, including weight loss. Amebiasis can cause infectious colitis but is not common in the United States unless patients have traveled outside of the country.

C. difficile

C. difficile has emerged as perhaps the most important cause of infectious colitis in North America. The elderly are particularly at risk because they are more likely to be hospitalized, live in an institutionalized setting, have outpatient procedures, and receive acid-suppressive therapy and/or antibiotics. It is unclear whether the acid suppression is the cause of the infection—because the organism is an anaerobic spore-forming bacterium that can survive the acidic pH in the stomach environment—or whether the acid suppression identifies a host who has multiple underlying problems and is at increased risk for the infection. The number of cases of *C. difficile* has markedly increased in the past decade. Initially, a more virulent strain of the bacteria was recently reported in Quebec among hospitalized patients in wards that housed multiple patients in one room. Soon afterward, reports of this more virulent strain were noted in hospitals in the United States as well.[2–4]

This more virulent strain of *C. difficile* was subsequently isolated and identified. Depending on the method of strain typing, this organism has been characterized as the B1 restriction enzyme analysis type, North American Pulsed-Field Type 1 (NAP1) and polymerase chain reaction ribotype 027. The organism is also a rare toxin type as described by the restriction enzyme analysis of the pathogenicity locus, toxin type III. B1/NAP1/027 *C. difficile* has been found to produce 16-fold more toxin A and 23 times more toxin B in vitro than other commonly isolated strains of the organism. In addition to being a high toxin producer, this strain has other features that make it a more virulent organism. The higher toxin production may be secondary to a frame shift mutation in the gene tcdC that downregulates toxin A and B in the pathogenicity locus. This strain also produces an as yet uncharacterized protein called binary toxin, which may also contribute to the increased virulence of this organism. It is believed that emergence of this particular strain is related to the ubiquitous use of fluoroquinolones, including moxifloxacin and gatifloxacin. Accordingly, the B1/NAP1/027 strain is believed to have now emerged because previously this organism was more sensitive to fluoroquinolones.

Transmission of the bacteria *C. difficile* to the patient in a healthcare setting usually occurs from the caregiver. Because the bacteria are spore formers, they have been found on hands, jewelry, bed rails, floors, and even the heating duct. It is believed that the organism colonizes the host and releases the toxin when the normal bowel flora is eliminated as a result of the widespread use of broad-spectrum antibiotics. Cases of community-acquired *C. difficile* infections are being increasingly reported. The source of such outbreaks may be from organisms recently found in colonized cattle and other antibiotic feed animals used for domestic consumption. Other sources may be from contact with the healthcare system, including visiting patients in hospitals and chronic care facilities. In addition, cases have been reported with no known risk factors for infection.

Clinical symptoms may range from mild diarrhea to severe abdominal pain with watery or bloody diarrhea to overt ileus with bowel wall edema in the frail elderly patient. Because *C. difficile* accounts for the majority of diarrhea and other acute changes in bowel habits seen in elderly acutely ill or hospitalized patients, physicians must have a high index of suspicion, particularly if the patient has been on an antibiotic, had a previous hospitalization, or presents with fever or leukocytosis. Abdominal pain with severe cramping may also be a common clinical presentation in the elderly, as well as bloody diarrhea that may mimic ischemic colitis.

In patients with known IBD, *C. difficile* has become a frequent cause of disease exacerbation. This is particularly a problem in older patients with IBD because I find that even high-dose vancomycin alone will not control the inflammation and infection and requires the addition of steroids, sometimes even with a short hospital stay for intravenous (IV) steroids. The use of steroids and other immunosuppressive agents may, in turn, predispose to CMV colitis, and this diagnosis should be considered in a patient who relapses with symptoms after initially responding to therapy for *C. difficile* and exacerbation of colitis. The severe abdominal pain often leads to the use of narcotic analgesics that may put the patient at risk for toxic megacolon or delayed organism clearance. Some patients diagnosed with *C. difficile* infection without IBD initially improve with vancomycin therapy, but the symptoms never completely abate or symptoms of diarrhea worsen. These patients often have clearance of the toxin production; however, flexible sigmoidoscopy demonstrates evidence of diffuse colonic inflammation that leads to the appearance of IBD. Further follow-up of these patients up to several years demonstrates that they indeed have IBD first diagnosed after an initial bout of *C. difficile* colitis.

Treatment in uncomplicated patients is usually accomplished by cessation of the underlying antibiotic use and a 10- to 14-day course of metronidazole 500 mg three times a day. More severely ill patients, particularly the elderly, intensive care unit patients, low albumin, fever, leukocytosis, those with renal compromise or the high toxin producing B1/NAP1/027 strain require the use of oral vancomycin. In patients with fulminant *C. difficile*, the addition of IV metronidazole and or vancomycin enemas should be instituted, and lastly, surgical management requiring colectomy if other measures fail. New treatment options are currently in clinical trials. Rifaximin therapy has been used, but the development of drug resistance in the B1/NAP/027 strain is a concern. Reports of systemic infection with

probiotics and the lack of clinical data dampen the enthusiasm for the use of probiotics. As mentioned previously, in patients with underlying IBD and *C. difficile* infection, a several weeks of steroids maybe necessary along with vancomycin to improve the colonic inflammation.

Editor's note (TMB): There are two chapters discussing *C. difficile* toxin diarrhea in patients with IBD in Volume 1.

Recurrent *C. difficile* Infection

Recurrent *C. difficile* infection occurs in up to 35% of patients and is often due to recurrent infection. Because *C. difficile* is a spore-forming organism, it can persist in any environment, including the colon, for many months. Infected patients are asked to clean their household bathrooms with a 10% hypochlorite solution. Alcohol-based hand cleaning solutions do not eliminate the organism; therefore, washing hands with soap and water is recommended after contact with the patient. Because elderly patients with and without IBD tend to be sicker than younger patients, I often retreat with vancomycin 250 mg four times daily for a 30-day period. There is seemingly less recurrence with this strategy. Others use 125 mg vancomycin and some use tapering doses of vancomycin over 6 weeks. The goal is to eliminate the spores that persist in the colon. Other strategies include adding a toxin-binding agent such as cholestyramine, long-term therapy with low-dose vancomycin, and the addition of a second antibiotic at the end of tapered therapy such as rifaximin. Large clinical studies for treatment of recurrent disease are lacking. Fecal enema transplant from uninfected patients has been a successful therapy in small studies but lacks the enthusiasm of the physician and the patient. Because infection with *C. difficile* is in part attributed to a poor antibody response to toxin A, case reports have documented success with the use of IV gamma globulin, but this therapy includes the inherent risks of using this agent.

Prevention

Primary prevention should be a goal of any hospital or institution. Strict hand washing after patient contact should be observed by all who care for patients. Infected patients should be isolated in separate rooms whenever possible. Avoidance of broad-spectrum antibiotics should be followed particularly with fluoroquinolones when an infection is not documented. Empiric antibiotic therapy in patients with Crohn's disease is common, particularly the use of ciprofloxacin, but should be avoided whenever possible. Even metronidazole, which is efficacious both for treatment of *C. difficile* and as empiric therapy in Crohn's disease, can actually lead to *C. difficile* colitis. Endoscopy should be avoided at the outset of disease to prevent the spread of the toxin in the endoscopy area. If endoscopy is needed to look for exacerbation of IBD or CMV, cases should be done as the last case in a room to avoid transmission of *C. difficile* infection. Ideally, universal cleaning should prevent this problem. In our IBD clinic, we noted a cluster of *C. difficile* infections, and this problem resolved after we asked our house cleaning team to clean our bathrooms and examination rooms immediately after we saw patients with suspected *C. difficile* colitis.

Diagnosis

Diagnosis requires a high index of suspicion and should be considered in all patients with new-onset diarrhea. We have found that most patients with IBD exacerbations have *C. difficile*. Instructions to patients for stool collection for immunoassays are important because there are proteins in the stool that degrade the toxin if stool stands at room temperature more than 4 hours. Patients with underlying IBD should be tested for the toxin whenever they present with an exacerbation of the disease. If the enzyme immunoassay is used for toxin detection, then at least two to three stool samples should be tested for both A and B toxin because of the lower sensitivity of this assay. Some laboratories use the rapid *C. difficile* antigen assay as the initial diagnostic test and then do a confirmatory assay. The cell culture tissue assay is the gold standard for diagnosis but requires at least 48 hours to perform.

Other Infections

Other infectious colitis may occur in elderly patients with and without IBD but are much less common. These infections may present with and without bleeding and, particularly in the elderly, may not always have systemic signs such as fever and leukocytosis. If bleeding is present, especially in the elderly patient, it is the job of the clinician to consider other forms of colitis such as ischemic colitis in the differential diagnosis. In diagnosing the etiology of bloody diarrhea, culture of the stool should be performed and include a request for *E. coli* O157:H7. In most laboratories, this organism must be requested specifically, or it is not included in the routine stool culture.

Although *Salmonella* is much less common in the United States, a recent outbreak occurred that was finally traced due to contamination of a large peanut processing factory. Large-scale recall of potentially infected products prevented further illness after the source was identified. In food-borne infections, it is important to notify the health department so that there is early identification and containment of the infection source. *Salmonella* is largely treated with supportive therapy because antibiotic therapy may prolong carriage of the organism unless systemic infection occurs. *Shigella* may require antibiotic therapy, but therapy can wait for culture results. *Campylobacter jejuni* needs antibiotic therapy if infection is not self-limited.

The reason to avoid early use of antibiotics in bloody diarrhea is the concern about development of hemolytic uremic syndrome in patients with *E. coli* O157:H7. Epidemics of this bacterium have been reported in the United States and elsewhere. Older patients may not mount a febrile response and lead to misdiagnosis and the use of antibiotics. Close follow-up is necessary along with supportive therapy with IV hydration. Deaths from this organism usually presents in clusters because of the food-borne nature of the illness and the fact that this form of colitis is commonly fatal in the young and the elderly. In addition, the organism is not included in routine stool cultures requested.

● NONINFECTIOUS COLITIS

Because diarrhea is a symptom of colonic inflammation, it can also be the result of other etiologies that may commonly affect the elderly. As previously mentioned, ischemic colitis early on in the clinical course may mimic an infectious diarrhea. However, in the majority of patients, there is pain, the episode is self-limited, and the symptoms resolve within 1 or 2 days. Rarely, the ischemia may become progressive and result in the need for surgical management.[5] Left-sided colon cancer may result in near complete colon blockage leading to acute onset of pain, overflow of liquid stools, and sometimes rectal bleeding. Medications may lead to diarrhea by various mechanisms, including bacterial overgrowth from antibiotics, alterations in bowel motility, microscopic colitis, osmotic agents such as magnesium, and direct mucosal toxicity among others. Careful history will elicit the report of a new medication, and the diagnosis will be secured by stopping the suspect medication.

Diverticular Colitis

Diverticular colitis was often believed to be the cause of non-infectious inflammation in the colon. Although patients with diverticulitis may present with findings, particularly on computed tomography (CT), and symptoms similar to patients with Crohn's disease, the clinical course and response to therapy certainly differ. Patients with mild diverticulitis may not require antibiotics, whereas those with severe inflammation require systemic antibiotics and sometimes periods of bowel rest and, in severe cases, surgery. This is a segmental disease that often involves the sigmoid or descending colon. Bleeding is not commonly seen with the clinical presentation. Right-sided diverticular disease rarely becomes inflamed and usually present with painless hematochezia. The clinical picture and CT along with endoscopy in the patient after their symptoms improve usually clinches the diagnosis. Endoscopy should not be performed in patients with suspected diverticulitis until the inflammation subsides to prevent perforation. The symptoms of chronic diverticulitis may mimic Crohn's disease by forming fistula to the skin or other organs because of the chronic nature of the inflammation that leads to a subacute bowel obstruction.

If an infectious etiology is not found and the other causes of acute diarrhea do not point to an etiology and if the diarrhea remains chronic, then other diagnostic considerations include microscopic colitis and *IBD*.

Crohn's Colitis

Crohn's colitis is the most common type of IBD with or without ileal involvement. Elderly patients may have classic presentations with diarrhea, weight loss, and bleeding. Bleeding may be hemorrhagic or may be absent entirely. However, they may present with a new-onset iron deficiency without any other symptoms, or IBD may be detected on screening colonoscopy without any signs or symptoms.[6] Older patients tend to have less stormy courses than patients presenting at younger ages and may do well on aminosalicylates alone, because these medications work best in colonic inflammation. In elderly patients who require immunosuppressive therapy, steroids tend to unmask hyperglycemia early even in nonobese elderly patients. Elderly patients are already at risk for hip fractures and other complications of steroids, so steroids should only be used short term to get the patient on other forms of medications such as immunomodulators and anti-tumor necrosis factor (anti-TNF) biologic agents if the patient has recurrent symptoms after steroid taper. Purinethol and azathioprine, hereafter referred to as mercaptopurines, are tolerated well by elderly patients and should be used preferentially because they have less infectious consequences than the anti-TNF biologics and long-term steroids. Patients with intermediate levels of thiopurine methyltransferase, the enzyme that metabolizes the mercaptopurine medications, achieve therapeutic levels of 6 thioguanine with lower doses. Older patients are more likely than younger patients to have been exposed to tuberculosis or have a remote history of hepatitis B infection. Screening for these diseases should be performed before initiating biologic therapy to prevent reactivation of latent disease. Patients on immunosuppressive therapy should also undergo yearly flu vaccination to prevent catastrophic illness. The medications for treatment of Crohn's disease in elderly are the same as those used to treat younger patients and have been thoroughly discussed elsewhere in this book.

Ulcerative Colitis

In elderly patients, ulcerative colitis is less common than Crohn's disease; however, with the recent increase in *C. difficile* infections in the elderly, there has been an increase in the number of cases of ulcerative colitis recognized immediately after infection with *C. difficile*. Mesalamine remains the drug of choice for ulcerative colitis in these patients, but in those who have multiple exacerbations of colitis, the mercaptopurines should be considered as the second-line therapy. Steroids may be necessary in severe colitis or treating a severe superimposed *C. difficile* colitis; however, the known side effects of steroids are magnified in the elderly who already have compromised immune functions, risk for osteoporosis, avascular necrosis, and cataracts. Infliximab is approved by the US Food and Drug Administration for treatment of ulcerative colitis, and the previous discussion of this medication for Crohn's disease applies to these patients as well.

Editor's note (TMB): There are chapters on ulcerative colitis therapy in Volume 1.

Other Colitides

Endoscopy is often helpful to diagnose IBD. Biopsies of the colon should be obtained even in the setting of a normal-appearing colon. *Microscopic colitis* may present in the elderly with profuse watery diarrhea and weight loss mimicking the symptoms of Crohn's disease. Endoscopy can also help differentiate patients with a partially obstructing left-sided colon cancer who have bloody or nonbloody diarrhea from overflow incontinence. It is important to get a history of NSAIDs use because many elderly patients take one or more NSAIDs. *NSAID-induced colitis* may mimic Crohn's colitis particularly with new-onset Crohn's when histologic evidence does not exhibit chronicity. Usually, stopping the NSAIDs clarifies the underlying cause. Just as important is the need to exclude infectious colitis in suspected new onset of IBD or in patients who present with an exacerbation of their underlying IBD. In patients who are already immunosuppressed and their colitis is not responding to conventional therapy, endoscopy should be performed with biopsies designated for immunohistochemical staining for CMV.

● TREATMENT OF THE ELDERLY

Treatment for both Crohn's disease and ulcerative colitis, as mentioned above, is similar in the elderly and young patients with IBD. There is the caveat that most elderly are on polypharmacy that will interact with the disease and with other medications. Specifically, *NSAIDs* have been shown to cause exacerbation of colitis in some patients, and the risks and benefits must be carefully weighed in each patient. Ciprofloxacin should be avoided to treat both Crohn's disease and urinary infections in older patients with IBD because of the risk of *C. difficile* colitis. *Allopurinol*, which is commonly prescribed to prevent gout, will increase thioguanine levels in patients on mercaptopurines and therefore purinethol and azathioprine should be reduced by about one fourth the dose. Because the biologic agents were initially approved for use in inflammatory joint disease, most of the severe infectious complications from the anti-TNF biologic agents have been reported in elderly patients with rheumatologic indications for the drug.

Microscopic Colitis

Microscopic colitis may present similar to IBD with sudden onset of profuse watery diarrhea and weight loss. Because microscopic colitis has been shown to be associated with the use of specific medications, a careful documentation of medications is needed, particularly with the over-the-counter status of *lansoprazole* and *omeprazole*, both of which have been reported to be associated with microscopic colitis. Microscopic colitis has been more frequently documented in patients older than 65 years, with a female predominance. Other than proton pump inhibitors, medications linked with IBD include NSAIDs, celecoxib, clozapine, entacapone, stalevo, simvastatin, flutamide, gold salts, ranitidine, and acarbose. Microscopic colitis has been seen in celiac and other autoimmune diseases. The etiology of this disorder is unknown; however, several lines of investigation include an association with the HLA-DR3-DQ2 locus (which is already associated with celiac disease), reduced expression of CD1d, a major histocompatibility complex class 1-like molecule, bile acid malabsorption, and various protein growth factors and polypeptides, such as basic fibroblast growth factor and albumin.[7]

● TREATMENT

Treatment of microscopic colitis should first focus on identifying any potential medications that can be stopped before initiating medical treatment. Many people start with an 8-week course of Pepto-Bismol four times daily. I have had a few patients develop gastric and duodenal ulcers on this high-dose therapy. Budesonide has been shown to be effective in double-blind randomized placebo controlled trial using 6 mg for 6 months. The problem with this medication is that it is costly, particularly compared with prednisone. I have found that a 10-mg dose of prednisone is effective in treating the symptoms, and this has been shown in uncontrolled studies in the literature. Mesalamine has been shown in nonrandomized uncontrolled studies to be effective in treating the disorder. In patients who

---

Editor's note (TMB): The next chapter is on Collagenous and Lymphocytic Colitis.

fail to respond to therapy, the clinician should consider biopsy of the duodenum to look for coexisting celiac disease.

● SUMMARY

The elderly are at risk for inflammatory conditions of the colon because of multiple underlying medical problems, the use of multiple medications, increased exposure to the healthcare system, and other institutionalized settings such as rehabilitation centers and chronic care facilities. A careful history, review of medications, and exclusion of infections can help with early diagnosis and treatment of patients with both classic symptoms and more cryptic presentations of colonic inflammation. Abdominal imaging and endoscopy can be useful when infection has been excluded to diagnose and treat inflammatory conditions of the colon.

References

1. Swaroop P. Inflammatory bowel diseases in the elderly. *Clin Geriatr Med.* 2007;23:809–821.
2. Gould CV, McDonald LC. Bench-to-bedside review: *Clostridium difficile* colitis. *Crit Care.* 2008;12:203–210.
3. Kelly C, La Mont JT. *Clostridium difficile*—More difficult than ever. *NEJM.* 2008:359:1932–1940.
4. Trinh C, Prabhakar K. Diarrheal diseases in the elderly. *Clin Ceriatr Med.* 2007;23:833–856.
5. Korotinkski S, Katz A, Malnic SDH. Chronic ischemic bowel diseases in the aged-go with the flow. *Age Ageing.* 2005;34:10–16.
6. Heresbach D, Alexandre JL, Bretagne JF, et al. Crohn's disease in the over-60 age group: a population based study. *Eur J Gastroenterol Hepatol.* 2004;16:657–664.
7. Tangri V, Chande N. Microscopic colitis: an update. *J Clin Gastroenterol.* 2009;43:293–296.

Collagenous and Lymphocytic Colitis and Enteritis | 162

Anne G. Tuskey and Mark T. Worthington

INTRODUCTION

Microscopic colitis (MC) is characterized by chronic, watery diarrhea and an endoscopically normal colon with chronic mucosal inflammation on biopsy. Because this is a microscopic disease, the normal appearance presents a problem for the endoscopist who does not consider the diagnosis at the time of colonoscopy. There are two histopathologic subtypes of MC: collagenous colitis (CC), which has a chronic mucosal inflammatory response with an associated subepithelial collagen band, and lymphocytic colitis (LC), which is similar in all respects, except for the lack of the collagen band. Lindström first described CC in 1976, whereas LC was described in 1989 by Lazenby et al.[1]

EPIDEMIOLOGY

Microscopic colitides are a common, accounting for 4% to 13% of patients with chronic diarrhea.[2] Most cases of MC have been reported from Europe and North America, but there are also cases in South America, Africa, and Australia.[1] The European annual incidence of CC and LC is 0.6 to 6.1 per 100,000 and 0.6 to 5.7 per 100,000, respectively.[2] The largest population-based study in the United States conducted from 1985 to 2001 estimated the incidence of MC as 8.6 per 100,000 person-years. During this study, the incidence increased from 1.1 per 100,000 in the beginning to 19.6 per 100,000 at the end.[3] A similar increase in incidence was seen in earlier Swedish studies, but whether this reflects an increased prevalence or improved disease awareness is not clear.

CC and LC are diseases of aging, with most cases presenting in the sixth to seventh decades, but can occur in all ages, including children. CC is associated with a female predominance, with female to male ratios as high as 20:1.[2] There is less of a female predominance in LC.

CLINICAL PRESENTATION

Microscopic colitides are typified by chronic or intermittent nonbloody diarrhea, abdominal pain, and weight loss. Patients typically have four to nine watery (and often nocturnal) stools a day, but dehydration is unusual. Associated fatigue, nausea, and fecal incontinence can impair quality of life. The presence of high fever, vomiting, and hematochezia suggests another diagnosis.[2] Abdominal pain, flatulence, and abdominal distension are common symptoms (>50% in most series) and initially suggest irritable bowel syndrome rather than an inflammatory colitis.

The clinical course of MC is variable, ranging from a single episode to intermittent flares or continuous symptoms. The etiopathogenesis of MC is not known, but the long-term prognosis is favorable for both CC and LC. In a 3.5-year follow-up study, 15% of patients with CC had spontaneous remission, whereas an additional 48% went into remission after treatment. In a study of 27 patients with LC, more than 80% of patients experienced normalization of stool frequency and histology within 4 months. In 25 patients with MC, all patients had symptomatic improvement at 47 months and only 29% required routine medications.[1,2] Unlike classical inflammatory bowel diseases (IBDs) such as Crohn's and ulcerative colitis, there seems to be no increased mortality or malignancy rate with MC.

LC and CC are colonic diseases, but ileal involvement has been described with ileal villous atrophy and subsequent bile salt malabsorption. Ileal atrophy has been reported with normal jejunal mucosa, unlike celiac disease where jejunal atrophy is diagnostic for that condition. Lymphocytic enteritis (LE) is discussed below. Because LC and CC can coexist with celiac disease as an overlap syndrome, and because MC can be similar to early Crohn's disease (CD), we consider the presence of ileal injury on colonoscopy as an indication that further evaluation of the small intestine is necessary before making the diagnosis of MC. Occasionally, changes in clinical findings require the diagnosis of MC to be reconsidered months or even years later, particularly if symptoms worsen or the disease becomes refractory to treatment.

Lymphocytic Enteritis

LE is a poorly characterized small intestinal disorder that, similar to celiac disease, can lead to duodenal and jejunal villous atrophy and chronic mucosal inflammation, but with negative celiac disease serologies. Like celiac disease, LE can occur in association with LC or CC (e.g., lymphocytic enterocolitis). A series of seven patients with LE with small intestinal villous atrophy that resolved spontaneously on a gluten-containing diet suggests that some cases are benign and self-limited.[4] The typical LE case is steroid responsive. Because both the proximal and the distal small intestine can be independently involved in MC with associated enteritis, small bowel biopsies using both upper endoscope and colonoscope are required to rule out small intestinal disease.

Distinction from celiac disease is critical because LE is a milder disease that does not require the elimination of gluten and has no associated increased risk of mucosal lymphoma. Because there are mild cases of celiac sprue where the peripheral blood serologies are negative, but there is intramucosal production of antitissue transglutaminase antibodies, a small number of patients with celiac disease will be missed if the diagnosis relies on peripheral blood serologies alone. Antibody testing on endoscopic biopsies is not commercially available, so an empiric trial of a gluten-free diet with repeat mucosal biopsies (and even a repeat gluten challenge) may be required to rule out mild celiac disease. A submucosal collagen band in celiac disease (collagenous sprue) has been described and is associated with more severe disease.

Association with Other Conditions

Extraintestinal symptoms such as arthritis, arthralgia, or uveitis can occur with MC and are related to other overlapping autoimmune diseases such as autoimmune thyroid disease, rheumatoid arthritis, diabetes mellitus, and bronchial asthma.[1,2] Increased erythrocyte sedimentation rates can occur. Stool studies positive for leukocytes, lactoferrin, and calprotectin have been described, but the percentages are low enough not to be diagnostically useful. Antinuclear and other autoantibodies have been described, although these usually reflect overlapping autoimmune disorders.[2] There are no diagnostic serologies, and only a compatible biopsy and clinical picture are required to make the diagnosis.

There is a strong association between MC and celiac disease: approximately one third of patients with celiac disease have evidence of MC on colonic biopsy, whereas 2% to 10% of patients with MC have small bowel mucosal changes consistent with celiac sprue.[2] Celiac disease without MC typically presents as an osmotic diarrhea, with the stool output decreasing with fasting. The inflammation in celiac disease promotes a net secretion of salt and water in the small intestine, but a physiologically normal colon is able to compensate for the increased salt and water load. When MC complicates celiac disease, the ability of the colon to adapt to the increased intestinal fluid is lost, resulting in a functional secretory diarrhea (i.e., diarrhea persists with fasting). Thus, MC should always be considered in patients with celiac disease with continued or unusual symptoms despite adherence to a gluten-free diet, just as the celiac disease should be considered in patients with refractory MC.

An evolution from MC to classical IBD (Crohn's or ulcerative colitis) has been reported in a few patients.[1] There are also those patients who represent an early diagnosis of classical IBD, typically CD, often identified on screening colonoscopies.

Complications in Microscopic Colitides

Severe complications in MC are rare, although there are several case reports of colonic perforation in CC, from both barium enema and colonoscopy.[1,5] Perforations in patients with CC tend to be right sided unlike the predominantly left-sided iatrogenic perforations in colonoscopy. In addition, endoscopic findings of longitudinal, linear ulcers in the right colon have been reported in patients with CC. Both these findings correspond to the apparent right colon predominance for CC.[5] The rate of colonic perforation in CC is estimated to be less than 1% of colonic procedures. Chronic MC is not associated with an increased risk for colon cancer.[1,2]

● DIAGNOSIS

Endoscopic and radiographic findings in patients with MC should be normal or display only subtle nonspecific changes such as edema, erythema, or abnormal vascular pattern. Colonic mucosal biopsy is required to diagnose MC, with the classic histologic feature of an intraepithelial lymphocytosis. Crypt architecture is usually preserved, but focal cryptitis may be present. Intraepithelial lymphocyte infiltration is more prominent in LC with more than 20 lymphocytes per 100 epithelial cells. Right colonic linear ulcers are not inconsistent with the diagnosis but are rare and might suggest other causes of colonic inflammation, such as CD or cytomegalovirus colitis.

CC is distinguished by an abnormal thickening of the subepithelial collagen band, which is normally 0 to 3 μm wide. This band is ≥10 μm wide in CC,[1] consisting of type VI collagen rather than the type IV collagen of the normal epithelial basement membrane.[6] The histologic changes in CC are typically limited to the colon, although thickened collagen bands have rarely been reported in the stomach, duodenum, and terminal ileum.[1] The severity of diarrhea in CC correlates with the amount of lamina propria inflammation rather than the size of the collagen band.[6] CC can have a patchy distribution. The severity of histologic changes also tends to decrease from the proximal to the distal colon; therefore, right colonic biopsies are essential.[1] We and others have seen several cases of LC only involving the right colon, suggesting that the only appropriate test to rule out either condition is a colonoscopy and not a flexible sigmoidoscopy. Biopsies from the terminal ileum and all colonic segments are strongly recommended to clearly characterize the disease and eliminate confounding diagnoses. Atypical forms of inflammation can involve giant cells, pseudomembranes, granulomatous changes, and inflammation that predominantly involves the crypts with limited intraepithelial lymphocytes. These atypical forms have symptoms similar to the more typical form. As previously discussed, small bowel biopsies from upper and lower endoscopy are necessary to make a diagnosis of LE.

● PATHOPHYSIOLOGY

The pathogenesis of MC is unknown and likely multifactorial, with bile acids, toxins, infectious agents, genetics, and drugs all suggested as possible causes. Of these, a clear link between specific drugs and MC has been established and will be explained below. Bile acid malabsorption can complicate MC, with 44% of CC cases associated with bile acid malabsorption.[7] Bile acids increase bacterial translocation, and luminal infusion of bile acids leads to epithelial damage and colitis in animal models.[2] A few familial cases of CC and LC have been reported, but associations with immunologic markers such as human leukocyte antigens, other than those seen in overlapping celiac disease, are inconclusive.[1] Specific genetic markers or susceptibility factors are not known.

Drugs and MC

There are many reports of drug-induced MC. An analysis of medications in those with MC found 17 drugs associated with a high or intermediate probability of causing these diseases (Table 162.1). Acarbose, aspirin, lansoprazole, ranitidine, sertraline, and ticlopidine were all associated with a high likelihood of inducing MC. Carbamazepine, flutamide, lisinopril, paroxetine, and simvastatin were associated with an intermediate likelihood of inducing MC.[1] Of note is the apparent association between nonsteroidal anti-inflammatory drugs (NSAIDs) and CC. A recent case-control study demonstrated strong associations between NSAIDs and selective serotonin reuptake inhibitors (SSRIs) for CC.[8] A strong association was also seen between LC and SSRIs, particularly sertraline, but no significant association was seen between LC and NSAIDs. Whether there is synergy between different medications in causing the disease is not known, although it is likely, particularly between NSAIDS that increase intestinal permeability and other agents that might act to create intestinal inflammation.

● TREATMENT

Therapy for MC should begin with the discontinuation of drugs associated with the disease, such as NSAIDs, SSRIs, and those listed in Table 162.1, and the elimination of other agents that

TABLE 162.1 Drugs Associated with Microscopic Colitis

High Likelihood of Association	Intermediate Likelihood of Association
Acarbose	Carbamazepine
Aspirin	Flutamide
Lanosoprazole	Lisinopril
NSAIDs	Paroxetine
Sertraline	Oxetorone
Ranitidine	Simvastatin
Ticlopidine	Tardyferon
	Vinburninr

From Nyhlin et al.[1] and Fernández-Bañares et al.[8]
NSAIDs, nonsteroidal anti-inflammatory drug.

exacerbate diarrhea (i.e., alcohol, caffeine, and dairy products). Over-the-counter NSAIDs are easily missed in the clinical history. Celiac disease should be treated if discovered by serology or duodenal biopsy. The diagnosis and treatment of bile acid malabsorption will require a therapeutic trial of a bile salt binder, discussed below. Although diarrhea may resolve within weeks with or without anti-inflammatory treatment, this is rare (fewer than 10%). Nonspecific antidiarrheals such as loperamide hydrochloride are generally well tolerated and can be effective, which makes them good first-line agents. We treat with 2 to 4 mg by mouth with the first diarrheal episode, then 2 mg with each diarrheal stool up to a maximum of 16 mg a day. Other antidiarrheals (e.g., diphenoxylate and atropine) can also be used.

Most patients will be offered an initial course of steroid with a prolonged taper after diagnosis, with the goal of any treatment to control symptoms before tapering medication. Unlike CD and UC, where immunomodulators and biologics (anti-tumor necrosis factor antibodies and natalizumab) can alter the natural history of the disease, the studies in MC have been primarily retrospective, and clear guidelines for selection of disease-modifying drugs do not exist. Studies for MC suffer from a lack of a standard scoring system for disease activity, such as the CDAI for CD.

Steroids

Oral budesonide, a synthetic corticosteroid with extensive first-pass metabolism and low systemic side effects, is our drug of first choice. Budesonide had high clinical and histologic response rates and improved quality of life in at least three randomized placebo-controlled trials for CC.[9] The data for budesonide in LC are more limited, but similar results were described in a randomized, controlled trial involving 42 patients.[10] We recommend initiation of budesonide 9 mg per day and consider tapering after 6 to 8 weeks assuming good symptom control. The formulation of budesonide in Entocort EC releases the medication predominantly to the ileum and right colon.

Like steroids in CD and UC, steroids such as budesonide do not seem to alter the natural history of the disease. Budesonide is an effective agent for the induction of remission; however, 61% to 80% of patients relapse after discontinuation.[1] Newer studies designed to evaluate the efficacy of budesonide as maintenance therapy in CC found a similar relapse rate after extended treatment with the medication. Thus, most patients with MC responding to budesonide will require long-term maintenance therapy with this or another drug.

Although minimally absorbed, long-term treatment with budesonide does have a slightly increased risk of steroid-related side effects such as diabetes, hypertension, weight gain, and metabolic bone disease, particularly in those taking drugs that inhibit the cytochrome P450 CYP3A4 enzyme, such as viral protease inhibitors (e.g., ritonavir), macrolide antibiotics (e.g., erythromycin), and azole antifungals (e.g., fluconazole). Each patient will have to be approached individually.

Prednisone is useful for those with disease unresponsive to budesonide, although there are a few studies supporting its use in MC. Like budesonide, there is a high rate of relapse after discontinuation of prednisone, and it is associated with a greater risk of systemic side effects. Therefore, we use it in refractory cases and often as a bridge to other agents. Because budesonide 9 mg each day is approximately equivalent to 20 mg of prednisone, patients advanced to prednisone will typically be treated with 30 to 60 mg per day in a slow taper (e.g., 5–10 mg a week), with the highest doses reserved for those with particularly intractable symptoms.

Immunomodulators

For patients with MC who are refractory to or dependent on corticosteroids, immunomodulators such as 6-mercaptopurine, azathioprine, and methotrexate are a logical next step, even though there are no placebo-controlled trials supporting their use. We define steroid dependence as those patients who require prednisone or another systemic steroid for more than 3 months a year.

Several small studies support the use of immunomodulators in MC. In one study, eight of nine patients with steroid refractory MC achieved complete or partial remission with azathioprine at a median dose of 2 mg/kg/day.[1] This is close to the standard 2.5 mg/kg/day of azathioprine prescribed for CD or ulcerative colitis in normal metabolizers of the drug (~90% of the population). In our practice, we assess TPMT enzymatic activity before initiating therapy with azathioprine and avoid using these drugs in the approximately 1 in 300 patients with no enzymatic activity because they are at high risk for bone marrow suppression. The approximately 10% of the population who are heterozygotes for azathioprine can be treated with 1 to 1.5 mg/kg/day of azathioprine. Serial complete blood counts and liver enzymes need to be followed. Whether lower doses are adequate at the outset is not known; because there is laboratory evidence that regulatory T cells (which inhibit inflammatory responses) may be more sensitive to certain immunosuppressive drugs, including steroids, than other immune cells, we prefer to achieve an adequate clinical response first, then taper the medication as we are able. Use of thiopurines like azathioprine and 6-mercaptopurine is treated extensively elsewhere in this book, including the clinical use of metabolite testing.

For those unable to take azathioprine, methotrexate is an alternative. Methotrexate is useful in CD at doses from 15 to 25 mg per week and can be administered orally, intramuscularly, or subcutaneously. An optimal dose or route in MC is unknown. A retrospective analysis of 19 patients with CC treated with methotrexate suggested a "good" response in 14, with the median dose of methotrexate as 7.5 mg/week, although doses of up to 25 mg per week were required in certain patients.[11] There was a suggestion that the clinical response to dose changes was faster than that seen in CD (2–3 weeks vs. 8 weeks). Folate 1 mg by mouth each day should be prescribed to every patient on methotrexate. This drug is pregnancy category X and is therefore not given to women of childbearing age or men with female sexual partners of childbearing potential without effective birth control.

Other Agents

Sulfasalazine and mesalamine are frequently used in MC despite a lack of randomized controlled trials. Retrospective studies report benefit in less than half of the patients treated,[2]

limiting our enthusiasm for these drugs despite a favorable side effect profile. The use of these drugs is therefore a personal decision and is addressed elsewhere in this book. If considered, we recommend using a colon-targeted mesalamine preparation at high dose (e.g., Asacol or Lialda at 4800 mg/day), with dose adjustments after a clinical response is achieved.

An unblinded trial of patients with CC treated with cholestyramine in combination with mesalamine demonstrated increased clinical response compared with patients treated with mesalamine alone. The increased efficacy of combination therapy with cholestyramine and mesalamine was not seen in patients with LC.[6] Because bile-acid malabsorption is more common in patients with CC, the major effect of a bile salt binder is likely to prevent additional colonic secretion by bile salts. Cholestyramine can also bind bacterial toxins. Bile salt malabsorption should be considered in refractory disease or if the stool frequency seems disproportionate to the degree of inflammation. We recommend cholestyramine 4 g in a large glass of water, starting at once a day and increasing to 4 times a day to control symptoms. Other drugs must be staggered with the dosing of cholestyramine, and a daily multivitamin to replace fat-soluble vitamins is recommended. Testing fat-soluble vitamin levels, particularly in MC associated with celiac sprue or microscopic enteritis, is recommended.

In a single, small, randomized trial on patients with MC treated with bismuth subsalicylate, most patients treated with bismuth improved clinically, and the majority demonstrated histologic regression.[1] Bismuth is generally well tolerated by patients, but there are toxicity concerns with chronic administration. It should not be given to aspirin-allergic patients or those already on aspirin. A typical dose is three 262 mg tablets three times a day. The standard over-the-counter Pepto-Bismol tablet is 262 mg of bismuth subsalicylate.

Other treatments with potential benefit include octreotide, cyclosporine, and antibiotics.

Nontraditional Approaches

Probiotics have shown mixed results in MC. A small, open-label study using the *Escherichia coli* strain Nissle demonstrated some benefit in patients with CC.[1] However, a placebo-controlled trial using *Lactobacillus acidophilus* and *Bifidobacterium animalis* failed to show a significant difference between the treatment and placebo groups.[1,9] An extract from the *Boswellia serrata* tree has anti-inflammatory properties. In a pilot study, *B. serrata* extract given in 400 mg capsules three times daily for 6 weeks improved symptoms but not quality of life or colonic histology in patients with CC.[1] It is not clear that current commercial formulations of *Boswellia* extract are comparable to the one in that series.

Surgery for MC

In patients with medically refractory disease, surgery may be considered. Surgical options, including ileostomy, sigmoidostomy, and colectomy, have been reported in patients with MC. In one series, split ileostomy was successfully performed in eight patients with severe, refractory CC. Postoperatively, diarrhea ceased in all patients, and the collagen layer was regressed to a normal thickness. However, clinical symptoms returned and the abnormal collagen layer recurred after closure of the ostomy.[12]

In summary, randomized controlled clinical trials to evaluate different treatment options are lacking and standardized definitions for clinical and histologic remission currently do not exist for MC and microscopic enteritis. Furthermore, the relapsing and remitting nature of these disorders makes interpretation of the efficacy of the various treatment options difficult. That said, our recommended treatment algorithm is as follows (Fig. 162.1).

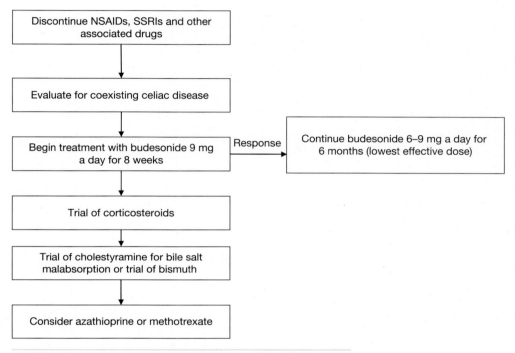

FIGURE 162.1 • Treatment algorithm for microscopic colitis.

References

1. Nyhlin N, Bohr J, Eriksson S, Tysk C. Systematic review: microscopic colitis. *Aliment Pharmacol Ther.* 2006;23(11):1525–1534.

2. Pardi DS, Smyrk TC, Tremaine WJ, Sandborn WJ. Microscopic colitis: a review. *Am J Gastroenterol.* 2002;97(4):794–802.

3. Pardi DS, Loftus EV Jr, Smyrk TC, et al. The epidemiology of microscopic colitis: a population based study in Olmsted County, Minnesota. *Gut.* 2007;56(4):504–508.

4. Goldstein NS. Non-gluten sensitivity-related small bowel villous flattening with increased intraepithelial lymphocytes: not all that flattens is celiac sprue. *Am J Clin Pathol.* 2004;121(4):546–550.

5. Allende DS, Taylor SL, Bronner MP. Colonic perforation as a complication of collagenous colitis in a series of 12 patients. *Am J Gastroenterol.* 2008;103(10):2598–2604.

6. Calabrese C, Fabbri A, Areni A, Zahlane D, Scialpi C, Di Febo G. Mesalazine with or without cholestyramine in the treatment of microscopic colitis: randomized controlled trial. *J Gastroenterol Hepatol.* 2007;22(6):809–814.

7. Münch A, Söderholm JD, Ost A, Ström M. Increased transmucosal uptake of E. coli K12 in collagenous colitis persists after budesonide treatment. *Am J Gastroenterol.* 2009;104(3):679–685.

8. Fernández-Bañares F, Esteve M, Espinós JC, et al. Drug consumption and the risk of microscopic colitis. *Am J Gastroenterol.* 2007;102(2):324–330.

9. Chande N, MacDonald JK, McDonald JWD. Interventions for treating microscopic colitis: a Cochrane inflammatory bowel disease and functional bowel disorders review group systematic review of randomized trial. *Cochrane Database Syst Rev.* 2008;16(2):CD003575.

10. Miehlke S, Madisch A, Karimi D, et al. Budesonide is effective in treating lymphocytic colitis: a randomized double-blind placebo-controlled study. *Gastroenterology.* 2009;136(7):2092–2100.

11. Riddell J, Hillman L, Chiragakis L, Clarke A. Collagenous colitis: oral low-dose methotrexate for patients with difficult symptoms: long-term outcomes. *J Gastroenterol Hepatol.* 2007;22(10):1589–1593.

12. Järnerot G, Tysk C, Bohr J, Eriksson S. Collagenous colitis and fecal stream diversion. *Gastroenterology.* 1995;109(2):449–455.

Chronic Immunodeficiency Syndromes Affecting the Gastrointestinal Tract

163

Lloyd Mayer and Jimmy Ko

The practicing gastroenterologist is frequently confronted with immune-related diseases such as Crohn's disease (CD), ulcerative colitis, celiac sprue, and pernicious anemia (PA). However, the role of the gastrointestinal (GI) tract as the body's largest lymphoid organ is often overlooked. In fact, the surface area of the GI tract could cover one tennis court, and within that surface is a rich supply of B and T lymphocytes, macrophages, and dendritic cells. The number of lymphocytes in the GI tract exceeds that in the spleen, but unlike other lymphoid organs, immune-associated cells in the GI tract are constantly confronted with antigen (mainly in the form of bacteria and food). Gut-associated lymphoid tissue, one component of the mucosa-associated lymphoid tissue, regulates immune responses in the intestine to maintain homeostasis. Without this tight regulation, inflammation would predominate in the GI tract. Therefore, it is not difficult to imagine how disease can result in the GI tract when immune regulation is disrupted.

The immune system in the GI tract, similar to that in the rest of the body, can be subdivided into two categories: cellular and humoral. T lymphocytes generally regulate cellular immune functions such as defense against viruses, intracellular bacteria, and proteins, whereas B lymphocytes produce immunoglobulins (Igs) to fight bacteria. Primary immunodeficiencies are the result of inherited defects in either or both the cellular or humoral branches of the immune system. In the GI tract, the major Igs are the secretory forms of IgA and IgM. These antibodies bind luminal antigens and form immune complexes, thus restricting bacterial and viral attachment to epithelium and decrease antigen burden on the mucosal immune cells. Antibody deficiency can lead to increased antigen uptake in the GI tract, as has been demonstrated with serum levels of dietary antigens after feeding.[1] However, it is interesting to note that, in the one disease exclusively restricted to B cells, X-linked agammaglobulinemia (XLA), there has been no significant predisposition to GI infection or disease.

CLASSIFICATION AND CLINICAL PRESENTATION OF PRIMARY IMMUNODEFICIENCIES

Predominantly Antibody Deficiencies

X-Linked Agammaglobulinemia

Also known as Bruton's disease, XLA is the prototypical antibody deficiency disease (Table 163.1). It is rare, occurring in 1 of 10^5 live births. The inherited defect has been localized to a gene on the long arm of the X chromosome encoding Bruton's tyrosine kinase (Btk). Defects in Btk lead to maturation arrest of pre-B cells, resulting in failure to generate mature B cells and a complete lack of all classes of Igs. XLA typically presents in young males as recurrent bacterial infections, especially with encapsulated bacteria such as *Streptococcus pneumoniae* and *Haemophilus influenzae*. Standard treatment is with IV Ig (IVIG) replacement.[2]

TABLE 163.1 Classification of Primary Immunodeficiencies

Predominantly antibody deficiencies
X-linked agammaglobulinemia
IgA deficiency
Combined or primary T-cell deficiencies
Common variable immunodeficiency
Severe combined immunodeficiency
Ataxia telangiectasia
DiGeorge syndrome
Wiskott-Aldrich syndrome

IgA Deficiency

IgA deficiency is the most common primary immunodeficiency and is found in an estimated 1 in 200 to 700 whites and less frequently in other ethnic groups. The overwhelming majority of people with IgA deficiency are healthy and do not exhibit any illness. Serum levels of IgA are less than 5 mg/dL with normal or increased levels of other Igs and normal B-cell numbers. If illness occurs, the most frequent disorders associated with IgA deficiency are recurrent sinopulmonary infections. Infections are typically caused by common bacterial or viral pathogens, and it is the frequency and repetition of these infections that often lead to assessing quantitative Ig levels and a workup. Autoimmune diseases, such as rheumatoid arthritis and lupus, and allergy have also been reported to be associated with IgA deficiency, and these subjects also commonly have autoantibodies.[3] IgA-deficient patients with concomitant IgG2 subclass deficiency tend to have more severe disease, and it is this subset of patients that has an increased frequency of GI manifestations, including celiac disease, inflammatory bowel disease (IBD), and giardiasis. There is a higher prevalence of IgA deficiency in patients with a family history of common variable immunodeficiency (CVID), suggesting a genetic link between the two diseases. Treatment with IVIGs is necessary only in patients with recurrent sinopulmonary infections and concurrent IgG2 deficiency. One caveat: some IgA-deficient patients have anti-IgA antibodies, which may increase the risk for anaphylactic reactions to blood products.[4]

Combined (B- and T-Cell) or Primary T-Cell Deficiencies

Common Variable Immunodeficiency

CVID is a diverse set of disorders but is characterized by low levels of at least two Ig classes and recurrent infections, most commonly of the upper and lower respiratory tract. With a prevalence of 1 in 50,000 (in Scandinavia), CVID is the primary immunodeficiency most often brought to clinical attention, frequently presenting in early adulthood.[5] Infection with encapsulated bacteria, such as *S. pneumoniae* and *H. influenzae*, reflects the defect in B-cell function. In addition to other T-cell–associated infections, fungal infections such as *Pneumocystis carinii* can be seen. Autoimmune diseases are relatively common (found in 22% of 248 patients in one series),[6] and an increased incidence of lymphoma and gastric carcinoma has also been reported.[7] Although GI manifestations are more common in CVID than IgA deficiency, the spectrum of disease is similar. Although Ig levels are low, B-cell numbers are generally near normal. However, defects in B-cell growth and differentiation, whether primary or secondary, are often found. Recurrent infections without treatment can lead to irreversible chronic lung disease with bronchiectasis and cor pulmonale. The probability of survival 20 years after diagnosis of CVID is 66% (compared with 93% for age-matched controls), which is likely a reflection of advanced progression of disease at the time of diagnosis. Although it has little effect on the GI disorders seen in CVID, the standard treatment of IVIG can help prevent recurrent sinopulmonary infections.[8]

Severe Combined Immunodeficiency

Severe combined immunodeficiency (SCID) is a group of congenital immune disorders in which both T-cell and B-cell development and function are disrupted. Several gene defects resulting in SCID have been identified, including mutations in the interleukin (IL)-2 receptor gamma chain, Janus kinase 3, adenosine deaminase, and recombinase-activating genes (RAG-1 and RAG-2). Because patients with SCID have few or no circulating B and T cells, they are susceptible to bacterial and opportunistic infections. Patients with SCID present in the first year of life with severe, recurrent bacterial and/or viral infections. Standard treatment is bone marrow transplant or enzyme replacement (in the case of adenosine deaminase deficiency).[9]

Ataxia Telangiectasia

Ataxia telangiectasia (AT) is an autosomal recessive disorder usually presenting between ages 2 and 5 with ataxia and telangiectasias of the nose, conjunctiva, ears, or shoulders. These patients have T-cell defects secondary to thymic hypoplasia, and IgA deficiency occurs in 50% of patients. A defect in the ATM gene, a protein kinase involved in cell-cycle control and DNA repair, is the culprit in this disorder and leads to the increased risk of malignancy.[9]

DiGeorge Syndrome

DiGeorge syndrome is the result of a congenital defect in migration of the third and fourth branchial arches, leading to thymic hypoplasia and other developmental abnormalities.[10] The severity of the T-cell defect corresponds to degree of thymic aplasia, and those with severe T-cell defects are susceptible to opportunistic infections, most commonly mucocutaneous candidiasis. *Wiskott-Aldrich syndrome* (WAS) is an X-linked recessive disorder resulting from a defect in the WAS protein, which is involved in intracellular signaling and actin polymerization. Patients usually present with eczema, thrombocytopenia, impaired T-cell function, and recurrent infections.[9]

● GI MANIFESTATIONS

GI disorders are common in primary immunodeficiencies, and at times, GI signs and symptoms, such as diarrhea or malabsorption, are the only manifestations of disease. Immune dysfunction in the GI tract can lead to infection, inflammatory disease, and malignancy; and these diseases are most prevalent in immunodeficiency states with combined B- and T-cell defects. Befitting its status as the most complex of primary immunodeficiencies, CVID has the broadest array of GI manifestations—the severity of which often leads to significant morbidity and mortality.

Common Variable Immunodeficiency

Both prospective and retrospective studies have shown a high rate of GI symptoms in patients with CVID (Table 163.2). A total of 40% to 60% of patients experience chronic diarrhea, which may be accompanied by steatorrhea or other signs of malabsorption.[6] Interestingly, infections with bacterial pathogens such as *Salmonella, Campylobacter,* and *Clostridium difficile* (from antibiotic use) are rare. Infections with the parasite

TABLE 163.2 Gastrointestinal Complications of Common Variable Immunodeficiency

Infectious

  Giardia lamblia

  Cryptosporidium

  Clostridium difficile

Inflammatory

  Sprue-like disorder

  Inflammatory bowel disease

  Pernicious anemia

  Atrophic gastritis

  Aphthous stomatitis

  Malakoplakia of the colon

  Ménétrier's disease

Malignancy and other (benign) lymphoproliferative

  Gastric adenocarcinoma

  Intestinal lymphoma

  Nodular lymphoid hyperplasia

Adapted from Sperber and Mayer.[12]

Giardia lamblia are more common. Inflammatory and malignant disorders of the GI tract also occur with increased incidence in patients with CVID.[6]

Giardia infection, although decreasing in frequency in recent years, is still an important infectious cause of diarrhea and malabsorption in patients with CVID. *Giardia* is transmitted as a cyst; typically, it is consumed with water or spread by person-to-person contact. Symptoms typical of giardiasis include watery diarrhea, abdominal cramping, and bloating. Stool examination demonstrating cysts or trophozoites is indicative of infection. However, duodenal biopsy is sometimes necessary for diagnosis. In patients with CVID, chronic or recurrent infection with *Giardia*, likely related to T-cell defects, is a real concern. Therefore, prolonged treatment with metronidazole is often required to eradicate infection and symptoms related to infection. Empirical treatment with metronidazole is often begun after the onset of diarrhea as a therapeutic trial, given the frequent difficulty in confirming the diagnosis of *Giardia* in patients with CVID. Other GI infections in CVID include *Cryptosporidium*, which was first described in a patient with CVID, and, less commonly, bacterial pathogens, such as *Salmonella* and *Campylobacter*; some authors have reported an increased in prevalence of bacterial pathogens in CVID.[12] In addition, infection with *C. difficile* should be considered in patients in whom antibiotics are used to fight recurrent infections, although high titers of antitoxin antibodies exist in IVIG preparations[16] so that this infection may be more easily controlled.

Inflammatory complications in the GI tract occur with increased frequency in patients with CVID. One of the most common is a celiac-like condition in which villous flattening in duodenal biopsy is found. Although the villous lesion appears similar to celiac disease, several important differences are found. Plasma cells are absent in patients with CVID, whereas patients with celiac disease have an abundance of plasma cells. Furthermore, antigliadin and antiendomysial antibodies are not found in patients with CVID. Finally, a gluten-free diet seems to have no effect on most patients with CVID with sprue-like villous atrophy.[13] Treatment for this condition includes steroids and immunomodulators such as azathioprine or 6-mercaptopurine (6-MP). Infectious complications are rare for patients given immunomodulators concomitantly with IVIG. Prolonged use of steroids in patients with CVID has led to reports of increased infectious complications. In one series from Mount Sinai, 4 of 248 patients receiving steroids had major complications, including *Pneumocystis* pneumonia and *Nocardia* brain abscess. The authors of that series suggest that prolonged immunosuppression be used with caution.[6]

IBD is also found with increased prevalence in patients with CVID. At Mount Sinai, 16 of 248 patients with CVID (6%) had an IBD-like illness.[6] It seems that patients with CVID and IBD have more severe T-cell defects than patients with CVID alone. Recently, Mannon et al.[17] studied the cytokine production patterns in the tissues of patients with CVID and IBD. They found that there was a marked increase in IL-12 and interferon gamma but not IL-17 (in contrast to conventional patients with CD). Both CD and ulcerative colitis typically respond to conventional treatment in patients with CVID. Treatment with 5-aminosalicyclic acid, azathioprine, or 6-MP can lead to long remissions. Oral steroids should be used with considerable care. Infliximab has been used in some cases, but this has been associated with infectious complications.

The last important inflammatory GI complication of CVID is PA. The diagnosis of PA is made at an earlier age in patients with CVID (20–40 years vs. 60 years in immunocompetent patients).[12] Plasma cells, anti-intrinsic factor antibodies, and antiparietal antibodies are absent in patients with CVID with PA, suggesting a T-cell–mediated mechanism. Treatment of PA in patients with CVID is the same as in immunocompetent patients: replacement of B12 systemically.

Other conditions associated with CVID include aphthous stomatitis, which frequently responds to sucralfate suspension treatment, and Ménétrier's disease. In addition, malakoplakia, a rare inflammatory disease characterized by granuloma formation (mostly in the bladder) and stricture formation in the bowel, can be found in CVID.

Malignancy is the leading cause of death in CVID, and two forms of cancer, gastric adenocarcinoma and non-Hodgkin's lymphoma (NHL), are found with increased frequency.[6] Gastric cancer is increased by 30-fold, whereas NHL is increased by 47-fold in patients with CVID compared with the general population.[7] Recent studies have suggested a role for *Helicobacter pylori* in gastric carcinogenesis in patients with CVID.[14] It is plausible that impaired B- or T-cell function can lead to compromised defense against *H. pylori*. Therefore, screening for *H. pylori* in symptomatic patients and monitoring of treatment in infected individuals are advised. Atrophic gastritis with or without PA has been noted in patients with CVID, and this association is also believed to play a role in the increased risk for gastric adenocarcinoma.

Benign lymphoproliferative disorders also occur with increased frequency in CVID with the main GI manifestation being nodular lymphoid hyperplasia (NLH). NLH is defined as multiple discrete nodules made up of lymphoid aggregates confined to the lamina propria and superficial submucosa. These nodules occur mostly in the small intestine and represent hyperplastic lymphoid tissue with prominent germinal centers. This hyperplastic response is believed to be a compensatory B-cell proliferative response to increase the pool of antibody-producing cell precursors. NLH occurs diffusely in the gut in 10% to 20% of patients with CVID. NLH was once believed to be secondary to *Giardia* infection, but antibiotic therapy does not result in resolution of nodules. Several reports suggest that NLH could be a premalignant condition leading to small intestine lymphomas.[13]

IgA Deficiency

The spectrum of GI disease in IgA deficiency is similar to that in CVID but is, in general, less severe. As in CVID, giardiasis, NLH, IBD, and celiac disease occur with increased frequency. These diseases occur almost exclusively in IgA-deficient patients with concomitant IgG2 subclass deficiency, which some authors, including this one, consider a disease distinct from selective IgA deficiency and more akin to CVID. Celiac disease in IgA-deficient individuals shares some features with the sprue-like illness in CVID: antibodies to gliadin and endomysium are not found, and IgA-secreting plasma cells are absent on small bowel biopsy. Otherwise, the clinical response in IgA-deficient patients with celiac disease differs in that many IgA-deficient patients with celiac disease will respond to a gluten-free diet. Giardiasis and NLH occur at a lower rate in IgA-deficient patients than in patients with CVID. Management of giardiasis and IBD in IgA deficiency is subject to the same caveats noted for patients with CVID. A recent study in Sweden and Denmark showed no increased risk for cancer in IgA-deficient patients, but it noted a nonstatistically significant increase (fivefold; 95% confidence interval, 0.7–19.5) in gastric cancer (2 of 386 cases).[15]

● GI MANIFESTATIONS IN OTHER PRIMARY IMMUNODEFICIENCY DISEASES

Other immunodeficiencies have been associated with GI disorders. Patients with XLA have intestinal biopsies that have a notable absence of lamina propria plasma cells. Giardiasis has been reported as a cause of chronic diarrhea, but GI complaints are rare in patients with XLA. Patients with SCID often have intractable diarrhea resistant to medical treatment, leading to failure to thrive. Children with SCID also present with oral candidiasis and viral infections, including rotavirus and adenovirus. Intestinal biopsy in patients with SCID shows villous atrophy and is devoid of lymphocytes. After bone marrow transplant, patients with SCID may develop graft-versus-host disease in the gut, leading to diarrhea and wasting.[8]

Patients with AT have an increased frequency of malignancy as noted above, although an increased risk for GI malignancy has not been reported in the literature. GI manifestations, including giardiasis, occur in the subset of patients with AT with IgA deficiency. In addition to oral candidiasis, GI manifestations are not frequently seen in DiGeorge syndrome. Chronic intestinal viral infections have been reported to cause diarrhea and necrotizing enterocolitis. The most prominent GI manifestation in WAS is intestinal hemorrhage caused by thrombocytopenia, although approximately 10% of these patients develop a mild colitis. Of note, the mouse model of WAS does develop significant colitis.

● CONCLUSION

Patients with primary immunodeficiencies often have GI manifestations. Therefore, in patients with recurrent giardiasis, celiac disease, NLH, and IBD, screening for CVID or IgA deficiency (plus IgG2 subclass deficiency) with serum Ig levels should be considered. Although treatment of inflammatory conditions with immunomodulators such as azathioprine and 6-MP does not lead to increased complications when given concurrently with intravenous Ig replacement therapy, use of chronic oral steroids in immunocompromised patients should be undertaken with extreme care. Given the increased risk of GI malignancy in CVID, periodic GI screening is warranted.

References

1. Cunningham-Rundles C, Brandeis WE, Good RA, Day NK. Milk precipitins, circulating immune complexes and IgA deficiency. *J Clin Invest.* 1979;64:270–272.

2. Ammann AJ, Ashman RF, Buckley RH, et al. Use of intravenous gamma-globulin in antibody immunodeficiency: results of a multicenter controlled trial. *Clin Immunol Immunopathol.* 1982;22(1):60–67.

3. Cunningham-Rundles C. Physiology of IgA and IgA deficiency. *J Clin Immunol.* 2001;21(5):303–309.

4. Burks AW, Sampson HA, Buckley RH. Anaphylactic reactions after gamma globulin administration in patients with hypogammaglobulinemia. Detection of IgE antibodies to IgA. *N Engl J Med.* 1986;314(9):560–564.

5. Spickett GP. Current perspectives on common variable immunodeficiency (CVID). *Clin Exp Allergy.* 2001;31(4):536–542.

6. Cunningham-Rundles C, Bodian C. Common variable immunodeficiency: clinical and immunological features of 248 patients. *Clin Immunol.* 1999;92(1):34–48.

7. Kinlen LJ, Webster AD, Bird AG, et al. Prospective study of cancer in patients with hypogammaglobulinaemia. *Lancet.* 1985;1(8423):263–266.

8. Cunningham-Rundles C, Siegal FP, Smithwick EM, et al. Efficacy of intravenous immunoglobulin in primary humoral immunodeficiency disease. *Ann Intern Med.* 1984;101(4):435–439.

9. Primary immunodeficiency diseases. Report of an IUIS scientific committee. *Clin Exp Immunol.* 1999;118(suppl):1–28.

10. DiGeorge AM. Congenital absence of the thymus and its immunologic consequences: concurrence with congenital hypoparathyroidism. *Birth Defects.* 1968;4:1116–1121.

11. Lai Ping So A, Mayer L. Gastrointestinal manifestations of primary immunodeficiency disorders. *Semin Gastrointest Dis.* 1997;8(1):22–32.

12. Sperber KE, Mayer L. Gastrointestinal manifestations of common variable immunodeficiency. *Immunol Allergy Clin North Am.* 1988;8:423–434.

13. Washington K, Stenzel TT, Buckley RH, Gottfried MR. Gastrointestinal pathology in patients with common variable immunodeficiency and X-linked agammaglobulinemia. *Am J Surg Pathol.* 1996;20(10):1240–1252.

14. Zullo A, Romiti A, Rinaldi V, et al. Gastric pathology in patients with common variable immunodeficiency. *Gut.* 1999;45(1):77–81.

15. Mellemkjaer L, Hammarstrom L, Andersen V, et al. Cancer risk among patients with IgA deficiency or common variable immunodeficiency and their relatives: a combined Danish and Swedish study. *Clin Exp Immunol.* 2002;130(3):495–500.

16. Leung DY, Kelly CP, Boguniewicz M, Pothoulakis C, LaMont JT, Flores A. Treatment with intravenously administered gamma globulin of chronic relapsing colitis induced by Clostridium difficile toxin. *J Pediatr.* 1991;118(4 Pt 1):633–637.

17. Mannon PJ, Fuss IJ, Dill S, et al. Excess IL-12 but not IL-23 accompanies the inflammatory bowel disease associated with common variable immunodeficiency. *Gastroenterology.* 2006;131(3):748–756.

Ulcerative Jejunoileitis | 164

Vivian Asamoah and Theodore M. Bayless

DEFINITION

Ulcerative jejunoileitis (UJI) is a description of multifocal ulcerating lesions in the jejunum and ileum, first described by Rosendahl[1] in 1927. Similar or identical cases have been published under the diagnosis of chronic nongranulomatous UJI or enterocolitis, unclassified sprue, and refractory sprue. The presentation is rare, and the true prevalence remains unknown. The majority of cases of UJI have been reported in patients with a refractory form of celiac disease, a gluten-sensitive enteropathy affecting genetically predisposed subjects characterized by villous atrophy and resulting in malabsorption. A few earlier cases have been described in patients with villous atrophy without a definitive diagnosis of celiac disease and a broad differential diagnosis must be considered in those situations. The discovery of highly sensitive and specific celiac serologic markers and improved histopathologic characterization has been strategic in facilitating the diagnosis of celiac disease and refractory cases.

Refractory Celiac Disease

Refractory celiac disease (RCD) has been defined as persistent or recurrent malabsorptive symptoms, and/or villous atrophy despite strict adherence to a gluten-free diet for at least 6 to 12 months in the absence of other causes of nonresponsive-treated celiac disease and overt malignancy.[2,3] The prevalence is rare, with an incidence of 0.6 per 100,000 person-years.[4] Complications of RCD include UJI, collagenous sprue, mesenteric lymph node cavitation syndrome, and enteropathy-associated T-cell lymphoma (EATL). RCD can be divided into two types: type 1 RCD shows normal intraepithelial lymphocyte (IEL) population, whereas type 2 RCD displays a predominantly aberrant IEL phenotype. UJI is believed to be a rare but severe manifestation of RCD type 2 and is strongly associated with the development of EATL, a fatal complication of RCD. UJI can be seen in patients with celiac disease in clinical remission on a strict gluten diet for years, or more commonly in patients who have been unresponsive to a gluten-free diet. In some cases, it can present simultaneously with a new diagnosis of celiac disease. It can also be the initial presentation of EATL in a patient with no history of celiac disease. The human leukocyte antigen (HLA; DQ2 and DQ8) in patients with UJI and EATL is identical to that found in celiac disease and supports the association of these two disorders.[5]

Pathogenesis

The exact role of gluten in the pathogenesis of UJI is unclear. It has been hypothesized that gluten-related mucosal damages and multifocal ulcers are a result of the cytotoxic capability of T cells in the setting of chronic inflammation. This chronic inflammatory state is what leads to phenotypically aberrant IELs, T-cell clonality in the ulcers and the development of EATL. Interleukin (IL)-15 is a cytokine thought to play a pivotal role in the regulation of IEL that characterize celiac disease and refractory celiac disease.[6]

CLINICAL MANIFESTATION

Majority of patients are in their fifth to seventh decade. Patients with UJI typically present with fatigue, low grade fevers, abdominal pain, nausea and vomiting, malabsorptive diarrhea, and weight loss. Complications include perforation, obstruction, intussception, and hemorrhage. Death from these complications is fairly common.[7]

DIAGNOSTIC EVALUATION

Careful history is important in assessing for viral or bacterial exposure, culprit medications, and prior history of malabsorptive disease (Table 164.1). In the case of a previously established diagnosis of celiac disease, it is important to determine strict adherence to gluten. Up to 50% of cases of nonresponsive celiac disease are secondary to poor adherence to the gluten-free diet.[8] Laboratory analyses should include cell blood count, comprehensive metabolic panel, and inflammatory markers (erythrocyte sedimentation rate, and C-reactive protein). Low hemoglobin, and hypoalbuminemia can be noted and may indicate poor prognosis in patients with refractory celiac disease.[9] Stool and blood cultures should also be preformed

TABLE 164.1 Causes of Small Bowel Ulcerations

Bacterial or viral enteritis
Parasitic infections
NSAID enteritis
Other drug-related enteritis
Ischemic enteritis
Polyarteritis
AIDS enteropathy
Adult onset autoimmune enteropathy
Hypogammaglobulinemia
Enteropathy-associated T-cell lymphoma

NSAID, nonsteroidal anti-inflammatory drug.

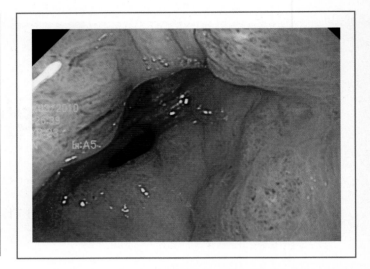

FIGURE 164.2 • Antral and duodenal ulcerations and edema.

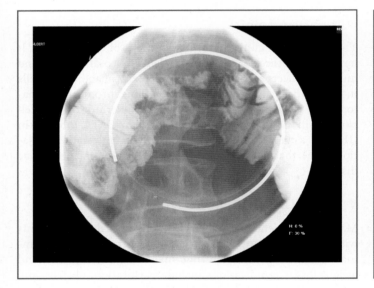

FIGURE 164.1 • Ulcerative jejunoileitis showing multiple short segments of abnormal "featureless" mucosa in the distal jejunum and ileum characterized by flattening of the circular folds and multiple small ulcerations.

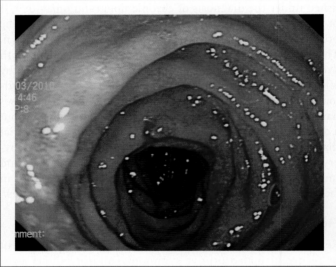

FIGURE 164.3 • Multifocal ulcers noted in proximal jejunum.

to rule out infection. Celiac serologies, transglutaminase Ab, and antiendomysial Ab, are useful. Most patients with RCD are likely to have negative serologic markers. However, positive serologies can be seen in 19% to 30% patients despite good compliance to gluten-free diet. It has been hypothesized that transglutaminase may be upregulated in the setting of severe inflammation with destructive lesion or in the presence of Ag-independent T-cell clones. HLA genotype may be helpful in excluding the diagnosis of celiac disease in patients with UJI as 98% of patients with CD are HLA DQ2 or DQ8 positive.[10] Imaging studies should include a small bowel follow-through that may reveal flocculation of barium, featureless mucosa,

stricture, and ulcerations or obstruction (Fig. 164.1). Upper gastrointestinal endoscopy with single- or double-balloon enteroscopy typically reveals multifocal small ulcerations or large ulcers greater than 1 cm involving the proximal jejunum, the most common site, and the ileum (Figs. 164.2 and 164.3). In patients with UJI, simultaneous gastritis and colitis has also been reported. Ulcerated nodular mucosa, occluding mass, or stricture, suggests malignant complications.[11] Computed tomography of the abdomen and pelvis and capsule endoscopy may provide information on the extent of the disease.[12] 18 F-fluorodeoxyglucose positron may be more sensitive for detection of EATL in patients with UJI.[13] In most cases, endoscopic or laparoscopic full thickness biopsy with flow cytometry will be critical in assessing for EATL.

Histopathology

The histopathologic features of the ulcers can be relatively non-specific. The ulcers vary in depth, penetrating into the muscularis propria in most cases with secondary vascular changes at the base of the ulcer. Acute inflammation of the lamina propria with submucosal edema can be observed. The nonulcerated mucosa can show other CD-like changes such as crypt hyperplasia, IEL infiltration, surface enterocyte irregularity, and lamina propria infiltrate with plasma cells, eosinophils, and neutrophils. Chronic inflammation, fibrosis, and muscular hypertrophy are also noted and can result in stricture formation. Varying degrees of villous atrophy can be observed both adjacent to, and remote from, areas of ulceration.[14] There is histological overlap with RCD, with distinctive features of RCD such as epithelial collagen deposition, and gastric metaplasia identified in patients with UJI. CD3/CD4 immunohistochemistry stains and T-cell receptor clonal rearrangement by polymerase chain reaction (PCR) are important for identification of abnormal cell types. Patients with UJI typically present with RCD type 2 histological features and have a significantly higher risk of developing EATL. In RCD type 2, abnormal populations of IELs are seen, characterized by (a) the loss of surface expression of CD3, CD4, and CD8 with preserved expression of intracytoplasmic CD3 (CD3ε) in more than 50% of IEL as evaluated by immunohistochemistry or more than 20% to 25% as determined by flow cytometry and (b) detection of clonal rearrangement of T-cell receptor chains (TCRγδ) by PCR.[15–17] Aberrant IELs may also be found in gastric and colonic mucosa and the blood of RCD type 2 patients, suggesting a diffuse gastrointestinal disease.[18] In RCD 1, the intraepithelial cells are phenotypically normal with a polyclonal population as in uncomplicated celiac disease. RCD 2, UJ, and EATL share immunohistochemical and molecular traits and are closely related. In the absence of proven etiology for small bowel ulcerations other than RCD, UJI should be considered a preneoplastic complication of CD. There is immunopathological and molecular evidence that most, if not all, cases represent early T-cell lymphoma complication of CD although a tumoriform infiltration is not often found.

● TREATMENT

Management of the UJI depends partly on the underlying cause. Presently, there is no curative therapy for UJI related to RCD type 2. Complications such as perforation and obstruction typically require urgent surgical intervention. Medical management includes a strict gluten-free diet, although the benefit in RCD is unknown, and supportive care with adequate hydration and supplemental nutrition. The use of steroids, prednisone 40 to 60 mg, or budesonide 9 mg daily is beneficial in patients with RCD type 1. However, minimal clinical or histological improvement has been observed in the UJI/RCD type 2 population.[19] Cases of steroid-precipitated perforation have also been reported and should be considered in a patient with an acute abdomen in setting of steroid initiation. Immunomodulatory drugs such as azathioprine or anti-tumor necrosis factor in combination

with steroids have been used and resulted in poor histological results with no impact on aberrant clonal IEL population.[20,21] Nucleoside analogues such as cladribine have been used with some success. Symptom improvement, mucosal recovery, and decrease of aberrant IEL have been reported in a few patients treated with cladribine.[22] Case reports of autologous hematopoietic stem cell transplantation in cases of RCD 2 have been described; however, it did not result in associated reduction in the population of abnormal T cells. Targeted therapy using IL-15 is promising and currently an area of active research.

● OUTCOME

The outcome of UJI is poor, notably because the complications are life threatening and the risk of progression to EATL is high. Poor prognostic factors of RCD include age greater than 65, albumin ≤ 3.2g/dL, and low hemoglobin ≤ 11 g/dL and total villous atrophy and UJI. The 5-year survival in patients with RCD type (typically UJI) has been reported at 40% to 58% compared with 95% in patients with RCD 1. This is largely explained by the higher incidence of EATL in patients with UJI. Fifty-two percent of patients with RCD type 2 will develop EATL within 4 to 6 years.[23,24]

● CONCLUSION

Significant progress has been made in our understanding of UJI and its association with refractory celiac disease. Nevertheless, the diagnosis remains challenging given its overlap with other causes of villous atrophy and the malabsorption syndromes. The complications are severe typically requiring surgical intervention and often resulting in death. Identification of phenotypically aberrant IEL and T-cell clonality has been key in identifying patients with premalignant and malignant lesions. The mortality for patients with UJI and EATL remains high in the absence of effective therapy. More research is needed for targeted treatment with a goal to reverse or suppress IEL aberrancy and clonality and to restore intestinal mucosa and gut absorption.

Editor's note (TMB): Review by Baer et al. helped put UTI and lymphoma in perspective (*Gastroenterolgy.* 1980; 79:754–765).

References

1. Rosendahl quoted by Bayless TM, Kapelowitz RF, Shelley WM, Ballinger WF, Hendrix TR. Intestinal ulceration—a complication of celiac disease. *N Engl J Med.* 1967;276:996–1002.

2. Biagi F, Corazza GR. Defining gluten refractory enteropathy. *Eur J Gastroenterol Hepatol.* 2001;13(5):561–565.

3. Leffler DA, Dennis M, Hyett B, Kelly E, Schuppan D, Kelly CP. Etiologies and predictors of diagnosis in nonresponsive celiac disease. *Clin Gastroenterol Hepatol.* 2007;5(4):445–450.

4. Di Sabatino A, Corazza GR. Coeliac disease. *Lancet.* 2009;373(9673):1480–1493.

5. Howell WM, Leung ST, Jones DB, et al. HLA-DRB, -DQA, and -DQB polymorphism in celiac disease and enteropathy-associated T-cell lymphoma. Common features and additional risk factors for malignancy. *Hum Immunol.* 1995;43(1):29–37.

6. Di Sabatino A, Ciccocioppo R, Cupelli F, et al. Epithelium derived interleukin 15 regulates intraepithelial lymphocyte Th1 cytokine production, cytotoxicity, and survival in coeliac disease. *Gut.* 2006;55(4):469–477.

7. Jewell DP. Ulcerative enteritis. *Br Med J (Clin Res Ed).* 1983;287(6407):1740–1741.

8. Abdulkarim AS, Burgart LJ, See J, Murray JA. Etiology of non-responsive celiac disease: results of a systematic approach. *Am J Gastroenterol.* 2002;97(8):2016–2021.

9. Rubio-Tapia A, Kelly DG, Lahr BD, Dogan A, Wu TT, Murray JA. Clinical staging and survival in refractory celiac disease: a single center experience. *Gastroenterology.* 2009;136(1):99–107; quiz 352.

10. Wolters VM, Wijmenga C. Genetic background of celiac disease and its clinical implications. *Am J Gastroenterol.* 2008;103(1):190–195.

11. Meijer JW, Mulder CJ, Goerres MG, Boot H, Schweizer JJ. Coeliac disease and (extra)intestinal T-cell lymphomas: definition, diagnosis and treatment. *Scand J Gastroenterol Suppl.* 2004;(241):78–84.

12. Daum S, Wahnschaffe U, Glasenapp R, et al. Capsule endoscopy in refractory celiac disease. *Endoscopy.* 2007;39(5):455–458.

13. Hadithi M, Mallant M, Oudejans J, van Waesberghe JH, Mulder CJ, Comans EF. 18F-FDG PET versus CT for the detection of enteropathy-associated T-cell lymphoma in refractory celiac disease. *J Nucl Med.* 2006;47(10):1622–1627.

14. Mills PR, Brown IL, Watkinson G. Idiopathic chronic ulcerative enteritis. Report of five cases and review of the literature. *Q J Med.* 1980;49(194):133–149.

15. Robert ME, Ament ME, Weinstein WM. The histologic spectrum and clinical outcome of refractory and unclassified sprue. *Am J Surg Pathol.* 2000;24(5):676–687.

16. Patey-Mariaud De Serre N, Cellier C, Jabri B, et al. Distinction between celiac disease and refractory sprue: a simple immunohistological method. *Histopathology.* 2000;37:70–77.

17. Verbeek WH, Goerres MS, von Blomberg BM, et al. Flow cytometric determination of aberrant intra-epithelial lymphocytes predicts T-cell lymphoma development more accurately than T-cell clonality analysis in Refractory Celiac Disease. *Clin Immunol.* 2008;126(1):48–56.

18. Verkarre V, Asnafi V, Lecomte T, et al. Refractory coeliac sprue is a diffuse gastrointestinal disease. *Gut.* 2003;52(2):205–211.

19. Al-Toma A, Verbeek WH, Mulder CJ. Update on the management of refractory coeliac disease. *J Gastrointestin Liver Dis.* 2007;16(1):57–63.

20. Goerres MS, Meijer JW, Wahab PJ, et al. Azathioprine and prednisone combination therapy in refractory coeliac disease. *Aliment Pharmacol Ther.* 2003;18(5):487–494.

21. Chaudhary R, Ghosh S. Infliximab in refractory coeliac disease. *Eur J Gastroenterol Hepatol.* 2005;17(6):603–604.

22. Al-Toma A, Goerres MS, Meijer JW, et al. Cladribine therapy in refractory celiac disease with aberrant T cells. *Clin Gastroenterol Hepatol.* 2006;4(11):1322–1327; quiz 1300.

23. Al-Toma A, Verbeek WH, Hadithi M, von Blomberg BM, Mulder CJ. Survival in refractory coeliac disease and enteropathy-associated T-cell lymphoma: retrospective evaluation of single-centre experience. *Gut.* 2007;56(10):1373–1378.

24. Malamut G, Afchain P, Verkarre V, et al. Presentation and long-term follow-up of refractory celiac disease: comparison of type I with type II. *Gastroenterology.* 2009;136(1):81–90.

Gastrointestinal Complications in Stem Cell Transplantation

165

Linda A. Lee and Georgia Vogelsang

Stem cell transplantation (SCT) is the standard of care for the treatment of many hematologic malignancies, pediatric solid tumors, inherited disorders, and aplastic anemia. It is also being used to treat many autoimmune disorders in experimental situations. Several patients with Crohn's disease and leukemia have remitted or remained in remission after allogeneic bone marrow transplantation. Complications related to SCT are becoming more widely recognized. Gastrointestinal (GI) complications of SCT result from preparative regimen toxicity, infection, and acute and chronic graft-versus-host disease (GVHD), which may be difficult to diagnostically separate and are therefore addressed in this chapter.

OVERVIEW OF SCT

The aim of SCT is to eradicate malignancy, a defective immune system, or disordered hematopoiesis by replacing stem cells with the patient's own (autologous) stored stem cells or those from a selectively matched human leukocyte antigen (HLA) donor (allogeneic transplant). The most common allogeneic transplant is still a matched sibling transplant; however, alternative donors with varying degrees of HLA mismatch from the donor are being performed more commonly. In pediatrics, the largest area of growth has been the use of partially matched cord blood transplants. Although GVHD and immunodeficiency occur more commonly after allogeneic transplantation, toxicity from the preparative regimen arises in both allogeneic and autologous transplants. Before transplantation, a preparative regimen is administered to rid the host of malignant or defective cells and to decrease the likelihood of donor stem cell rejection in allogeneic SCT. One of the largest areas of growth in transplantation has been the use of nonmyeloablative (often referred to as reduced intensity transplants or RITs) allogeneic transplants. These RITs rely on the antitumor effects of the allogeneic immune response rather than an intensive, myeloablative preparative regimen for their effectiveness. The use of RIT

has allowed the expansion of allogeneic transplants into older patients: patients who have had previous autologous transplants and patients with other significant medical issues.

Protocols for SCT vary, depending on the disease, but often include total body irradiation (TBI) and chemotherapy. The day of stem cell infusion into the host is designated as day 0, whereas the days before infusion, during which the preparative regimen is administered, are designated day 4, day 3, and so on.

TOXIC INJURY

Most transplant centers change the preparative regimen based on the disease, the donor source, and if the transplant is full (myeloablative) or an RIT. Thus, the expected toxicity of the preparative regimen depends on the combination of agents administered, the dose intensity of those agents, and the overall condition of the patient.

Protocols often include cyclophosphamide, busulfan, melphalan, fludarabine, and TBI (1100–1400 cGy), which, in combination, injure the intestinal mucosa. TBI at high doses (>1200 cGy) induces damage to DNA, particularly in rapidly dividing cells that are found in the crypts. The impaired regenerative capacity of the crypt epithelium leads to villous blunting and loss of brush-border enzyme activity; the patient may become lactose intolerant. If the regenerative capacity is severely impaired, ulceration may develop and lead to fluid and electrolyte losses. High doses of TBI have been associated with an increased likelihood of developing intestinal GVHD in animal models. The chemotherapy may itself induce mucositis, diarrhea, and, rarely, hemorrhagic colitis. Diarrhea related to toxicity induced by the preparative regimen may last until day 15 after SCT. To eliminate superimposed bacterial infection in the evaluation of diarrhea, stool cultures should be obtained. Once infectious etiologies are ruled out, antidiarrheal agents, such as loperamide, may be initiated. Nausea, vomiting, and anorexia occur commonly during the preparative regimen. Prophylactic antiemetics are routinely given, and the 5-hydroxytryptamine-3 serotonin receptor antagonists, such as granisetron, seem to offer significant protection against radiation-induced vomiting. If mucositis, nausea, and vomiting are severe, total parenteral nutrition must be frequently instituted. Studies are underway to determine whether addition of glutamine to enteral or parenteral feedings alters morbidity from SCT.

The more widespread use of the immunosuppressant, mycophenolate mofetil (MMF), as prophylaxis for GVHD, especially in the RIT setting, has also raised the issue of GVHD prophylaxis as a cause of GI toxicity. MMF may cause nausea, vomiting, diarrhea, and anorexia. Histologic changes in the GI tract consist of crypt architectural disarray and loss, increased crypt apoptotic bodies, flattened epithelial lining, intraluminal neutrophils, cryptitis, and reactive gastropathy changes. Some of these histologic findings may also be associated with acute GVHD. These symptoms have not correlated well with MMF levels. Because the symptoms overlap with those for GVHD, CMV, and many other processes, it is common practice to hold the drug for a few doses to see whether symptoms improve. Some patients respond to different dosing schedules, although some patients, for unclear reasons, tolerate the drug poorly.

● INFECTION

Evaluation of posttransplant diarrhea, which affects 43% of patients after day 20, must prompt a consideration of infectious etiologies. Although GVHD remains the most common cause of diarrhea after day 20 in allogeneic SCT, viral and bacterial pathogens must be sought in all patients. The most likely bacterial pathogen is *Clostridium difficile*, and despite the variables that contribute to the infection, namely use of broad-spectrum antibiotics and an immunocompromised state, the infection usually responds to standard therapy with metronidazole or vancomycin. Parasites are rarely found in patients with SCT, although case reports of amebiasis and giardiasis exist.

Viral infection, particularly that caused by cytomegalovirus (CMV), significantly affects mortality in this patient population. Although some transplant groups use prophylactic ganciclovir, the side effect of marrow toxicity has made this a difficult practice. Many groups now use serologic detection of CMV early antigen as an indication to initiate ganciclovir therapy, even before overt CMV disease develops in CMV-seropositive patients. In the absence of prophylaxis, CMV may occur 30 to 100 days after SCT in 70% of seropositive recipients and in up to 40% of seronegative recipients, but it is rare in seronegative patients maintained on seronegative blood products. CMV may infect epithelial and endothelial cells anywhere in the GI tract and cause diarrhea, abdominal pain, or GI bleeding. Ulceration may occur, probably as a result of local ischemia induced by CMV infection of endothelial cells and vasoconstriction. The most sensitive methods for the diagnosis of CMV involvement of the gut are centrifugation culture, polymerase chain reaction, and in situ hybridization using biopsy specimens.

Routine histology may be insensitive, and routine viral culture may take 2 weeks to provide a result. Other viruses, such as adenovirus, rotavirus, and astrovirus, have been identified as pathogens in patients with SCT. Adenoviral infection, with its poor prognosis, manifests as a multisystemic disease, with pneumonitis, cystitis, and enteritis occurring concurrently. No adequate treatment is currently available. Rotavirus infection may be diagnosed by enzyme-linked immunosorbent assay of the stool or by electron microscopy. Frequently, it is a self-limited infection, but administration of intravenous immunoglobulin in children with refractory infection has led to reports of therapeutic response. The significance of astrovirus as a pathogen remains unclear but was the virus identified most frequently in patients with SCT in one study. Finally, visceral varicella zoster infection may cause abdominal pain, diarrhea, nausea, vomiting, abnormal liver function tests, and fever. It is unclear from the case reports that whether the symptoms always arise from true viral infection of tissues of the gut or whether the symptoms really stem from compromise of GI motility secondary to disseminated viral infection. However, electron microscopy positively identified the presence of varicella zoster viral particles in the gastric biopsy specimen in one report. Abdominal pain may be the presenting symptom of disseminated varicella zoster infection and can be so severe that it has sometimes resulted in exploratory laparotomy. Abdominal pain may precede the vesicular skin eruption by up to 2 weeks, which contributes to the difficulty in making the diagnosis. The symptoms of visceral varicella zoster infection respond to acyclovir. Neutropenic enterocolitis, or typhlitis, may occur in recipients of SCT. Although the pathogenesis remains ambiguous, typhlitis is believed to arise from cytotoxic injury to the mucosa of the terminal ileum, cecum, or right colon, followed by superimposed bacterial or fungal infection. Infection may lead to perforation and an acute abdomen. Symptoms and physical signs may be nonspecific, but the diagnosis should be performed in any patient with fever, neutropenia, and abdominal pain.

Abdominal radiography and computed tomography demonstrate thickening of the right side of the colon and possibly pneumatosis intestinalis. Typhlitis may be managed conservatively with broad-spectrum antibiotics. Development of peritoneal signs warrants surgical consultation and intervention.

● GI BLEEDING

Significant GI bleeding may occur posttransplant and contributes to higher mortality associated with SCT. GI bleeding is most significant in the upper GI tract. More specifically, the site of bleeding is the antrum where there is generalized hemorrhage from the mucosa, but rarely is ulceration seen. Biopsies have demonstrated a chemical gastropathy characterized by foveolar hyperplasia, reactive epithelial changes, edema, and vascular congestion. Bipolar electrocoagulation is of limited efficacy, and significant quantities of blood products are required to support the patient. Gastric vascular ectasia (watermelon stomach) frequently has been reported in these patients and may be amenable to laser therapy. Occasionally, bleeding occurs as a consequence of GVHD or peptic ulcer disease.

● GRAFT-VERSUS-HOST DISEASE

At its simplest level, GVHD arises from the recipient's immune recognition of antigenic differences between donor and recipient. In those who obtain severely lymphocyte-depleted grafts, GVHD is rare. Increased numbers of infused lymphocytes, increased disparity between donor and host (as in unrelated donor transplants), and inflammatory cytokine production (as in sepsis) increase the risk for GVHD. Acute GVHD presents after the patient engrafts and arises from activation of donor T cells in response to host. Both tissue damage from the preparative regimen and T-cell activation contribute to the release of inflammatory cytokines, such as interleukin(IL)-2 and tumor necrosis factor-alpha (TNF-α) and TNF-γ. Cytokines, in turn, trigger a cascade of more intense inflammatory events. In the presence of these cytokines, natural killer and cytotoxic T cells mediate injury to three organ systems: skin, gut, and liver. Skin is the organ most commonly involved in GVHD. Gut or liver involvement usually is seen with skin disease, but it is possible to have isolated organ involvement.

In patients receiving RIT, because the preparative regimen is less toxic, there is much less cytokine release. Engraftment is generally later so that the onset of GVHD is also later. This is an extremely important point because most patients receiving RIT are not staying at the transplant center. They often present to their local healthcare facilities with their initial symptoms of GVHD. GVHD seen in RIT is the same as after a full allograft, although onset, because engraftment is a more gradual process, in often delayed.

CLINICAL MANIFESTATIONS

Patients with gut GVHD present with abdominal pain, nausea, and vomiting or diarrhea. The physical examination or history may reveal rash or serum elevations in alkaline phosphatase and direct bilirubin, which are consistent with GVHD involvement of the skin and liver. Initially, the rash involves the hands, feet, and ears. It initially may resemble a drug-related eruption, but as the GVHD progresses, it becomes confluent and, in severe cases, leads to blisters. The abdominal pain seen in gut GVHD usually is severe. It often is associated with cramping, requiring narcotics for control of the pain. Nausea and vomiting may indicate gastric involvement, whereas diarrhea suggests small bowel or colonic involvement. Patients with limited upper GI GVHD (i.e., nausea and vomiting as the only manifestations) do well with treatment and have a much better prognosis than those with lower GI involvement. A secretory diarrhea, at times in excess of 3 L/day, results from defects in salt and water resorption in the distal small bowel and colon. Careful attention to fluid and electrolyte replacement is required, especially in small children. When mucosal sloughing is present in the most severe form of gut GVHD, the diarrhea may be described as "stringy" and composed of protein exudates. Acute GVHD is graded by several clinical criteria, one of which is the volume of diarrhea. Volumes less than 500 mL/day usually are associated with grade 1, whereas those in excess of 1500 mL are characteristic of grade 3 GVHD. Significant GI blood loss may result from mucosal ulceration associated with GVHD and, as mentioned, is associated with a poor prognosis. Abdominal bloating, gastroparesis, and gastroileitis may occur and are indicative of severe injury. Abdominal radiography may show dilatation of the small

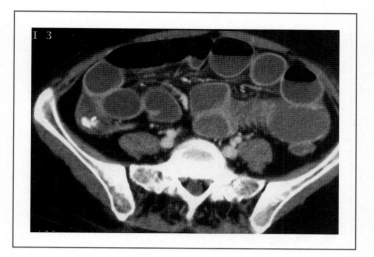

FIGURE 165.1 • Radiologic appearance of advanced acute graft-versus-host disease in the gut. Computed tomographic scan showing dilatated loops of small bowel with thickened walls and air-fluid levels.

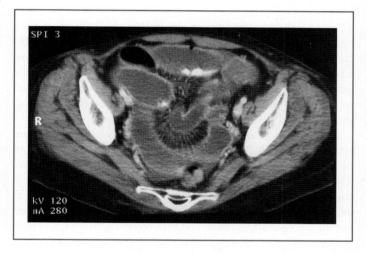

FIGURE 165.2 • Computed tomographic scan showing thickened bowel wall, fluid accumulation, and mesenteric changes.

bowel with air–fluid levels. A characteristic "ribbon sign" observed on computed tomography of the abdomen reflects widespread mucosal edema, small bowel dilatation, and loss of normal gut topography (Figs. 165.1 and 165.2). Because of the gut denudation, these patients are at extreme risk for disseminated bacterial infection. Most groups treat such patients with empiric antibiotic coverage for gram-negative and anaerobic organisms. Occasionally, clinically significant GI bleeding may result from mucosal ulceration.

HISTOLOGIC DIAGNOSIS

The diagnosis of GVHD is optimally made by histology. There is some debate in the literature as which biopsy site is most likely to yield the diagnosis. In our experience, acute GVHD typically involves the entire GI tract and where biopsies are taken is

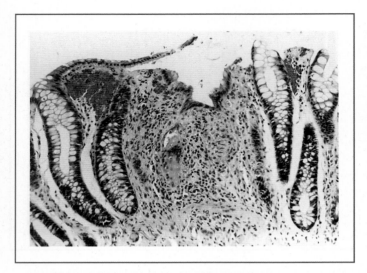

FIGURE 165.3 • Histologic appearance of graft-versus-host disease in the sigmoid colon. Apoptotic cells and vanishing crypts are characteristic features.

guided by the principal symptom. In those patients presenting chiefly with diarrhea, distal colonic biopsies are usually sufficient for diagnosis. In those with abdominal pain and diarrhea, a colonoscopy might be considered if there is concern for CMV infection, because colonic involvement may be focal as opposed to diffuse. If the presenting symptom is nausea and vomiting, duodenal and gastric biopsies typically suffice.

Thrombocytopenia may dissuade the endoscopist from obtaining biopsies of the mucosa, but biopsies probably can be safely obtained if platelet counts are more than 50,000/mm². The endoscopic appearance of the gastric or intestinal mucosa may be normal or demonstrate nonspecific erythema or edema. With mild GVHD, there is poor correlation between the endoscopic appearance and histology; endoscopically normal mucosa may yield significant histologic changes of GVHD. In more advanced cases, ulceration that progresses to frank mucosal sloughing can be seen. Histology of the gastric mucosa demonstrates apoptotic cells, or in the intestinal mucosa, apoptotic cells within the crypt epithelium, vanishing crypts, and some times crypt abscesses (Fig. 165.3). A lymphocytic infiltration of the lamina propria usually is present. Antral biopsies correlate well with the severity of GVHD in the duodenum and the colon, even if the presenting symptom is diarrhea. However, because CMV and other infections may coexist with acute GVHD, evaluation of the colon is extremely important in patients with diarrhea.

● MANAGEMENT

Treatment of acute GVHD consists of increasing immunosuppressive therapy. All patients, except for recipients of markedly lymphocyte-depleted grafts, are started on prophylactic cyclosporine or tacrolimus at the time of the SCT. If GVHD occurs, patients usually receive solumedrol 2 mg/kg/day intravenously, initially for 3 to 7 days, and then are placed on a steroid taper. Oral beclomethasone, a topically active steroid,

when used in conjunction with oral prednisone or intravenous prednisolone has been reported to improve anorexia, nausea, vomiting, and diarrhea in small studies of patients with mild intestinal GVHD. A large phase III trial (ENT00–02) of 129 patients examined beclomethasone dipropionate (BDP) as a prednisone-sparing therapy for GI GVHD. This study suggested that oral BDP prevented GVHD relapse and was associated with better survival compared with placebo after prednisone taper.

Editor's note (TMB): Beclomethasone is now available commercially and has been approved for this usage.

Oral budesonide is a nonabsorbable corticosteroid that undergoes rapid hepatic metabolism resulting in fewer systemic side effects compared with other corticosteroids when used in the treatment of inflammatory bowel disease. Although there are case reports and its potential use is attractive, there are no large studies examining its efficacy in the treatment of GI manifestations of acute GVHD. Buccal administration of budesonide has been somewhat effective in the treatment of oral chronic GVHD.

If there is no improvement with steroids, repeat endoscopy and biopsy should be considered before second-line treatment is initiated, because the risk of opportunistic infection is high. In addition, in patients with severe gut damage from GVHD, extensive mucosal injury certainly will require weeks to heal, during which time, diarrhea may persist. Unfortunately, most immunosuppressive agents are associated with an increased risk for opportunistic infection, and GVHD itself is immunosuppressive. Investigational drugs directed at controlling cytokine-induced effects include pentostatin, anti-IL-2, and anti-TNF-α. Salvage therapy until recently in GVHD has been disappointing.

Diarrhea Management. The control of symptomatic diarrhea can be difficult in these patients. Antidiarrheal agents initiated at high doses often are ineffective in reducing the volume of diarrhea. In a nonrandomized pilot study, octreotide at 500 μg intravenously every 8 hours for 7 days has been reported to induce complete resolution of diarrhea in 71% of patients with grade 3 or 4 GVHD. Patients were treated with an intense immunosuppressive regimen simultaneously. The high rate of response was attributed in part to the early initiation of therapy. Octreotide is believed to act by stimulating water and electrolyte absorption, a process that can take place only if the gut epithelium has not sloughed. A possible complication of long-term use of octreotide is gallbladder stasis and predisposition to gallstone formation.

● CHRONIC GVHD

Chronic GVHD affects 40% of patients. Chronic GVHD affects skin, liver, eyes, mouth, and gut, and the clinical manifestations differ from those seen in acute GVHD. Chronic GVHD arises from a dysregulation in autoimmunity, similar to that seen in collagen-vascular disease, which it clinically resembles. Damage to the ethymus may predispose to the development of autoreactive cells. Chronic GVHD of the gut most commonly presents with anorexia, cachexia, nausea, and vomiting. Oral involvement with chronic GVHD is one of the most common manifestations. Patients may have extensive leukoplakia, ulceration, and dysphagia. Dry mouth is common, especially in patients who also have dry eyes. Secondary viral and fungal infections are common and often present with an increase in pain without a clinically significant change in appearance of the mouth. In addition to treatments of oral infection, treatment of isolated oral GVHD should start with local therapy. In many cases, decadron swishes will contain the process. Oral beclomethasone and budesonide, as discussed above, have also been used in small studies with some efficacy. Liquid cyclosporine swishes, intraoral psoralen plus ultraviolet A, and intralesional injection with steroids also have been used alone or in conjunction with systemic therapy for patients with multisystem disease.

Late posttransplant diarrhea often is ascribed to chronic GVHD. In the current era of lymphocyte depletion and immunosuppression, actual active gut involvement is rare. However, infection and drug-induced inflammation, particularly that attributable to mofetil, occur frequently and should be sought aggressively. Malabsorption from pancreatic enzyme deficiency may also present after transplantation because TBI has been noted to induce chronic pancreatitis. As in the case of diarrhea immediately after transplantation, ascertaining an etiology of malabsorption is the first step in treatment. Oral chronic GVHD may contribute to anorexia and weight loss because it may cause ageusia, difficulty swallowing, and an inability to open the mouth. Anorexia and weight loss may also be mediated in part by high levels of circulating TNF-α, but it is important to exclude structural and functional abnormalities of the gut. Gastroparesis and gallbladder disease should be considered in the differential diagnosis of nausea, vomiting, and anorexia in stem cell transplant recipients.

Patients may have scleroderma-like gut involvement and present with esophageal, gastric, and small bowel dysmotility secondary to submucosal fibrosis, esophageal reflux, and proximal esophageal web formation. Small bowel strictures may lead to delayed small bowel transit, bacterial overgrowth, and steatorrhea. Biopsies may show changes suggestive of inactive inflammatory disease and usually do not possess the pronounced inflammatory infiltrate seen in acute GVHD. Focal fibrosis in the submucosa and serosa may occur. Biopsy of gut mucosa is not as informative in acute GVHD, and, therefore, barium studies may prove more useful. Esophageal webs and strictures respond to endoscopic dilatation. Systemic treatment thus far has been aimed primarily at the skin manifestations, which commonly include joint contractures, hypo- and hyperpigmentation, and sclerodermatous changes. Administration of anti-TNF-α antibody, as is used in rheumatoid arthritis and Crohn's disease, may one day prove effective in treating some of the GI symptoms related to chronic GVHD. Increasing immunosuppression to address the skin and oral changes may likewise improve the GI disease.

Editor's note (TMB): There is an excellent follow-up report of stem cell transplantation for patients with refractory Crohn's disease by Burt RK, Craig RM, et al. in Blood 2010;110:6123–6132.

Additional Reading

1 Hockenbery DM, Cruickshank S, Rodell TC, et al. A randomized, placebo-controlled trial of oral beclomethasone dipropionate as a prednisone-sparing therapy for gastrointestinal graft-versus-host disease. *Blood.* 2007;109(10):4557–4563.

2 Ibrahim RB, Abidi MH, Cronin SM, et al. Nonabsorbable corticosteroids use in the treatment of gastrointestinal graft-versus-host disease. *Biol Blood Marrow Transplant.* 2009;15(4):395–405.

3 Bordigoni P, Dimicoli S, Clement L, et al. Daclizumab, an efficient treatment for steroid-refractory acute graft-versus-host disease. *Br J Haematol.* 2006;135(3):382–385.

4 Bobak D, Arfons LM, Creger RJ, Lazarus HM. *Clostridium difficile*-associated disease in human stem cell transplant recipients: coming epidemic or false alarm? *Bone Marrow Transplant.* 2008;42(11):705–713.

5 Cruz-Correa M, Poonawala A, Abraham SC, et al. Endoscopic findings predict the histologic diagnosis in gastrointestinal graft-versus-host disease. *Endoscopy.* 2002;34(10):808–813.

6 Parfitt JR, Jayakumar S, Driman DK. Mycophenolate mofetil-related gastrointestinal mucosal injury: variable injury patterns, including graft-versus-host disease-like changes. *Am J Surg Pathol.* 2008;32(9):1367–1372.

7 Eagle DA, Gian V, Lauwers GY, et al. Gastroparesis following bone marrow transplantation. *Bone Marrow Transplant.* 2001;28(1):59–62.

8 Abbott B, Ippoliti C, Bruton J, Neumann J, Whaley R, Champlin R. Antiemetic efficacy of granisetron plus dexamethasone in bone marrow transplant patients receiving chemotherapy and total body irradiation. *Bone Marrow Transplant.* 1999;23(3):265–269.

9 Cox GJ, Matsui SM, Lo RS, et al. Etiology and outcome of diarrhea after marrow transplantation: a prospective study. *Gastroenterology.* 1994;107(5):1398–1407.

10 David DS, Tegtmeier BR, O'Donnell MR, Paz IB, McCarty TM. Visceral varicella-zoster after bone marrow transplantation: report of a case series and review of the literature. *Am J Gastroenterol.* 1998;93(5):810–813.

11 Ippoliti C, Champlin R, Bugazia N, et al. Use of octreotide in the symptomatic management of diarrhea induced by graft-versus-host disease in patients with hematologic malignancies. *J Clin Oncol.* 1997;15(11):3350–3354.

12 McDonald GB, Bouvier M, Hockenbery DM, et al. Oral beclomethasone dipropionate for treatment of intestinal graft-versus-host disease: a randomized, controlled trial. *Gastroenterology.* 1998;115(1):28–35.

13 Nevo S, Enger C, Swan V, et al. Acute bleeding after allogeneic bone marrow transplantation: association with graft versus host disease and effect on survival. *Transplantation.* 1999;67(5):681–689.

14 Ponec RJ, Hackman RC, McDonald GB. Endoscopic and histologic diagnosis of intestinal graft-versus-host disease after marrow transplantation. *Gastrointest Endosc.* 1999;49(5):612–621.

15 Snover DC. Graft-versus-host disease of the gastrointestinal tract. *Am J Surg Pathol.* 1990;14(suppl 1):101–108.

16 Song HK, Kreisel D, Canter R, Krupnick AS, Stadtmauer EA, Buzby G. Changing presentation and management of neutropenic enterocolitis. *Arch Surg.* 1998;133(9):979–982.

Gastrointestinal Behçet's Disease | 166

Eric Vasiliauskas

Behçet's disease (BD) is a chronic relapsing multisystem immune-mediated inflammatory disorder characterized by recurrent oral ulcers and numerous other potential manifestations, including genital ulcers, ocular disease, skin lesions, neurologic disease, vascular disease, and arthritis. The spectrum of clinical involvement is broad, and the severity of disease varies from individual to individual; some live somewhat normal lives; others may become severely disabled. The incidence of gastrointestinal tract involvement in BD shows remarkable geographic variation, the reported frequency being highest along the eastern rim of Asia, including Korea and Japan (50–60%), while significantly lower rates are seen in the United States (8%), Turkey (5%), and other Mediterranean countries.[1,2] To optimally care for a patient with gastrointestinal BD (GIBD), it is important to have an understanding not only of the complex potential gastrointestinal issues but of the full compliment of systemic manifestations as well.

Editor's note (TMB): We have elected to include more information on BD than provided in most other chapters because this is a unique condition in some parts of the world. The differential diagnosis from Crohn's disease is sometimes quite difficult and the author, Eric Vasilauskas, has provided us with a masterful review.

The first description of what is now known as BD is attributed to Hippocrates in the 5th century BC when he referred to an endemic disease in Asia Minor characterized by a constellation of oral ulcerations, "many ulcerations about the genital parts," and "watery ophthalmies of a chronic character...which destroyed the sight of many persons."[3] In the early 1930s, the Greek ophthalmologist Benediktos Adamantiades published a case of a patient with recurrent iritis with hypopyon in both eyes that led to blindness, recurrent oral aphthous ulcers, scarring scrotal ulcers, and a sterile arthritis of both knees.[3] Several years later the Turkish dermatologist, Hulusi Behçet, described the classic triad of recurrent oral ulceration, genital ulceration, and ocular inflammation as a unique disease entity.[3]

BD is more common along the ancient international trading route known as "the Silk Road," which extends from eastern Asia to the Mediterranean.[4] The prevalence of Behçet's is highest in Turkey (110–420 cases per 100,000), ranges from 13 to 20 per 100,000 in Japan, to only 1 to 2 per 100,000 in the United Kingdom and the United States.[5] While the proportion of men and women affected is similar in the areas where BD is more common, women are more commonly affected in northern Europe and the United States. BD tends to manifest in the third to fourth decades of life, but may present at any age. Clinical manifestations are similar in children and adults.[5] BD has been observed to be more severe in young males and those living in Middle Eastern and Far Eastern regions.[5]

HISTOPATHOLOGY

BD is a systemic necrotizing vasculitis that affects blood vessels of all sizes—small, medium, and large—on both the arterial and venous sides of the circulation. Histologic examination of involved Behçet's lesions frequently reveals vasculitis, though this may not be seen in all specimens. Features found in "classic" Behçet's lesions include perivascular lymphocytic and monocytic cellular infiltration, with or without fibrin deposition in the vessel wall.[5] Significant neutrophil infiltration is also seen.[5] Inflammation results in blood vessel wall thickening, fibrosis, or necrosis destroying blood vessel architecture, which may cause ischemia by decreasing or permanently interrupting blood flow to tissues, ultimately leading in transient or irreparable end-organ damage.

ETIOPATHOGENESIS

The etiopathogenesis of BD has yet to be fully elucidated. Similar to Crohn's disease and ulcerative colitis, what is now collectively termed "Behçet's disease" is likely not a single disease process, but rather a spectrum of diseases that present with similar overlapping clinical manifestations, the specific phenotype being influenced by the interplay between genetic, immune, and environmental factors.

While many cases of BD have been described to be sporadic, familial clustering has been observed.[4] Having a first degree relative with BD increases the risk of developing the disease.[5] Genetic anticipation has been suggested. The genetic predisposition is likely polygenic and includes human leukocyte antigen (HLA) and non-HLA genes.[5] While genetic testing is not yet being used clinically for diagnostic, predictive, or treatment purposes, research suggests that certain genetic profiles are associated with disease aggressiveness and severity.[4]

As with other immune-mediated disorders, the immune abnormalities in Behçet's may be triggered in genetically susceptible individuals by environmental stimuli, including infectious agents and medications. A link between infection and certain manifestations of BD has been proposed.[4] Studies suggest a possible pathogenic role of molecular mimicry between specific infectious agents and the host in the initiation, perpetuation, and/or exacerbation of BD.[4,5] Supporting the contribution of environmental stimuli is the observation that Turkish and Japanese emigrants have been shown to have significantly lower risk of developing BD.[5]

Polymorphonuclear leukocytes activation contributes to BD. Upregulation of surface adhesion molecule expression may mediate enhanced neutrophil binding to the vascular endothelium thereby facilitating neutrophil migration beyond affected vessels.[4] Increases in neutrophil apoptosis have been demonstrated in patients with active BD.[3] Similar to Crohn's disease and rheumatoid arthritis, a T helper cell type 1-predominant response has been observed in many studies in patients with Behçet's.[4,5] Humoral immune activation also contributes to disease pathogenesis. Increased numbers of circulating B lymphocytes, believed to be antigen driven, have been observed.[4] Autoantibodies against host self antigens have been described against a number of targets.[5] Elevated levels of serum immune complexes have been demonstrated in about one-half of patients with BD, particularly those with active cutaneous, ocular, or neurologic manifestations. Immune complex deposition can be identified in some Behçet's lesions.[3]

● CLINICAL MANIFESTATIONS

Most of the clinical features in BD are believed to be related to vasculitis. The most common clinical manifestation in BD is the presence of recurrent and usually painful mucocutaneous ulcerations. The other clinical manifestations are more variable. *Minor disease manifestations* are those that interfere significantly with patients' quality of life, but do not threaten vital organ function (i.e., arthritis and mucocutaneous disease). *Major disease manifestations* may result in significant organ morbidity, potentially even death (i.e., certain ocular and neurological manifestations, venous thrombotic disease, complications of large-vessel arteritis, intestinal perforation).

Oral Behçet's

Oral involvement is usually considered separately from the other gastrointestinal manifestations in BD. Repeated episodes of oral ulcerations precede the development of other Behçet's manifestations by 1 to 8 years in most patients.[4] Oral ulcers most often occur in crops, but may occur singly. The most common sites of involvement in order of frequency are the inner lips, buccal mucosa, tongue, gums, palate, tonsils, and oropharynx.[4] Aphthous ulcerations may be grossly and histologically similar to common "canker sores," but they tend to be more numerous,

more frequent, and often larger and more painful. Oral ulcers usually start as slightly raised, erythematous lesions that progress to ulceration within 48 hours and may be clinically indistinguishable from those seen in patients with inflammatory bowel disease (IBD).[4] Ulcers are rounded, usually have an erythematous border and the surface may be covered by yellowish pseudomembrane. Minor ulcers are shallower and defined as less than 10 mm in diameter; major ulcers are deeper and range from 1 cm to over 2 cm in diameter.[5] Oral BD may also manifest as recurrent crops of hundreds of tiny, painful herpetiform ulcerations, which may become confluent. In some cases, oral BD can manifest as a striatic pattern resembling lichen planus.[4] Oral Behçet's ulcers are characteristically painful and may limit eating. Smaller ulcerations typically resolve spontaneously and heal completely without treatment within 1 to 3 weeks, though they persist in some patients. Larger ulcers may be more persistent and can result in permanent scaring, which may present as dysphagia and even laryngeal stenosis.[4]

Extra-Oral Gastrointestinal BD

Vasculitis involving the gastrointestinal tract is usually part of a broader systemic process although the signs and symptoms may initially be limited. Inflammation and ulceration may occur anywhere from the mouth to the anus. In one study, 45% of BD patients presented with gastrointestinal manifestations.[4] An important consideration is that a significant number of individuals with GIBD do not satisfy the conventional criteria of systemic BD at the time of initial presentation with intestinal involvement, and only later go on to develop the additional systemic symptoms to fulfill diagnostic criteria.[1]

Upper Gastrointestinal Tract

Patients with symptoms of substernal pain, dysphagia, odynophagia, epigastric pain, anorexia, vomiting, hematemesis, and melena should be evaluated for possible upper gastrointestinal tract involvement of BD. Esophageal BD is uncommon and is more frequent in males.[6] The mid-esophagus is most commonly involved. There are no typical esophageal Behçet's lesions; they may take the form of erosions, discrete aphthous, linear, or perforating ulcerations or wide-spread esophagitis. Dissection of the mucosa, varices, and severe stenosis may also occur. Over half of the individuals with esophageal Behçet's have additional gastrointestinal disease elsewhere. Gastroduodenal involvement varies with the population; rates as high a 43% have been reported.

Small Bowel and Colonic Disease

The ileocecal region, including the ascending colon, has historically been described as being the most commonly affected portion of the bowel in GIBD. While the rest of the colon may be involved, the rectum is frequently relatively spared. Recent wireless capsule endoscopy (WCE) studies suggest that the incidence and extent of small bowel involvement may be significantly underestimated. In a British study, WCE identified small intestinal ulcers scatter throughout the ileum in 10 of the 11 BD patients whose gastrointestinal symptoms remained unexplained with conventional studies.[7] Erythrocyte sedimentation rate (ESR), C-reactive protein (CRP), and CT scans were normal in all. Small (<5 mm) superficial ovoid punched out ulcerations with surrounding areas of erythema were the dominant type of lesion. In a Brazilian cohort of BD patients with abdominal complaints, WCE revealed multiple small and widespread lesions in all ten subjects, the most frequently involved segment being the jejunum where lesions were identified in 80%.[8]

The typical lesions of GIBD have been described as large, discrete, round, ovoid punched-out-appearing, or excavated mucosal ulcerations. Behçet's ulcerations may be broadly classified into three types based on their macroscopic appearance: volcano-type (well-demarcated penetrating ulcers), geographic (shallow ulcers of variable shape), and aphthoid (shallow, ovoid ulcers).[9–11] Typical colonoscopic findings in GIBD are single large ulcerations measuring 1 cm to over 3 cm in diameter, or a few deep ulcers with discrete margins in the ileocecal area or anastomotic site.[9] While pancolitis may be seen in BD, in many cases the colonic lesions are confined to one segment of the colon. Areas of denuded mucosa may also be seen. GIBD presenting as an inflammatory mass in the ileocecal region has been described. Anal involvement is rare, but may occur.[12]

Signs and Symptoms

The spectrum of clinical signs and symptoms of GIDB may include diarrhea, abdominal pain, bloody stools including melena, abdominal masses, nausea, vomiting, anorexia, weight loss, fever, and constipation. Symptoms can be debilitating and may be related to either more acute vasculitic local gut inflammation and ulceration or to chronic mesenteric ischemia. Patients with chronic mesenteric ischemia resulting from a low flow state may give a history of chronic abdominal pain or postprandial abdominal pain ("intestinal angina"), nausea, vomiting, and/or diarrhea.

Patients with GIBD may complain of pain that is out of proportion to findings on abdominal exam before intestinal infarction occurs. Thus, in patients with chronic vasculitis-associated intestinal ischemia, it is important to be vigilant for potential bowel infarction, perforation, and peritonitis, particularly in the setting of steroids which can mask fever and pain. Fistula formation, hemorrhage, or perforation may occur in up to half of patients with GIBD. Other more severe complications such as intestinal stenosis or structuring with resultant small bowel obstruction, massive gastrointestinal hemorrhage secondary to aneurysm formation, and persistent bleeding due to gastric, duodenal, or other gastrointestinal ulcerations can also lead to significant morbidity and may be potentially life-threatening.[1]

Prognosis

There are few reports on the long-term prognosis of GIBD. "Volcano-like" ulcerations have been noted to be more medically refractory, more likely to perforate and require surgery, and have a higher recurrence rate when compared to the shallower "geographic" type or "aphthous" type ulcers.[1,11] Patients with GIBD who are able to achieve complete remission are less likely to require operation than those who do not. However, the probability of recurrence of GIBD following medically induced complete remission is reported to be 25% at 2 years and 49% at 5 years.[13]

Perforation

In one report, two thirds of children with GIBD underwent surgery for indications that included intestinal stenosis and perforation.[14] Intestinal perforations may be more common in Far East populations, where large deep ulcers have been described to be more common.[1] One quarter of patients underwent surgery for perforation, in a Korean study of adults with GIBD, the most common site of perforation being the ileocecal region (51.5%).[1] Perforation occurred within 3 years of diagnosis in 44.4% of patients, between 3 and 5 years of diagnosis in 22.2%. Gross perforation was noted in 60.6% and microperforation in the remaining 39.4%. Multiple perforations were observed in over half the cases. The authors indentified three independent risk factors to be associated with predisposition to bowel perforation: diagnosis of GIBD before age 25 years, history of prior laparotomy, and deep volcano-shaped intestinal ulcers.[1]

Anastomtoic Recurrence

Following bowel resection, excessive postoperative infiltration of inflammatory cells into the anastomotic region has been observed and can result in leakage at the anastomotic site, prompting the practice of administering intermediate doses of corticosteroids for several days postoperatively in an attempt to prevent this complication.[2] This phenomenon has been postulated to originate from the similar pathogenesis of pathergy reaction. Postoperative recurrence adjacent to or at the anastomotic site seems to be a relatively common complication in resected intestinal BD and historically has lead to multiple operations with eventual short bowel syndrome in some.[1] Because of this, some investigators have advocated right hemicolectomy and more extensive surgical resection, as much as 60 to 100 cm of ileum, for perforating intestinal BD. Others have found that the length of ileal resection and whether or not hemicolectomy was performed has no significant effect on the recurrence or reoperation rate, and thus, suggest a more conservative approach, resecting only grossly affected bowel segments.[1,13]

Postoperative recurrence is variable, but has been reported to be as high as 87.5% in a Japanese cohort.[15] Seventy-five percent recurred within 2 years of surgery; 37.5% of the patients required repeat surgery for intestinal obstruction because of ulcers at the site of anastomosis. In a Korean cohort, patients who had undergone intestinal resection for perforation or fistula were noted to have a higher probability of postoperative GIBD recurrence than those in whom resection was performed for other reasons (59% vs. 33% at 2 years; 88% vs. 57% at 5 years).[13] Patients treated with postoperative azathioprine (AZA) maintenance therapy had a lower probability of requiring reoperation than those who did not (7% vs. 25% at 2 years; 25% vs. 47% at 5 years).[13]

Other Gastrointestinal Considerations

Ischemic hepatitis, ischemic pancreatitis, ischemic cholecystitis, and appendicitis may occur.[3] Although celiac disease is not more common in patients with BD, the two diseases have been shown to coexist and thus needs to be considered when evaluating patients with gastrointestinal involvement.

In patients who experience gastrointestinal symptoms, the possibility that the symptoms might be secondary to medications prescribed for the various BD manifestations also need to be considered. Gastrointestinal toxicity is common with nonsteroidal anti-inflammatory drugs (NSAIDs), colchicine, pentoxifylline, mycophenolate mofetil (MMF), and interferon therapy. In addition to *Clostridium difficile* and other enteric infections, immunosuppression-associated infectious complications, including candidal, herpes, or cytomegalovirus (CMV), may occur.

Urogenital Disease

About 55% to 94% of patients develop genital ulcerations at some point in their disease course.[4] In men, these typically occur on the scrotum and can affect the penis; in women the vulva, but may affect the vagina and cervix and result in dyspareunia. Groin, perineal, and perianal ulcers occur in both sexes and may be accompanied by secondary infection. Genital ulcers generally start as papules or pustules that then rapidly mature into rounded or oval erosions or ulcers with a yellow fibrinoid base and surrounding red halo. They are similar in appearance to oral ulcers, but tend to be larger and deeper. They are usually painful and may be associated with dysuria and difficulty walking.[4] Urogenital ulcerations heal more slowly and typically recur, though less frequently than oral ulcerations. Scarring over time from these lesions is not unusual. Urethritis, epididymitis, salpingitis, and urethral fistulae occur less commonly.[4]

Cutaneous Lesions

Skin lesions are expressed in more than 75% of patients with BD. BD-associated papules and pustules appear to be the most common cutaneous manifestation and visually resemble ordinary resembling acne or folliculitis, but occur at any age, and may appear nearly anywhere on the body.[4] These lesions are frequently not sterile and may harbor *Staphylococcus aureus* and *Prevotella* spp. BD-associated erythema nodosum (EN) often represents a medium-vessel vasculitis and usually affects the lower limbs. EN lesions are painful and may resolve spontaneously. BD-associated EN lesions frequently ulcerate and may heal with scarring or resolve leaving deeply hyperpigmented areas. Superficial thrombophlebitis is fairly common and presents as painful, often migratory, erythematous nodules, usually on the lower extremities that may be confused with EN.[4] The spectrum of dermatologic manifestations also includes erythema multiforme-like lesions, pseudofolliculitis, palpable purpura, and cellulitis-type lesions.

Ocular Disease

As many as 85% of patients with BD exhibit eye involvement, which usually becomes evident within 2 to 3 years of disease onset and is the presenting feature in 10% to 20% of patients.[4] Ocular BD is both more common and tends to be more severe in men than in women.[5] Ocular sequelae are not always fully reversible and a subset of BD patients experience progressive vision loss to the point of blindness despite aggressive therapy. Uveitis is the most common feature and is typically bilateral and episodic, may not resolve completely between exacerbations. Uveitis may be classified as anterior or posterior, though involvement of the entire uveal tract (panuveitis) is not uncommon. *Anterior uveitis* (iridocyclitis) is inflammation of the iris and anterior chamber. This manifests clinically as pain, blurry vision, light sensitivity, tearing, or redness of the eye. Many such patients will have associated retinal vasculitis. Severe anterior

uveitis can result in the formation of hypopyon, a characteristic sign of ocular BD seen in roughly one third of patients, in which the inflammatory exudate forms a visible layer of pus or a pus-like fluid in the anterior chamber of the eye.[5] Left untreated, episodes of anterior uveitis may subside spontaneously; however, repeated attacks result in progressive irreversible structural changes, such as deformity of the iris and secondary glaucoma. *Posterior uveitis* (chorioretinitis) is the inflammation of the choroid and retina. This form of uveitis is considered more vision-threatening; it often causes fewer clinical symptoms while damaging the retina. Patients usually experience a painless, bilateral decrease in visual acuity. BD may be complicated by optic neuritis, retinal vein occlusion, inflammation-induced retinal neovascularization, vitreous hemorrhage, glaucoma, scleritis, episcleritis, secondary cataracts, keratitis, conjunctival ulceration, and sicca syndrome.[4] Conjunctivitis is rare.[5]

Neurologic Disease

Central nervous system (CNS) manifestations occur in 2% to 30% of patients with BD.[4] Neurologic involvement typically presents within the first 5 years of disease onset and is more common in men than women.[5] The most common abnormalities are focal parenchymal lesions, demyelination of the cerebrospinal tract, and complications of arterial or venous vascular thrombosis.[4,5] Cerebral venous thrombosis, dural sinus thrombosis, and cerebral artery thrombosis have all been described. Behçet's lesions can affect the corticospinal tract, brainstem, periventricular white matter, spinal cord, and basal ganglia; cerebellar involvement is uncommon. Neurologic BD may manifest as aseptic meningitis, aseptic encephalitis or meningoencephalitis, or arterial vasculitis that may lead to ischemic strokes, aneurysmal dilatation, dissection, and subarachnoid hemorrhage. Depending on the type of neurologic involvement, patients may present with headaches, fever, neck stiffness, papilledema, cranial nerve palsy, confusion, behavioral or personality change, psychiatric disorders, and motor disturbances, including coordination difficulty, hemiparesis, pyramidal signs, and sphincter disturbance.[3,4] CNS involvement may be chronic. Repeated cycles of exacerbations and remissions lead to progressive and irreversible disability over time, including dementia. Neurologic disease-related mortality is estimated at 5% to 10%.[5] Peripheral neuropathy is uncommon. Importantly, the side effects of cyclosporine, which is used to treat some BD manifestations, may not only be indistinguishable from the Behçet's CNS involvement but may actually accelerate the development of neurological involvement in this disease and should thus be avoided in BD patients with CNS involvement.[4,5]

Large Vessel Vascular Disease

This BD manifestation affects up to approximately one-third of patients. Acute or chronic relapsing episodes of perivascular and endovascular inflammation may lead to hemorrhage, stenosis, aneurysm formation, thrombotic occlusion of major veins, and arteries, which may result in varices or organ infarction or failure.[4] Aneurysmal rupture may be fatal.

Pulmonary Involvement

Pulmonary vascular lesions, including thrombosis, aneurysm, and fistula, cause recurrent episodes of dyspnea, cough, chest pain, and hemoptysis. The most common pulmonary vascular lesion of BD is pulmonary artery aneurysm involving the large proximal branches of the pulmonary arteries.[4] This process is rarely seen in any condition other than BD. Hemoptysis is a common presenting symptom and may be due to pulmonary arteriobronchial fistulae which are often associated with venous obstruction elsewhere. Pulmonary arteriography is diagnostic, whereas ventilation-perfusion scan findings can be misleading. Other lung manifestations include pulmonary infarction, hemorrhage, both organizing and eosinophilic pneumonias, pleural effusion, pulmonary arteritis or venulitis, bronchial stenosis, abscess, obstructive airway disease, chronic bronchitis, and pulmonary fibrosis.[4]

Cardiac Disease

Symptomatic Behçet's-associated cardiac disease is infrequent though pericarditis, myocarditis, coronary arteritis, atrial septal aneurysm, conduction system disturbances, ventricular arrhythmias, endocarditis, endomyocardial fibrosis, mitral valve prolapse, and valvular insufficiency have all been described.[3]

Nephropathy

Compared to other vasculitis, renal involvement in BD is not only less frequent but also tends to be less severe and may present as secondary (AA) amyloidosis, glomerulonephritis, renal arterial aneurysms, renal microinfarction, and/or interstitial nephritis.[4] Patients may present with proteinuria, hematuria, nephrotic syndrome, or mild renal insufficiency. Progression to renal failure is rare.

Arthropathy

About 16% to 93% of Behçet's patients experience arthritis or arthralgias, most commonly of the medium and large joints.[4] Joint symptoms occasionally precede other BD manifestations. Behçet's arthropathy is usually nonerosive and nondeforming, but can be quite debilitating. The knees are most frequently affected, followed by the wrists, ankles, and elbows. Joint involvement is typically asymmetric and most often pauciarticular or monoarticular, much less often polyarticular. Though symptoms may be more persistent, joint pains, swellings, and stiffness are often intermittent, lasting 1 to 3 weeks. The coexistence of ankylosing spondylitis and sacroiliitis has been reported.[3]

Constitutional Symptoms

Patients with active BD may experience nonspecific symptoms, including significant fatigue, generalized malaise, and/or weight loss. Children are more likely to manifest recurrent fevers.[5]

● DIAGNOSTIC EVALUATION AND MONITORING CONSIDERATIONS

At present, there are no definitive laboratory tests or blood test panels to diagnose BD; the diagnosis is made on the basis of the clinical findings. Most individuals presenting with gastrointestinal manifestations will have already been diagnosed with Behçet's, or will have a history of other systemic findings suggestive of the underlying systemic vasculitic disease.

Editor's note (TMB): The astute pathologist may be the first to suggest or confirm this diagnosis. Visiting Korean pathologists have increased the awareness for this diagnosis in our institution.

The phenomenon of *pathergy* has been shown to be highly specific for BD.[4] Pathergy refers to the inflammatory process triggered by a minor trauma such as a bump or bruise that leads to the development of skin lesions or ulcers that may be resistant to healing. Pathergy may be induced by a blood draw, a peripheral IV line, or a surgical incision. A positive pathergy test is characterized by erythematous induration with an erythematous papular or pustule-like response in the center of the lesion that appears at the site of the needle stick 48 hours after skin prick by a 20- to 21-gauge needle.[3] The pathergy phenomena, when present, is helpful in diagnosing BD, for it is seen in only a few other conditions such as pyoderma gangrenosum, Sweet's syndrome, and in about 8% of IBD patients. The limitation is that while pathergy may be seen in 50% to 75% of BD patients in more endemic areas such the Middle East and Japan, it is only seen in 10% to 20% of North European and North American patients with BD. Also, pathergy has been observed to be a dynamic phenomenon which can appear and disappear during the course of the disease; it is less common in patients on BD-directed therapy; and the positivity of the test diminishes in those who have had disease longer than 5 years.[4] Pathergy should be distinguished from dermographism, a response in which the skin becomes raised and inflamed to light scratching of the skin which may be also be present in some patients with BD, but is seen in about 4% to 5% of the general population.

A variety of clinical criteria have been proposed to characterize BD. Importantly, the accepted classifications were designed to ensure comparability between international research studies, not for use in establishing the diagnosis of Behçet's in individual patients.[16]

The international criteria put forth and published in 1990 by the International Study Group for BD require the presence of recurrent oral aphthous or herpetiform ulcerations (observed by physician or reported reliably by the patient) with at least three episodes in any 12-month period PLUS at least two of the following (in the absence of other systemic diseases)[16]:

- Recurrent genital aphthous ulceration or scarring (observed by physician or reliably reported by the patient)
- Eye lesions (including anterior or posterior uveitis, cells in the vitreous on slit lamp examination, or retinal vasculitis documented by an ophthalmologist)
- Skin lesions (including EN-like lesions) observed by physician or reliably reported by the patient, pseudofolliculitis, papulopustular lesions *or* acneiform nodules consistent with BD—observed by a physician and in postadolescent patients not receiving glucocorticoids
- A positive pathergy test (a papule 2 mm or more in size developing 24 to 48 hours performed with oblique insertion of a 20-gauge or smaller needle under sterile conditions 5 mm into the skin, generally performed on the forearm) read by a physician at 24 to 48 hours

These criteria have been subsequently validated across several populations and appear to be relatively sensitive and specific.[16] Of note is that because of the very low prevalence of pathergy in some populations, some have proposed that in those populations other manifestations of BD might be substituted for pathergy.

Blood Tests

There is no single clinical or laboratory parameter, which consistently and reliably reflects the level of intestinal inflammation in intestinal BD.[4] Circulating immune complexes are almost always elevated in patients with active vasculitis; however, while sensitive, these markers are also nonspecific. Autoantibodies such as rheumatoid factor, antinuclear antibody, and antineutrophil cytoplasmic antibody are usually negative in BD.[4,5] Data regarding anti-*Saccharomyces cerevisiae* antibodies are conflicting—elevated levels have been reported on some populations including, healthy family members of BD patients, but not in others.[17]

Nonspecific biochemical markers of inflammation such as neutrophilic leukocytosis, anemia, the ESR, and CRP may be useful in following disease activity, but may not be elevated in some patients and may be normal despite significant active oral, genital, ocular, CNS, or gastrointestinal disease.[4] While there may be a potential role for fecal calprotectin testing in GIBD, this has not been formally studied. The utility of specific genetic and cytokine profiles has not been clearly enough defined at this time to be clinically utilized in the diagnosis or management of BD.

Serum lactate levels may be helpful in evaluating patients with suspected mesenteric ischemia; however, normal values do not exclude this condition. Serial monitoring for acidosis and bandemia should be considered for patients with acute gastrointestinal manifestations.

Radiographic Imaging Studies

The role of traditional upper gastrointestinal and small bowel follow-through series using barium or gastrografin, MR, and CT enterography are similar to their respective role for evaluating the gastrointestinal complications of Crohn's disease. The appearance of large, discrete, nodular lesions with central ring-like collections of barium in the terminal ileum has been reported to be a specific manifestation of intestinal BD.[18] Nuclear medicine scanning using white blood cell markers such as Indium-111 may assist in localizing bowel inflammation, though its clinical utility in BD is uncertain. Conventional angiography, MR angiography, and CT angiography may be useful in diagnosing and defining the extent of vasculitis and vascular complications.

Endoscopic Evaluation

While the endoscopic and histologic findings are important for the diagnosis, assessment of disease extent and severity of GIBD, and to exclude other non-Behçet's gastrointestinal complications, such as NSAID-induced ulcerations, CMV infection, hemorrhoidal bleeding, and so on, it has been suggested that endoscopy should be performed with great caution in BD because of the risk of perforation, especially in the setting of potentially ischemic bowel. Consideration should be given to using carbon dioxide (CO_2) instead of air when possible during endoscopic procedures, and wireless capsule video endoscopy when appropriate. Given the sensitivity limitations of noninvasive biochemical markers and traditional radiographic studies and the potential for clinically significant, yet clinically silent active GIBD lesions, WCE may prove to be useful, not only to diagnose gastrointestinal involvement in BD but also to monitor intestinal disease activity in selective cases, as well as to guide therapeutic decisions, especially when considering changes in maintenance therapy in patients with GIBD.

Gastrointestinal Disease Activity Index for BD

The Korean IBD Study Group recently developed a disease activity index, the Disease Activity Index for BD (DAIBD), to objectively and numerically quantify clinical GIBD disease activity.[19] The total cumulative score is based on eight clinical variables that can theoretically range from 0 to 325, with higher scores reflecting greater disease activity. The DAIBD was designed to be easily administered in the outpatient clinical setting. Cheon and colleagues validated the DAIBD in a second BD patient cohort and reported that the DAIBD correlated well with the physicians global assessment score and performed better than the Crohn's Disease Activity Index for longitudinal follow-up of GIBD.[19] The utility of DAIBD in the clinical office setting and in the formal clinical trials has yet to be determined. Importantly, the DAIBD does not rely on a symptom diary and does not include laboratory data or endoscopic findings and thus may underestimate residual gastrointestinal disease.

● DIFFERENTIAL DIAGNOSIS

The differential diagnosis in BD varies with each patient's particular clinical features or constellation of features. GIBD and Crohn's disease can not only have similar gastrointestinal manifestations but share similar extraintestinal features as well. The intestinal ulcerations in BD tend to be more focally distributed and are more commonly round or oval with more discrete margins compared to the more segmental and diffuse involvement with stellate and more longitudinal ulcerations of Crohn's disease.[2] There is less inflammation surrounding ulcers in BD than in Crohn's. The presence of granuloma is usually considered a distinguishing factor; however, a substantial number of patients with Crohn's disease do not have granuloma and granuloma have occasionally been identified in biopsy specimens of patients with known BD.[15] Thus, differentiation of GIBD from Crohn's can be challenging, particularly when there is incomplete disease expression in BD.

The differential diagnosis of recurrent oral ulcers is quite broad and includes IBD, benign oral aphthosis, herpes simplex, Stevens-Johnson syndrome, cyclic neutropenia, PFAPA syndrome (periodic fever with aphthous pharyngitis and adenitis), MAGIC syndrome (mouth and genital ulcers with inflamed cartilage), other systemic rheumatic diseases such as systemic lupus erythematosus, pemphigoid, pemphigus vulgaris, cicatricial pemphigoid, lichen planus, and linear IgA disease, trauma secondary to dental prosthetics or oral hygiene products, and side effect of medications including methotrexate and thiopurines.[4]

The constellation of cutaneous vasculitis, inflammatory eye disease, neurologic disease, vascular disease, arthritis, and/or unexplained systemic illness seen in BD needs to be distinguished from other causes, including systemic lupus erythematosus, Crohn's disease, ulcerative colitis, celiac disease, microscopic enterocolitis, sarcoidosis, reactive arthritis, psoriatic arthritis, ankylosing spondylitis, juvenile arthritis, familial Mediterranean fever and other periodic febrile syndromes, other vasculitides, multiple sclerosis, systemic infections including tuberculosis (TB), human immunodeficiency virus, CMV, syphilis, as well as malignancies. With certain BD manifestations, Sweet's syndrome, Reiter's syndrome, and Stevens-Johnson syndrome need to be considered. Importantly, some of these may coexist in patients with established BD.

TREATMENT OVERVIEW

The optimal management of BD remains uncertain, since symptoms wax and wane with time, and the spectrum of individual clinical manifestations and disease severities are so varied. Although the etiology of BD remains unclear, most interventions are directed at modifying the inflammatory response by downregulating the immune system. Many therapies are directed toward treatment of specific manifestations of the illness. Treatment choices depend not only on the organ system affected but also by the severity of disease within that particular organ system. When more than one organ system is involved, treatment is usually influenced by the degree of disease severity of the organ with the most potential morbidity.

Glucocorticoids have been, and remain, a cornerstone of treatment for many of the manifestations of BD, particularly those with moderately severe to severe disease activity. High IV doses may be required for acute life- or organ-threatening disease and lower doses for less acute or severe disease. Though they are frequently effective in treating acute BD exacerbations, symptoms may recur as the dose is tapered and dependency on steroids may result. Steroid side effects are significant and include osteopenia, osteoporosis, avascular necrosis, adrenal suppression, growth retardation, impaired wound healing, cataracts, glaucoma, hypertension, weight gain, edema, Cushingoid habitus, moon face, acne, striae, skin atrophy, hirsutism, alopecia, myopathy, insomnia, emotional lability, psychosis, glucose intolerance, hyperlipidemia, atherosclerosis, headache, pseudotumor cerebri, fatty liver, and increased susceptibility to infections, including opportunistic infections. Importantly, even low steroid doses may mask fever and pain, which are important signs of deterioration (such as perforation or peritonitis) or infectious complications. Arthralgias and fatigue associated with the withdrawal of steroids must be distinguished from recurrence of disease activity.

The literature addressing pharmacological intervention in BD is composed predominantly of case reports and small case series. Randomized controlled trials that have been performed tend to focus on one particular disease manifestation of BD, though some allow for broader conclusions. Published treatment approaches and duration of treatments are diverse and the lack of comparability across trials precludes the pooling of data. With respect to individual BD manifestations and to Behçet's overall, there is little quality long-term outcome data upon which to draw firm conclusions. Many current nonsteroid approaches used in treating BD are derived from extrapolations of potentially promising medications in other inflammatory conditions. Following a systematic review of the literature through 2006, the European League Against Rheumatism (EULAR) put

forth official recommendations for the management of BD, but concluded, "Recommendations related to the eye, skin-mucosa disease and arthritis are mainly evidence based, but recommendations on vascular disease, neurological and gastrointestinal involvement are based largely on expert opinion and uncontrolled evidence from open trials and observational studies."[4] Of interest is that the EULAR multidisciplinary expert committee task force did not include a gastroenterologist. Importantly, there are considerable differences in the practical approaches to treatment, which remains largely empirical, and is often strongly influenced by the perspective and experience of the subspecialist who is managing the patient.

TREATMENT BY ORGAN SYSTEM
Luminal Gastrointestinal Disease

The approach to managing the gastrointestinal manifestations of BD is largely based on case reports and small, uncontrolled series, and extrapolations based on successes in other similar conditions. The assessment strategies and decision-making processes used for the management of the luminal aspects of BD are similar to treatment approaches used for luminal Crohn's disease. Importantly, the observations that attainment of complete remission is associated with a better short- and medium-term prognosis suggests that a shift toward aggressive early intervention and more prolonged ongoing maintenance therapy may improve longer-term outcomes.

Systemic *glucocorticoids* have been the mainstay for acute exacerbations of GIBD, the dose and route depending on the severity of the involvement. It is best to treat aggressively early on, including escalating to IV steroids early in those who fail to adequately respond to initial oral therapy, rather than incrementally "stepping up" the dose. The historical approach has been to continue the initial dose of 0.5 to 1 mg/kg/day for at least 1 month or until symptoms improve before beginning to taper. The dose is then slowly decreased over the 2 to 3 months to 10 mg/day and the subsequent tapered to discontinuation over an additional 2 months if disease control is maintained. Steroids should not be used as monotherapy for GIBD. Long-term maintenance therapy should be initiated early on, rather than waiting until steroids are tapered.

For many years, *sulfasalazine* had been used as part of the treatment regimen for luminal BD.[5] In recent years, the newer non–sulfa containing 5-aminosalicylic acid (5-ASA)-containing derivatives are being used more frequently, as they allow for more targeted delivery of the active 5-ASA ingredient and higher dosing of 5-ASA with fewer side effects. The use of these compounds to treat GIBD is widespread, but not well-studied formally and is often adjunctive, being used in combination with more traditional or newer biologic immunosuppressive therapies.

Although there are no randomized trials specifically focusing on the efficacy of thiopurine analogs in GIBD, several decades of clinical experience with *6-mercaptopurine and AZA* suggest beneficial effects. Both are generally well-tolerated and continue to be widely utilized for maintenance of remission and for steroid-sparing effects. They remain a cornerstone of BD therapy despite the introduction of the newer class of biologic therapeutics. Because of their very slow onset of action of 1 to 9 months, thiopurines should be initiated early on and continued long-term to sustain remission, given the recurring nature of GIBD once therapy is discontinued. Thiopurine methyl transferase genotyping and thiopurine metabolite level monitoring allow for identification of metabolic subgroups and may facilitate improved optimization of thiopurines therapy in BD.

Anti-TNF-α biologics are being increasingly used in GIBD to induce and maintain remission, and for steroid-sparing effects. In a March 2010 review, the authors identified 88, 12, and 13 primary articles from 20 countries on the off-label use of infliximab, etanercept, and adalimumab in BD, reporting on 325, 37, and 28 patients, respectively.[20] Improvement in acute GIBD symptoms was described in 29 of 32 (91%) patients who received infliximab and all three who were treated with adalimumab. Rapid responses ranging from 1 to 10 days were reported for intestinal manifestations. Tapering of background steroid treatment was possible in most patients. Relapses were common after cessation of anti-TNF-α treatment, but remission was generally achieved upon reinitiation of therapy.

The short-term effects of the chimeric anti-TNF-α monoclonal antibody *infliximab* have been reported in several case reports and small case series.[10,11,20–22]

Editor's note (TMB): As stated in the text, the use of anti-TNF agents for the treatment of Bechet's disease has not been approved by the FDA.

Infliximab doses of 3, 5, 7.5, and 10 mg/kg have been described. There was a tendency to use the typical dosing regimen used in IBD with 5 mg/kg IV infusion induction at weeks 0, 2, and 6, followed by maintenance doses of 5 mg/kg every 8 weeks, other described episodic dosing. Infliximab was reported to rapidly and effectively suppress early postoperative recurrent ulcers following ileocecectomy.[22] Of patients with refractory gastrointestinal involvement including potentially life-threatening situations, such as extensive bleeding, 91% responded to infliximab.[20] Healing of a perianal fistula has been reported.[10] Twelve patients with GIBD have been enrolled in prospective studies with infliximab; improvement was noted in all, 83% achieving complete remission. All 10 who continued maintenance monotherapy with infliximab experienced sustained response.[20]

A total of four patients with GIBD are reported in the literature to have been treated with subcutaneous *adalimumab*.[20,23–25] Acute response to adalimumab induction was seen in three; one patient failed to respond to the adalimumab after responding and then attenuating to infliximab.[23,24] All three acute responders continued to do well on adalimumab 40 mg subcutaneous every other week maintenance therapy, one of whom at 22 months remains in complete clinical, endoscopic, and histologic remission on adalimumab monotherapy.[23,24] The standard adalimumab dosing regimen used for Crohn's disease could be considered for GIBD; induction with 160 mg followed by 80 mg 2 weeks later, then maintenance with 40 mg every other week.

To date, there are no published articles on the use of *certolizumab pegol* (a pegylated humanized Fab fragment of a humanized anti-TNF-α monoclonal antibody) or *golimumab* (another fully human anti-TNF-α monoclonal antibody) in BD. While the soluble TNF receptor etanercept has been shown to benefit in randomized clinical trials in controlling mucocutaneous and articular manifestations of BD, there is no published data concerning the effect of etanercept on GIBD.[20]

Given the variable and limited success of other interventions in BD and the mounting data that strongly suggest that anti-TNF-α therapy leads to rapid and effective suppression of almost all BD manifestations, this class of therapeutic shows great promise in BD, at least in the short-term. Host immunogenicity to monoclonal antibody therapy may impact retreatment and the longitudinal use of these types of agents. Anti-TNF-α therapies have been used as primary maintenance monotherapy for GIBD or as a bridge to an alternate maintenance immunosuppressive therapeutic, such as a thiopurine or thalidomide. The latter strategy puts patients at risk for host antitherapeutic antibody formation, which may affect that particular monoclonal antibodies effectiveness and tolerability should the patient require that in the future for the same or different, and perhaps more severe BD manifestation. Host antitherapeutic antibody formation is one of the major concerns associated with monoclonal antibody therapies for it can lead to undesirable outcomes such as attenuation of effect with time, serum-sickness-like reactions, and immediate infusion reactions, including anaphylaxis, fevers, hives, or local injection site reaction.

Editor's note (TMB): Although the adverse events with anti-TNF agents are described in chapters 14, 62, 107, 108, 109, 110, 113, this is a very complete listing and was included.

Other side effects of anti-TNF-α biologics include worsening of heart failure; drug-induced psoriasis; exacerbation of multiple sclerosis; neuropathy, increased incidence of leukemia, lymphoma, including hepatosplenic T-cell lymphoma; and other malignancies. The development of anti-double-stranded DNA antibodies and elevated ANA is common, but only rarely results in a clinical drug-induced lupus-like syndrome. *Pneumocystis carinii* pneumonia, *Legionella pneumophila* pneumonia, de novo or reactivation of TB, hepatitis B virus reactivation, cryptococcal meningitis, varicella zoster infection, and CMV colitis have all been described in BD patients on anti-TNF-α therapies.[20] Appropriate screening for TB and hepatitis B is warranted prior to initiation of anti-TNF-α therapy.

The best dose and dosing regimen to both enhance efficacy and avoid immunogenicity has not been determined. Because BD is a lifelong disease, single "immunizing" doses of biologic therapies should be avoided. Again, these are off-label uses of anti-TNF agents.

A few case reports suggest a potential role for *thalidomide* in patients with refractory BD. Thalidomide is an immunomodulator that decreases TNF-α production and inhibits interleukin-12 production and of chemotaxis of both lymphocytes and neutrophils. Improvement with thalidomide is often evident within 1 to 2 weeks of initiating treatment. Mucosal healing of GIBD lesions has been described.[2] The dose of thalidomide may in part depend on the severity of disease. Some reports describe starting at higher doses of 300 to 400 mg per day, then once remission is achieved, tapering thalidomide to 100 mg/day, though it may be possible to reduce the maintenance dose to 50 mg/day to 50 mg twice a week in some cases.[26] There is a report of an infant whose refractory GIBD responded well to thalidomide 10 mg/kg/day.[12] Symptoms have been observed to eventually recur upon discontinuation.[10] Infliximab transition to thalidomide maintenance therapy has been described.[10] Seven juvenile-onset patients, aged 7 to 19 years, with severe, recurrent GIBD were reported to have "dramatic" responses to 0.5 to 3 mg/kg/day of thalidomide; all then successfully discontinuing steroid therapy.[27] An advantage of thalidomide over monoclonal antibody therapies is that it can be given in episodic doses for flares.[10] Because of its sedative effects, thalidomide is generally dosed at bedtime. The most concerning side effect is teratogenicity, which can occur even with a one-time exposure. Peripheral neuropathy is often dose-dependent, but in some cases may be irreversible and thus warrants careful monitoring. Other side effects include skin rash, leukopenia, anemia, elevated liver enzymes, mood changes, constipation, diarrhea, nausea, and impotence. Thalidomide has been considered for selected refractory patients with GIBD.[27]

Colchicine is an anti-inflammatory agent that interferes with the initiation and amplification of inflammation predominantly through its effects on neutrophils. While it has been widely used for Behçet's-associated EN and oral ulcerations, there is a paucity of published data with respect to its effectiveness for extraoral GIBD.[4] In one case report, a patient's gastrointestinal and other systemic BD symptoms resolved with 0.6-mg oral colchicine twice daily.[28] Potential side effects include oligozoospermia and gastrointestinal complaints.

MMF is an immunosuppressive agent with anti-inflammatory properties that suppresses B- and T-cell proliferation and inhibits the release of TNF-α. A case report describes that MMF rapidly reduced clinical symptoms and eventual mucosal healing in a patient with AZA-refractory, steroid-dependent Behçet's ileocolitis.[29] While more experience is needed, MMF may represent a potential option for patients who have limited access to biologic therapeutics.

Nonmyeloablative high-dose *cyclophosphamide* therapy without stem cell rescue has been employed with success in the treatment of patients with refractory systemic lupus erythematosus and other systemic rheumatologic disorders. Although quality published data are limited, cyclophosphamide administered as weekly or monthly high-dose IV pulse dosing or in oral doses of 1 to 2.5 mg/kg/day has been used in patients with severe cutaneous, ocular, and CNS BD manifestations and/or systemic vasculitis. There is little published on the use of cyclophosphamide for GIBD. A recent report describes the case of a woman with severe infliximab- and adalimumab-refractory BD, who required multiple courses of high-dose IV steroids for flares of oral, genital, and GIBD, despite maintenance therapy with prednisone, hydroxychloroquine, colchicine, and sulfasalazine who was treated with cyclophosphamide 200 mg/kg IV divided over 4 consecutive days.[25] Following a transient pancytopenia, her oral, genital, and gastrointestinal manifestations rapidly subsided and she remained in steroid-free clinical remission of all immunosuppressive therapy 2 years later. There are several case reports that include descriptions of GIBD failing to respond to cyclophosphamide.[12,18] Potential side effects include infertility, hematological dyscrasias, and malignancy.[4] Cyclophosphamide *may be an option* for selected patients with refractory GIBD.

Lymphocyte-depleted *autologous stem cell transplantation* (ASCT) following high-dose immunosuppressive therapy was described in a child with severe/refractory Behçet's ileocolitis whose intestinal disease had failed to be adequately controlled with high-dose oral and IV steroids, sulfasalazine, AZA, cyclosporine, tacrolimus, methotrexate, cyclophosphamide, and bowel rest with total parenteral nutrition. Two years after undergoing ASCT, the child was reported to still in complete, steroid-free, medication-free clinical, and endoscopic remission.[30]

Anti-CD52 antibody therapy (CAMPATH 1-H)–induced T-cell depletion induced acute and sustained remission in 72% of 18 patients with BD, including some with gastrointestinal manifestations.[31]

Additional therapeutics have been used by clinicians and researchers to treat nongastrointestinal manifestations of BD, including pentoxifylline, chlorambucil, cyclosporine, antimalarials, tacrolimus, interferon-α, IV immunoglobulin, and methotrexate, though the efficacy and potential role of these latter agents in GIBD is not well defined. Methotrexate may be more effective in controlling IBD when given parenterally, than orally. Whether the same is true of GIBD remains to be determined.

Intestinal Vasculitis

The approach to intestinal vasculitis involves treating the underlying inflammatory disease, usually with immunosuppressive agents, addressing specific gastrointestinal symptoms, and monitoring for and addressing mesenteric ischemic issues when present. Surgical intervention is warranted in patients with mesenteric infarction or intestinal perforation.

Oral and Genital Ulcerations

For patients with acute or very intermittent lesions, a short-term "pulse" therapy approach is successful in some. While topical therapy in the form of rinses, gels, ointments, pastes, or creams may be tried, systemic therapy is usually needed to effectively treat and suppress the oral and genital lesions in Behçet's.[4] Topical glucocorticoid preparations are more likely to relieve ulcer-related pain than topical anesthetics. Triamcinolone acetonide cream 0.1% in Orabase, prednisolone mouthwashes, or topical sucralfate suspension may be used to reduce pain, healing time, and frequency of oral and genital ulceration occurrence. Long-term use of topical glucocorticoid therapy may lead to skin atrophy. Topical 5-ASA suspensions have been used to treat both oral and genital ulcerations. Intralesional injection of large ulcers with a glucocorticoid preparation such as triamcinolone 5 to 10 mg/mL may be considered.

Systemic glucocorticoids such as prednisone may be used for more refractory mucocutaneous lesions. If there is no major disease manifestation, doses as low as 15 mg/day may work. Once lesions resolve, in some cases prednisone can then be successfully tapered and discontinued altogether over 2 to 3 weeks. While *colchicine* is used to treat oral BD, published data on the effectiveness of colchicine for minor oral ulcers or genital lesions are mixed.[4] It is generally well-tolerated at a dose of 1 to 2 mg/day, though gastrointestinal intolerance may occur at doses higher than 1.5 mg/day.

Patients with recurrent or more refractory ulcerations may require longer courses of steroid therapy, though doses of prednisone as low as 5 mg/day may successfully control symptoms. In such patients, consideration should be given to escalating to maintenance therapy, usually *AZA*, which has been shown to be beneficial in placebo-controlled trials.[5] Infliximab, cyclosporine, interferon-α, dapsone, and thalidomide have all shown potential benefit in controlled studies.[4,5] A controlled trial of etanercept found it to be beneficial for the oral, but not the genital ulcerations in BD.[20] Anecdotal reports suggest that pentoxifylline and chlorambucil may be treatment options.[4,5]

Smoking has been described to have a beneficial effect on the symptoms of BD, while cessation of smoking may activate or aggravate the disease, in particular mucocutaneous lesions.[32] Nicotine-patch therapy and resumption of smoking has been shown in case reports and small series to improve or induce complete regression of oral aphthae and other mucocutaneous lesions, while other manifestations of BD do not respond.[32]

EN and Pyoderma Gangrenosum

Treatment of Behçet's-associated EN and PG requires special considerations. In BD, it is particularly important to consider the possibility of an underlying significant vasculitis in those presenting with EN. While colchicine is frequently used as a first-line agent, glucocorticoids and other immunosuppressive medications should be considered if it is ineffective.[4,5] Confirmation of the presence of a medium-vessel vasculitis through biopsy or by ulceration of the EN lesions is an indication for IV or oral systemic glucocorticoid treatment combined with another immunosuppressive agent, such as AZA. BD-associated PG is often complicated by the pathergy phenomenon; thus, debridement of cutaneous lesions is discouraged for it can aggravate PG lesions and lead to local expansion. While not studied in BD, consideration may be given to interventions that have been reported to be useful to treat non-BD-associated pyoderma, including IV cyclosporine, infliximab, thalidomide, and hyperbaric oxygen therapy.

Editor's note (TMB): These uses have not been approved by the FDA.

Venous Thrombosis

Venous thrombotic events in BD are believed to arise from endothelial inflammation leading to thrombosis rather than from inherent problems with coagulation. Some such as pulmonary vein thrombosis, cerebral sinus thrombosis, and cerebral vein thrombosis hold high potential morbidity and can be life-threatening. Treatment of venous thrombotic events must be individualized, but in general consists of suppressing systemic inflammation, anticoagulation, and may include local thrombolysis.

Arthropathy

While arthritis and arthralgias can be debilitating, the intensity of therapy is often determined by the other manifestations of BD. Colchicine at a dose of 1 to 2 mg/day in divided doses has been shown to effectively control arthritic symptoms.[4] Joint complaints not controlled by colchicine may respond to low-dose (5–10 mg/day) prednisone. Sulfasalazine may also be considered. *AZA* has also been demonstrated in clinical trials to be effective and may serve as a steroid-sparing agent.[4] Sulfasalazine, methotrexate, anti-TNF-α biologics, and interferon-α may be effective.[4,5] NSAIDs have been used to treat residual joint complaints. While some patients may respond, NSAIDs are generally considered to be of little benefit for Behçet's-associated arthropathy. They should be used with caution, particularly in those with GIBD, since they can cause gut injury. While the potential disease-aggravating effect of NSAIDs is not known in BD, both NSAIDs and COX-2 inhibitors have been observed to be potential triggers for the initial presentation and of disease exacerbation and ongoing inflammation of some patients with IBD and microscopic colitis.

SPECIAL CONSIDERATIONS

Intestinal manifestations and resultant resections may affect nutrient absorption and overall oral intake, resulting in nutritional deficiencies and malnutrition. It is important to identify and address deficiencies such as those of iron, vitamin B12, folate, and vitamin D to avoid additional preventable complications. Bone health should be assessed and monitored in those at risk for disease-, diet-, and medication-related bone loss.

In patients on immunosuppressive regimens, including steroids alone, mononucleosis, varicella, herpes zoster, opportunistic infections (such as CMV, herpes simplex, and Pneumocystis carinii), and EBV-related lymphoproliferative disorders can be potentially life-threatening and mandate early recognition, expedient evaluation, and prompt aggressive treatment to avoid morbidity and even mortality.

Immunization issues thus warrant consideration, as some infections are preventable. Live viral vaccines are to be avoided in the setting of immunosuppression, and immunosuppressive therapies may blunt the response to attenuated vaccines. Given that many, if not most patients with Behçet's will eventually require treatment with steroids and other immunosuppressive therapies, thought should be given early on to assessing each individual's current and future potential vaccination needs and addressing those early on, ideally before a patient needs to begin those common therapies. Given the increasing likelihood that anti-TNF therapy may be warranted at some point during a patient's disease course, consideration should be given to assessing for TB and hepatitis B ahead of time, thereby potentially avoiding later delay in initiation of biologic therapy in the setting of an acute exacerbation of a more serious BD manifestation.

PROGNOSIS

The course of BD is highly variable and is characterized by exacerbations and remissions of the various manifestations of the disease. The types of BD manifestations and their aggressiveness vary with population, gender, age, duration of disease, and decisions on maintenance therapy. Delay in diagnosis is common in nonendemic areas and likely increases morbidity and mortality. Gastrointestinal, neurologic, ocular, and large vessel arterial or venous disease are associated with the greatest morbidity and mortality. Mucocutaneous, ocular, and articular involvement tend to be more prominent early in the disease course. While disease activity of many manifestations may decline with time, the overall disease burden may rise due to cumulative vascular, ocular, or neurologic damage, blindness and neurological disease being the major cause of permanent disability.[5] Genome-wide studies in BD and related conditions should eventually allow for identification of specific genes that can then be linked to specific systemic manifestations and to specific disease mechanisms, setting the stage for more targeted mechanism-based treatment approach in the future.

● CONCLUSIONS

An improved strategic approach to treating and following gastrointestinal manifestations of BD over time is clearly needed. BD is a long-term disease and is one of the best examples of a condition that should be ideally treated with coordinated multidisciplinary approach with close and effective communication among the various specialists, especially when therapeutic changes are being weighed. Medication choices should ideally cover as best as possible all the various systemic manifestations expressed by the individual patient, to avoid over immune suppression and to minimize side effects while addressing maintenance across the spectrum of that specific patient. Biologic therapies show great promise, particularly for acute severe flares, but immunogenicity, cost, and potential side effects remain substantial concerns. The concepts of treating mucosal healing, true long-term maintenance therapy, and combination therapy deserve consideration.

Despite a growing recognition of gastrointestinal involvement in BD, the natural history of GIBD is not well defined. The postoperative disease course in GIBD, including the clinical and endoscopic recurrence risks, the influence of more structured postoperative recurrence assessment, and therapeutic intervention strategies, needs to be further studied in a rigorously prospective manner. Given the reality that GIBD is relatively uncommon, and that clinical courses and associated BD manifestations are variable amongst patients, it is unlikely that adequately powered prospective placebo-controlled studies will be undertaken to any significant degree in the near future. Perhaps an alternate strategy of large coordinated international BD registries could fill gaps in understanding on how to best approach, not only each individual manifestation but BD disease as whole.

References

1. Moon CM, Cheon JH, Shin JK, et al. Prediction of free bowel perforation in patients with intestinal Behçet's disease using clinical and colonoscopic findings. *Dig Dis Sci*. 2010;55(10):2904–2911.

2. Sayarlioglu M, Kotan MC, Topcu N, Bayram I, Arslanturk H, Gul A. Treatment of recurrent perforating intestinal ulcers with thalidomide in Behçet's disease. *Ann Pharmacother*. 2004;38(5):808–811.

3. Kaklamani VG, Vaiopoulos G, Kaklamanis PG. Behçet's disease. *Semin Arthritis Rheum*. 1998;27(4):197–217.

4. Tunes R, Santiago M. Behçet's syndrome: literature review. *Curr Rheumatol Rev*. 2009;5:64–82.

5. Marshall SE. Behçet's disease. *Best Pract Res Clin Rheumatol*. 2004;18(3):291–311.

6. Chung SY, Ha HK, Kim JH, et al. Radiologic findings of Behçet syndrome involving the gastrointestinal tract. *Radiographics*. 2001;21(4):911–924; discussion 924.

7. Hamdulay SS, Cheent K, Ghosh C, Stocks J, Ghosh S, Haskard DO. Wireless capsule endoscopy in the investigation of intestinal Behçet's syndrome. *Rheumatology (Oxford)*. 2008;47(8):1231–1234.

8. Neves FS, Fylyk SN, Lage LV, et al. Behçet's disease: clinical value of the video capsule endoscopy for small intestine examination. *Rheumatol Int*. 2009;29(5):601–603.

9. Lee SK, Kim BK, Kim TI, Kim WH. Differential diagnosis of intestinal Behçet's disease and Crohn's disease by colonoscopic findings. *Endoscopy*. 2009;41(1):9–16.

10. Travis SP, Czajkowski M, McGovern DP, Watson RG, Bell AL. Treatment of intestinal Behçet's syndrome with chimeric tumour necrosis factor alpha antibody. *Gut*. 2001;49(5):725–728.

11. Kim JS, Lim SH, Choi IJ, et al. Prediction of the clinical course of Behçet's colitis according to macroscopic classification by colonoscopy. *Endoscopy*. 2000;32(8):635–640.

12. Shek LP, Lee YS, Lee BW, Lehman TJ. Thalidomide responsiveness in an infant with Behçet's syndrome. *Pediatrics*. 1999;103(6 Pt 1):1295–1297.

13. Choi IJ, Kim JS, Cha SD, et al. Long-term clinical course and prognostic factors in intestinal Behçet's disease. *Dis Colon Rectum*. 2000;43(5):692–700.

14. Tabata M, Tomomasa T, Kaneko H, Morikawa A. Intestinal Behçet's disease: a case report and review of Japanese reports in children. *J Pediatr Gastroenterol Nutr*. 1999;29(4):477–481.

15. Naganuma M, Iwao Y, Inoue N, et al. Analysis of clinical course and long-term prognosis of surgical and nonsurgical patients with intestinal Behçet's disease. *Am J Gastroenterol*. 2000;95(10):2848–2851.

16. O'Neill TW, Rigby AS, Silman AJ, Barnes C. Validation of the International Study Group criteria for Behçet's disease. *Br J Rheumatol*. 1994;33(2):115–117.

17. Monselise A, Weinberger A, Monselise Y, Fraser A, Sulkes J, Krause I. Anti-*Saccharomyces cerevisiae* antibodies in Behçet's disease–a familial study. *Clin Exp Rheumatol*. 2006;24(5 suppl 42):S87–S90.

18. Lim HK, Wang TE, Chen TL, et al. Perforation of an ileal ulcer in a patient with Behçet's disease. *J Intern Med Taiwan*. 2003;14:89–94.

19. Cheon JH, Han DS, Park JY, et al.; Korean IBD Study Group. Development, validation, and responsiveness of a novel disease activity index for intestinal Behçet's disease. *Inflamm Bowel Dis*. 2011;17(2):605–613.

20. Arida A, Fragiadaki K, Giavri E, Sfikakis PP. Anti-TNF agents for Behçet's disease: analysis of published data on 369 patients. *Semin Arthritis Rheum*. 2010.

21. Hassard PV, Binder SW, Nelson V, Vasiliauskas EA. Anti-tumor necrosis factor monoclonal antibody therapy for gastrointestinal Behçet's disease: a case report. *Gastroenterology*. 2001;120(4):995–999.

22. Byeon JS, Choi EK, Heo NY, et al. Antitumor necrosis factor-alpha therapy for early postoperative recurrence of gastrointestinal Behçet's disease: report of a case. *Dis Colon Rectum*. 2007;50(5):672–676.

23. van Laar JA, Missotten T, van Daele PL, Jamnitski A, Baarsma GS, van Hagen PM. Adalimumab: a new modality for Behçet's disease? *Ann Rheum Dis*. 2007;66(4):565–566.

24. Ariyachaipanich A, Berkelhammer C, Nicola H. Intestinal Behçet's disease: maintenance of remission with adalimumab monotherapy. *Inflamm Bowel Dis*. 2009;15(12):1769–1771.

25. Henderson CF, Brodsky RA, Jones RJ, Levine SM. High-dose cyclophosphamide without stem cell rescue for the treatment of

refractory Behçet's disease. *Semin Arthritis Rheum.* 2011. [Epub ahead of print].

26. Sandborn WJ, Hanauer SB, Katz S, et al. Etanercept for active Crohn's disease: a randomized, double-blind, placebo-controlled trial. *Gastroenterology.* 2001;121(5):1088–1094.

27. Yasui K, Uchida N, Akazawa Y, et al. Thalidomide for treatment of intestinal involvement of juvenile-onset Behçet disease. *Inflamm Bowel Dis.* 2008;14(3):396–400.

28. Raynor A, Askari AD. Behçet's disease and treatment with colchicine. *J Am Acad Dermatol.* 1980;2(5):396–400.

29. Kappen JH, Mensink PB, Lesterhuis W, et al. Mycophenolate sodium: effective treatment for therapy-refractory intestinal Behçet's disease, evaluated with enteroscopy. *Am J Gastroenterol.* 2008;103(12):3213–3214.

30. Rossi G, Moretta A, Locatelli F. Autologous hematopoietic stem cell transplantation for severe/refractory intestinal Behcet disease. *Blood.* 2004;103(2):748–750.

31. Lockwood CM, Hale G, Waldman H, Jayne DR. Remission induction in Behçet's disease following lymphocyte depletion by the anti-CD52 antibody CAMPATH 1-H. *Rheumatology (Oxford).* 2003;42(12):1539–1544.

32. Ciancio G, Colina M, La Corte R, et al. Nicotine-patch therapy on mucocutaneous lesions of Behcet's disease: a case series. *Rheumatology (Oxford).* 2010;49(3):501–504.

Index

Note: Page references followed by "*f*" and "*t*" denote figures and tables, respectively.